STANDARD METHODS
FOR THE EXAMINATION OF
DAIRY PRODUCTS

17th Edition 2004

Edited by

H. Michael Wehr, PhD
Joseph F. Frank, PhD

American Public Health Association
800 I Street, NW
Washington, DC 20001
www.apha.org

American Public Health Association
800 I Street, NW
Washington, DC 20001–3710
www.apha.org

Georges C. Benjamin, MD, FACP
Executive Director

APHA Committee on Laboratory Standards and Practices (CLaSP)
Liaison: Carl H. Blank, PhD

Printed and bound in the United States of America
Set In: Palatino and Franklin Gothic
Interior Design and Typesetting: Susan Westrate
Cover Design: Joseph R. Loehle
Printing and Binding: Victor Graphics, Inc., Baltimore, MD

ISBN 0-87553-002-8
5M 6/04

Contents

DEDICATION

Carl H. Blank, PhD
March 16, 1927 – May 4, 2002

Dedicated to the memory of Carl H. Blank, PhD, a member of the American Public Health Association for over 40 years; former chair of APHA's Laboratory Section (1977–1978); a long time member and former chair of APHA's Committee on Laboratory Standards and Practices (CLaSP); and CLaSP liaison to the Technical Committee for this 17th edition of Standard Methods for the Examination of Dairy Products.

Technical Committee

H. Michael Wehr, PhD, Chair
U.S. Food and Drug Administration
Washington, DC 20204

Edward A. Arnold, Jr.
Land O'Lakes/R. Tech Laboratories, Inc.
Arden Hills, MN 55126

Mary Bulthaus
Dairy Quality Control Institute
Moundsview, MN 55112–1400

John C. Bruhn, PhD
Department of Food Science and Technology
University of California
Davis, CA 95616–8598

James E. Fitts
Division of Milk Control
New York Department of Agriculture and Markets
Albany, NY 12235

Joseph F. Frank, PhD
Department of Food Science and Technology
University of Georgia
Athens, GA 30602–7610

Robert T. Marshall, PhD
Department of Food Science and Nutrition
University of Missouri
Columbia, MO 65211

Larry A. Maturin, PhD
U.S. Food and Drug Administration
Laboratory Quality Assurance Branch
Summit Argo, IL 60501–1957

APHA Committee on Laboratory Science and Practice (CLaSP) Liaison
Carl H. Blank, PhD

APHA Project Liaison
Ellen T. Meyer
Director of Publications

Contributors

Edward A. Arnold, Jr., Land O'Lakes/R. Tech Laboratories, Inc., Arden Hills, MN 55126

David M. Barbano, Department of Food Science, Cornell University, Ithaca, NY 14853–7201

Robert L. Bradley, Jr., Department of Food Science, University of Wisconsin, Madison, WI 53706

Mary Bulthaus, Dairy Quality Control Institute, Moundsview, MN 55112–1400

Genevieve L. Christen, Department of Food Technology and Science, University of Tennessee, Knoxville, TN 37901–1071

W. Clark

P. Michael Davidson, Department of Food Science and Technology, University of Tennessee, Knoxville, TN 37901–1071

Gary L. Davis

Susan E. Duncan, Food Science and Technology, Virginia Polytechnic Institute and State University, Blacksburg, VA 24061

Randy L. Dyer, Ice Cream Unit, Nestle USA, Solon, OH 44139

Amr Fatouh, Department of Food Science and Technology, University of Georgia, Athens, GA 30602–7610

James E. Fitts, Division of Milk Control, New York Department of Agriculture and Markets, Albany, NY 12235

Russell S. Flowers, Silliker Laboratories Group, Inc., Chicago Heights, IL 60411

Joseph F. Frank. PhD, Department of Food Science and Technology, University of Georgia, Athens, GA 30602–7610

Sonya A. Gambrel–Lenarz, Regulatory Affairs, 3M, St. Paul, MN 55144

Thomas E. Graham, PhD, Center for Food Safety & Applied Nutrition, U.S. Food & Drug Administration, Summit Argo, IL 60501

David R. Henning, PhD, South Dakota State University, Brookings, SD 57006–4071

Paul J. Hickey, Wadsworth Center for Laboratories and Research, New York State Department of Health, Albany, NY 12201

Roger Hooi, Morningstar Foods, Inc., Dallas, TX 75201

Elizabeth M. Johnson, Columbia, SC 29223

David T. Laird, PhD, Laboratory Quality Assurance Team, U.S. Food & Drug Administration, Summit Argo, IL 60501–1957

Diane Lewis, Market Access & Regulatory Affairs, U.S. Dairy Export Council, Arlington, VA 22201

Larry J. Maturin, PhD, U.S. Food and Drug Administration, Laboratory Quality Assurance Team, Summit Argo, IL 60501–1957

J. Sue McAllister, 3M Health Care, 3M Center, St. Paul, MN 55144–1000

Paul Nierman, Dairy Quality Control Institute, Moundsview, MN 55112–1400

Ravinder Reddy, PhD, Laboratory Quality Assurance Team, U.S. Food & Drug Administration, Summit Argo, IL 60501–1957

Raoul Reiser, PhD, Toxin Technology Inc., Sarasota, FL 8012

R.M. Rocco, PhD, Center for Biomedical Laboratory Science, San Francisco State University; Science Consultant, Los Altos, CA 94023

Lawrence A. Roth, Food Lab, Alberta Agriculture, Edmonton, Alberta, Canada T6H 4P2

Eliot T. Ryser, PhD, Department of Food Science and Human Nutrition, Michigan State University, East Lansing, MI 48824–1224

Fran M. Scher

Michelle A. Smith, U.S. Food & Drug Administration, Washington, D.C. 20204

Duane R. Spomer, Standards & Grading Dairy Program, Agricultural Marketing Service, USDA, Washington, D.C. 20250

Susan S. Sumner, Food Science & Technology, Virginia Polytechnic Institute and State University, Blacksburg, VA 24061

H. Michael Wehr, PhD, U.S. Food & Drug Administration, Washington, DC 20204

B.R. Yaun

Ahmed E. Yousef, PhD, Food Science & Technology, Ohio State University, Columbus, OH 43210–1097

Consensus Reviewers

Most contributors were involved in the concensus review and made appropriate suggestions for improvement. In addition, the following volunteers were provided drafts of one or more chapters in areas of their expertise and invited to suggest modifications to the Technical Committee. We gratefully acknowledge Arnold W. Appelt, Jeff Bloom, M. Gretha Davis, Lynelle Ford, Melodee Kelly, Thomas Kitsmiller, Doug McDougal, Robert Salter, Eileen Q. Sanders.

Preface

Standard Methods for the Examination of Dairy Products (SMEDP) serves as the primary analytical reference for the sampling and testing of dairy products in the United States. The publication has had a long and distinguished use by those involved in dairy product analysis—government, industry and commercial laboratories. It has come to be recognized as the preeminent source of information in the field.

As with any technical reference, advances and changes to the field occur. Within the dairy industry, while many classical methods continue to be used, new advances in both microbiological and chemical procedures have taken place. Rapid test kits for the detection of microorganisms and antibiotic residues have seen significant advances in the past few years. In some cases, new concerns have arisen that require attention, such as the emergence of new strains of Enteropathogenic *E. coli.*

The business and regulatory environment also creates change. The new Hazard Analysis and Critical Control Point (HACCP) system to ensure the safety of foods has had an impact on the dairy industry. Additionally, the passage of the Uruguay Round Sanitary and Phytosanitary (SPS) and Technical Barriers to Trade (TBT) Agreements are also influencing how industries, including the dairy industry, operate in both the international and domestic arenas.

Changes included in this 17th Edition are outlined in Chapter One.

History

It has been over 100 years since Sedgwick and Batchler published a report of the bacteriological examination of Boston's milk supply (*Boston Med. And Surg. J.* 126:25:1892), which emphasized the importance of dairy sanitation. The 1905 report of S.C. Prescott on "The Need for Uniform Methods in the Sanitary Examination of Milk" prompted the American Public Health Association (APHA) to appoint a committee; that committee's 1910 report entitled "Standard Methods of Bacterial Milk Analysis" was the beginning of a series of "Standard Methods" books, of which this is the 17th edition. The reader is referred to the 12th and earlier editions for excellent historical records.

Process

The Technical Committee responsible for the present edition was appointed by the APHA Committee on Laboratory Standards and Practices (CLaSP). Members were chosen to represent developers and users of methods. Included were two representatives of the U.S. Food & Drug Administration (FDA) who have a working knowledge of the regulatory application of standard methods.

The Technical Committee nominated, and CLaSP approved, chairs and members of chapter committees. Individual members of the Technical Committee served in a liaison capacity with the chapter committees. Chapter committees were encouraged to review the status of all applicable methods and to include those methods that provide the greatest utility to the users.

Revised chapters were submitted to the Technical Committee for review. When that committee recommended significant changes, manuscripts were returned to the chapter committees for revision. After being edited by the chair of the Technical Committee, chapters were sent to consensus reviewers, who were asked to justify any changes they recommended. The Technical Committee was the final authority that determined the status of methods.

Acknowledgments

The major portion of this work was done by committees that revised the chapters, and the Technical Committee is especially thankful for their efforts. We also gratefully acknowledge the contributions of our CLaSP liaison, the late Carl Blank, who faithfully attended meetings of the Technical Committee and generously shared his considerable knowledge of laboratory standards and practices. Thanks also to Ellen Meyer, APHA Director of Publications, for her coordination of the Technical Committee's meetings and for her oversight of the development and production processes for this volume.

Chapter 1

Standard Methods

H. M. Wehr

1.010 Introduction

Standard Methods for the Examination of Dairy Products (*SMEDP*) is designed for regulatory, industry, and commercial laboratories that need to assess the safety and quality of dairy products. It is also a compendium of microbiological, chemical, and physical methods for analyzing milk and dairy products. The focus of *SMEDP* is on tests for hidden attributes that can only be detected by laboratory procedures. These include test methods and procedures that may be applied routinely for the laboratory evaluation of products and complex nonroutine methods, such as those for foodborne pathogens and vitamin content analysis.

Some test methods are not included in *SMEDP*, although the references may provide sources for readers interested in additional analysis. Tests for specific pesticide residues, radionuclides, and nutrient constituents, with the exception of tests for vitamins A and D, are not included. Qualities of dairy products that are discernible by the consumer are generally not included. By and large, subjective tests for such variables as body, texture, and flavor are not adaptable to *SMEDP*.

The 17th edition of *SMEDP* provides the dairy industry, associated research organizations, and the governmental bodies charged with ensuring the safety and wholesomeness of dairy products with validated methodology to ensure that harmful levels of organisms and other substances are absent and that the nutritive qualities, flavor, and appearance of products meet established specifications. An aim of *SMEDP* is to provide a system for the uniform testing of dairy products that will become a critical component of both government and industry analytical programs. The presentation of methods in *SMEDP* is designed to foster uniformity by providing sufficient information on key test procedures so that analysts have a clear set of procedures when performing each method.

1.020 Function of Standard Methods

SMEDP has long been recognized as a highly credible source of validated methods for dairy product analysis. This edition of *SMEDP* is specifically designed to serve multiple purposes and to be a source of:

1. Microbiological, chemical, and physical analytical methods for the uniform analysis of milk and milk products for use in U.S. regulatory control programs, both those regulated under the U.S. Pasteurized Milk Ordinance[11] for manufacturing grade milk and for tests carried out on behalf of U.S. Department of Agriculture milk marketing programs.
2. Analytical methods for the analysis of milk and milk products for use by industry to ensure product compliance with governmental regulations and for quality control purposes.
3. Information on dairy products for international trade purposes.
4. Background information on test methods including information important to the interpretation of analytical results.
5. Information on product sampling and laboratory quality assurance programs.
6. Information on compositional specifications and regulatory requirements for dairy products.

1.030 Organization

This edition begins with chapters on laboratory quality assurance and safety and the sampling of dairy and related products. The balance of the remaining chapters are primarily analytical methodology. Individual chapters cover longstanding key dairy product test areas including: standard plate count (SPC), coliform and other indicator bacteria, direct microscopic methods for bacteria or somatic cells, methods to detect abnormal milk, the detection of antibiotic drug residues in milk and dairy products, alkaline phosphatase methods, and microbiological tests for equipment and containers. This edition also includes chapters on methods for detecting foodborne pathogens in milk, microbiological tests specific for groups of dairy products, and chemical and physical analytical methods.

1.040 Changes in This Edition

Significant changes have been made to this edition of *SMEDP* to make it a more useful and comprehensive reference.

In addition to the routine updating of methodology, comprehensive revisions have been made to the chapters on antibiotic drug residues and chemical and physical methods. Rapid changes in antibiotic residue testing methodology have replaced methods in earlier editions. New and updated instrumentation in the field of chemical and physical testing have also resulted in multiple changes to chapter 5, although classical test methods still form the backbone of the chapter. Similarly, changes in current technology necessitated significant changes to chapter 11. Chapter 4 has also been significantly revised to focus on media preparation.

As detailed below, new method classes have been added to recognize the method validation carried out by the AOAC® International Research Institute and by the U.S. National Conference on Interstate Milk Shipments (NCIMS).

To focus on currently used and validated standard methods, method classes C (unproved methods that have been proposed as useful) and D (outdated or unused methods) have been deleted from this edition of *SMEDP*.

Recognizing the lack of readily available information, a chapter on compositional standards and regulatory requirements for milk and milk products has been included in this edition of *SMEDP*.

Additionally, the growing importance of international trade is recognized. Selective reference to International Dairy Federation (IDF) methods has been incorporated into various chapters of this edition.

1.050 Standard Methods for International Trade

International trade in food products, including milk constituents and dairy products, is increasing significantly. Furthermore, international trade agreements[14] arising from the GATT Uruguay Round of trade discussions, particularly the World Trade Organization (WTO) Agreement on the Application of Sanitary and Phytosanitary Measures (SPS agreement) and Agreement on Technical Barriers to Trade (TBT agreement), have moved the world toward the international harmonization of food product standards. In this regard, the work of the Codex Alimentarius Commission (Codex) is particularly important.

1.051 *Codex Alimentarius*

Codex is an international intergovernmental body that develops science-based food safety and commodity standards, guidelines, and recommendations to promote consumer protection and to facilitate world trade.[2] Codex is a subsidiary body of two United Nations organizations, the Food and Agriculture Organization (FAO) and the World Health Organization (WHO). Codex currently has 167 member countries. Under the statutes of the Codex Alimentarius,[2] Codex is charged with developing food standards for member countries. The Codex Alimentarius is a collection (comprised of 14 volumes) of international food standards adopted by the Codex Alimentarius Commission. The purpose of these standards is to protect the health of consumers and facilitate fair practices in food trade.[2] Codex texts are specific food standards, codes of practice, and recommendations. The scope of the Codex Alimentarius includes standards for all principle foods, whether processed, semi-processed, or raw, that will be distributed to consumers. Materials used for further processing of foods are included in a standard, to the extent necessary, to achieve the purpose of the standard. The Codex Alimentarius includes provisions for food hygiene, food additives, pesticide residues, contaminants, labeling, and methods of analysis and sampling. It also includes advisory provisions such as codes of practice, guidelines, and recommended measures.

Codex is important today because it is recognized in the WTO's SPS agreement.[14] The SPS agreement requires countries to base their sanitary and phytosanitary measures on international standards, guidelines, or recommendations unless they can scientifically justify a more stringent standard. It also states that, for food safety, the standards, guidelines, and recommendations established by the Codex Alimentarius Commission shall be recognized as international standards under the agreement and that products conforming to these standards shall be presumed to be consistent with agreement. While Codex standards are voluntary, countries have an obligation to base their own food safety standards on the work of Codex.

Additionally, products produced in accordance with Codex standards essentially have safe harborage in international trade.

Codex is also important within the context of the TBT agreement that deals with product specifications not related to safety including commodity composition, packaging, and certain labeling standards. The TBT agreement also requires countries to use international standards. While Codex is not specifically referenced in the TBT agreement, the WTO has recognized Codex standards as preferential in resolving technical trade disputes.

Codex thus becomes a true international focal point for food safety and quality with major impact on international trade and, potentially, on domestic food regulations. Its importance has therefore increased significantly.

Codex undertakes its work through the Codex Alimentarius Commission and a series of horizontal general subject committees, vertical commodity committees, and regional coordinating committees. Horizontal committees are those committees whose work applies to multiple commodities, such as the Codex Committee on Food Hygiene. Vertical committees are those that deal with a single commodity type or single commodity group, such as the Codex Committee on Milk and Milk Products. The structure of Codex is shown in Figure 1.1. Readers are referred to the *Codex Procedures Manual*[2] for specific terms of reference for all Codex committees.

Codex uses an 8-step procedure to elaborate on and to adopt standards and other texts.[2] This process is a purposefully deliberative one that ensures all member countries are given an opportunity to consider the issues coming before any individual Codex committee. New work must be approved by the commission or by the executive committee and the commission must approve the adoption of all standards. Steps 1 and 2 of the Codex procedure are the initial development processes for the elaboration of Codex texts. Step 3 involves the initial submittal of the document to member countries for review and comment. Step 4 is the first formal review of the proposed standard or text by the assigned Codex committee, while step 5 is the first review by the full commission. At step 6, the now revised standard, including any comments made by the commission, is sent to all member countries for a second review. Step 7 is the second opportunity for the assigned Codex committee to review the revised proposed Codex standard or text. Step 8 is the second and final review by the Codex commission. The commission has the option of adopting the standard at this point, amending and adopting the standard, sending the standard back to committee for further work, or rejecting the proposal. Normally, this review results in the adoption of the standard. The desire in Codex is for decisions to be reached by consensus, although provisions exist within the formal Codex operating procedures for voting on proposed standards and texts. An accelerated procedure is provided for in which steps 6 and 7 are omitted. Thus, steps 5 and 8 are combined and the proposed Codex standard or text may be adopted at the first consideration by the commission.

Most important to the dairy industry is the Codex Committee on Food Hygiene (CCFH), the Codex Committee on Milk and Milk Products (CCMMP), and the Codex Committee on Methods of Analysis and Sampling (CCMAS).

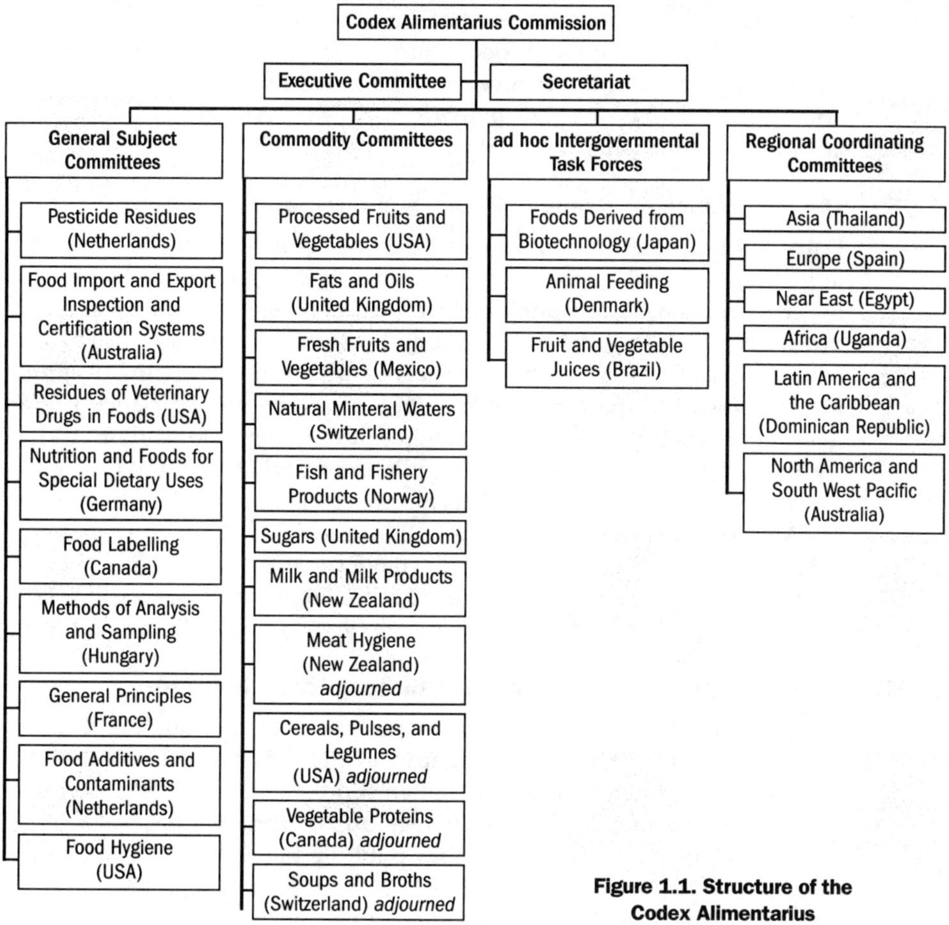

Figure 1.1. Structure of the Codex Alimentarius

CCFH has the primary responsibility for food hygiene matters within Codex.[2] Food hygiene generally encompasses the areas of the hygienic portion of good production, manufacturing, distribution, and marketing practices, the hazard analysis and critical control point (HACCP) system, microbiological criteria for foods, microbiological risk assessment, and risk management. The terms of reference for CCFH include the development of codes of hygienic practice for various commodity types and the review the hygiene sections of the various Codex standards for specific commodities. One of the most important codes of hygienic practice currently under development by Codex is the Code of Hygienic Practice for Milk and Milk Products.[3]

CCMMP develops individual standards for various dairy products,[2] including cheese, butter, milk and cream powder, sweetened and condensed milk, and milkfat products. Each of these standards contains basic compositional requirements for the product type and references other Codex texts for requirements in pesticide residues, food additives, food hygiene, labeling, and methods of analysis.

CCMAS has the primary responsibility to review and approve methods of compositional analysis of food commodities including dairy products.[2] CCMAS is not currently involved in the field of microbiological methods; however, it does have responsibility for such areas as product sampling and laboratory assessment procedures.

1.052 *The Importance of Standard Methods in International Trade*

Dairy product analysis and standard methods of analysis are as important in the international arena as they are domestically. Governments involved in certifying and/or accepting dairy products must have analytical procedures on which they can rely. Trading partners have similar needs. The widespread acceptance of the analytical methods and procedures outlined in *SMEDP* are of considerable value when assessing dairy products traded internationally. Recognizing the changes in the international dairy industry, the technical committee for this edition of *SMEDP* included reference to selected methods of the IDF. This information should be helpful to users of *SMEDP* who are involved with the international dairy product trade. Additionally, Codex compositional standards for major dairy product types have been included in chapter 16. This chapter outlines compositional standards and regulatory requirements for milk and milk products.

1.060 Adopting New Methodology and Uniformity of Methods

Methods in *SMEDP* often have quasi-legal status even though procedures used to designate a method as standard are often far removed from the legal process. U.S. regulatory ordinances often stipulate that *SMEDP* procedures be used to determine whether a product satisfies certain aspects of the regulations. Within the U.S., the methods published in *SMEDP* may be recognized by the NCIMS for the testing of milk shipped interstate and subject to the provisions of the Pasteurized Milk Ordinance. These methods are incorporated into the U.S. Food and Drug Administration (FDA) Form 2400 series used by the FDA and individual states to describe methods and to evaluate laboratories operating under the NCIMS program.

Decisions to change *SMEDP* have been made only after interested parties and consensus reviewers have had an opportunity to study and react to the proposal(s). The American Public Health Association (APHA) requires publication of proposed methods in a peer-reviewed scientific journal and widespread use of the method in the dairy industry before accepting a new method or modifications of old methods. Certain method classifications require a successful method validation study.

Standard methods, especially those used by government bodies to determine compliance of dairy products with applicable laws and regulations, should be validated. That is, the performance of the method must be clearly and statistically shown to be appropriate for the intended purpose of the method.

As noted in the method classification system described below, this edition of *SMEDP* recognizes several types of method validation.

The most rigorous validation is that of the Official Methods of Analysis of the Association of Analytical Communities (AOAC)® International. These methods are subjected to a collaborative study as described by Horwitz.[8]

This approach incorporates the following elements:

1. A minimum of 8 collaborators.
2. A minimum of 5 test samples in duplicate. Test samples should cover the expected concentration range of the analyte(s).
3. Estimates of experimental error.
4. Estimates of variation between laboratories.

Official Methods of Analysis of AOAC® are validated only for specific analytes in specific products. Application of AOAC® methods beyond the matrices for which they are validated requires, as with any nonvalidated method, development of sufficient statistical data to show that the method may be successfully used in a specific application.

This edition of *SMEDP* also recognizes the Performance Tested™ validation of the AOAC® Research Institute, methods validated through a program of the NCIMS, and method validation performed by the IDF. Users of this book are encouraged to contact these organizations for particular details on their method validation programs.

Emphasis must also be placed on the uniformity of testing procedures used by laboratories.[5] If products are moved from one plant to another, or from one regulatory jurisdiction to another, uniformity of procedures is essential to ensure a reasonable degree of agreement among laboratories. Minor variations in technique can cause significant changes in analytical results. The U.S. Food and Drug Administration's (FDA) Laboratory Quality Assurance Branch, in cooperation with each individual state, has been an important factor in standardizing laboratory procedures. Elements of this FDA program are incorporated in the chapter on laboratory quality assurance and safety.

1.070 Classification of Methods

The classifications of methods in this edition of *SMEDP* are presented below. These classifications generally follow the APHA's Committee on Laboratory Standards and Practices (CLASP) designation of methods described in the categories of methods prepared for APHA publications. This unpublished report provides guidance for classifying new methods and phasing out older technology.

SMEDP method classifications are defined as follows:

1.071 *Class O*

A method or procedure that has been subjected to a thorough evaluation, has been widely used, and has thereby demonstrated its value by extensive application, but that may not have been formally and collaboratively tested or otherwise validated. This classification includes methods that are referred to as standard methods in prior editions of *SMEDP* or other APHA publications; essentially it is a grandfather clause.

1.072 *Class A1*

A method or procedure that has been subjected to thorough evaluation, has demonstrated its application for a specific purpose on the basis of extensive use, and has been successfully and collaboratively studied. AOAC® International official final action methods are included in this class.

1.073 *Class A2*

A method or procedure that has been subjected to a thorough evaluation and has been successfully and collaboratively studied. AOAC® International official first action methods are included in this class.

1.074 *Class A3*

A method or procedure that has been evaluated as prescribed by NCIMS and has been approved for use by NCIMS on milk that is produced and shipped under provisions of the U.S. Pasteurized Milk Ordinance.

1.075 *Class A4*

A method or procedure that has been subjected to an evaluation as prescribed by the AOAC® International Research Institute and has been granted Performance Tested™ status.

1.076 *Class B*

A method that has been used successfully in research or other situations; devised or modified explicitly for the routine examination of dairy product samples; published in a scientific journal that uses a peer review process; has current widespread use in the dairy industry, but has had limited evaluation; and has not been subjected to a collaborative study. This may include, but is not limited to, methods or procedures given AOAC® International Peer-Verified™ status.

IDF methods, if given in detail, are given a letter designation, if applicable.

SMEDP users should note that method classes C (unproved methods that have been proposed as useful) and D (outdated or unused methods) that appeared in earlier editions have been omitted from this edition of *SMEDP*. Users are referred to the 16th edition of *SMEDP* for definitions of these two method classes.

1.080 Chapter and Method Formats Used in This Edition

A format for chapters and methods is used in this edition of *SMEDP* to clarify methods, to make future revisions easier, and to make the book more consistent with other method references, particularly those used internationally.

This new format uses different numbering systems for chapter headings and for headings of the individual method sections.

Chapter headings use a numbering system that has three places after the decimal point. For example:

4.000 MEDIA AND REAGENT PREPARATION
- 4.010 Introduction
- 4.020 Preparation of Dilution Water
  - 4.021 Stock Phosphate and Magnesium Chloride Solution
  - 4.022 Phosphate Dilution Water
- 4.030 Water Toxicity Tests
  - 4.031 Dilution Water Toxicity Tests
  - 4.032 Water Quality Test

For methods, while the specific title of the method is a chapter heading and therefore follows the above format, the various sections of the method are numbered independently:

1. Scope
2. References
3. Definitions
4. Principle
5. Reagents
6. Apparatus and Glassware
7. Sampling
8. Preparation of Test Sample
9. Procedure
10. Expression of Results
11. Precision and Performance Parameters
12. Test Report and Interpretation
13. Bibliography

Sections that may require explanation:

A. ***Scope:*** A short statement describing the field of application (products) for which a method may be used.

B. ***References:*** This is *not* the list of cited references. Cited references are listed in the bibliography section. The reference section provides supplementary guidance for the conduct of the method found elsewhere in this book (e.g., the sampling chapter), or in another technical standards or reference (e.g., the U.S. FDA Bacteriological Analytical Manual for Foods).

C. ***Definition:*** A technical explanation of the analyte to be determined. If other terms in the method need to be defined, these definitions are also placed here.

D. ***Principle:*** A brief statement of the technical explanation of how a method works, or the basis for a procedure.

E. ***Sampling:*** This is additional information on sampling that is *not* included in chapter 3.

F. ***Procedure:*** Includes any precautions needed in performing the procedure.

G. ***Precision and performance parameters:*** Most performance parameters can be found in section 1.11 and reference to this section. If it is important that performance parameters be in the chapter (e.g., if analysts will routinely need to compare performance of multiple methods given in SMEDP prior to determining which method to use), the performance parameters will appear here.

H. ***Bibliography:*** Publications cited in the method description.

1.090 Method Selection

All classes of methods are applied throughout the dairy industry. The purpose for which the analytical result will be used (e.g., product regulation, quality assurance) and sampling requirements and analytical costs will be among factors that dictate the type and class of method to be used. Methods classified as A 1 to 4 or O are usually necessary whenever legal or regulatory considerations are involved. Methods with only a B classification may be well suited for use in quality assurance programs.

Laboratory procedures to evaluate dairy products cover materials of widely different physical and chemical composition. They include products in which certain milk constituents are concentrated in some instances and diluted in others. Furthermore, constituents that may be added in the formulation of certain products can complicate examination procedures. Details of procedures for test sample preparation and/or analysis applicable to one product may be unsuitable for another. Therefore, the final product and the individual materials used to make the final product must be considered when selecting a test method. Methods are normally validated only for certain analytes in certain commodities, so application to other matrices removes them as standard and/or validated methods for these purposes.

Proper selection of a specific analytical method is important. Considering whether it is best to determine the analyte of concern directly, as is done normally in chemical determinations, or whether it is best to use a test that is an indicator for a specific entity of concern, such as is often done in the field of microbiology, is imperative. For microbiological methods, the impact of processing, holding conditions, and other factors may influence which tests are best to use. The presence of yeast and molds, the total bacterial population, or the numbers of thermoduric, thermophilic, or psychrotrophic bacteria in a product may be of greater significance in some circumstances than others. In this edition, presentations are made for different products with cross references to basic procedures.

Method selection will differ depending on whether the test is for regulatory purposes, or for some other purpose such as quality assurance. For regulatory purposes, a method must be chosen that matches the regulatory standard to be applied. That is, the method must be sufficiently sensitive to be able to detect the analyte at the regulatory criterion set for the product. The statistical performance of the method must be such that it will not permit unsafe product to go undetected while, at the same time, preventing unnecessary rejection of product. For other purposes, a more flexible policy may be appropriate. For example, it may be adequate to consider a method that allows the following judgments to be made regarding a product: 1) it has good margins of safety or quality; 2) it falls just within acceptable limits; 3) it marginally violates standards; or 4) it is unacceptable. In each case, determinations on individual test samples by any one method should be interpreted solely on the merits of that method.

1.100 Split-Sample Test Program

Within the U.S., the NCIMS approved a provision in 1950 that individual states may accept the results of local laboratories that comply with *SMEDP* and that check closely with results on split samples[4,9,10] at least once a year.

The split-sample program[12] entails annually sending split samples to be analyzed by all laboratory methods for which the analysts of accredited laboratories are certified. The test samples represent the major types of milk and milk products. They include replicate samples yielding a normal range of results as well as results above and below the normal range and official limits. The program allows administrators to determine whether work is being done satisfactorily by analysts under their supervision. Systematic errors can easily be identified and eliminated and random errors can be minimized.

Coordination of the split-sample program is a function of the U.S. Food and Drug Administration under agreements with NCIMS. Some of the precision parameters included in this chapter [1.11] were obtained through this test program.

1.110 Precision Parameters

Precision parameters are measures of the variability of analytical methods. In practice, all methods generally demonstrate some differences in repeated measurements. Duplicate portions of the same test sample will rarely yield the exact analytical value. Only rarely can two analysts using the same test method and sample obtain the same analytical result. These differences (between duplicate samples and between different analysts) represent the variability in the application of test procedures.

All new statistically validated quantitative and qualitative methods will have published precision parameters, just as do many older methods that initially were not subjected to statistical validation studies. Precision parameters available for statistically validated methods appearing in this book are summarized in Tables 1.1 and 1.2.

The following discussion of precision parameters is provided for those analysts who may have a more detailed interest in how such parameters are determined and used.

Relationships among performance parameters, mean (X), repeatability (within laboratory) variance (S^2_r), reproducibility (between laboratory) variance (S^2_R), repeatability relative standard deviation (RSD_r) and reproducibility relative standard deviation (RSD_R), are detailed in the AOAC® International guidelines for collaborative studies.[8]

The mean (X) is the average of multiple analytical results (i.e., the sum of the results divided by the number of analyses performed). The repeatability variance (S^2_r) measures variation within laboratories or among independent replicate analysis of one test unit (e.g., a sample of milk). Reproducibility variance (S^2_R) represents the sum of replicate repeatability variance and variation between laboratories on the same test sample.

For repeatability relative standard deviation, the formula is:

$$RSD_r = (S_r / X) \cdot 100.$$

In other words, the repeatability relative standard deviation (RSD_r) equals 100 times the repeatability standard deviation (S_r) divided by the average (X) of all results used to estimate the S_r. The S_r is the square root of the repeatability variance (S^2_r). Thus, if the RSD_r and X are known, the S_r and S^2_r can be computed. The same is true for the reproducibility parameters RSD_R, S_R, and S^2_R.

1.111 *Description of Tables*

Tables 1.1 and 1.2 summarize some of the published data relating to collaborative or proficiency studies on methods in the current text. Data in Table

Table 1.1. Summary of Precision Parameters for Class A1, A2, B, and O Methods of Testing for Microorganisms and Abnormal Milk

Test	SMEDP Chap/Sec	Method[a] Class	Method[a] Name	Product	Reference[b]		Assays (N)	Determination[c] (N)	Mean ± S[d] Log_{10} (Count)	RSD_r ± S[e] (%)	RSD_R ± S[e] (%)
Total Microbial Count	6.020	O	SPC	Raw milk	JAOAC	69:671;1986	3	36	5.080±0.543	3.6±1.6	15.3±3.4
				Raw milk	JAOAC	71:343;1988	3	60	8.466±0.412	3.0±2.1	9.7±4.2
				Raw and homog. milk	JAOAC	69:527;1986	8	176	3.349±0.204	1.5±0.5	2.1±0.3
				Homog. milk	JAOAC	71:343;1988	3	60	8.219±0.283	5.1±1.4	12.1±0.9
				Milks	JFP	43:729;1980	46	1380	4.699[g]	1.5	2.0
				Milks	JFP	47:707;1984	12	120	6.197±0.640	1.1±0.8	2.5±0.7
				Milks	—	[f]	33	13512	4.783±0.705	1.2±0.6	1.5±0.6
				Chocolate milk	JAOAC	72:312;1989	4	86	2.390±0.383	5.7±3.1	7.4±3.3
				Cream	JAOAC	71:343;1988	3	60	7.844±0.413	2.4±1.1	9.3±3.4
				Evaporated milk	JAOAC	72:312;1989	3	66	2.303±0.623	10.5±9.7	10.6±9.6
				Nonfat dry milk	JAOAC	72:312;1989	4	88	3.376±0.355	3.0±0.4	5.0±1.4
				Cheese	JAOAC	71:343;1988	3	60	8.048±0.510	4.4±2.7	12.7±7.5
				Cheese	JAOAC	72:312;1989	3	64	3.213±0.797	4.2±1.2	5.9±0.7
	6.030	O	PLC	Milks	JFP	43:729;1980	45	630	5.221[g]	1.2	1.8
				Milks	—	[f]	15	906	5.176±0.097	1.2±0.4	2.0±0.9
	6.050	A2	PGPC	Cream	JAOAC	71:343;1988	3	60	8.106±0.273	1.7±0.8	6.7±2.5
				Raw milk	JAOAC	71:343;1988	3	60	8.711±0.315	2.9±2.5	8.5±2.6
				Homog. milk	JAOAC	71:343;1988	3	60	8.638±0.131	5.0±3.1	7.5±0.3
				Cheese	JAOAC	71:343;1988	3	60	8.037±0.771	3.4±0.9	10.1±4.8
	6.040	A1	PAC	Raw and homog. milk	JAOAC	69:527;1986	8	176	3.377±0.183	1.2±0.4	1.8±0.5
				Chocolate milk	JAOAC	72:312;1989	4	86	2.354±0.314	4.3±1.7	6.8±2.0
				Evaporated milk	JAOAC	72:312;1989	3	66	2.320±0.659	8.9±7.3	9.2±6.9
				Ice cream	JAOAC	72:312;1989	4	84	2.606±0.461	6.2±5.9	8.2±5.7
				Nonfat dry milk	JAOAC	72:312;1989	4	88	3.319±0.523	4.6±1.2	7.0±2.0
				Cheese	JAOAC	72:312;1989	3	64	3.149±0.656	3.1±1.2	3.6±0.8
	6.060	A2	SPLC	Milks	JFP	40:462;1977	5	60	4.934±0.603	1.4±0.4	1.7±0.5
Coliform	7.081	O	VRB	Raw and homog. milk	JAOAC	69:527;1986	7	154	1.356±0.235	7.1±3.1	8.1±2.8
				Milks	JFP	43:729;1980	45	540	2.301[g]	4.4	5.5
				Raw milk	JAOAC	72:936;1989	6	66	4.459±1.557	1.4±2.5	2.1±3.3
				Chocolate milk	JAOAC	72:312;1989	3	66	1.806±0.589	7.1±1.0	11.2±2.0
				Evaporated milk	JAOAC	72:312;1989	3	66	1.502±0.515	13.8±7.3	18.1±4.0
				Ice cream	JAOAC	72:312;1989	3	66	1.602±0.661	9.3±10.3	18.4±11.8
				Nonfat dry milk	JAOAC	66:897;1983	5	168	4.525±0.597	5.6±2.9	6.7±1.9

			Nonfat dry milk	JAOAC	72:312;1989	3	60	2.341±0.359	9.8±3.3	13.1±6.3
			Cheese	JAOAC	72:312;1989	3	66	2.088±0.720	8.4±8.3	10.0±9.8
			Cheese powder	JAOAC	72:936;1989	3	72	1.821±0.448	20.3±7.2	21.6±6.5
7.071	A1	PCC	Raw and homog. milk	JAOAC	69:527;1986	7	154	1.338±0.236	5.8±7.9	5.2±8.8
			Chocolate milk	JAOAC	72:312;1989	3	66	1.787±0.667	9.2±4.2	14.5±6.3
			Evaporated milk	JAOAC	72:312;1989	3	66	1.734±.0.569	12.6±6.1	14.2±7.0
			Ice cream	JAOAC	72:312;1989	3	66	1.974±0.567	4.4±1.3	6.9±1.7
			Nonfat dry milk	JAOAC	72:312;1989	3	60	2.335±0.391	8.5±4.9	22.4±13.0
			Cheese	JAOAC	72:312;1989	3	66	2.119±0.768	11.3±12.6	11.7±12.2
7.072	A2	PHSCC	2% Milk	JAOAC	80:505;1997	8	864			
			Low level					0.681	8.4±0.058	14.9±0.101
			Medium					1.576	4.3±0.067	5.2±0.082
			High					2.437	2.9±0.071	4.5±0.109
			Chocolate milk							
			Low level					0.612	39.4±0.241	39.4±0.241
			Medium					1.637	5.4±0.088	5.5±0.09
			High					2.602	4.4±0.114	4.5±0.116
			Cream							
			Low level					0.638	39.9±0.255	39.9±0.255
			Medium					1.661	2.8±0.046	4.3±0.071
			High					2.679	3.0±0.081	3.5±0.095
			Vanilla ice cream							
			Low level					0.147	138.1±0.203	141.2±0.208
			Medium					1.098	13.3±0.146	16.2±0.178
			High					1.899	4.6±0.087	9.0±0.17
			Cottage cheese							
			Low level					1.42	9.8±0.139	13.0±0.185
			Medium					2.41	4.7±0.112	5.4±0.131
			High					3.361	3.4±0.115	3.7±0.125
			Cheddar cheese							
			Low level					0.311	17.7±0.055	17.7±0.055
			Medium					1.633	6.4±0.105	11.0±0.18
			High					3.122	2.3±0.071	7.2±0.226
7.080	A1	PGPC	Raw milk	JAOAC	72:298;1989	3	108	1.594±0.737	8.5±6.9	11.7±6.4
			Homog. milk	JAOAC	72:298;1989	3	108	1.744±0.613	8.3±3.8	12.2±2.9
			Cream	JAOAC	72:298;1989	3	108	1.673±0.799	42.2±60.1	50.7±67.1
			Sour cream	JAOAC	72:298;1989	3	120	1.800±0.654	8.6±5.1	14.0±7.8
			Yogurt	JAOAC	72:298;1989	3	120	1.656±0.762	11.2±9.8	23.3±17.9
			Cottage cheese	JAOAC	72:298;1989	3	120	1.677±0.599	8.3±3.8	19.1±12.9

Table 1.1. Continued

Test	SMEDP Chap/Sec	Method[a] Class	Method[a] Name	Product	Reference[b]		Assays (N)	Determination[c] (N)	Mean ± S[d] Log_{10} (Count)	RSD_r ± S[e] (%)	RSD_R ± S[e] (%)
	7.080	A1	PGPC	Cheddar cheese	JAOAC	72:298;1989	3	120	1.085±0.754	129.8±111.3	138.1±196.9
Yeast and mold count	8.110	A2	PDA	Cheese, nonfat dry milk	JFS	47:930;1982	10	140	5.11[g]	1.8	2.
	8.115	A2	DRF	Yogurt	JAOAC	80:806;1997	15	540			
				Low level					2.34	6.90±0.16	31.81±0.75
				High					3.21	13.45±0.43	15.70±0.50
Direct microscopic count (bacteria)	10.02	O	DMC/MB	Nonfat dry milk	JDS	46:810;1963	6	276	7.773±0.421	2.0±1.1	3.9±2.5
			DMC/LW	Nonfat dry milk	JDS	46:810;1963	6	276	7.864±0.444	1.6±0.5	3.7±2.0
Abnormal milk	11.031	O	DMSCC	Raw milk	JFP	40:456;1977	9	108	6	1.9	2.4
				Raw milk	JAOAC	67:615;1984	6	60	5.788±0.057	0.4±0.2	4.9±0.7
				Raw milk	JMFT	34:285;1971	20	520	6.170±0.198	1.6±0.3	2.0±0.3
			Field strip	Raw milk	JMFT	34:285;1971	20	520	6.045±0.217	1.7±0.5	3.2±0.3
				Raw milk	—	[f]	16	5364	5.805±0.368	0.9±0.3	1.3±0.3
				Raw milk	JFP	43:729;1980	32	960	5.845[g]	0.9±0.1	1.9±0.4

a *SPC* = standard plate count, *PLC* = plate loop count, *SPLC* = spiral plate count, *PAC* = Petrifilm aerobic count, *PGPC* = pectin gel plate count, *VRB* = violet red bile, *PCC* = Petrifilm coliform count, *PDA* = potato dextrose acid agar, *DMC/MB* = direct microscopic count/methylene blue, *DMC/LW* = direct microscopic count/Levowitz-Weber, *DMSCC* = direct microscopic somatic cell count, and *DRF* = dry rehydratable film.

b *JAOAC* = *Journal of the Association of Official Analytical Chemists*, *JFP* = *Journal of Food Protection*, *JFS* = *Journal of Food Science*, *JDS* = *Journal of Dairy Science*, and *JMFT* = *Journal of Milk and Food Technology.*

c Number of determinations before outliers are deleted.

d S = Estimate of variation among multiple assays.

e *RSD* = Relative standard deviation: *r* = within laboratories, *R* = within and among laboratories, and *S* = standard deviation for a given study.

f Peeter, J.T.; Messer, J.W.; Leslie, J.E.; Houghtby, G.A. Precision parameters for FDA milk split samples: 1983–1987. Unpublished data.

g Data on individual results cannot be determined in the paper.

Table 1.2. Summary of Performance Parameters for Class A1, A2, and O Methods of Chemical Analysis

Test	SMEDP Chap/Sec	Method[a] Class	Method[a] Name	Product	JAOAC Reference	Assays (N)	Determination[a] (N)	Mean ± S (%)	$RSD_r \pm S$[b] (%)	$RSD_R \pm S$[b] (%)
Acidity	15.021	O	Titratable	Evaporated milk	34:239;1951	4	40	0.3±0.02	1.0±0.3	1.3±0.3
Ash	15.041	O	Gravimetric	Evaporated milk	34:239;1951	4	40	1.5±0.04	0.6±0.2	2.3±1.0
					23:454;1940	4	40	1.6±0.1	0.7±0.4	2.3±0.9
				Standard H_2SO_4 solution	24:631;1941	1	12	0.1[c]	0.1	0.2
Chloride	15.051	O	Mohr	Butter	49:518;1966	6	84	1.8±0.6	1.1±0.7	2.3±0.7
	15.052	A1	Volhard	Standard H_2SO_4 solution	24:631;1941	1	12	0.1[c]	0.1	0.1
				Cheese	20:339;1937	1	33	1.4	1.5	2.0
Fat	15.081	A1	Babcock	Raw milk	55:488;1972	10	90	3.7±0.9	–[d]	0.7±0.5
				Raw milk	56:1401;1973	15	270	4.0±0.7	–	1.2±0.7
				Raw milk	58:949;1975	10	180	3.5±0.4	0.5±0.2	1.2±0.2
				Raw milk	80:845;1997	9	162	4.11	0.901±0.037	1.147±0.047
				Homog. milk	50:537;1967	8	95	3.2±0.8	2.1±0.9	2.9±1.2
	15.082	A1		Cream	79:907;1996	9	180	38.209	0.548±0.209	0.712±0.272
				Cream	80:845;1997	9	162	37.555	0.687±0.258	0.94±0.353
	15.085	O	Ether extraction	Dried milk	IDF;1988[e]	10	100	26.4±0.9	0.5±0.3	0.6±0.2
				Dried milk	IDF;1988[e]	15	120	19.3±6.9	0.3±0.2	0.5±0.3
				Dried milk	15:524;1932	8	112	27.9±0.6	0.5±0.2	1.8±0.2
				Homog. milk	50:537;1967	8	96	3.2±0.8	0.6±0.6	1.2±0.4
				Chocolate milk	50:537;1967	4	48	2.6±0.7	1.3±0.8	1.7±0.5
	15.085	A1	Mojonnier	Raw milk	72:719;1989	9	156	3.9±0.67	0.26±0.05	0.38±0.05
				Cream	79;907;1996	9	180	37.932	0.33±0.125	0.398±0.151
	15.121	A1	Infrared	Raw milk	55:488;1972	5	50	3.7±0.9	–	0.6±0.4
				Pasteurized milk	55:488;1972	5	40	3.8±0.1	–	1.6±0.3
				Whole milk	61:1015;1978	66	792	3.6±0.7	0.6±0.3	1.9±0.6
				Retail milk	61:1015;1978	14	168	2.5±0.6	0.8±0.4	3.0±1.0
	15.122	A2	Near Infrared	Raw milk	56:1401;1973	30	540	3.9±0.7	–	1.1±0.6
	15.123	O	Kohman	Butter	35:194;1952	6	324	81.3±0.1	0.06±0.02	0.4±0.1
Lactose	15.121	A1	Infrared	Raw milk	55:488;1972	10	180	4.7±0.1	–	2.8±0.8
Protein	15.121	A1	Infrared	Raw milk	55:488;1972	10	90	3.3±0.3	–	2.2±0.3
				Whole milk	61:1015;1978	66	792	3.1±0.2	0.4±0.2	1.1±0.3
				Retail milk	61:1015;1978	22	264	3.2±0.05	0.4±0.2	1.9±0.5
	15.131	A1	Kjeldahl	Milk (Hg)	55:488;1972	10	70	3.3±0.3	–	2.2±0.7
				Milk (Cu)	71:893;1988	6	216	3.2±0.8	0.6±0.2	1.0±0.1

Table 1.2. Continued

Test	SMEDP Chap/Sec	Method[a] Class	Method[a] Name	Product	JAOAC Reference	Assays (N)	Determination[a] (N)	Mean ± S (%)	$RSD_r \pm S^b$ (%)	$RSD_R \pm S^b$ (%)
Protein continued										
				Cheese (Cu)	112:317;1987[f]	6	108	22.4±3.1	1.4±0.7	1.8±0.6
				Milk	52:126;1969	12	384	2.9±0.3	1.4±0.6	2.8±0.5
Nonprotein nitroge	15.135			Raw milk	81:763;1998	9	180	0.762	1.287±0.01	2.146±0.016
Casein (indirect)	15.136			Raw milk				2.585	0.56±0.015	0.841±0.022
Casein (direct)	15.137							2.575	0.597±0.015	0.988±0.025
Moisture	15.111	O	Vacuum oven	Cheddar cheese	60:1392;1977	6	72	38.2±0.5	0.3±0.1	0.7±0.3
				Colby cheese	60:1392;1977	6	72	40.3±0.6	0.3±0.1	0.8±0.3
				Monterey Jack cheese	60:1392;1977	6	72	41.3±2.1	0.3±0.1	0.8±0.3
				Swiss cheese	16:584;1933	1	33	36.2	0.2	0.7
				Cheddar cheese	52:117;1969	3	72	41.1±2.6	0.6±0.5	2.5±1.4
				Cheddar cheese	32:303;1949	4	50	37.2±1.3	0.5±0.3	0.8±0.3
				Evaporated milk	23:453;1940	4	68	26.6±0.3	0.13±0.03	0.68±0.38
	15.114	A1	Forced air	Raw milk	72:712;1989	9	180	12.7±0.7	0.15±0.06	0.33±0.05
			Forced air: steam predry	Raw milk	72:712;1989	9	154	12.7±0.7	0.14±0.04	0.37±0.04
Freezing point	15.032	A1	Cryoscope	Canned milk	51:816;1968	1	38	–0.497°C	0.29	0.96
				Milk	IDF;1986[g]	2	240	–0.516°C	0.29	1.35

a Numbers of determinations before outliers are deleted.
b *RSD* = Relative standard deviation: *r* = within laboratories, *R* = within and among laboratories, and *S* = standard deviation for a given study.
c 0.1N solution.
d Estimate of replicate error could not be computed from data given in reference.
e Hopkin E. International Dairy Federation letter, March 22, 1998, Reference 2/233 to Members of Group E30-Statistics of Analytical Methods—"Roese-Gottlieb method for determinations of the fat content: report of collaborative and/or comparative studies."
f Analyst 112, 317 (1987).
g International Dairy Federation, IDF Standard 108A:1986 (cyroscopic method) Bulletin 207/chapter B.

1.1 cover procedures and precision parameters for testing for microorganisms and abnormal milk. Table 1.2 gives precision parameters for the chemical analysis of milk. Both tables are arranged to show the analyte (e.g., fat) or test category (e.g., abnormal milk), current *SMEDP* chapter and section number, class and acronym for the method, and product(s) used in the study. The reference column shows where the data are located. For example, JAOAC 67:615; 1984 means that the article can be found in the *Journal of the Association of Official Analytical Chemists*, volume 67, in 1984 starting on page 615. The number of assays performed (on replicate samples) and the total number of determinations observed before data were corrected for outliers and missing data are also given. The data, as published, often do not reflect recent decisions by the AOAC® International[7,8,13] for statistical analysis. Therefore, most of the data have been reanalyzed to ensure a common basis of comparison. An explanation of these statistical analyses is given elsewhere.[9] The precision parameters are RSD_r and RSD_R. An estimate of variation among multiple assays, or standard deviation (S), is also presented. The range to which these estimates apply is approximated by taking the mean ± 3 standard deviations (±3S).

Because there are multiple studies on some methods, data from methods for which more than 15 assays were performed are summarized in Tables 1.3 and 1.4. The mean, median (middle value), and 90-percentile intervals (range including 90 of values) are presented for RSD_r and RSD_R. A median RSD_R means that 50% of all of the RSD_R values lie below the RSD_R value and 50% are higher than the RSD_R value. Using ether extraction of fat as an example, Table 1.4 shows that the low RSD_R value for the 90-percentile interval (0.3 to 2.1) is 0.3, or the 5 percentile point. That is, 95% of the RSD_R values are larger than 0.3 and 5% are smaller. The upper limit is 2.1, or the 95% percentile point. Accordingly, 5% of the RSD_R values are higher than 2.1 and 95% are lower.

1.112 *Use of Tables*

The tables present published precision information on quantitative tests. These parameters can be used to determine the precision of the tests listed, or to compare precision parameters of tests being used, or are in consideration by laboratories. The method of analysis used by laboratories is often specified in a legal standard, and some methods have special requirements not specified in the tables. In some cases, the differences between studies are considerable. Caution should be used in interpreting results and when choosing a data set as a standard against which to compare a laboratory's results. For example, data for the ether extraction of fat in Table 1.2 shows that: 1) the studies were performed many years apart; and 2) the concentration range is from 2.6% to 27.9% fat. If the RSD_r is considered, the values are relatively constant above the fat concentration of 2.6%. Table 1.4 shows that the median RSD_r for the ether extraction method is 0.5 and the 95% percentile point is 2.0.

Also to be considered are comparative data between a new procedure and the standard or reference test. As an example, consider data in Table 1.1 for the standard plate count (SPC) and for alternate methods to the SPC. For

Table 1.3. Statistical Parameters Characterizing Selected[a] Microbiological Methods

Test	SMEDP Chap/Sec	Method Name[b]	Studies (N)	Assays (N)	RSD_r Mean (%)	RSD_r Median (%)	RSD_r 90 Percentile Interval (%)	RSD_R Mean (%)	RSD_R Median (%)	RSD_R 90 Percentile Interval (%)
Total microbial count	6.02	SPC 1[c]	4	61	1.3	1.1	0.5- 2.8	1.8	1.8	0.9- 3.5
		2[d]	3	20	4.2	3.9	1.1-10.4	10.6	10.9	4.1-18.8
	6.03	PLC	2	22	1.2	1.1	0.7-1.9	1.8	1.9	1.3- 3.6
Abnormal milk	11.031	DMSCC	5	70	1.3	1.2	0.4-2.3	2.4	2.1	1.1- 4.7

[a] Based on having at least 15 assays reported.
[b] SPC = standard plate count, PLC = plate loop count, and DMSCC = direct microscopic somatic cell count.
[c] Studies performed with seeded analytical samples.
[d] Studies performed with natural flora in analytical samples.

Table 1.4. Statistical Parameters Characterizing Selected[a] Chemical Methods

Test	SMEDP Chap/Sec	Method Name[b]	Studies (N)	Assays (N)	RSD_r Mean (%)	RSD_r Median (%)	RSD_r 90 Percentile Interval (%)	RSD_R Mean (%)	RSD_R Median (%)	RSD_R 90 Percentile Interval (%)
Fat	15.081	Babcock	4	43	1.2	0.8	0.3-3.5	1.4	1.2	0.0-2.9
	15.085	Ether extraction	4	45	0.6	0.5	0.1-2.0	1.0	0.9	0.3-2.1
	15.121	Infrared	2	98	0.6	0.6	0.2-1.2	2.2	2.0	0.8-4.8
	15.122	Near infrared	1	30	–	–	–	1.1	0.9	0.6-2.2
Protein	15.121	Infrared	2	106	0.4	0.4	0.2-0.8	1.5	1.3	0.8-2.7
	15.131	Kjeldahl	4	22	1.2	1.1	0.3-2.6	1.8	1.6	0.8-2.9
Moisture	15.111	Vacuum oven	4	25	0.4	0.3	0.1-1.3	1.2	0.9	0.4-3.8

[a] Based on having at least 15 assays reported.

homogenized milk, the average RSD_r of the pectin gel plate count (PGPC) is 5.0 [6.05, line 3 in Table 1.1] and the average RSD_r for the SPC, from the same study, is 5.1 [6.02, line 4]. This compares unfavorably with the RSD_r values of 1.1 to 1.5 reported for the SPC in proficiency studies performed by milk laboratories [6.02, lines 3, 5, 6, and 7]. The larger RSD_r and RSD_R for the PGPC may be due to variation among analysts; however, these results may also be due to the use of natural samples in the study, whereas seeded samples were used in the proficiency studies.

Another factor to consider, when comparative results are available, is the difference between the means. Again, using for an example the data in Table 1.1, the mean SPC for homogenized milk is 8.219 [6.02, line 4], whereas the mean of the PGPC is 8.638 [6.05, line 3]. When the antilog of these means is taken, the latter count is seen to be almost 3 times higher than the former count: 4.35×10^8 as compared to 1.66×10^8. Thus, when comparing methods, both means and performance parameters should be considered. Comparing the means and precision parameters without knowledge of studies may lead to incorrect conclusions as to the comparison of the tests.

Tables 1.3 and 1.4 show typical published levels of performance of specific methods averaging over assays and studies. If the repeatability performance observed for 50% of the assays is being sought, the median value should be chosen. For the ether extraction of fat method, this is $RSD_r = 0.5$ [Table 1.4]. On the other hand, an analyst may wish to see what the upper limit of variability might be. For the ether extraction method, the 95 percentile point (the upper value of the 90-percentile limit) would be chosen: $RSD_r = 2.0$. Two examples are given below to illustrate the possible application of these numbers:

A. ***Example 1:*** An analyst using the ether extraction of fat method wants to determine an upper limit of the difference between results of duplicate tests of the same sample. The expected fat content of the product is 3.25% (g/100g). The analyst decides to use the median $RSD_r = 0.5$. One suggested algorithm for determining a limit for duplicate values is to compute the repeatability value $(r) = (0.028)(X)(RSD_r)$. This is the absolute (always positive) difference between the results of each duplicate measurement, which is expected to be below r in 95% of the assays. For the present example, $RSD_r = 0.5$ and X = 3.25. Thus, $r = (0.028)(3.25)(0.5) = 0.046$, and so duplicate fat determinations should not differ by more than 0.046% (g/100g).

B. ***Example 2:*** The analyst has performed a series of replicate measurements using the ether extraction of fat method. The results are expressed as percent fat (g/100g) and a variance (S^2) has been computed. What is a typical variance for this product when the mean percent fat is 3.25%? The variance can be computed from the equation noted above. Again choosing the median $RSD_r = 0.5$, we solve for S_r:

$$S_{\mathrm{r}} = RSD_r \bullet \mathrm{X} / 100 = (0.5)(3.25) / 100 = 0.0163$$

The variance is the square of S_r, or S^2_r; therefore, $S^{\mathrm{r}}_2 = (0.0163)^2 = 0.00026$.

Analysts should be aware that regulatory testing laboratories often participate in proficiency programs that reduce variation within and among laboratories. These programs may require performance that is more precise than that obtained in method validation studies; that is, the level of required performance may be near the median. In other cases, analysts may wish to verify that a method performs adequately in their hands, in which case the 95-percentile estimate may be a suitable choice. The tables display published data on both good and poor performance.

For further information on how method validation studies can be performed, refer to references 1, 6–8, and 13.

1.120 Cited References

1. ANDREWS, W.H. Recommendations for preparing test samples for AOAC collaborative studies of microbiological procedures for foods. JAOAC **70**: 931-936; 1987.
2. CODEX ALIMENTARIUS COMMISSION. *Procedural manual*, 12th ed. Rome: Food and Agriculture Organization of the United Nations; 2001:150.
3. CODEX ALIMENTARIUS COMMISSION. *Draft Proposed Code of Hygienic Practice for Milk and Milk Products*, CX/FH 98/5. Rome: Food and Agriculture Organization of the United Nations; 1998.
4. DONNELLY, C.B.; PEELER, J.T.; BLACK, L.A. Evaluation of state central milk laboratories by statistical analysis of standard plate counts. J. Milk Food Technol. **29**: 19-24; 1966.
5. FAULKNER, J.D.; TAYLOR, D.W; SCHLAFMAN, I.H. The USPHS method of rating milk supplies and its use in the interstate milk shipper program. J. Milk Food Technol. **26**: 277-281; 1963.
6. GINN, R.E.; BENGSCH, H.K.; BRAZIS, A.R.; BULTHAUS, M.M.; CASE, R.; FUQUA, R.G.; GILMAN, C.R.; HEADY, J.; HICKEY, P.J.; KELLEY, W.N.; KOENIG, E.K.; MESSER, J.W.; WEHR, H.M.; WHALEY, K.W.; ZIMMERMAN, A.F. NCIMS informational statements for developers of dairy product analysis methods. J. Food Prot. **49**: 760-762; 1986.
7. HORWITZ, W. Committee on interlaboratory studies. JAOAC **70**: 352-356; 1987.
8. HORWITZ, W. Guidelines for collaborative study procedure to validate characteristics of a method of analysis. JAOAC **71**: 160-171; 1988.
9. PEELER, J.T.; HORWITZ, W.; ALBERT, R. Precision parameters of standard methods of analysis for dairy products. JAOAC **72**: 784-806; 1989.
10. RUPPERT, E.L; TAYLOR, D.W; SCHLAFMAN, I.H. The interstate milk shipper certification program; a cooperative accomplishment. J. Milk Food Technol. **28**: 379-382; 1975.
11. UNITED STATES DEPARTMENT OF HEALTH AND HUMAN SERVICES, PUBLIC HEALTH SERVICE, FOOD AND DRUG ADMINISTRATION. *Grade A Pasteurized Milk Ordinance*. Washington, DC: U.S. Govt. Print Off; 1995 Rev.
12. UNITED STATES DEPARTMENT OF HEALTH AND HUMAN SERVICES. *Evaluation of milk laboratories*. Washington, DC: U.S. Govt. Print Off.; 1985 Rev.
13. WEHR, H.M. Official Methods Board. JAOAC **69**: 314-315; 1986.
14. WORLD TRADE ORGANIZATION. *Results of the Uruguay round of multilateral trade negotiations*. Geneva, Switzerland: The Legal Texts; 1995.

Chapter 2

Laboratory Quality Assurance and Safety

R. Reddy, T. E. Graham, D. T. Laird, and L. J. Maturin
(E. Arnold, Tech. Comm.)

2.010 Introduction

This chapter is an overview of dairy laboratory quality assurance and covers laboratory equipment and supply requirements, analysis, and record keeping. Laboratory safety is also discussed. Most of the information presented is applicable to all laboratories; however, portions of the material may be applicable only to those doing diversified microbiological and chemical analyses. The topics discussed in this chapter, when combined with close attention to standard methods of analyses, form the basis of good laboratory practice (GLP).

Quality assurance is a vital component of laboratory operations. Without proper attention to laboratory quality assurance, the validity of analytical results can be questioned. Quality assurance is a systems approach to achieve quality results. Quality control encompasses a number of components, including analysis and record keeping, of a quality assurance system. Therefore, quality assurance is the sum of all activities designed to ensure that information generated by a laboratory is valid.

Initiatives for hazard analysis and critical control points (HACCP) systems are being prepared for food safety. Recommendations relevant to laboratory quality assurance, including government-initiated systems for accrediting state and private laboratories testing food products for contaminants, are discussed. Other recommendations include long-term strategies for food laboratory evaluation and the establishment of international harmonization of laboratory quality programs.[1,16,22]

The International Standardization Organization (ISO)[23,28,29] defines quality as "the totality of features and characteristics of a product or service that bear on its ability to satisfy stated or implied needs."[29] Baldwin[2] equated quality with credibility, a term that connotes trust, believability, reliability, and dependability, and stated that "scientific data must be able to withstand the careful scrutiny of all interested parties, be they consumers, manufacturers, scientists, lawyers, bureaucracy, judges, media, Congress, and many others."

Requirements for accurate and precise results, whether the results are generated to monitor quality systems or are being used for regulatory purposes by government agencies, are needed in dairy laboratory analysis. From a public health point of view, the only presupposition is the expectation of reliable analytical results.

For food safety or for achieving a company's specifications, a laboratory must produce quality data to justify its cost and existence. The process of ensuring the quality of dairy laboratory data begins by answering several questions. The 3 critical parameters in this context are: 1) the determination of reasons for inadequate quality of analytical results; 2) the determination of requirements, methods, and means to generate quality analytical results; and 3) the ability and method of demonstration of a laboratory's capability of producing quality data consistently.

Inadequate planning and/or the lack of human resources are primary reasons for not achieving a quality analysis.[31] Other reasons may include improper sampling, sample handling during transportation and storage, analytical method, analyst performance, reporting errors, lack of traceability, and analyst training.[17]

2.011 *Various Stages of Laboratory Analysis and Probable Point(s) of Error*

A. **Sampling** (sampling technique, collection of homogeneous samples, aseptic technique, sufficient sample for analysis).

B. **Sample storage and transportation to laboratory** (proper conditions for storage and transport, protection from contamination, time and temperature concerns, protection from tampering, chain of custody).

C. **Sample receipt** (condition of samples, determination of suitability for analysis).

D. **Laboratory handling and storage of samples** (condition of storage until analysis performed, time and temperature concerns, protection from contamination, protection from tampering).

E. **Sample preparation** (improper preparation, contamination, homogenous subsamples).

F. **Analysis** (suitability of method and equipment, specificity, sensitivity and validity of method, calibration of equipment, use of suitable controls, standards and external assessment, analyst proficiency, training and skill).

G. **Results** (record of analytical results, documented, proper record keeping, results reviewed for accuracy).

H. **Reports** (results accurately transcribed, timely issue of reports).

I. **Traceability of analysis** (from initial sample collection through the completion of analysis and the issuance of the report).

ISO has developed a comprehensive set of requirements for testing and calibration laboratories.[28] ISO requirements are suitable for any testing irrespective of the type of industry. The basis of the ISO requirements is for a competent laboratory to organize its analysis in a systematic way, based on the principles of quality assurance, to preclude problems from arising. A systematic approach requires an agreement on the order in which tasks should be performed to assure that the analytical service provided is fit for its intended purpose. It is possible to set up a system that clearly sets out what must be done and makes provision to monitor day-to-day operation to ensure that the specified work has been completed.[24]

Achieving quality laboratory results includes employing and retaining well-trained and motivated technologists, using improved technologies and scientific methods, developing a quality manual, implementing adequate quality control procedures, participating in external and internal proficiency testing programs, and maintaining a deep commitment to improve quality from top management to bench analysts. When well-trained and motivated technologists use high-quality assays according to standard operating procedures, the end result is usually highly accurate and precise. Because unacceptable results are sometimes produced even by the best systems, protocols must be established to detect and correct error situations.[5]

A laboratory must demonstrate to its customers (e.g., dairy producers, processors, regulators, consumers) that it is capable of generating quality data by achieving recognition either through registration, accreditation from an independent organization, or demonstration of conformance to certain guidelines. Accreditation confirms the competency of the laboratory to perform tasks consistent with stated goals. In the current global marketplace, international trade is dependent upon laboratory competency. Currently there are a number of accreditation programs run by government and private agencies. Each of these programs contains common elements. The National Institute of Standards and Technology (NIST) has developed criteria for the evaluation of many of these programs.[4]

2.020 Quality Management System

2.021 *Introduction*

In the day-to-day operation of a dairy laboratory, many independent and interdependent functions are carried out. Each of these operations must be clearly defined. For example, if equipment (e.g., analytical balances, pH meters, or thermometers) is not calibrated, different dependent laboratory functions may be affected. Yet if the calibration of equipment is taken as an entity then all calibration-related problems can be solved. Therefore, a systematic approach is needed for a laboratory to generate quality data. A detailed understanding of the term system is needed to formulate a quality assurance system in an analytical laboratory. Early[9] described the term system as:

A. A system is an organization of discrete components (some of which are subsystems).

B. A system performs an identifiable task of set of tasks.

C. The components of a system each contribute to the overall tasks.

D. The components of system interrelate and interact.

E. The removal or breakdown of a component in a system will result in failure of the system.

F. The system is contained within a boundary.

G. During the operation of the system inputs are made to the system and outputs are gained from the system.

Ensuring the quality of data generated by a laboratory involves two principle parts: quality assurance (QA) and quality control (QC).[23,29] ISO defines QA as "all those planned and systematic actions necessary to provide adequate confidence that a product will satisfy given requirements for quality" and QC as "the operational techniques and activities that are used to fulfill requirements for quality."

A quality management system (QMS) is defined by ISO as "the organizational structure, responsibility, procedures, and resources for implementing quality management." A dairy laboratory should carefully study the definition of quality. Quality, as defined earlier in this chapter, is the fulfillment of stated or implied needs. Therefore, a laboratory needs to state its objectives regarding quality from the outset. The statement of quality objectives sets the stage for establishing and implementing a QMS.

2.022 *Features of a Quality Management System*

A. Common features incorporated into a QMS include[9]:

1. A systems approach to quality management.
2. Operation through documented procedures.
3. Focus on continuous satisfaction of customers through compliance with specifications.
4. Orientation on product and service.
5. Requirement for personnel to be trained for involvement.
6. Involvement of only the personnel concerned with a product or service.
7. Recognition of achievement through registration to ISO 9000, through an independent accreditation service, or through approval by regulatory agencies.
8. Being driven by routine surveillance by the accreditation body.

B. **Goals of QMS:** In its simplest form the quality objective of a dairy laboratory is to produce accurate, precise, and reproducible results and to have a system of traceability to monitor sample and data flow. The QMS is used to achieve these goals. Some of the typical goals of laboratories are summarized below. Each laboratory may have a distinct set of priorities, and typical objectives may include some or all of the following goals:

1. Satisfy accreditation, certification, and/or legal requirements.
2. Improve reliability of analytical service.
3. Fulfill the company's public health responsibilities.
4. Provide a safe working environment for the employees.
5. Incorporate improved technologies rapidly and efficiently.
6. Reduce the cost of operations.

7. Provide a historical basis for laboratory performance.
8. Monitor trends or patterns of a process.
9. Evaluate methods.
10. Ensure sample integrity.
11. Improve employee morale and sense of accomplishment.
12. Ultimately improve overall quality of the organization.

2.023 *Establishing a Quality Management System*

A. Steps involved in establishing a QMS[41]:

1. Develop guideline requirements used for the basis of the QMS that will satisfy current as well as near future needs.
2. Develop goals and objectives to fulfill all QMS requirements. Employers should be familiar with and resolve all QMS, regulatory, and safety requirements from the start. Resolve any cost-benefit conflicts.
3. Develop a quality structure and a quality manual. Examine all of the quality elements such as facilities, analysis, and management, etc., and form quality circles and review the quality manual for accuracy and methods.
4. Appraise the current system.
5. Implement the new system.
6. Monitor and audit the new system.
7. Develop a system to periodically review and implement new developments for improved quality.

A dairy laboratory QMS will have several subsystems or elements. The elements relevant to the selected QMS, or for a specific laboratory, should be identified. Garfield,[17] Wilson & Weir,[41] ISO/DIS 17025,[28] and others[13-15,26,27] have listed most of the quality elements relevant to a laboratory QMS. Some of the quality elements of a laboratory, and their significance in successful implementation of a QMS, are outlined in the following sections.

Quality elements must be incorporated into a written document in a structured and easily comprehensible manner so that the document becomes the primary source for stated objectives of quality and a reference source for implementation of the QMS.

2.030 Quality Elements

2.031 *Quality Assurance Policy Statement*

A quality assurance policy statement establishes the general principles, policies, and guidelines under which the dairy laboratory operates. It should reference such things as the Grade A Pasteurized Milk Ordinance,[36] applicable state and federal codes, and any other manuals or sources of information to be used, such as ISO documents.[28,34] This section also needs to contain specific and detailed information on management's commitment to quality assurance in the laboratory and activities and/or processes to maintain the program. The laboratory's quality goals, procedures, and remedial actions must be clearly outlined in the quality manual. The importance of strict adherence to the quality manual both by management and technicians must be emphasized.

The dairy laboratory must be committed to a QA plan. This document outlines what is expected of all parties involved—from management to the analysts. This includes a commitment and appropriate support from management and proper analysis from analysts. ISO has numerous documents that outline and define the roles of all parties involved.[24,25,41] Laboratory management should maintain a policy that provides for the scope, type, and amount of testing it undertakes in conjunction with the assurance that the level of performance will be maintained. The plan specifies guidelines to ensure valid results. These include areas such as procedures/samples, supplies/equipment, records, audits, corrective/preventive actions, personnel, and management.[14,15,26,27]

2.032 *Quality Assurance Manual*

The quality assurance manual is the single most important element of any QMS. A quality manual is often interchangeable with a standard operating procedure (SOP), which may cause confusion. Each element of quality could have a standard operating procedure such as sampling, reporting compliance, or an instrument calibration technique. A quality manual brings together all the elements of the quality management system. It is a standard operating procedure for achieving quality. The preparation of a quality manual requires a major commitment from management in terms of time and cooperation. For many laboratories, developing a quality manual is a beneficial experience and may uncover many operational errors.

This plan (the terms "plan" and "manual" will be used interchangeably) outlines the policies and procedures a dairy laboratory uses to produce valid, uniform, and reproducible analytical results.[14,15,28] The plan contains quality control measures and details how the laboratory is administered and monitored. A well detailed plan that is adhered to (and is not open to interpretation or choice) leaves little room for error, question, or interpretation, and results in uniformity. The ISO/DIS 17025 standard defines the quality manual as a document stating the quality policy, quality system, and quality practices of an organization.[28] Definitions of relevant terminology, laboratory quality assurance principles, objectives, and their role in improving data reliability will be outlined.

2.033 *Laboratory Organization*

The organization of a dairy laboratory is important to its successful operation. Of the many possible organizational structures for a laboratory, the most common center on either projects or functions.[11,21]

Project organizational structure concentrates on the type of work being done for the laboratory's clients, irrespective of the technology being employed. Examples include methods development groups, quality control laboratories, and special project groups and can involve both chemical and microbiological analyses.

Functional organizational structure is developed around similarities of techniques, procedures, and instrumentation. A project can be divided so that each function (e.g., sample receiving, preparation, microbiological analysis, gas chromatographic analysis) is done by a separate section of the laboratory and/or analyst.

Each approach offers advantages and disadvantages.[17,41] Project organizational structure maximizes project control by concentrating all aspects of the project within a single laboratory operating unit, but requires various project groups to either share or duplicate equipment. Organization by function concentrates services into specialized groups whose equipment and personnel are dedicated to a specific technology, but makes management and control of individual projects more difficult because responsibility is usually spread over several laboratory sections.

Laboratory organizational structure is really a function of the philosophy of the managers and of the nature or type of work being performed. Organizational structures cannot be static. As the nature of the work changes over time, managers need to reevaluate their laboratory's organizational structure.

2.034 *Laboratory Staffing, Personnel Selection, and Training*

Staffing is a function of the dairy laboratory organization, structure, and diversity of operations being performed. Personnel selection should be based on a written position description for each individual employed within the organization. This allows both the applicant and the laboratory to understand exactly what is required for the job and whether the applicant is qualified. The position description details the position title, reporting relationships, position responsibilities, and qualifications desired (e.g., education, experience, special needs of the position).

Once a position is filled, it is management's responsibility to ensure that personnel are properly trained to perform the specific functions for which they are responsible. Formal training, whether performed within or outside the laboratory, is essential and can be accomplished in one of two ways. New employees may be trained by working with an experienced individual or with a staff trainer who is familiar with the responsibilities of the position. Alternatively, training may be conducted through use of written descriptions of methods of analyses, instrument operating manuals and procedures, policy and procedural texts, and audio visual technique programs; however, this would depend on the individual's experience.

In practice, good training employs both an individual and a written approach. The new employee should not be allowed to work without close supervision until the training process is completed, and the position's responsibilities have been comprehended and mastered. Management must ensure that the new hire demonstrates an ability to perform the job before discharging responsibilities to that person. On-the-job activities of the new employee need to be monitored until it is obvious that the quality of his or her work is satisfactory. If a problem arises, the employee needs to be informed and shown again how to properly perform that specific responsibility.

Initial training, as well as periodic retraining, should be well documented in the employee's personnel records. Such a requirement is an essential aspect of the laboratory's quality assurance program. Not only does this requirement ensure that management is performing its training responsibility, but it also allows supervisors to review the qualifications and specific experience levels of personnel in unfamiliar departments.

The section or group leaders (supervisors) should make training activities, and their documentation, part of each employee's overall performance evaluation. The laboratory manager should similarly review the section or group leaders' performances, in part noting their attentiveness to, and effectiveness in, training activities of their respective employees.

2.035 *Methods*

Dairy laboratories should use validated methods and procedures accepted by the entity submitting the sample or reviewing the sample results. Any method modification used must be appropriately documented and validated in the QA plan. The laboratory should maintain a copy of current publications or references that are industry standards. The laboratory's QA plan should contain documentation for reporting results and a protocol when the results are unexpected. Unexpected results could be due to several factors, including a procedural failure, or analyst or equipment error.[8,14,15,17,28,38,41]

Procedures routinely fall into the following general divisions: policy, administrative, technical operations, equipment operation, and analytical methods. Procedural documentation, such as glassware washing, balance calibration, maintenance, and analytical assay procedures, is essential to the overall control of laboratory quality. Laboratory personnel should have written, approved, and accepted procedures for all aspects of laboratory work readily available. These need to be reviewed and updated regularly. Inaccurate or outdated procedures may cause severe quality control problems.

Laboratory analytical methods are of 2 types: 1) standard or official methods such as Class A or O methods and 2) methods developed or modified by the laboratory or taken from the literature, such as Class B methods. The need for methods that have been modified by the laboratory, such as Class B methods, arises because method compendiums do not always have methods for an analysis that the laboratory has been requested to perform, or the laboratory cannot use the compendium method due to circumstances (e.g., equipment availability). Whether official methods or other methods are employed, the laboratory must be able to demonstrate, with historical validation data, that it can perform the analytical determination described by the method. Validation data should be evaluated for precision, both within a trial and between trials. In addition, recovery or standard-addition studies should be performed whenever appropriate.

When a modified method is employed, the responsibilities of the laboratory go beyond the validation requirement. The laboratory in this instance must demonstrate that the modified method and the reference methods are equivalent. Equivalence is determined by demonstrating, with statistically evaluated data, that the modified method is capable of generating data with precision and accuracy that are equal to or exceed those generated by the reference method. This is especially important if the modified method will be used to produce results for regulatory purposes. All validation data, equivalence data, and written procedures should be reviewed periodically by management and quality assurance personnel. Procedures should not only be reviewed for technical content, but also for format and clarity. The review process should be repeated on a regular basis to ensure that the written procedures accurately reflect the laboratory's current practices.

2.036 *Records and Reports*

Records and QA/QC are a necessity for a dairy laboratory, for without them none of the results are valid. The use of standardized QC forms makes record keeping simpler for the user. The process of record keeping, outlined in a QA plan, allows the laboratory to present data and results to various parties with assurance that the results are valid. In addition, this demonstrates that the laboratory and analysts have done everything possible to assure that the QA plan was followed.[8,9,17,28,36,37,41]

The following is taken from the FDA 2400 Series forms (cultural procedures)[37] used to evaluate NCIMS Grade A milk laboratories. It illustrates record keeping and emphasizes corrective actions.

2. d. Records written in ink or other indelible substance. Pencil or erasable ink not allowed.
   e. Corrections to quality control records, bench sheets, and reports follow the requirements below:
      1. Make a single line through the incorrect information.
      2. Write in the correct information next to the incorrect information.
      3. Person making the correction initials the information.
      4. If not obvious, include reason for correction.
   f. Requirements for electronic/computer records:
      1. Software must be well documented.
      2. Protocols and policies must be clearly documented.
      3. Records must be indexed and cross referenced to allow easy review, or must be printed and made available.
      4. Records must be secure from unauthorized access and changes.
      5. When corrections are necessary the old information must be retained, and the person making the correction must be identified and the reason for the change recorded.
      6. If records are not available at time of audit, facility will be cited for not having records and will be subject to penalties.

A system for cataloging records by department, sample number, date, or assay should be developed so that records may be located easily when the need arises (e.g., audit) and to ensure that review and ultimate disposal may be accomplished in an orderly fashion. Raw data should be stored in clearly labeled, record-retention boxes and housed in a vermin-free area. Raw data include all recorded data such as microbial colony counts, optical densities, peak heights, strip charts, and calculations (i.e., all support material and information). All data that are necessary to reconstruct a reported result can be considered raw data. The laboratory must establish a records-retention policy that clearly defines the period of time for which records will be kept. This period is not only a function of the laboratory's needs, but may also be specified by state and federal regulations.

Many final reports are now computerized. These reports are often based on original raw data that are in paper form. Raw data in paper form, such as microbial colony counts and computations, must be kept in an archive and indexed (by box number, shelf number, etc.) by the computer system using the sample number or other criterion. Original raw data may be captured directly by the computer. Special care must be taken to guard against loss of original data. Where practical, original raw data should be printed on hard copy as early as possible and archived as described above. Original raw data are required in case a question later arises as to the accuracy of computer processing and a total reconstruction has to be carried out. Copies of final analytical reports also need to be kept as a permanent record of results sent to clients. Copies may be kept on diskette, tape, microfiche, or other suitable longterm storage medium. Security against tampering and loss is of paramount importance. Prevention of alteration of QC and/or final results, while not losing corrected or changed information, is also of utmost importance. Computer systems should be equipped with a variety of security software and hardware. Computer security requirements vary with the type of computer and operation systems used. Computer hardware and software vendors should be consulted for security information.

The end product of dairy laboratory analysis is the report of results. While maintaining the original and/or copies of a final report and supporting material is sufficient, the laboratory must be organized in such a manner as to keep these items together, not separate, and have the ability to tie-in all associated information to the report. The format of the report should assure that data are clearly presented. At a minimum, the analysis report must contain the following information: laboratory name and address, laboratory sample number, time-date-temperature of sample collection, person collecting sample, time-date-temperature of sample receipt and analysis, date of final report, sample description, assay name(s), assay result(s)/unit(s), and analyst signature/initials. Incoming sample logs, section logs, laboratory worksheets, the final analytical report, and other pertinent forms should provide sufficient information to document the chain of custody from sample collection through receipt, analysis, storage, and disposition. The ISO/DIS 17025 standard requires an entire report be reissued if any changes are made.[28]

An incoming log for samples must also be maintained. This log should include the dates and times that samples were received, who received the samples, the type of samples, from whom/where the samples were received, collection information, and the incoming sample temperature (when appropriate). It should also list any sample and/or report numbers, and assigned laboratory numbers. Additional information may include the condition of the samples when received and, if appropriate, the section of the laboratory to which it was assigned.

Individual laboratory section logs are recommended. These logs may indicate much of the same information shown in the incoming sample log, but additionally should show the date(s) analysis was initiated (with time(s) and temperature(s) as appropriate), analysis used, when analysis was completed, and all test results (including raw and computed data).

Analytical worksheets for sample analysis must be maintained. Worksheets must show all raw data and calculations needed to determine precisely how the analytical results were obtained. These worksheets should be kept with the final report.

The laboratory must also have a secure records archive in which its original, raw data and reported analysis are maintained. The laboratory must also have a policy, if one is not specified by a regulatory agency, for how and for how long records should be maintained.

2.037 *Analytical Quality Control*

Analytical quality control ensures that dairy laboratory personnel are performing the analyses in a manner so that the accuracy and precision of the method are as good as the method is capable of providing.[38] Additionally, the laboratory needs to ensure that, as analysts change over time, the precision and accuracy of results do not change appreciably. Variation in technique such as pipeting, use of volumetric glassware, weighing, colony counting, peak measurement, etc., can exist among analysts, thereby leading to differences in final results. Training, onsite audits, proficiency test samples, etc., can minimize these variations.[28] The laboratory should establish a daily routine quality control program that monitors assay/analyst quality by generating data or instrument performance and analysis results[20] based on known control samples, sterility controls, dilution buffer blanks, known additions, etc. Quality tools such as charts can be used to decide whether the data are acceptable. The acceptance or rejection of laboratory results of unknown samples can be made based on the results obtained from a quality control program. Quality control data must be preserved historically.

2.038 *Proficiency Testing*

Laboratory proficiency testing must be used on a periodic basis. Proficiency samples can, in some instances, be obtained externally. When no such samples are obtainable, the laboratory can prepare its own proficiency samples, either by pooling samples or preparing samples of known quantities of test compounds by standard additions. In the case of self-prepared samples, the laboratory must generate sufficient data to be statistically significant, reflecting precision within the analytical technique and between/among analyses. A special type of proficiency testing commonly employed is the split-sample program.[34] Samples are split by a laboratory, and results are obtained by different analysts within that laboratory, or between/among laboratories. Data are analyzed statistically to determine which analysts and/or laboratories are yielding data that are significantly different. It is essential that all analysts clearly understand that the procedure specified should be followed uniformly. Although this caution appears obvious, it is probably the most serious and largest obstacle to obtaining comparable data among laboratories in split-sample programs.

2.039 *Sample Control and Preparation*

It is axiomatic that a laboratory result is only as good as the sample obtained for analysis [chapter 3]. Proper sample control involving identification, preparation, storage, and disposal is important to maintaining the integrity of the sample and, thus, to the ultimate generation of reliable analytical results. Written procedures for sample receipt, identification, subsampling, preparation, storage, distribution, retention, and ultimate disposal must be standardized.[6,17,21,38,39] All of the many approaches to sample control that exist in various laboratories have several factors in common.

The process of sample control begins with collection. Key factors that affect sample quality include the age of the sample(s); temperature control; agitation; proper collection; refrigeration; shipment of samples; contamination during shipment due to improper packaging, leakage, or breakage during shipment; contaminated or improper sample containers; or inadequate sample identification. Standards for sample identification and supporting instructions should be established.

Examples of sample information that may be required include: sample description; approximate sample size (at shipment); sample collector, time, date and temperature of collection (when necessary); safety precautions; stability information (heat, light, air, etc.); analysis requested; specific method(s) to be employed (optional); client contact and phone; date results needed; and where results should be sent. The sample receipt function is primarily one of inspection to ensure that all the required sample information is present and that the sample is in acceptable condition. Special attention should be directed to the sample size at shipment, shipping conditions required, safety precautions, and stability information. Time of receipt at the laboratory may also be important. If anything unusual is observed in any of these areas, the client and/or the sender should be notified immediately.

If the sample has been properly received with sufficient information to perform the analyses requested, the laboratory has to translate the request into a format that is acceptable to the laboratory. If the laboratory analysis request form is properly designed, it should be sufficient to accompany the sample for analyses. The system employed should be developed with the needs of the analytical laboratory in mind.

Many laboratories identify samples using unique sample numbers. These numbers are assigned and placed on samples at receipt. In addition to sample numbers, some laboratories also list sample descriptions, storage conditions, and abbreviated analysis requests. This information may be placed on a worksheet or on labels placed on the samples. Since a label may not provide sufficient space for detailed information, the laboratory must have a system to match label information (e.g., sample number) with the analysis request form or worksheet.

If samples must be subdivided, it is most efficient and appropriate to do so in a centralized, sample preparation area by qualified personnel. Samples must be mixed well before any portion is removed. If more than one preparation technique is employed on the same sample because of differing analyses, subsamples must be clearly identified as to the analysis intended. Microbiological sampling, when necessary, should precede chemical sampling. Laboratory workers should be aware of differences between subsamples and honor label/worksheet designations.

Laboratory analysts should have the responsibility of ensuring that samples are maintained within the laboratory under specific conditions and are analyzed within a specified time frame (criteria for samples in and out of specification specified in QC system/manual). For example, if samples requiring refrigeration should, for any reason, warm above the allowable maximum temperature they must be discarded and recorded as not tested due to a laboratory accident and not simply placed back into a refrigerator until they cool and then analyzed. If a sample must be kept frozen before analysis and multiple analyses should be performed on the sample, the laboratory should request individually frozen subsamples or require that all analyses are started with the initial thawing of the sample. Multiple thawing and refreezing of samples can adversely affect sample stability and homogeneity and can affect chemical and microbiological results. The above examples point to the need for dairy laboratories to design stringent sample control procedures that are evaluated periodically and modified to meet the needs of each laboratory and its clients. Because mistakes will happen, the laboratory should also maintain a reserve portion of the sample (preferably unaltered from its original state) for reanalysis, if that is required due to a problem encountered by the laboratory.[28] This reserve sample can also serve as the laboratory retention sample. Analysis time constraints and regulatory requirements may preclude the use of reserve samples and may require that new samples be obtained.

The sample tracking system within laboratories is of critical importance to efficient laboratory operation and image. A significant amount of time can be wasted if samples are stored haphazardly. If samples are coded upon receipt with a chronological number, tracking can be facilitated. Samples can thus be stored in refrigerators in numerical order. If laboratory analysts place samples into their appropriate positions after use, the system can be selfsustaining. Responsibility for monitoring the orderliness of the sample storage area should be assigned to someone in the laboratory. This individual should also be responsible for removing samples from the storage area for disposal as required.

2.0310 *Facilities and Environment*

This section details the laboratory work environment.[3,7,12,17,38,41] A floor plan must be included with detailed information on specifications (dimensions, usable space, counter space, special equipment areas, electrical and plumbing, air quality, ventilation, lighting, etc.), content (nonmovable and movable equipment), location of safety equipment, use of the space, and duties performed in each area. This section should also include general and specific housekeeping practices as well as monitoring procedures (including records) to assure proper functioning and upkeep.

Laboratory work areas should meet the following criteria for microbiological testing purposes.

Laboratories must be well-ventilated and free of dust and drafts. Temperatures should normally be maintained between 16° and 37°C (60.8° and 80.6°F); extremes must be avoided. Laboratory lighting should be even, screened to reduce glare, and provide adequate working illumination (minimum of 50 footcandles, preferably 100 footcandles). The work area should contain a table, bench, or other rigid support surface that is level and has ample space to accommodate analysis being performed (6 linear feet excluding equipment for each analyst working). Separate areas should be established for instruments for microscopy and plate counting as well as for computer usage, or writing space. Bench tops should be of stainless steel, epoxy plastic, or other smooth, impervious material that is inert, corrosion resistant, and able to be sanitized. Particleboard construction is not recommended. There should be minimal seams.

Adequate storage space should be provided for laboratory supplies. Storage areas should be kept clean and orderly and should be adequate for the protection of glassware or other laboratory supplies or apparatus. Flammable solvent areas must be well ventilated and temperature controlled. Additionally, such areas must be equipped with an appropriate fire retardant system and be posted to indicate storage of flammable materials. Electrical grounding connections should be available for use where flammable solvents are transferred. Acids and bases must be stored separately in dry, well-ventilated areas on lower shelves below eye level. Care must be exercised so that organic and inorganic chemicals are not stored next to each other. All chemicals and reagents must be stored as specified in their material safety data sheets (MSDS). Safety showers, eye wash fountains, and other protective equipment (face masks, rubber aprons, etc.) must be available and operable according to Occupational Safety and Health Administration (OSHA), local, state, and federal regulations. Radioactive materials, if used, must be stored in conformity to their MSDS, or, if applicable, as required by the laboratory's Nuclear Regulatory Commission (NRC) licensing requirements.

Adequate utilities should be available for all laboratory operations and may include grounded electrical connections of proper voltages, hot and cold water, gas, air, vacuum, and steam as needed. All utility connections must meet all local, state, and federal codes.

High standards of cleanliness are essential in laboratory operations. Unclean and disorderly laboratories may affect analysis and the safety of employees.

In chemical laboratories, hazardous or flammable solvents must be restricted to (properly functioning) hoods. Chemical storage areas must be well ventilated to the outside.

In microbiological laboratories, when plating is conducted, the microbic density of air should be determined. When plating throughout the day, prepare 1 plate for samples plated in the morning and 1 for samples plated in the afternoon, preferably with each set of plates pre-prepared. The number of microorganisms (e.g., bacteria, yeasts, molds) in the air in the plating area should not exceed 1 colony per square foot per minute. This is equivalent to 1 standard petri plate completely exposed for 15 minutes with no more than 15 colony-forming units after incubation. Maintain records of all air quality tests. Steps to correct excessive air contamination include: 1) improve laboratory cleanliness, especially dust removal; 2) close windows and reduce drafts; and 3) replace air filters or otherwise clean the air-handling system.

Although specific space requirements for routine analyses are difficult to define because of differing functions among laboratories, it is essential that adequate area be provided for analytical functions, support equipment, and related activities. The recommended bench space per analyst is 6 linear feet exclusive of space devoted to support equipment or specialized activities. Specialized analyses may require additional space per analyst.

Precautionary measures for pathogen testing must be taken to avoid cross-contamination of pathogenic organisms from laboratories to processing areas. The FDA recommends that the actual analysis for pathogenic organisms be done in a separate laboratory isolated from any dairy processing areas.[1] A separate building for the laboratory is preferable. If this is not possible, the laboratory should be accessible only through an outside, locked entrance. There must be no direct access to processing areas. In dairy plant laboratories testing for pathogens, the ventilation system must also be separate from the rest of the plant.[40] Once an individual has entered the pathogen testing area, he or she cannot reenter the plant until proper decontamination procedures have been taken.

2.0311 *Supplies and Equipment*

This section lists supplies and equipment typically used by a laboratory. For supplies, it is necessary to maintain storage, use, safety concerns, performance testing, disposal, and resupply records. Product information sheets and copies of MSDS sheets may be included. [Note: There are special OSHA regulations concerning MSDS sheets that must be observed.] For equipment, it is necessary to maintain use, safety concerns, performance criteria, and maintenance records (including calibration, QC, routine use). Copies of equipment manuals may be included.

Written procedures should be established for monitoring equipment performance and preventive maintenance, including assignments of personnel responsibilities. All laboratory equipment must be properly maintained through regular inspection and servicing. Records of repairs and service must be kept. Regular maintenance of laboratory facilities should be provided to prevent unnecessary disruption of, or damage to, air handling equipment, and electrical and other utilities. Painted or finished surfaces should be maintained to prevent peeling or cracking.

Laboratories must have all equipment and supplies necessary for the accurate performance of test methods. Routine functions (daily monitoring) or calibration of equipment/supplies may be required by the laboratory's QA policy and/or by the party receiving the report. An equipment/supply list and calibration data should be maintained. This includes the identification, location, and serial number of equipment. Additional information includes the manufacture instructions, dates of calibration and/or service (preventive maintenance or repair), routine compliance checks, and replacement.[38]

2.0312 *Audits and Reviews*

Audits are reviews of QA protocols and laboratory tests, and may consist of internal and/or external reviews.[2,9,18,20] Audits identify problems so the laboratory can correct them. Internal audits should occur on a predetermined schedule to verify that operations comply with the QA plan or standard operating procedures (SOP). The audit should be conducted by qualified personnel, preferably from outside of the audited area.[28] Outside or external audits involve the complete review of documentation, supporting data, and other related activities to ensure the validity of the results from the laboratory, and for compliance and accreditation. External audits are conducted less often than internal audits. External audits are conducted by an independent third party that is either private or government based.

Corrective actions are a response to a deviation in a laboratory's QA Plan or SOP. Re-occurrences of deviations mean that a response to a problem was not sufficient or did not correct the problem. Corrective actions are a response to a cause. Preventive actions are a proactive approach to solving problems before they occur. Taking corrective actions involves more than just a response to a problem, but requires knowledge of the factors/problems that may affect a system. Preventing and correcting problems require continual evaluations through inside and outside reviews.[32]

For the NCIMS Grade A Milk Laboratory Program responses to findings of onsite surveys or audits and proficiency test performance reports must be maintained (as with ISO guidelines). The consequences of unsatisfactory performance within program criteria must be clearly detailed and documented along with corrective actions.[32]

2.0313 *Inventory Control*

Inventory control records must be maintained for microbiological media, reagents, and other chemicals. Each container (and packing box if the container is stored in its box) must be marked with the date of receipt. Open containers must be marked with the date of opening. If verification of any reagents or other laboratory supplies is necessary, verification should be conducted immediately after receipt into the laboratory. If the results are not acceptable, then the laboratory should return the reagent/media to the supplier. Inventory control assists in the use of media before expiration dates, prevents over- or under-ordering, and prevents excessive degradation of sensitive chemicals. Inventory control for other supply items, including disposable and reusable glassware and plasticware, is also recommended.

2.0314 *Quality Manual*

Listed below are elements of a quality manual used by an ISO-9002 certified analytical laboratory.[25] Elements can be added or eliminated to suit the needs of the laboratory.

A. **Quality policy statement:** A typical laboratory quality policy statement indicates management's commitment to follow ISO-9002 standards to pursue continuous improvements in the quality of both products and services. This may also include a mission statement for both the company and laboratory. It is the responsibility of each individual in the laboratory to support and comply with the quality policy and with ISO-9002 standards.

B. **Company background:** An introduction to the company, its function, and goals, as well as some background information. The purpose and function of the laboratory are also described.

C. **Management responsibility:** A statement of the management's philosophy and functions. The responsibility of management includes (but is not restricted to) periodic reviews of the quality policy, quality assurance reports, subcontractor performance, customer service information, resource allocation, and results of audits.

D. **Quality system:** The quality system and documentation include a quality assurance plan, position descriptions, and specific procedures and methods. The quality manual provides information regarding the quality system, including a quality assurance policy and descriptions of the components of the quality system. The quality assurance plan describes the quality control measures used by the laboratory and includes information on organization and responsibility, facility and environment, sample handling, quality control measures, analytical testing, equipment, calibrations and standards, data handling, verification and reporting, corrective actions, and performance and system evaluations.

E. **Contract review:** A contract review process provides a documented agreement between the customer and the laboratory. This section does not apply to all laboratories.

F. **Design control:** Design controls are generally not applicable to a laboratory.

G. **Document and data control:** The document and data control process used by the laboratory. It is the responsibility of laboratory personnel to generate, review, and revise laboratory documents as assigned by laboratory management.

H. **Purchasing:** The process for purchasing services and supplies for the laboratory.

I. **Control of customer-supplied products:** Control of customer-supplied products generally is not applicable to a laboratory.

J. **Sample and report identification and traceability:** The policy and mechanism for identification and traceability of samples and reports. This is a critical function in a laboratory.

K. **Process control:** Laboratory processes that directly affect quality and define the plan to provide controlled conditions under which these processes are performed. Procedures, sometimes called standard operating procedures (SOP), are written documentation of detailed laboratory processes that directly affect quality. Methods document all aspects of analysis, including quality control, records, and method references.

L. **Inspection and testing:** The in-process and final inspection and testing of data generated by the laboratory. In-process inspection of data consists of evaluating the QC data generated against established guidelines. Final inspection consists of the review of all data for approval prior to a report being issued.

M. **Inspection and measuring of test equipment:** The requirements for control, maintenance, and calibration of equipment used in the laboratory

N. **Inspection and test status:** The inspection process by which the status of tests and data are monitored in the laboratory. This section includes information on how data and reports are identified and tracked throughout the laboratory.

O. **Control of nonconforming product (reports):** Procedures to prevent the unintended use of data and reports that did not pass all quality control measures, or were otherwise found to be unacceptable. This section discusses control of nonconforming data and reports including identification, documentation, evaluation, segregation, disposition, and notification to those concerned.

P. **Corrective and preventive action:** Company response to customer complaints and nonconforming product/quality control/analysis/data/reports. This corrective action process is used to identify, document, and follow up on corrective action issues. The preventive action section describes the preventive action process for gathering and review of available data in order to identify, analyze, and eliminate potential causes of nonconformities.

Q. **Handling, storage, packaging, preservation, and delivery:** The handling, storage, packaging, preservation, and delivery of samples as well as results and product reports.

R. **Control of quality records:** A company's policy on how records should be maintained and reviewed.

S. **Internal quality audits:** The process for performing internal audits such as scheduling, selecting the audit team, preparing the final report on the audit results, and initiating corrective actions.

T. **Training:** The type and frequency of laboratory personnel training.

U. **Servicing:** The servicing needs of a company. This section is generally not needed for the laboratory.

V. **Statistical techniques:** Identifies the statistical techniques required for establishing, controlling, and verifying process/testing capabilities and product/data characteristics.

2.040 Common Dairy Laboratory Equipment and Supplies

2.041 *Autoclaves*

A. **Equipment:** Autoclaves should be of sufficient size and construction as to prevent crowding of the interior and provide uniform temperatures within the chamber of at least 120° ± 1°C (sterilization point). Autoclaves must also be equipped with a pressure gauge, a properly adjusted safety valve, a properly functioning timer, and thermometer or temperature recorder-controller (properly located to register the minimum temperature within the sterilizing chamber, usually on the exhaust line).

B. **Quality control:** Verify chamber temperature at least quarterly (preferably weekly) using a maximum registering thermometer (MRT) calibrated at 120°C. Place MRT in a vessel of water in the center of the load while running a 15-minute liquid media cycle. Sterility should be checked and confirmed weekly using commercially available sterility check ampoules or strips containing *Bacillus stearothermophilus* spores. Position the ampoule in a vessel of liquid or place the strip near the exhaust drain in the autoclave. Run the autoclave using a 15-minute liquid media cycle. Incubate the ampoule or strip using the manufacturer's instructions along with a non-autoclaved ampoule or strip (positive control). Verify timer accuracy quarterly. Use temperature indicator (tape, ampoule, card, etc.) with each run.

C. **Maintenance:** The laboratory should have a policy in place in case of problems and keep a record of the corrective actions taken. For safe and adequate operation, autoclaves must be periodically inspected and serviced by qualified service representatives. It is highly recommended that a service contract be maintained on the autoclave.

D. **Records:** Keep records of each sterilization cycle. Records should include items treated (including waste), date, start-up time, temperature and time temperature reached, length of time at temperature, time item(s) were removed, and operator identification. Automatic recording devices can capture most of these parameters; however, any parameter not captured, such as items autoclaved and operator, must be manually recorded. Since charts may not accurately reflect the information needed, this information must either be written directly on the chart or in a separate written record. If automatic recorders are used, charts or tapes recording use must be maintained. Keep records of all quality control checks, including MRT temperatures, sterility checks, and timer verification. Records of all repairs and maintenance on the autoclave must also be kept.

2.042 *Balances*

A. **Equipment:** Electronic balances with a sensitivity of 1.0 mg (0.001 g) or greater with a 10-g load should be used when weighing 2 g or less. For larger quantities, a balance with a sensitivity of 100 mg (0.1 g) at a 200-g load should be used. The balance sensitivity must be sufficient for the accuracy required.

B. **Quality control:** Balances should be checked monthly with a set of certified weights (S or S-1, or ANSI/ASTM 1, 2 or 3) or weights traceable to NIST. Use weights that encompass the normal use of the balance being checked. Balances and weights should be cleaned as necessary after each use. Weights should be protected from the atmosphere, manual contact, and corrosion. If weights are subjected to abusive conditions, have the weights rechecked to ensure they meet specifications.

C. **Maintenance:** Balances must be serviced and checked for accuracy at least annually by a qualified maintenance representative.

D. **Records:** Keep records of each monthly balance check. The laboratory should have a certificate on file verifying the class of weights used. Keep records on all repairs and maintenance performed on each balance. Keep records of annual checks since stickers may be removed or covered.

2.043 *Centrifuge*

A. **Equipment:** Centrifuge, rotors, baskets, and tubes suitable for intended use. Centrifuge should be operated as per manufacturer's instruction and on a level surface away from any vibration-sensitive equipment such as balances.

B. **Quality control:** Verify speed on a periodic basis (recommend monthly or quarterly). Check and calibrate variable speed indicator. Verify that timer is accurate.

C. **Maintenance:** Centrifuges should be routinely serviced by a qualified maintenance representative.

D. **Records:** Keep records on all speed and timer checks as well as on all repair and maintenance performed.

2.044 *Colony Counters and Tallies*

A. **Equipment:** Quebec-type darkfield or equivalent colony counter that provides adequate lighting and magnification and has sufficient visibility to allow accurate colony counts. Grid plates should not be excessively scratched or etched and the grid should be clearly visible. Some grid plates are painted and wear down with excessive use. This should be avoided by flipping the grid over so that the painted side is on inside. Noninstrumental enumeration of colonies must use a hand tally.

B. **Quality control:** Hand tallies should be checked periodically to ensure accuracy. If instrumental colony counters are used, they should be evaluated periodically to provide results equivalent to manual counts.[37]

C. **Maintenance:** Internal mirror placement and cleanliness should be checked periodically to ensure optimal illumination.

D. **Records:** Keep records on any quality control and maintenance preformed on counters and tallies. Keep record of quality checks on instrument counters. Perform and keep monthly visual count comparisons to instrument counts [chapter 5].

2.045 *Dilution Bottles*

A. **Equipment:** Dilution bottles (capacity of about 150 mL) should be made of borosilicate glass, polysulfone, polycarbonate, polypropylene, or other autoclavable, non-toxic plastic material. Dilution bottles should be marked indelibly (preferably etched) at 99 ± 1 mL graduation level. Premarked bottles obtained from the manufacturer should be standardized at the 99 ± 1 mL level and re-etched as warranted (do not assume that the bottles are accurately marked). Dilution bottles should be closed with Escher-type stoppers or screw caps. Use friction-fit liners in screw caps to make sure the closure is leak-proof.

B. **Quality control:** Fill dilution bottles to contain 99 ± 2 mL dilution buffer after sterilization. Following sterilization, standardized dilution bottles (at room temperature) may be visually surveyed using the 99 ± 1 graduation mark and those appearing to be under or overfilled discarded. Check the volume of 1 of every 25 remaining dilution bottles with a NIST class A graduate or equivalent. If any of these dilution bottles are <97 or >101 mL, then the entire batch must be discarded.

New bakelite type plastic caps and closures with friction-fit liners must be treated before use to remove toxic residues. This may be accomplished by autoclaving them twice at 120 ± 1°C for 15 minutes or boiling twice for 15 minutes while they are submerged in microbiologically suitable water. Be sure to change the water after the first boiling. Toxic residues can be evaluated using a *B. stearothermophilus* type assay on the second autoclaved rinse water or boiling water.[37]

Perform detergent suitability test as described in section 2.0412 if glass petri dishes or other glassware are not used for this test. Substitute dilution bottles for the dishes. Samples and agar may be pipeted into the treated dilution blanks, laid on their side, and incubated.

C. **Records:** Keep records for each batch of dilution bottles prepared. Keep records of each new lot of caps that are tested for toxic substances. Record results of detergent suitability test if performed with dilution blanks.

2.046 *Dispensing Apparatus*

A. **Equipment:** Use a dispenser suitable for the laboratory's needs with an appropriate, clean dispensing tube to fill dilution blanks.

B. **Quality control:** The accuracy of a dispensing apparatus should be checked with a NIST Class A graduated cylinder at the start of each volume change and periodically thereafter.

C. **Maintenance:** Moving parts should be lubricated according to the manufacturer's recommendations. Leaks, loose connections, or malfunctions must be immediately corrected. Clean as necessary.

D. **Records:** Keep records of all quality control volume checks and any maintenance performed on this piece of equipment.

2.047 *Hoods and Laminar Flow Cabinets*

A. **Equipment:** Fume hoods, laminar flow cabinets, and exhaust systems should be fabricated of corrosion resistant material and, except for balancing dampers, should possess no airflow restrictive devices. Hoods and laminar flow cabinets should be located away from room exits and traffic corridors as a fire safety measure and because traffic movement can disrupt hood face velocity. Fume hood face velocity must be at least 30.5 linear meters per min (100 cu. ft. per min.) for hoods and 23 m per min (75 cu. ft. per min.) for Class II type A cabinets.[33] Air discharge points should be located away from building air intakes to prevent reentry of discharged air/fumes.

B. **Quality control:** Hoods and cabinets should be checked periodically with an accurate airflow measurement device. Sterilization lamps, if provided, should be checked quarterly with a short-wavelength, ultraviolet meter and replaced if output falls below 80% of rated value.

C. **Maintenance:** Adjust flow as necessary. Filters should be checked monthly for plugging or dirt accumulation and cleaned or replaced as needed. Perform any routine maintenance recommended by the manufacturer.

D. **Records:** Keep records of all flow checks, filter replacement, and UV light monitoring. Maintain records of all routine maintenance and repairs performed.

2.048 *Glassware*

A. **Equipment:** Laboratory glassware must be free of scratches, chips, cracks, bubbles, or other defects. Graduations on pipets, dilution bottles, and other measurement items must be clearly, distinctly, and indelibly marked with a contrasting color. Calibrations on certified Class A glassware must be reliable, and the glassware can be used without recalibration.

B. **Quality control:** Routinely inspect glassware. Damaged and worn glassware should be discarded. After washing reusable glassware, the presence of residual traces of acid or alkali on each batch of glassware cleaned should be determined using 0.04% bromthymol blue indicator.

Perform detergent suitability tests as described in section 2.0412 if glass petri dishes or dilution bottles are not used. Substitute pieces of glassware for the dishes.

C. **Records:** Results of all residual pH tests should be recorded and kept. Record results of detergent suitability test if performed with glassware.

2.049 *Incubators*

A. **Equipment:** Incubators or incubator rooms should be properly constructed and temperature controlled and be of sufficient size to prevent crowding of the interior. Incubator rooms, if used, must be well insulated, equipped with properly distributed heating units, and have forced-air circulation. An incubator is of sufficient size if when it is completely filled there is at least 2.54 cm (1.0 in.) of space between adjacent stacks of plates and between walls and stacks.

B. **Quality control:** Keep incubators in rooms where temperatures are within the range of 16° to 27°C. The temperature within the incubator[37] must not vary more than the specification allowed by the test being performed (32° ± 1 °C, 35° ± 0.5 °C, 64° ± 2 °C, etc.). Chamber temperatures should be measured by no fewer than 2 thermometers, 1 on the upper and 1 on the lower shelf of use.[37] Thermometer bulbs should be submerged in water or appropriate liquid using 20- × 150-mm stoppered test tubes (or in an appropriate size sealed container). Test points should be increased proportionately in walkin incubators. Temperatures should be recorded twice daily (in the morning and again in the afternoon). Do not take readings during or immediately after excessive opening of the incubator. If excessive use is anticipated, take readings prior to any excessive opening or allow the incubator to recover after it has been closed for a while. Optionally, automatic temperature devices of predetermined accuracy for controlling and recording temperatures may be used to track temperatures in incubators and/or incubator rooms. Check the accuracy of these devices weekly by comparing readings with those from accurate thermometers and record the results. When standard thermometers are used, minimum and maximum registering thermometers may be placed in each incubator to indicate undetected gross temperature deviations. Do not depend on readings from these special thermometers for daily records of temperatures. As necessary, adjust thermoregulators to maintain proper temperatures.

Determine acceptable moisture loss of standard plate count (SPC) agar plates (10 to12 mL of agar) from 10 plates distributed throughout the incubator (recommended at least 2 plates on each shelf to be used). Laboratories using 3M Petrifilm™ may use Petrifilm™ aerobic count films to determine moisture loss, substituting 10 films for the 10 agar plates. Moisture loss should not exceed 15% after 48 hours of incubation at 32° ± 1°C. Corrective action must be taken and documented whenever the weight loss exceeds 15%. Moisture loss can be corrected by placing pans of water in the incubator or by reducing airflow in forced air incubators. Moisture loss should be determined quarterly.

C. **Records:** Record and keep temperatures daily, or weekly when using an automatic temperature device. Record and maintain moisture loss determinations and corrective actions.

2.0410 *Microscopes*

A. **Equipment:** Binoculars with 1.8-mm oil immersion objective, rack and pinion substage, condenser with iris diaphragm, Huygenian or wide-field oculars, 10 × (or 12 × or 12.5 ×), lamp, suitable mechanical stage for the examination of slides, and have a microscopic factor or 600,000 or less. Stage micrometer ruled in 0.1-mm and 0.01-mm divisions, hand tally, and immersion oil with a refractive index of 1.51 to 1.52 (at 20°C).

B. **Maintenance:** When not in use, keep microscopes covered with a dust cover. After each use, clean the optical surfaces with 70% isopropyl alcohol. Periodically wipe the lamp bulb and lens with alcohol-moistened lens paper. Keep the gears and slideways lubricated. Have the microscope inspected and cleaned by factory-authorized personnel annually.

C. **Records:** Keep records of all maintenance and repairs performed.

2.0411 *Microwave Ovens*

A. **Equipment:** Microwave of suitable size and power for laboratory needs. It is recommended that laboratories use a microwave specifically designed for laboratory use since power output varies greatly with different brands of microwave ovens designed for home use.

B. **Quality control:** Determine the optimal time(s) to melt media. Media melts at different rates depending on the power of the unit and the location of bottles in the microwave. Each bottle should be watched carefully to prevent the medium from boiling over. Experience will determine the location of bottles and power level for best results. Extreme care must be exercised when removing hot media from the microwave as it may abruptly overflow or erupt from the container, especially if swirled. Gloves must always be worn when removing the bottles from the microwave.

C. **Records:** Keep records of all maintenance and repairs performed.

2.0412 *Petri Dishes*

A. **Equipment:** Use petri dishes with bottoms with at least an 80-mm inside diameter (exception for BsDA, 86.1 to 87.0 mm), 12 mm deep, with interior and exterior surfaces of the bottoms free from indentations, bubbles, scratches, or other defects. Petri dishes may be made of glass or nontoxic, sterilized plastic.[37] Petri dish containers made of nontoxic stainless steel or aluminum, with covers, are preferred. Char-resistant sacks of high-quality sulfite pulp Kraft paper may also be used. Single-service petri dishes should be stored in their original sterilized plastic sleeves until used. Prepared plates should be place in containers or the original sterilized plastic sleeves and stored as required by the media.

B. **Quality control:** Glass petri dishes should be tested annually for toxic substances using the detergent suitability test. Using 3 dishes, wash 1 using castile soap, wash another dish with the detergent used to wash dishes, and dip the third dish into a solution of the detergent used (do not wash). Rinse the dish washed with castile soap several times with microbiologically suitable water and allow to dry. Rinse the dish washed with detergent (normal laboratory procedure), and allow to dry. Do not rinse the third dish dipped in detergent; simply allow it to dry. Once all 3 dishes are dry, plate all 3 with a sample having an expected bacterial count of 100 to 200. Incubate the plates for 48 hours at 32° ± 1°C. Determine the count on each plate. If the dishes washed normally or the dishes dipped in detergent give counts ≤20% of the plate washed with castile soap, then the detergent is not suitable. Replace detergent and repeat test if unacceptable.

C. **Records:** Record and keep results of detergent suitability test.

2.0413 *pH Meters*

A. **Equipment:** Electronic pH meters, accurate to at least 0.1-pH units, should be used to determine pH values of media and reagents. Electrode must be suitable for pH meter, preferably double-junction reference.

B. **Quality control:** Measure pH at room temperature only. The instrument must be standardized before each series of measurements using reference solutions approximating pH 4.0, 7.0, and 10.0.[37] Buffer solutions should be used 1 time only and discarded. Slope determination should be made each time the pH meter is calibrated, either by using a built-in function or by using millivolt (mV) readings of the buffers. Slope is a function, reported as percent, of the actual millivolt reading divided by its theoretical value. The expected slope should be about 95 to 102%.

C. **Maintenance:** Periodically clean electrode with commercially available electrode cleaner, or use 0.1 N NaOH. Store in-use electrode in a liquid pH 7.0 buffer or, preferably, in commercially available storage solution. Refillable electrodes must be kept full with the appropriate solution recommended by the manufacturer. Empty and replace filling solution if crystals appear. The plastic collar on refillable electrodes must be removed from the filling hole when taking pH readings. Replace collar after pH readings have been taken to prevent evaporation and accelerated crystal formation.

D. **Records:** Keep records of pH meter calibrations, slope determination, and date electrodes are put into service. Record all media pH measurements and maintenance performed on the meter. Keep records on all maintenance and repairs performed.

2.0414 *Pipets*

Pipeting by mouth is not allowed for any operation within the laboratory.

A. **Equipment:** Pipets[37] may be made of glass or plastic and operated manually (e.g., bulbs) or mechanically (e.g., pipeters). They should be nontoxic, conform to specifications, be marked to contrast sharply with milk,

Table 2.1.* Bacteriological transfer pipets.

- **Delivery 1 mL;**
- **Delivery 1.1 mL in 0.1- and 1.0-mL amounts;**
- **Delivery 1.1 mL in 0.1-, 1.0-, and 0.5-mL amounts;**
- **Delivery 2.2 mL in 0.1-, 0.1-, 1.0-, and 1.0-mL amounts; and**
- **Delivery 11.0 mL.**

Capacity/Graduation (mL)		Tolerance (mL)
0.1	.01	± 0.0025
0.2	.01	± 0.004
1.0	.10	± 0.01
2.0	.10	± 0.01
5.0	.10	± 0.02
10.0	.10	± 0.03
17.6	.10	± 0.05
25.0	.10	± 0.05

Bacteriological transfer pipets should conform to the following accuracy specifications:

Pipet Size (mL)	Accuracy* (mL)
1.0	± 0.025
1.1	± 0.025
2.2	± 0.040
11.0	± 0.20

*All pipets calibrated to deliver with stated accuracy at 20°C. Volumes delivered in 2 to 4 seconds, with the last drop of undiluted milk blown out, or last drop of diluted milk touched off, 1.0-mL tolerance ± 0.025 mL. To allow for residual milk and milk dilutions on walls and in tip of the glass pipet under rapid transfer techniques, pipets shall be calibrated to contain 1.075 mL of water at 20°C. If the pipet is of styrene plastic, it should be calibrated to contain 1.055 mL of water at 20°C.

and be undamaged. If for manual use, they must have straight walls.

If glass, tips should be ground or fire polished or otherwise designed to ensure volume delivery. Disposable pipets should be used 1 time only; however, if disposable glass pipets can be cleaned and resterilized without losing their graduation marks, these may be reused. For microbiological examination of milk, use only pipets calibrated for bacteriological use. Classical transfer pipets must conform to APHA specifications (Table 2.1).

1. **Pipet containers:** Stainless steel or aluminum pipet containers are preferred. Copper containers should not be used. Char-resistant, high-quality sulfite pulp Kraft paper may be used. Sterile plastic or paper pipet covers are satisfactory for single-service plastic pipets.
2. **Pipet aids:** Various safety bulbs, pipet fillers, dispensers, and pumps are available and must be used to eliminate potential contamination hazards associated with pipeting by mouth.

B. **Pipet tolerance values:** Several tolerance specifications exist to describe pipet accuracy. When accuracy of measurements is critical in chemical determinations, only Class A pipets with the following tolerance limits must be used (reference NIST specifications for Mohr measuring pipets, Class A Volume Tolerances Circular 602, and Federal Specification NNN-P-350). Tolerances are certified by the supplier/manufacturer;

there is no requirement for laboratories to check the volumes of pipets, unless a problem is suspected.

C. The major types of laboratory pipets are calibrated according to the method of draining.

1. **To deliver (TD) pipets:** TD pipets are designed to release the calibrated amount when the pipet tip is held against the receiving vessel wall until draining stops. Certain types of serological pipets are calibrated for "blowout" or, in other words, they deliver the indicated volume with a small amount of liquid remaining in the tip after free delivery has ceased or been blown out. These pipets may be marked with a wide opaque ring, 2 narrower opaque, or 2 printed rings near the top.

2. **To contain (TC) pipets:** TC pipets are calibrated to hold or contain the amount specified. They must be completely emptied to provide the stated volume. These pipets are used in many operations where accurate dilutions are made by rinsing the pipet after initial delivery with dilute solution.

   The ISO designation for "to deliver" is "EX" and "to contain" is "IN."

3. **Pipets used in testing milk:** Pipets are calibrated to deliver the correct volume of undiluted milk when the small amount remaining in the tip, after free delivery has ceased, is gently expelled and added to the free delivery volume. However, for diluted milk, the correct volume is delivered by touching the pipet to a dry area after free delivery has ceased.

2.0415 *Mechanical and Electronic Pipeters*

A. **Equipment:** Numerous types of pipeters exist that can be used in analyses. These may be mechanical or electronic devices. While pipeters can be purchased with adjustable or fixed volumes, it is preferable to use calibrated fixed volume pipeters for laboratory analysis (thus, the need for adjustable pipeters for regulatory analysis may be precluded). Sterile disposable tips exist, which can make them adaptable to microbiological techniques. The volume delivered should be verified prior to utilizing a pipeter.[10] If not marked with a serial number, permanently mark each pipeter with a unique identification.

B. **Quality control:** When accuracy cannot be readily determined by measuring volume using class A graduate cylinders (this is usually the case with pipeting devices ≤ 1.0 mL) use the following procedure to determine accuracy by weight. This procedure is recommended for all pipeters with dispensing volumes ≤ 1.0 mL.

1. **Calibration of pipeters:** This test is used to determine the weight of water delivered by an instrument. The equipment and test water should be placed in the test environment of 19° to 24°C (66° to 75°F) for at least 2 hours prior to testing.

2. **Test procedure**

   a. Place a lightweight container, petri dish lid, or weigh boat on analytical balance and record its weight.

b. Have a 50-mL beaker of tempered deionized water available for measuring.
c. If the pipeter is used to transfer samples without diluting the sample in the pipeter tip, aspirate water from beaker equal to the quantity of sample to be pipeted and expel it back into the same container and record the weight. This should be done in the same manner that samples are routinely pipeted (i.e., if wetting the tip is routine, then wet the tip prior to discharging to the container).
d. If 1.0 mL of a 1:10 dilution should be made in the pipeter tip, aspirate water from beaker equal to the quantity of sample (0.1 mL) and diluent (0.9 mL) to be pipeted and expel it into the same container and record the weight. Next, repeat the process but do not take up the sample volume. Finally, repeat the process for the sample volume only. The difference with this pipeter is there will be 3 weights. These are 1.0 mL, 0.9 mL, and 0.1 mL. This should be done in the same manner that samples are routinely pipeted.
e. Repeat steps a through c, or a, b, and d as appropriate for the number of weighings to be examined (normally 10) and divide by the number of measurements to obtain the average value.

3. **Tolerances** (based on weight of water at 19° to 24°C)
   a. 0.1 mL should weigh 0.0975 to 0.1025 g.
   b. 0.9 mL should weigh 0.890 to 0.910 g.
   c. 1.0 mL should weigh 0.990 to 1.010 g.
4. **Test frequency:** Perform a measurement following a change of any removable parts. Routinely perform 10 consecutive measurements quarterly, or more frequently depending on use or requirements.

C. **Maintenance:** Routinely examine the end of the barrel for fouling. Clean as necessary. Prior to each use, repeatedly depress plunger to distribute lubricant and to ensure smooth action. Have pipeters that fail calibration testing adjusted and repaired by a qualified technician.

D. **Records:** Keep records of each calibration check and for all maintenance and repair work performed.

2.0416 *Refrigerators and Freezers*

A. **Equipment:** Refrigerators to cool and maintain samples must be of sufficient size to prevent crowding and maintain samples, media, and reagents between 0° and 4.4°C. Refrigerator temperatures should be measured using at least 2 thermometers with bulbs submerged in 50% glycerin water (suitable liquid) in 20 × 150 mm stoppered test tubes (or other suitably sized sealed containers) on the upper and lower shelves of use.

Freezers should have sufficient storage capacity to maintain dairy samples or reagents at –15°C or below. Nonfrost-free freezers are recommended to prevent damage to samples or reagents due to the thawing cycle of frost-free freezers. If frost-free freezers are used, it may be necessary to place sensitive items inside small styrofoam containers within the freezer. Determine temperatures by placing thermometers submerged in antifreeze in a sealed vessel.

Refrigerated and frozen materials must be stored to avoid contamination of items (e.g., liquid samples for analysis are not to be stored above prepared media). Flammable solvents must be stored in explosion-proof or flammable-storage refrigerators.

B. **Quality control:** Keep refrigerators and freezers in rooms where temperatures range between 16° and 27°C. The temperature within the refrigerator or freezer[37] must not vary more than the specification allowed (0° to 4.4 °C for refrigerators, –15 °C or less for freezers). Chamber temperatures should be measured by no fewer than 2 thermometers, 1 on the upper and 1 on the lower shelf of use.[37] Thermometer bulbs should be submerged in water or appropriate liquid using 20 × 150 mm stoppered test tubes (or in an appropriate size sealed container). Test points should be increased proportionately in walkin coolers. Temperatures should be recorded twice daily (in the morning and again in the afternoon). Do not take readings during or immediately after excessive opening of the refrigerator or freezer. If excessive use is anticipated, take readings prior to any excessive opening or allow the refrigerator or freezer to recover after it has been closed for a while. Optionally, automatic temperature devices of predetermined accuracy for controlling and recording temperatures may be used to track temperatures in refrigerators, coolers, or freezers. Check the accuracy of these devices weekly by comparing readings with those from accurate thermometers and record the results. When standard thermometers are used, minimum and maximum registering thermometers may be placed in each refrigerator or freezer to indicate undetected gross temperature deviations. Do not depend on readings from these special thermometers for daily records of temperatures. Adjust thermoregulators to maintain proper temperatures as necessary.

C. **Maintenance:** Clean and sanitize refrigerator periodically. De-ice non-frost-free freezers to help maintain proper temperature. Adjust, as necessary, to maintain required temperatures.

D. **Records:** Adjusted temperatures taken in the morning and afternoon must be recorded daily and records kept. Do not take temperatures during or immediately after repeated opening and closing of a refrigerator or freezer. Take temperatures prior to heavy use, or allow sufficient time for temperature recovery before taking the temperature. Maintain records on any maintenance or repairs performed.

2.0417 *Sterilizing Ovens*

A. **Equipment:** Sterilizing ovens should be of sufficient size to prevent crowding and be constructed to give uniform and adequate sterilizing temperatures throughout the chamber with vents suitably located to ensure prompt and uniform heat penetration. Ovens should be equipped with an accurate thermometer of an adequate range (to 220°C) with its bulb in sand suitably located to register minimal temperatures. To achieve sterility, operate the oven at a minimum of 170°C for 2 hours or more.

B. **Quality control:** Oven sterilization performance should be tested quarterly using commercially available *B. subtilus* spore strips. Caution: Do not place ampoules with liquid spore suspensions in the oven as these may explode. Position the strip in the center of the load. Run the oven at 170°C for 2 hours. Exceeding 2 hours may char the strip, making it unusable. Incubate the strip according to the manufacturer's instructions along with a nonheated strip (positive control). Use temperature indicator (tape, ampoule, card, etc.) with each run.

C. **Records:** Records must be kept for each sterilization cycle and include date, start-up time, temperature reached, length of time at temperature, time item removed, items sterilized, and operator. Keep records of each run, sterility check, and maintenance and repairs performed.

2.0418 *Stomacher*

A. **Equipment:** A stomacher may be used to mix and prepare dilutions of semisolid and solid samples.

B. **Maintenance:** Keep paddle faces clean. Lightly oil the paddle shafts every 6 months. Annually inspect the flexible couplings between the motor connecting rods and paddle shafts. Replace if signs of deterioration are evident. Check the security of all fasteners annually. Adjust the forward limit of the paddle strokes when necessary.

C. **Records:** Keep records on all maintenance and repairs performed.

2.0419 *Thermometers*

A. **Equipment:** Thermometers of appropriate range may be glass, mercury-filled, or have a distinctively colored fluid (with a freezing point lower than –1.0°C), or be electronic or digital. Thermometers should have graduation intervals that do not exceed 0.5°C in the 0° to 100°C range or not to exceed 1.0°C < 0° or > 100°C.

B. **Quality control:** Unless otherwise specified, accuracy should be checked before initial use and at least annually against a thermometer certified by the NIST or one of equivalent accuracy. Dial thermometers (not allowed for laboratory use) should be checked more frequently, including before initial use and at least once every 6 months.

Thermometers may be checked where they are normally used or by placing them in a water bath, either partially or totally immersed in the water, according to the way they will be used in the laboratory. The NIST-traceable thermometer should be placed along side of the thermometer being checked. Most, but not all, NIST thermometers are calibrated for total immersion. Vigorous stirring of the water in the bath is essential to ensure uniform temperature during thermometer calibration. Calibration instruments are available and may be used. Laboratories also have the option to send thermometers out to have calibrations checked.

Check the calibration by comparing the temperature reading on the certified thermometer with that of the laboratory thermometer at or very near the temperature the thermometer will be used to measure (e.g., an incubator thermometer should be checked at 32°C because this is the temperature of interest).[37] If the thermometer is to be used for several purposes, it should be checked at the different temperatures of use. If there is a difference in the temperature reading between laboratory and certified thermometers (after the reading of the certified thermometer has been corrected as indicated by the certificate), indicate the correction needed to obtain an accurate measurement of temperature on a tag attached to the laboratory thermometer. This correction must not exceed 1°C.

The NIST thermometer or equivalent must be checked at the ice point at least annually.

C. **Records:** Tag all thermometers with the date of calibration check, identification, and correction factor (0 if none required). Records of thermometer calibration checks, including the NIST ice point check, should be maintained. The NIST thermometer or equivalent must have a certificate of calibration.

2.0420 *Water Baths*

A. **Equipment:** Water baths must be of an appropriate size for the required workload with a suitable water level maintained. Baths should be thermostatically controlled at the appropriate temperatures. Recirculators are necessary to prevent temperature stratification.[37] For holding melted media, the bath must be maintained at 45° ± 1°C. Temperatures should be monitored by maintaining an accurate thermometer partially immersed in the water bath. Only racks constructed of stainless steel, rubber, plastic, vinyl coated substances, or other corrosion-proof material should be used.

B. **Maintenance:** Maintain suitable water level for items in water bath. Change water periodically. A solution to suppress microbial growth in the bath water may be used.

C. **Records:** Maintain records of temperatures and any maintenance or repairs performed.

2.0421 *Water Stills, Reverse Osmosis Units, and Deionizers*

A. **Equipment:** Water distillers, reverse osmosis (RO) units, and deionizers capable of producing laboratory quality water should be available to the laboratory. Water may be purchased, provided it meets the requirements of the laboratory.

B. **Quality control:** Monitor water quality at least monthly. Test methods should be those specified in *Standard Methods for the Examination of Water and Wastewater.*[6] Total residual chlorine should be ≤0.1 ppm. The standard plate count must be <1,000/mL. Conductivity must be <2.0 µohms/mL. Laboratory water should be analyzed for trace metals annually and contain <0.5 mg/L Cd, Cu, Cr, Ni, Pb, and Zn and <1.0 mg/L total for these metals.[38]

C. **Maintenance:** Units should be cleaned, and/or have cartridges replaced at intervals recommended by the manufacturer or as indicated by control test results. Since RO units remove only about 90% of impurities, water from an RO unit should not be used for microbiological or other analyses sensitive to water quality. The principal use of RO units should be initial cleanup of water before deionization or distillation.

D. **Records:** Records of water quality test results should be maintained. Maintain records on all maintenance performed.

2.050 Laboratory Safety

2.051 *Introduction*

Laboratory safety is an essential element of any laboratory operation. A vigorously enforced safety program is critical for the protection of laboratory personnel, visitors, and the facility. Prevention of laboratory accidents should be the goal of any safety management plan. Safety management has evolved over the years as a result of experience. An important aspect of safety management is the documentation of incidents. This helps plan future preventive measures. Aspects of safety management include laboratory design, availability of safety equipment, employee awareness and training, and a commitment to safety by management.

A laboratory safety program must be established by management and made available by manual to everyone in the laboratory. This action program must be reviewed and amended as required to meet the changing needs of local, state, and federal codes, and supplemented by specific procedures and policies for individual departments and projects. Thus, different policies may exist for different laboratory areas and projects.

Some of the general areas of laboratory safety that should be considered when preparing a written safety program are described below. This is not an all-encompassing treatment of the subject. Texts on laboratory safety should be consulted for additional information.[19,30,33,42,43]

Creating and maintaining a successful program requires daily commitment from every individual to 5 basic aspects of safety: 1) prevent accidents; 2) deal quickly and efficiently with accidents that do occur; 3) establish cause, where possible, and disseminate information to all to prevent reoccurrence; 4) provide employees with safety information and education; and 5) ensure that safety procedures are closely followed.

Regular evaluation of personal safety practices and housekeeping procedures in the work area are essential to ensure laboratory safety. This evaluation involves a safety committee review. It is recommended that members be rotated to allow new members on the committee.

An overall policy regarding laboratory safety should be established and incorporated into the quality system. Because safety results from employees' attitudes as well as from physical or engineering factors, good results depend upon the efforts of each individual to eliminate unsafe acts and conditions. Continuing safety requires a genuine interest in safety from all employees, at all levels of responsibility.

A laboratory's safety policy must charge employees to follow safe work methods and to be concerned about the safety of their fellow workers as much as their own.

2.052 *Right-to-Know*

As part of the Super Fund Amendments and Reauthorization Act of 1986, the Emergency Planning and Community Right-to-Know Act established reporting procedures for hazardous and toxic chemicals.

These provisions, also known as Title III, were designed to provide the public, government agencies, and emergency responders with information concerning the use, storage, and release of chemicals in local communities.

The act has 4 important sections: 1) emergency planning; 2) emergency notification; 3) community right-to-know reporting requirements; and 4) toxic chemical release reporting. The emergency planning section calls for a state emergency response commission and local emergency planning committees. The primary responsibility of the local committee is to develop an emergency plan to respond to potential chemical releases. According to the emergency notification section, any manufacturer or importer should immediately inform both local and state emergency teams when an amount above the reportable quantity of a listed hazardous substance is released into the environment. Under the community right-to-know reporting requirements, facilities (primarily manufacturers and importers) should provide copies or a list of material safety data sheets (MSDS) and other pertinent information for all chemicals used or stored to the local emergency planning committee, the state emergency response commission, and the local fire department. The toxic chemical release reporting section requires facilities that use more than the established quantities of listed hazardous chemicals to submit toxic chemical release forms to the Environmental Protection Agency (EPA) and the state emergency response commission. Later these forms will be used by the National Academy of Sciences (NAS) to develop a national toxic chemical release program to determine the amount of toxic chemicals released into the environment every year.

2.053 *Occupational Safety and Health Standards*

Two important federal standards apply to safety and health of laboratory workers. The regulations describe risks associated with laboratory work and assign responsibilities for protecting workers.

A. **Hazard communication standard:** The Hazard Communication Standard (29 CFR 1910.1200; *Federal Register*, Vol. 52, No. 163, Aug. 24, 1987, p. 31877) has been implemented by federal and state governments to protect workers who use chemicals. The standard instructs employers to inform their employees of the hazards of chemical exposure. It is aimed at specific Standard Industrial Classifications (SIC) that are most prevalent in the manufacturing sector. However, nationwide employee health concerns are contributing to expansion of the Hazard Communication Standard into the nonmanufacturing sector.

Employers affected by the standard must meet several requirements. For example, each employer needs a written hazard communication program that defines provisions for compliance with all aspects of the Hazard Communication Standard.

In the written program, employers should identify the specific ways in which they will assess chemical hazards. To do this, they should evaluate the processes being conducted at the site and the chemical hazards involved. Other components required for the written program include labels and warnings, material safety data sheets (MSDS), and employee training and information.

1. **Labeling:** Labels need to be affixed to all containers of chemicals and chemical products. The labels should include the name of the chemical, a list of the ingredients in the chemicals or products, and the appropriate hazard warnings for the chemical and ingredients. All containers should have labels distinctly displayed and written in English. Additional labeling in other languages may be affixed to the containers.
2. **Material safety data sheets:** Material safety data sheets are used by manufacturers, importers, and other producers to supply standard health and safety information to the employees and consumers who use their products. Every MSDS should contain health and safety information including the identifier, names of hazardous constituent(s), physical information, fire and explosion information, health hazard data, spill information, and special protection and precautions. Emergency first aid information and telephone number(s) of the producer(s) should also be listed. Employers should keep all MSDS current and readily available to employees during work hours.
3. **Employee training:** The Hazard Communication Standard requires that employers properly communicate health and safety information to their employees. The training program should include information concerning the ways in which the working environment is monitored for hazards, proper work practices, appropriate personal protective equipment, and emergency procedures.

B. **Occupational exposure to hazardous chemicals in laboratories:** This standard (CFR 1910.1450; *Federal Register*, Vol. 55, No. 21, Jan. 31, 1990, p. 3327) applies to all employers engaged in the laboratory use of hazardous chemicals. Some of the general principles of this regulation follow.

Because few laboratory chemicals are without hazards, general precautions for handling all laboratory chemicals should be adopted rather than specific guidelines for particular chemicals. Skin contact with chemicals should be avoided as a cardinal rule. One should assume that any mixture of chemicals will be more toxic than its single most toxic component and that all substances of unknown toxicity are toxic.

Responsibility for chemical hygiene rests at all levels of management—from the chief executive officer, who has the ultimate responsibility, to the laboratory worker. The laboratory supervisor is assigned the following particularly important responsibilities:

1. Ensure that laboratory workers know and follow the chemical hygiene rules, that protective equipment is readily available and in working order, and that appropriate training has been provided.
2. Provide regular and formal chemical hygiene and housekeeping inspections, including routine inspections of emergency equipment.
3. Know the current legal requirements concerning regulated substances.
4. Determine the required levels of protective apparel and equipment.
5. Ensure that facilities and training for use of any material being ordered are adequate.

C. **Radioactive materials:** The Nuclear Regulatory Commission (NRC) regulates the use of radioactive materials in laboratories. The possession and/or use of radioactive material is allowed only when covered by a state and/or federal license, except when procedures call for use of small exempt quantities of radioactive materials. Such a license specifies the type and quantity of radioactive material, the conditions of use, required test programs, and the conditions of storage and disposal. Possession, use, or disposal by any means other than those specified in the license is a violation of federal law and is punishable by fine and/or imprisonment.

A requirement for obtaining the license is to have appointed a radiation safety officer for the laboratory. This person should be responsible for all laboratory use of radioactive materials and sources of radiation. The specific radioactive safety program for the laboratory needs to be designed and monitored by the radiation safety officer.

Laboratories conducting pesticide residue, antibiotic, or other analyses in which radioactive materials may be employed, either in detector devices or radioactive chemicals, must be familiar with the safety and operating requirements for their usage.

D. **Personnel practices in microbiological laboratories:** The following guidelines may serve as a basis for developing a microbiological laboratory safety program:

1. Working surfaces should be disinfected immediately before and after use.
2. Laboratory clothing must be worn at all times in the work area. Laboratory coats or gowns should be removed prior to entering non-laboratory areas.
3. Hands and exposed areas of the arms of the analyst should be washed immediately before and after handling potentially dangerous microbiologic materials.
4. Spills of contaminated materials must be flooded immediately with disinfectant solutions and cleaned up promptly. Large spills may require that an official report be made.
5. All labware containing incubated culture material known or suspected to contain pathogens must be autoclaved at 120° ± 1°C for 30 minutes prior to being washed or discarded. Containers of primary dilutions made from milk or dairy products need not be sterilized unless there is reason to suspect the presence of pathogens.
6. Materials should not be placed in autoclaves overnight anticipating autoclaving the next day.
7. Contaminated glass from broken laboratory ware should be picked up with forceps, autoclaved, and then disposed of properly. Contaminated glassware must be autoclaved prior to being discarded in a "sharps" container.
8. Centrifuging should be done only in suitable, closed tubes.
9. Contaminated pipets should be placed, immediately after use, in a tray or pipet jar containing a suitable disinfectant.
10. Flamed loops and needles must be allowed to cool before introduction into inoculated media.

11. All filter flasks should be fitted with a trap to prevent escape of contaminated material into the vacuum system.
12. All broth, agar, or suspensions, whenever inoculated from suspect material, should be considered hazardous.
13. Contaminated materials and toxin-producing cultures must not be removed from the laboratory except under controlled conditions.
14. Laboratory clothing that is contaminated with potentially dangerous microorganisms should be sterilized before laundering.
15. Surgical gloves should be worn when working with pathogens if the analyst has noticeable skin cuts, lesions, or abrasions.
16. Sniffing unknown cultures may result in infection. Do not sniff inoculated media.
17. Do not mouth pipet. Various pipet aids may be used to provide a vacuum.

2.054 *Pathogenic Organisms*

Pathogen testing is technique-dependent and more specialized than routine analysis of dairy products. It should only be undertaken by well-trained and proficient analysts. Appropriate health department personnel should be consulted for additional information regarding the handling of pathogens. Some states or localities may have additional regulations and/or recommendations regarding the handling of pathogens.

Laboratory facilities in dairy plants testing for pathogens are discussed in section 2.0310. Disposable laboratory coats, shoe covers, and eye protection should be worn while in the pathogen area and properly disposed of prior to leaving the area.

There should be limited access to stock cultures to prevent their unauthorized removal from the laboratory. Stock cultures should be kept in a locked cabinet or refrigerator with 1 or 2 individuals accountable for usage.

2.055 *Microbiology Laboratory Safety*

A. **General:** Studies have documented laboratory-associated infections of laboratory workers. Most of these have been pathogen laboratories; however, a number of cases were due to unknown sources. Less than 20% of the cases were attributed to laboratory accidents. There has been a very low rate of secondary infection outside of laboratories.

B. **Principles of biosafety**[33]

1. **Laboratory practice and technique** *(specified in* Biosafety/QA Manual*):* Individuals properly trained in technique, safety, and knowledge of the handling of potential and known infectious agents. Strict adherence to laboratory practices and techniques is the most important way to prevent contamination.
2. **Safety equipment** *(primary barriers):* Equipment used to minimize exposure to infectious agents (e.g., biological safety hoods). Safety equipment also includes personal protective items such as lab coats, safety glasses, masks, and respirators.
3. **Facility Design** *(secondary barriers):* The design of the laboratory is important to provide a barrier to protect those working inside and

outside the laboratory and to prevent an accidental release of organisms into the environment.

C. **Biosafety levels**

1. **Biosafety level 1:** This level of safety is sufficient for laboratories that are working with organisms not generally known to cause human disease and present minimal hazard to laboratory personnel. Work is generally conducted on open benches with only standard microbiological practices employed. The laboratory does not need to be isolated from general traffic, nor are special containment equipment and facilities required. Workers should be trained and supervised by someone who has general training in microbiology. Containment is by adherence to standard microbiological practices.
2. **Biosafety level 2:** Laboratories in this category work with known pathogens that possess moderate health risks. Requirements are similar to level 1 except laboratory workers have been trained to work with pathogens and are supervised by someone competent to work with these organisms. Access to this laboratory is restricted while work is conducted. In addition to standard microbiological practices, special precautions are observed by laboratory personnel to prevent accidental infection. Containment equipment and facilities are required.
3. **Biosafety level 3:** Laboratories in this category work with known pathogens that possess serious health risks. Laboratory workers must be trained to work with these pathogens and be supervised by someone competent to work with these organisms. Access to this laboratory is restricted. In addition to level 2 precautions, special precautions are observed by laboratory personnel to prevent accidental infection. Containment equipment and facilities are required. These laboratories must be isolated from other areas or buildings with negative airflow.
4. **Biosafety level 4:** Laboratories in this category work with serious known pathogens that either can be transmitted by aerosol or are life threatening. Laboratory workers must have specific and thorough training to work with these extremely hazardous pathogens and are supervised by someone competent to work with these organisms. Access to this laboratory is restricted. Special precautions are observed by laboratory personnel to prevent accidental infection. Specialized containment equipment and facilities are required. Laboratories must be completely isolated from other areas or buildings. The laboratory must have negative airflow with dedicated air handling and decontamination systems.

Most milk laboratories fall into biosafety level 1 criteria. Many state laboratories and commercial laboratories, however, fall into biosafety level 2, although not due to the routine analysis of milk. A few industry laboratories may also fall into biosafety level 2 if they test for pathogens.

A very few milk laboratories fall into biosafety level 3. Level 3 labs are primarily health department laboratories that also do clinical work. There are no milk laboratories in biosafety level 4.

These categories do not always completely encompass the work done

CFSAN LABORATORY INSPECTION CHECKLIST

Office/Division/Branch:________________________ Building/Room:________________________

Inspector:__________________________________ Date:_____________________________

Use this checklist as a guide when conducting routine and quarterly inspections. This list is not all inclusive. The list contains items that may be the responsibility of the Center, the Division, the Researcher, the Safety Office, or the Facilities Section. The purpose of the list is to document deficiencies and initiate corrective action regardless of responsibility. Y = Yes, N = No, NA = Not Applicable. Refer to CFSAN Staff Manual Guide 2130.4 for additional policies and procedures governing CFSAN's Laboratory Safety Inspection Program. Contact the CFSAN Safety Office if you have any questions or comments.

	A. Emergency Contacts and Egress	Y	N	N/A
1.	Emergency contacts and phone numbers posted on each lab and storage area.	☐	☐	☐
2.	Exits are free of obstructions and stored materials.	☐	☐	☐
3.	Emergency exits not locked with slide bolts, dead bolts, padlocks, etc.	☐	☐	☐

	B. Fire Extinguisher	Y	N	N/A
1.	Accessible.	☐	☐	☐
2.	Locations clearly visible or marked.	☐	☐	☐
3.	Monthly and annual inspections current.	☐	☐	☐
4.	Mounted.	☐	☐	☐
5.	Charged and seals intact.	☐	☐	☐
6.	Correct for hazards present.	☐	☐	☐

	C. Safety Shower and Eyewash	Y	N	N/A
1.	Not blocked.	☐	☐	☐
2.	Locations clearly marked.	☐	☐	☐
3.	Weekly inspections and flushings current and documented.	☐	☐	☐
4.	Protective caps in place on eyewash.	☐	☐	☐

	D. Housekeeping	Y	N	N/A
1.	Counters and floors clean and clear of clutter.	☐	☐	☐
2.	A minimum of 28" egress is maintained.	☐	☐	☐
3.	Lab is free of trip hazards.	☐	☐	☐
4.	Equipment on benches stable or secured.	☐	☐	☐
5.	Supplies stored in a stable and secure manner.	☐	☐	☐
6.	Sharps disposal container provided and clearly labeled.	☐	☐	☐
7.	No storage within 18 inches of sprinkler heads.	☐	☐	☐
8.	Hallways and exits are clear.	☐	☐	☐
9.	Moving parts on machinery guarded.	☐	☐	☐
10.	Caution, warning signs and emergency phone numbers are posted on lab door windows to caution strangers of hazardous work. Other vision obstructing material is <u>not</u> posted.	☐	☐	☐
11.	Compressed gas cylinders are transported with regulators removed and cylinder caps in place.	☐	☐	☐
12.	Heat producing appliances are used only on non-combustable surfaces. Bunsen burners have an 18 inch radius clear area. Flames are never left unattended.	☐	☐	☐
13.	Pressurized glass vessels are shielded.	☐	☐	☐
14.	Water or other suitable liquid is maintained in the traps of cupsinks.	☐	☐	☐
15.	Laboratory stools are in good condition.	☐	☐	☐
16.	No food storage in chemical areas.	☐	☐	☐
17.	No chemical storage in food areas.	☐	☐	☐
18.	Refrigerators for food storage labeled "Lunch Food Only" or "FDA Food Samples Only."	☐	☐	☐
19.	Emergency phone numbers are visible near every telephone.	☐	☐	☐
20.	Temperature log of refrigerator, oven, incubator, etc., are maintained. Temperatures are given.	☐	☐	☐

	E. Electrical	Y	N	N/A
1.	Electrical equipment is double insulated or grounded (3 pronged).	☐	☐	☐
2.	Electrical cords and plugs in good condition.	☐	☐	☐
3.	Circuits feeding potentially wet areas have GFCI protection.	☐	☐	☐
4.	Electrical panels closed and not blocked.	☐	☐	☐
5.	Extension cords <u>not</u> used as a permanent means of wiring.	☐	☐	☐
6.	Pigtail adapters are <u>not</u> used.	☐	☐	☐
7.	Hot water/constant temperature bath units are independently grounded.	☐	☐	☐
8.	Laboratory equipment, such as dryers, variacs, blenders, mixers, etc., are properly grounded with a three prong grounded plug.	☐	☐	☐
9.	Water and vacuum pumps, electric stirring machines, and electric motors have a suitable belt guard, or are enclosed in an instrument.	☐	☐	☐
10.	Metal desk lamps are not used on metal surfaces near water sources.	☐	☐	☐

	F. Chemical Hygiene and Storage	Y	N	N/A
1.	Appropriate hazard warning signs posted on door and door and storage areas (e.g., Cancer Agent).	☐	☐	☐
2.	CFSAN Chemical Hygiene Plan present in Laboratory.	☐	☐	☐
3.	All containers labeled legibly with content and hazard warning.	☐	☐	☐
4.	Storage containers in good condition: no rust, leakage, dents, or crystallization.	☐	☐	☐
5.	Glass storage containers are limited to 1 gallon size or smaller.	☐	☐	☐
6.	Peroxide forming chemicals labeled and dated upon receipt and opening.	☐	☐	☐
7.	Peroxide forming chemicals disposed of within 3-12 months after opening depending up on the compound.	☐	☐	☐
8.	Manufacturer expiration dates observed.	☐	☐	☐
9.	Acid and bases are stored separately.	☐	☐	☐
10.	Acids and bases stored separately from solvents. Exception: store acetic acid with solvents.	☐	☐	☐
11.	Water reactive chemicals stored away from water and water vapor.	☐	☐	☐
12.	Corrosive and flammable chemicals are stored below eye level.	☐	☐	☐
13.	Chemical containers are not stacked.	☐	☐	☐
14.	No more than 10 gallons of flammable liquid stored outside of flammable storage cabinet.	☐	☐	☐
15.	No more than 40 gallons of flammable liquid stored per lab.	☐	☐	☐
16.	Explosion resistant refrigerators and freezers used for flammable liquids.	☐	☐	☐
17.	All refrigerators and freezers labeled to indicate their suitability for flammable storage.	☐	☐	☐
18.	Carcinogenic and highly toxic chemicals stored in main compartment of refrigerator instead of the door.	☐	☐	☐

F. Chemical Hygiene (continued) Y N N/A

19. Carcinogens, reproductive toxins, and highly toxic chemicals stored and used in a designated and labeled area. No open bench storage. □ □ □
20. Food and drink are not stored in laboratory refrigerators. No eating or drinking in the laboratory is allowed. □ □ □
21. Laboratory chemicals are not stored on floors. □ □ □
22. Chemical hood ventilation has been checked within the past year and arrows indicating adequate air flow are affixed to the sash. □ □ □
23. Toxic materials are centrifuged in a hermetically closed centrifuge with safety cups. □ □ □
24. Toxic materials are personally taken to the autoclave and seen that they are sterilized immediately. Proper records are maintained. □ □ □
25. Mechanical pipeting devices are used. NEVER PIPET BY MOUTH – anything. □ □ □
26. Chemicals with a limited shelf life are receipt dated and disposed of when shelf life expires. □ □ □
27. Chemical spill cleanup kits are available in every laboratory. □ □ □

G. Compressed Gases

1. Cylinders secured in place. □ □ □
2. Protective caps in place when not in use. □ □ □
3. Oxygen and flammable gases stored separately. □ □ □
4. Manual shutoff valves provided at all points of supply and use. □ □ □
5. Corrosive gases stored no more than 6 months. □ □ □
6. Pressure gauges and regulators are in place as appropriate. □ □ □

H. Ventilation

1. Hood sash is in working order – not stuck, broken, or removed. □ □ □
2. Airfoils are not altered or removed. □ □ □
3. Equipment and materials are positioned and used at a minimum of 6" from the front of the hood. □ □ □
4. Equipment or materials do not obstruct air flow. □ □ □
5. Hood interior is clean, uncluttered, and not used as permanent storage. □ □ □
6. Annual hood certification present indicating face velocity is 100-120 fpm. □ □ □
7. Arrows indicating the correct sash height. □ □ □
8. Hood low flow alarms present and operational. □ □ □
9. Perchloric acid hoods labeled "For Perchloric Acid Operations Only." □ □ □

I. Personal Protective Equipment

1. Safety glasses available. □ □ □
2. Lab coats and aprons available. □ □ □
3. Face shields available for operations with appreciable slash hazards (e.g., handling acids). □ □ □
4. Appropriate shoes worn (e.g., no sandals). □ □ □
5. Appropriate gloves available. □ □ □
6. Lab coats and safety glasses are worn at all times. Eye Hazard areas are posted. □ □ □
7. Fire blankets are available nearby. □ □ □
8. Employees working alone in the laboratory after hours or on weekends should arrange a "buddy system" whereby one or more people know of his/her whereabouts. □ □ □

J. Biosafety Y N N/A

1. Annual certification of biosafety cabinet present. □ □ □
2. Appropriate hazard warning signs posted on door and storage areas (e.g., Biohazard – Legionella pneumophila). □ □ □
3. All containers labeled as to content and hazard. □ □ □
4. Sharps containers provided and clearly labeled. □ □ □
5. Biological waste containers labeled. □ □ □
6. Municipal trash containers free of biohazardous waste. □ □ □

K. Chemical Waste Management

1. CFSAN Hazardous Waste Plan present. □ □ □
2. Waste containers labeled with contents. Start date included for DC labs. □ □ □
3. Waste stored less than 90 days (DC Labs only). □ □ □
4. Waste containers closed and in good condition. □ □ □
5. Secondary containment of wastes stored outside hood. □ □ □
6. Municipal trash containers free of chemical waste. □ □ □

L. Office Space

1. Extension cords not used as a permanent means of wiring. □ □ □
2. Office free of tripping hazards (e.g., cables, loose tiles, damaged carpet). □ □ □
3. Workstation set-up provides a minimum of 28" egress. □ □ □
4. Electrical cords and plugs in good condition. □ □ □
5. Office supplies stacked in a stable and secure manner. □ □ □
6. Hallways and exits are clear. □ □ □
7. No storage within 18 inches of sprinkler heads. □ □ □
8. Fire extinguisher mounted, accessible, and inspected. monthly and annually. □ □ □
9. Coffee pots not placed in or near combustible material. □ □ □

M. Special or Unique Hazards

1. ______________________ □ □ □
2. ______________________ □ □ □
3. ______________________ □ □ □
4. ______________________ □ □ □
5. ______________________ □ □ □

Additional Comments:

____

____

____

____

____

____

____

____

in laboratories. For example, there is a potential that pathogens may be present at laboratories testing raw milk. While raw milk is generally considered safe and may be disposed without any special precautions, any incubated plates should be handled as potentially hazardous. In this case, the laboratory falls under biosafety level 2 criteria.

D. **Standard microbiological practices**

1. Access to the laboratory is limited or restricted at the discretion of the laboratory director when experiments are in progress.
2. Persons wash their hands after they handle viable materials and animals, after removing gloves, and before leaving the laboratory.
3. Eating, drinking, smoking, handling contact lenses, and applying cosmetics are not permitted in the work areas. Persons who wear contact lenses in laboratories should also wear goggles or a face shield. Food is stored outside the work area in cabinets or refrigerators designated for this purpose only.
4. Mouth pipeting is prohibited. Mechanical pipeting devices are used.
5. All procedures are performed carefully to minimize splashes or aerosols.
6. Work surfaces are decontaminated at least once a day and after any spill of viable material.
7. All cultures, stocks, and other regulated wastes are decontaminated before disposal by an approved decontamination method, such as autoclaving. Materials to be decontaminated outside of the immediate laboratory should be placed in a durable, leak-proof container and closed for transport from the laboratory. Materials to be decontaminated offsite from the laboratory are packaged in accordance with applicable local, state, and federal regulations before removal from the facility.
8. An insect and rodent control program is in effect.
9. Emergency planning and community right-to-know reporting is enforced.

2.056 *Disposition of Milk or Dairy Products*

The practice of allowing individuals in the laboratory to perform organoleptic evaluation of milk and dairy products is common. While this in and of itself is not an unsafe practice, it has the potential of being unsafe. Storage of the samples prior to distribution for consumption should be confined to a refrigerator that does not contain potentially toxic chemicals or hazardous microorganisms.

Since nonsterile procedures and glassware may be used, samples that have been tested must be discarded immediately. Often samples are left at room temperature for long periods of time, allowing the number of bacteria present to significantly increase. An alternative practice would be to transfer a portion of the sample from the original container to a separate container using sterile glassware or implements.

Most laboratories have developed policies requiring that all samples submitted for analysis be discarded after the necessary retention period, if any, and are not allowed to be consumed. This is a recommended practice.

2.057 *Laboratory Safety Inspection Checklist*[35]

See pages 37–40.

2.060 Cited References

1. ANONYMOUS. *Food safety from farm to table. A national food safety initiative: a report to the President.* Washington, DC: U.S. Govt. Print. Off.; 1997.
2. BALDWIN, R. A. QA/QC agenda: When is enough science, enough? Food Testing & Analysis **3**:1; 1997.
3. BARKER, J. H.; BLANK, C. H.; STEEVE, N. V. *Designing a laboratory*. Washington, DC: APHA; 1989.
4. BRIETENBERG, M.A. *The ABC's of the U.S. conformity assessment system: NIST IR 6014.* Gaithersburg, MD: Office of Standards Services, National Institute of Standards and Technology; 1997.
5. CEMBROWSKII, G. S. Thoughts on quality control system: a laboratorian's perspective. Clin. Chem. **43**(5): 886-892; 1997.
6. CLESCERI, L.S.; GREENBERG, A.E.; EATON, A.D, eds. *Standard methods for the examination of water and wastewater,* 20th ed. Washington, DC: APHA; 1998.
7. CODE OF FEDERAL REGULATIONS. *Good laboratory practices for non-clinical laboratory studies*, Title 21, Part 58. Washington, DC: U.S. Govt. Print. Off.; 1997.
8. DYBKAER, R. Quality assurance, accreditation, and certification: Needs and possibilities. Clin. Chem. **40**(7): 1416-1420; 1994.
9. EARLY, R. *Guide to quality management systems for the food industry*. New York, NY: Blackie Academic Professional; 1995.
10. FELLAND, H.S.; NADIG, J.W. A comparative study of the volumetric deliveries from glass and plastic pipettes. J. Milk Food Technol. **28**:124-126; 1965.
11. FISCHBECK, R.D. Good laboratory practice regulations and their impact on laboratory organization and operation. Amer. Lab. **12**(9): 125-130; 1980.
12. FLICKINGER, B. Defining and designing the modern QC laboratory. J. Food Quality. **1**(7): 33-38; 1995.
13. FLICKINGER, B. Microbiology lab performance. J. Food Quality. **2**(4): 21-28; 1996.
14. FOOD AND AGRICULTURE ORGANIZATION OF THE UNITED NATIONS. *Quality assurance in the food control microbiological laboratory.* Manual of food quality control. Rome: Food and Agriculture Organization of the United Nations; 1990. 1:12.
15. FOOD AND AGRICULTURE ORGANIZATION OF THE UNITED NATIONS. *Quality assurance in the food control chemical laboratory.* Manual of food quality control. Rome: Food and Agriculture Organization of the United Nations; 1990. 1:14.
16. FOOD TESTING & ANALYSIS. Special focus: putting together the regulatory puzzle: an update on the rules and regulations affecting the food industry. Food Testing & Analysis **4**:5; 1998.
17. GARFIELD, F. M. *Quality Assurance principles for analytical laboratories*. Arlington, VA: AOAC International; 1991.
18. GRIMM, D. QA/QC agenda: Internal QA audits for the micro lab. Food Testing & Analysis. **3**:1; 1997.
19. HEINDEL, G.D. *Introduction to chemical laboratory safety.* Washington, DC: American Chemical Society; 1991
20. HUBBARD, M. R. *Statistical quality control for the food industry.* New York, NY: Van Nostrand Reinhold; 1990.
21. INHORN, S.L., ED. *Quality assurance practices for health laboratories*. Washington, DC: APHA; 1978.
22. INTERNATIONAL COMMISSION ON MICROBIOLOGICAL SPECIFICATIONS FOR FOODS OF THE INTERNATIONAL UNION OF MICROBIOLOGICAL SOCIETIES. *HACCP in Microbiological Safety and Quality*. Cambridge, MA: Blackwell Scientific Publications; 1992.
23. INTERNATIONAL ORGANIZATION FOR STANDARDIZATION: ISO 840. *Quality Management and Quality Assurance—Vocabulary.* Geneva, Switzerland: ISO; 1994
24. INTERNATIONAL ORGANIZATION FOR STANDARDIZATION: ISO 9001. *Quality systems—Model for quality assurance in design, development, production, installation and*

servicing. Geneva, Switzerland: ISO; 1994.

25. INTERNATIONAL ORGANIZATION FOR STANDARDIZATION: ISO 9002. *Quality systems—Model for quality assurance in production, installation and servicing*. Geneva, Switzerland: ISO; 1994.
26. INTERNATIONAL ORGANIZATION FOR STANDARDIZATION: ISO 9004-1. *Quality Management and Quality System Elements—Part 1 Guidelines*. Geneva, Switzerland: ISO; 1994.
27. INTERNATIONAL ORGANIZATION FOR STANDARDIZATION: ISO 9004-4. *Quality Management and Quality System Elements—Part 4 Guidelines for Quality Improvement*. Geneva, Switzerland: ISO; 1994.
28. INTERNATIONAL ORGANIZATION FOR STANDARDIZATION: ISO/DIS 17025. *General requirements for the competence of testing and calibration laboratories*. Geneva, Switzerland: ISO; 1998.
29. INTERNATIONAL ORGANIZATION FOR STANDARDIZATION: ISO/IEC Guide 2. *General terms and their definitions concerning standardization and related activities*. Geneva, Switzerland: ISO; 1996.
30. NATIONAL RESEARCH COUNCIL. *Biosafety in the laboratory: Prudent practices for the handling and disposal of infectious materials*. Washington, DC: National Academy Press; 1989.
31. TAMINI, N.; SEBASTIANELLI, R. Barriers to total quality management. Quality Progress. **31**(6): 57-60; 1998.
32. TAYLOR, C.M. Preventive action vs. corrective action: the horse, the barn, and the apple. Quality Progress **31**(3): 66-71; 1998.
33. U.S. DEPARTMENT OF HEALTH AND HUMAN SERVICES. *Biosafety in Microbiological and Biomedical Laboratories*, 4th ed. Govt. Print. Off. Washington, DC: HHS; 1999: CDC 93-8395.
34. U.S. DEPARTMENT OF HEALTH AND HUMAN SERVICES. *Evaluation of milk laboratories*. Washington, DC: FDA; 1995.
35. U.S. DEPARTMENT OF HEALTH AND HUMAN SERVICES. *Food and drug administration—CFSAN safety manual*. Washington, DC: FDA; 1997.
36. U.S. DEPARTMENT OF HEALTH AND HUMAN SERVICES. *Grade "A" pasteurized milk ordinance*. Washington, DC: FDA; 1995.
37. U.S. DEPARTMENT OF HEALTH AND HUMAN SERVICES. *Milk laboratory evaluation forms*. Cincinnati, OH: FDA; 1987.
38. U.S. ENVIRONMENTAL PROTECTION AGENCY. *Handbook for analytical quality control in water and wastewater laboratories*. Cincinnati, OH: EPA; 1979. EPA-600/4-79-019.
39. U.S. ENVIRONMENTAL PROTECTION AGENCY. *Microbiological methods for monitoring the environment, water and wastes*. Cincinnati, OH: EPA; 1978. EPA-600/8-78-017.
40. U.S. FOOD AND DRUG ADMINISTARTION; MILK INDUSTRY FOUNDATION; INTERNATIONAL ICE CREAM ASSOCIATION. Recommended guidelines for controlling environmental contamination in dairy plants. Dairy Food Sanitation **8**(2):52-56; 1987.
41. WILSON, S.; WEIR, G. *Food and drink laboratory accreditation: a practical approach*. New York, NY: Chapman & Hill; 1995.
42. YOUNG, J.A. *Improving safety in the chemical laboratory: a practical guide*, 2nd ed. New York, NY: Wiley-Interscience; 1991.
43. YOUNG, J.A.; KINGSLEY, W.K.; WAHL, G.H. Jr. *Developing a chemical hygiene plan*. Washington, DC: American Chemical Society; 1990.

Chapter 3

Sampling Dairy and Related Products

T. Graham
(L. Maturin, Tech. Comm.)

3.010 Introduction

The proper collection, transportation, and storage of milk and milk product samples are critical if the laboratory analysis of the samples is to be valid. The best analytical technique cannot overcome a sample that has been compromised during collection or storage during transportation to a laboratory.[6] The perishable nature of milk compounds the problem. Even under the best conditions, microorganisms survive and grow, and chemical and physical changes can occur. It is essential that authorized sample collectors be trained to be continually aware of potential problems that can occur during the initial collection and delivery of samples to the laboratory.[7,18,21]

Because it is expected that a sample is representative of the entire mass that was sampled, the initial concern is adequate mixing. Samples taken from insufficiently mixed milk or milk products may not be representative of the entire mass, even if collection and transport were conducted under ideal conditions. During the collection of the sample, the collector must ensure that contamination, microbial and chemical, is not introduced into the sample. After samples are collected, they must be protected from contamination and maintained under specified conditions (depending on the sample and the microbiological, chemical, and physical analysis to be performed) so that when the samples are delivered to the laboratory they are essentially the same as when collected. Maintaining proper temperature is essential to preventing microbial growth and ensuring that there are no chemical or physical changes in the samples until they are analyzed. Under ideal conditions, analysis of the samples should begin within 24 hours and, in most cases, no later than 48 hours after original collection (not from an intermediate pick up/transfer location). Collectors must also ensure that all pertinent information is recorded and delivered to the laboratory.[7,18,24] This includes sample identification information, date, time, and temperature of collection, and who collected the sample. Due to the legal nature of the process, when collecting samples for regulatory purposes, a chain of custody should always be established to ensure only those with the proper authority handled the samples.[18]

It is not realistic to assume that a single sample will always accurately reflect the composition of the represented mass, especially if the mass is large and is not properly mixed just prior to sampling, or if samples are not randomly selected. Proper mixing or randomizing is difficult to determine in the laboratory. Chemical composition, especially if it is compared to historical information, may determine the likelihood that a mass was adequately mixed prior to sampling. Collection of multiple samples statistically increases the probability of a sample result reflecting the condition of the mass.[19]

The physical nature of a sample (fluid, viscous, semi-solid, solid, dry) dictates how samples are taken, held, and transported. Different products require different sampling procedures.[7,18] Conditions may also dictate how samples should be taken. Public health considerations are an overriding concern when taking samples. Other considerations include information for the producer and plant, and payment for the milk. No one method can cover all of the types of samples that must be collected. Basic information on sampling methods is available from publications listed in the reference section [3.010, No. 2]. The bibliography section [3.130] contains all publications cited in this chapter.

1. **Scope:** This chapter provides information on the collection and transportation of milk and milk product samples to a laboratory for analysis. The information in this chapter is for general reference and not intended to be all inclusive. Specifically, this information does not supersede any regulatory requirements; however, it is expected that the information reflects good practices that would meet regulatory requirements.
2. **Definitions**
   A. **Sample:** Portion of a mass, or unit of a lot, taken for inspection and/or laboratory analysis.
   B. **Sample collector:** Person authorized, trained, and recognized to take samples.
   C. **Sample form:** Document or report submitted with samples that contains all necessary information on the samples delivered to a laboratory [3.041].
   D. **Sampling plan:** Plan that sets forth the number and frequency of samples that will be taken for analysis or inspection based on risk and/or regulatory requirements [3.020].
   E. **Universal sample:** Single sample taken for the purpose of a number of analyses, typically a regulatory sample.

3.020 Sampling[5,6,11,13-15]

3.021 *Sampling Plans*

The concept of sampling plans is presented below. Readers are directed to IDF Standard 113A: 1990 and ISO 2859 for additional information. The information below is summarized from these documents.

Sampling plans or strategies should be set up to ensure adequate consumer and producer protection. These plans are a final check that ensures that products are of the expected quality. Depending on the nature of the material to be sampled and the level of certainty that is desired or necessary, the required number of samples can be determined. Samples can be taken from several sources at one time or from different lots of the material at different times. Health and economic considerations often dictate the advantage of one of these arrangements over the others. For example, some sampling methods are destructive while others leave the samples unharmed. The cost added by destructive sampling is one economic consideration. Current practices in sampling are often a compromise between the desire to achieve a high level of consumer protection and the cost of providing service. When a sampling plan for inspection of items or units is being devised, the services of a statistician should be obtained.

It must be determined what level of safety or quality is desired, which if maintained will result in the acceptance of most of what is produced. Selecting a sampling plan requires that critical, major, and minor defects be defined and understood.

Simply put, a *critical defect* is one that makes a product unacceptable. In other words, it is likely to be (not could be) hazardous or unsafe, or render the product unusable. In the case of milk, adulteration with a toxic substance would be considered a critical defect. Selection of a defect as critical must be done with care, since if found this will result in the rejection of an entire lot. In the case of critical defects, there is no minimal level of acceptance.

A *major defect* is an item that will most likely make a unit unfit for sale to consumers. These may include composition defects (microbiological, chemical, or physical), presence of inhibitors, packaging problems, or visible contamination. Sampling plans are based on the number of defects found per number of units in a lot. Typically a plan specifies the number of units to be tested and the maximum number of defects that can be found and still have the lot acceptable and the minimum number of defects, that if found, will reject a lot.

A *minor defect* generally refers to a failure to meet a specification, but does not make a product unsafe or unusable. For example, this may involve appearance or a level of a component, such as milk solids. Generally sampling plans designed to detect minor defects have a lower level of concern and require fewer units to be inspected or analyzed.

All sampling plans require samples to be randomly collected (i.e., each unit has exactly the same probability of being chosen). This may not occur if someone arbitrarily selects units. There is the possibility a person will unknowingly be biased (e.g., select more units from one area than another), especially if collection is difficult. It is preferable to use a randomization protocol to select the units, such as using a random number table.

3.022 *Critical Defects*[13]

By definition critical defects are unacceptable under any circumstance. The best plan is to sample 100% of a lot with acceptance set when no critical defects are found. This is possible only when a nondestructive inspection takes place. In this type of inspection scheme if a critical defect is found, the whole lot is discarded. Ideally this also stops production so a determination can be made as to where the problem occurred so that corrective actions can be instituted. This drastic action is meant to prevent a reliance on the inspection to find critical defects. The producer of a product may; however, institute inspection and sorting as part of the process prior to final inspection.

If it is believed that a product does not warrant this type of inspection, then consideration should be given to changing the status of the defect to major instead of critical. Selecting a defect as critical, and then deciding that finding one or more critical defects should not result in rejecting the lot, defeats the purpose of the designation.

If only destructive inspection is possible, or the cost of 100% inspection is prohibitive, then 100% inspection is not an option. A decision would have to be made on a sampling plan that would have a high probability of detecting a single defect present in a lot and establish a risk for failing to find that defect. Typically this requires a large number of samples to be taken.

An alternate approach may be an option in some cases. This would involve a safety margin. If a defect is critical at one level, but only major at another, it may be possible to use the more stringent level, but inspect with a major defect sampling plan. This approach requires in-depth knowledge of the product and defect(s) concerned and confidence that the risk level will ensure that no critical defects go undetected. While this approach may indeed provide the safety and quality desired, consumers may perceive the milk product as less than safe.

3.023 *Sample Size and Defective Units*

Experimental data indicate that at least 10 units are necessary for a representative sampling when a large lot or a large number of units is to be sampled. Large lots often exceed 10,000 test units (e.g., single-service, nonsterile, leak-proof containers). Table 3.1 shows the relationship between the number of test units and the risk of accepting 5% defective units in a lot. The sampling plan assumes that (*N*) units are tested and that all tests are negative for the defect under consideration.

A sampling plan for *Salmonella* testing demonstrates how the number of samples taken for analysis is used to achieve different levels of safety.[6] In this plan, food is classified in 3 categories:

A. **Food category I:** Foods that would not normally be subjected to a process lethal to *Salmonella* between the time of sampling and consumption are intended for consumption by the aged, the infirm, and infants.

B. **Food category II:** Foods that would not normally be subjected to a process lethal to *Salmonella* between the time of sampling and consumption.

C. **Food category III:** Foods that would normally be subjected to a process lethal to *Salmonella* between the time of sampling and consumption.

Each of these categories requires a different number of samples to be tested per lot. For example, food category I requires 60 samples, food category II requires 30 samples, and food category III requires 15 samples. Based on the food category type, a lot is acceptable only if all samples test negative for *Salmonella*. This plan demonstrates progressive sampling based on the need

Table 3.1. Relationship of Sample Size to the Probability of Accepting a Lot with 5% Defective Units, when (*N*) Test Units are Negative

Test Units From a Lot (*N*)	Probabilities of Accepting a Lot When 5% of the Units are Defective
10	0.61
20	0.37
50	0.08
100	0.01

Note: Table adapted from the International Commission on Microbiological Specifications for Foods.

for increased safety. The probability of accepting a lot contaminated with *Salmonella* decreases as the number of units (*N*) increases. It is assumed that samples are chosen randomly.

Apart from the vulnerabilities of the target population, other considerations may enter into the statement of risk. These may include pathogens or toxins that can use milk or milk products as the vehicle of transmission, the frequency and distribution with which the pathogens or toxins occur, and the severity (including secondary factors) of the disease state they cause.

To reduce the laboratory workload, an alternative to sampling at least 10 units out of a large lot is to composite groups of samples within a lot or series of units. Compositing is acceptable when the microbiological method is capable of detecting a single viable microorganism in the composite sample. The lot is rejected if the microbial limit is exceeded. No retest is allowed.

3.030 Equipment

3.031 *Thermometers*[22–24]

A. **Glass:** Filled with mercury (thermometer encased in Teflon/plastic) or a distinctively colored fluid. Must be checked for accuracy initially and annually thereafter. Graduations must not exceed 1°C (2°F).

B. **Electronic:** Must be checked for accuracy initially and annually thereafter. Recommended for use when glass thermometers are likely to break, for example, with farm bulk tanks and in processing plants. Graduations must not exceed 1°C (2°F).

C. **Dial:** Must be checked for accuracy initially and rechecked every 6 months thereafter as these thermometers tend to lose calibration quickly. May be used when glass thermometers are likely to break, for example, with farm bulk tanks and in processing plants (excluding the laboratory). Graduations must not exceed 1°C (2°F).

D. **Tests for Accuracy:** Tests for accuracy must be made against a thermometer certified by NIST (formerly National Bureau of Standards [NBS]), or a thermometer traceable to an NIST thermometer [chapter 2]. Thermometers must be accurate to within ±1°C (±2°F) (± 1 division/graduation). Do not use thermometers that are not accurate to within ±1°C (±2°F) [e.g., > 1°C (> 2°F)]. Each thermometer must be tagged (for dial thermometers label cases) for identification, the date checked, the temperature at which it was checked, and any correction factor. Thermometers must be checked at or near the temperature(s) of use. Records of thermometer accuracy must be maintained.

3.032 *Sample Transfer Instruments*[12,22,23]

These instruments are typically made of seamless stainless steel or some other suitable material that will not cause any changes to the sample or affect analysis or inspection. Typically sample transfer instruments have smooth surfaces and rounded corners that can not trap sample material. They may be sterile, and should be easily cleanable, sterilizable, or sanitizable. For chemical and physical analysis, the instruments need only be clean and dry.

A. **Sample transfer instruments**

1. Auger.
2. Chisel.
3. Coring tube/bit.
4. Cork borers.
5. Dippers (with long handles silver soldered to the bowl, capacity 10 mL or greater).
6. Forceps.
7. Hatchet.
8. High-speed drill.
9. Knives (with a pointed blade).
10. Scalpel or scissors.
11. Screw cap vials/tubes (sterile).
12. Sediment sampler.
13. Spatulas.
14. Spoons.
15. Strainer.
16. Swabs (sterile).
17. Syringes (sterile with 16-gauge or larger needle, capacity 20 mL or greater).
18. Tongue depressors (sterile).
19. Triers.
20. Tubes (individually wrapped, sterile, single service, or sanitized stainless steel).

3.033 *Sample Containers*[6,12,22,23]

The construction and the materials used the make sample containers and closures must protect the sample from contamination and not alter the sample in a way that affects the analysis. The size and shape of the container must be suitable for the sample taken and, depending on the sample and the analysis to be performed, the container may also need to be opaque (e.g., vitamin analysis).

A. **Multiple-use containers:** Sterile, made of glass or food-grade, sterilizable plastic with nontoxic, leak-proof closures (not made of or containing cork if microbial analysis to be performed).

B. **Single-service containers**

1. Sterile, made of nontoxic food-grade plastic.
2. Nonsterile, made of nontoxic food-grade plastic—for raw milk and cream only—assuming the following conditions are met:

a. Maximum viable microbial counts in rinse tests of 60 containers per lot do not exceed 1 per milliliter of capacity. The lot is accepted only if all containers tested are in compliance. The probability of accepting a lot with 5% defects is less than 0.05 if all 60 containers are in compliance [Table 3.1].
b. Closures are designed so that the container can be easily opened and closed without contaminating the lip of the container or the inner surface of the closure.
c. Government agencies have the authority to inspect and certify manufacturers to ensure the fabrication process and materials are acceptable for single-service containers.
d. One of 2 methods listed below are used to verify that sample containers of a lot do not leak.

C. **Sampling plans to verify that sample containers of a lot do not leak**

1. **Method I:** Select 14 containers at random from the lot of containers to be tested. Fill each container ¾ full with powdered sugar or a color-indicating desiccant that has been dried. Cap the containers, making certain the closure is properly positioned.

   Secure the containers upright in racks using a wire cover or other means. Place the racks into a case containing ice water (0° to 1°C) and a dye or indicator solution and submerge the containers for at least six hours or overnight. Place enough weight on top of the containers to keep them under the solution.

   Remove the racks from the ice water solution and examine the containers for leakage. Using paper towels or other absorbent material, carefully remove the water on the outside of the containers and especially around the rim of the closure to prevent water accidentally entering the containers when opened. Carefully open the containers and inspect their contents for signs of water entry and record the number of containers that leaked. The lot will be accepted if no defective containers are observed.
2. **Method II:** Select 24 containers at random from the lot of containers to be tested. Fill each container ¾ full with raw milk. Cap the containers, making certain the closure is firmly and completely positioned.

   Invert containers in racks and refrigerate (0° to 4.4°C) for at least 15 hours. Transfer inverted containers to an incubator and warm the containers and their contents to 40°C. If any containers leak, the lot is rejected. If no containers leak, return them to an upright position and shake 25 times in 7 seconds with a 30-cm movement. If no containers leak, the lot is accepted.
3. **Results:** Results of all tests conducted on each lot must accompany that lot when marketed.
4. **Defects:** When frequencies of testing are 14 containers (Method I) or 24 containers (Method II) and the number of units in the lot is large (i.e., $N = 10{,}000$), there is 1 chance in 20 that a lot will be accepted with more than 21.4% or 12.5% defects, respectively. Conversely, the probability of accepting lots with more than 21.4% defects (Method I) or 12.5% defects (Method II) is less than 0.05.

3.034 *Sample Case*[12,22,23]

A. **Construction:** The sample case must be constructed of rigid metal or opaque plastic, be corrosion resistant and insulated, and have a tight cover. The case must not affect or alter the samples and must be capable of withstanding expected conditions to which it may be exposed. Cases may need to be lockable if they contain legally sensitive samples.

B. **Space:** Ample space must exist for ice or other refrigerants to maintain samples at the required temperature. The case should not be adversely affected by the refrigerant.

C. **Testing:** The case should be tested for suitability under the conditions that it will be exposed. The case should be able to maintain samples in the required temperature range for the time period the samples will normally be held. Procedures for testing cases are described in IDF Standard 50C:1995.[12]

D. **Cooling mechanism:** When a mixture of ice and water is used, the case must provide racks, compartments, or baffles to 1) hold the sample containers vertically, 2) keep the tops of the containers above the surface of the cooling medium at *all* times, and 3) maintain the cooling medium at a level slightly above that of the liquid in the sample containers.

E. **Moisture:** To protect samples from moisture, sample containers may be placed in a moisture-proof metal box or can or in a sealed plastic bag.

3.035 *Shipping Cases*[22,23]

A. **Primary case:** When samples are transferred to a laboratory from a receiving station, plant, or other point of collection via a common carrier, the outer shipping case must be provided with a tamper-evident sealing and locking device (for regulatory use) and handles. Attach a "This Side Up" label on the top of the shipping case.

B. **Secondary case:** When an inner shipping case is needed to protect samples, provide boxes just large enough to hold containers upright and to prevent container breakage when the box is placed in a larger shipping case. Boxes must have tightly fitted covers.

3.036 *Agitators*[12]

A. **Mechanical agitators:** The 3-A Sanitary Standards[8-10] specify types of equipment or mechanical agitators acceptable for use in bulk milk operations, weigh tanks, vats, and storage tanks. Air systems used for agitation must comply with the applicable 3-A Sanitary Standards for odor-free, oil-free, filtered air.[12]

The following methods may be used to agitate milk in tankers or storage tanks:

1. A mechanical agitator built into the tank. Based on the construction of the tank and product, the mechanical agitator must be adequate to mix the mass in the tank. Agitators must have sufficient surface area to adequately mix the tank contents.
2. A propeller or agitator placed through the manhole with the agitator suspended in the milk. Ideally the propeller should reach to about ¾ the depth of the tank fill height with the stirrer angled at about 5° to 20° or as allowed by the tank design.

3. An oil-free, filtered, 3-A quality air supply injected through a quick coupling device on the rear of the tanker or through a sanitary air hose inserted through the manhole of the tanker.
4. An approved sanitary tank washer or air agitator system, permanently installed in the tank, through which 3-A quality air enters and agitates the milk. This method of agitation is not recommended unless an approved clean-in-place (CIP) system [3.084] has been installed.
5. The milk transfer hose, which, when attached both to the tanker unloading pump and to the manhole, permits recirculation and mixing of the milk.

B. **Manual agitators**[12,22,23]
1. Stainless steel scoop or plunger (about 15 cm or 6 inches in diameter) on the end of a stainless steel rod long enough to reach the bottom of the container.
2. Bowl-type agitator-sampler consisting of a stainless steel handle welded to the outside of the bowl with a pouring spout (silver soldering of the handle to bowl is acceptable).

3.037 *Cleaning, Sanitizing, and Sterilizing Equipment*

A. **Cleaning:** All multiple-use equipment must be cleaned with a suitable dairy cleaner and rinsed thoroughly before sanitization or sterilization.

B. **Sanitizing**[20]
1. **Hot water sanitization:** Use 2 stainless steel containers of approximately 40-L or 10.5-gal. capacity (or 2 37.85-L (10-gal.) milk cans in good condition) equipped with threaded fittings to provide metal inlets for steam and water connections. Do not substitute rubber hose. The first container is for a cold-water rinse of the agitator and sampling instruments. The second container, with a bottom inlet for steam under pressure, is for hot-water treatment (not less than 82°C or 180°F) of instruments. Equip the second container with a thermometer immersed in the water. Minimal exposure time at 82°C is 1 minute. Use equipment immediately after treatment. Minimize the risk of burns and excessive noise by installing a steam coil with a condensate trap on the exhaust side.

   To ensure against possible back-siphonage into potable water lines, the cold-water lines should terminate not less than 2.54 cm (1 inch) above the lip of the can or be equipped with an approved anti-siphon device.
2. **Chemical sanitation:** Use 2 containers as above. In the second container, however, replace the hot water with a solution of an approved germicide that is at all times bactericidally equivalent to 200 mg/L (200 ppm) or more of available chlorine as hypochlorite. Submerge sampling equipment for at least 1 minute in the chemical sanitize. Dry and use equipment immediately after treatment. Sampling dippers carried on bulk-tank milk trucks should be stored in a tightly stoppered tube-type container of sanitizer solution.[20,22,23]

   Other chemical sanitizers, such as some quaternary ammonium compounds at 200 ppm (depending on the quality of the water used), iodine compounds at 25 ppm, and some detergent sanitizers, may also be effective to sanitize equipment.[20]

Check sanitizer strength regularly for potency.[22,23]

3. **Sterilizing**[4,6,12,24]
   a. **Hot-air sterilizing:** Glassware and metal equipment may be sterilized by holding at a temperature not lower than 170°C for not less than 2 hours. Instruments may be stored under proper conditions after treatment for later use [chapter 4].
   b. **Autoclave (steam) sterilization:** Glassware, metal, and some plastic equipment may be steam sterilized by holding at 120° ± 1°C for not less than 20 minutes. Equipment must be dry before use. Instruments may be stored under proper conditions after treatment for later use [chapter 4].
   c. **Other:** In addition to the above methods, especially if the above are not possible, other methods exist for treatment of equipment. Not all are suitable for all situations and they do not guarantee sterility. In each of the following treatments, use equipment immediately after treatment. These methods include flaming (allow to cool before use), immersion in 70% (v/v) ethanol, and a combination of dipping in 96% (v/v) ethanol then flaming or exposure to 100°C steam for 1 hour. Commercial, single-use items may also be sterilized using γ-irradiation or ethylene oxide treatments (may be stored in original, unopened packages until needed; once opened, use immediately).

Consideration should be given to ensure the sanitizing or sterilization method(s) used does not affect the analysis of the samples. For microbial and organoleptic analyses hot air, autoclaved, or commercially sterilized instruments are best.[4,12]

3.038 *Sanitizing Sampling Cocks and In-Line Sampling Points*

A. **Sampling cocks:** Prepare a sanitizing solution containing 200 mg/L (200 ppm) of available chlorine such as hypochlorite, or another equivalent strength sanitizer (see Section 3.037.B2). Submerge the sampling cock by fitting a bag of the sanitizer solution over and around it. While holding the tip of the bag of sanitizing solution tightly around the body of the sampling valve, flush the sanitizer in and out of the sampling cock for at least 1 minute. Prepare an adequately sized sanitized container to catch the flush milk. Then purge the sampling cock valve with at least 2 liters (≈ half gal.) of milk, which may be caught in a sanitized container and retained for reprocessing when handled aseptically.

B. **In-line points:** Swab the gasket or rubber sampling nipple with 200 ppm of available chlorine solution or equivalent and expose the area for 1 minute before wiping away excess sanitizer with a clean, single-service towel.

3.040 General Requirements

3.041 *Records*[12,22-24]

A. **Acceptable information:** The following information should accompany all samples to a laboratory:

1. Date and time samples were collected. This refers to when a sample is originally collected. There are situations when samples may be delivered to an intermediate location. When a sample collector picks up samples from an intermediate location this does not constitute the date and time when the samples were collected.
2. Product(s) sampled.
3. Temperature of product(s) sampled.
4. Location sampling took place.
5. Number of samples in group.
6. Name of person who took the sample or identifier.
7. Interim transfer point: Date, time, and temperature of each temperature control when sample was received or shipped.
8. Additional information may be required for regulatory purposes.[12,24]

B. **Sample submission form:** A sample submission form (also may be called a sample report or sample collection report) is essential in the sampling process. All information necessary to identify and to ensure all requirements have been met must be captured so that the final sample analysis report will be complete. Some information may be recorded directly on the sample container.

3.042 *Agitation*[12,22,23]

Collection of representative samples requires proper agitation of the milk, especially when the milk is held in bulk storage tanks and transportation tanks. With inadequate agitation of bulk tank milk (i.e., milk from farm tanks, tank trucks, or plant storage tanks), samples taken from the top of the tank contain more bacteria, somatic cells, and milkfat than samples taken lower in the tank.[2] Rising fat globules "sweep" microorganisms and somatic cells toward the surface, thus concentrating them in the cream layer.

A mass that has been quiescent for a period of time will require longer agitation (the time varies with product, temperature, and tank design) to completely mix the mass to give a representative sample. Also, tanks that are completely filled may require more agitation.

A. **Farm bulk tanks:** Agitate milk stored in a farm holding, cooling tank for at least 5 minutes immediately prior to sampling if the tank has been filled within 30 minutes of collection of the sample. Agitate contents of tanks of more than 3,800 liters (1,000 gallons) for at least 10 minutes, or as specified by the tank manufacturer.[9] Tanks that have been standing for more than 30 minutes after filling need to be agitated for at least 15 minutes before they are sampled.

B. **Mobile tank trucks** *(farm pickup and over-the-road tankers)* **and dairy plant storage tanks:** Time required to agitate a tank of milk until homogeneous is determined by the size and shape of the tank; volume and type of the product held; type, location, and number of agitators on the tank; force of the agitator; and time allowed for creaming before starting agitation. For each individual tank, it is necessary to determine how much agitation time is needed to ensure homogeneity of its contents. Pronounced creaming requires mechanical agitation.

Agitation time for milk storage tanks and milk tank trucks may be determined by taking a series of milkfat samples at specified intervals (e.g., every 3 to 5 minutes) during mixing until at least 5 milkfat tests stabilize at a definite value. From a full tank, when possible, take samples from the top and bottom and from points near and far from the source of agitation. Where the construction of a tank does not permit direct removal of subsamples, draw samples through an outlet valve or sampling cock while the agitator is running (purge at least 2 L of milk through the valve before taking the sample. [3.050]).

Adequate agitation[9,12] is that degree of agitation that, in a full tank, will result in the milkfat content of the product in the tank varying by not more than 2 standard deviations from the mean. For example, if the mean is 3.5%, differences between tests of individual samples should not vary by more than 0.08% (based on estimates of the reproducibility standard deviation [SR] in chapter 1).

When the appropriate time of agitation has been determined for each stationary and mobile tank, record and use it for proper agitation time for samples from that specific tank.

C. **Milk cans and weigh tanks:** Agitate milk in cans for at least 7 seconds, with at least 7 pulls stirring from the bottom up.

3.043 *Cooling*

Cool and maintain samples at 0° to 4.4°C by immediately placing the samples into ice or in with another refrigerant capable of holding this temperature. For rapid cooling, place the samples into an ice-and-water mixture; however, avoid completely submerging the samples below the ice-and-water mixture to prevent possible contamination. An ice-and-water mixture cools samples more quickly than ice alone. Do not freeze refrigerated samples or allow them to freeze, as this affects the microbial content and may also affect the chemical and physical characteristics of the samples.

3.044 *Temperature Control*

A temperature control sample must be collected at 1) the first sampling point on each farm route, 2) each sampling point for raw milk in dairy plants, 3) each over-the-road tanker (by sampling through the dome immediately after filling), and 4) each location pasteurized products are sampled. The size of the temperature control, in most cases, should be the same size as the largest sample, but in no case less than half the size of the largest sample collected. For example, a half-gallon or gallon could be used when gallon samples are collected.

3.045 *Storage and Transportation*[12,22,23]

The condition of the samples at collection must not be significantly altered by storage or transportation. Time and temperature must be considered together. It is important to get the samples to the laboratory as quickly as possible, preferably in less than 24 hours.

A. **Refrigerated samples**

1. Use ice or some other refrigerant at all times to cool and hold samples

at 0° to 4.4°C. Keep the ice level in the sample case and slightly above the level of the milk in the sample containers, but below the top of the containers. Maintaining the samples so that the level of the milk stays below the ice level but the tops of the containers are above the ice is difficult, especially on samples that are shipped and not hand delivered to laboratories. It is recommended that samples be placed in waterproof bags so that the samples can be submerged in the ice without concern for contamination from the ice. Do not freeze fluid samples before or during shipment to the laboratory. The laboratory may not test milk for bacteria, antibiotics, or somatic cells if the sample(s) are received frozen. Do not rely on winter air temperatures to keep samples cold. Ice water is necessary to prevent freezing of samples in very cold weather and to prevent warming of samples in warm weather.

2. Protect samples from contamination. Contamination by ice water in the sample case may be prevented by using racks, compartments, sealed plastic bags, or other means. Ice water is to be only slightly higher than the level of milk in the sample containers. Do not bury the tops on container in ice unless samples are in a sealed plastic bag. Laboratories may refuse to officially analyze samples that are received submerged in ice water unless they are protected by a sealed plastic bag.
3. Promptly deliver all samples to the laboratory. Tests for somatic cells (nonpreserved samples) by the direct microscopic cell count (DMSCC) method and microbiological counts in all samples must begin within 48 hours of initial collection (not from pickup at a transfer location). Initial analysis of milk for antibiotics and drugs should also begin within 48 hours. Analysis of samples for electronic somatic cell counts (not direct somatic cell counts) must begin within 72 hours.
4. Ensure that samples shipped to a laboratory by a common carrier are packed in a shipping case with a tamper-evident seal. The case must have a "This Side Up" label on top. Ensure samples are protected, preferably in a sealed plastic bag so they arrive without being contaminated by the refrigerant or case.

B. **Frozen samples:** Use an appropriate refrigerant, preferably dry ice, to maintain samples in a frozen state (preferably –18°C or 0°F if not colder)[12] until they are delivered to the laboratory. Maintain semi-frozen products (mixes, soft serves, etc.) as described above. These samples must be promptly delivered to the laboratory.

C. **Dry samples:** These samples may be shipped without refrigeration; however, they should be protected from moisture and temperature extremes.

3.046 *Preservatives*[3,4,12]

Preservatives may be added to some samples, but they may not be used when they may interfere with the analysis to be performed, or if the samples are going to undergo sensory evaluation. Preservatives may not be used in any samples collected for microbiological analysis when the test involves microbial growth. After samples are received in a laboratory, and after microbiological testing has been initiated, they may be preserved (e.g., to extend time to allow electronic somatic cell counting [ESCC] at another laboratory). If preservatives are added prior to submission to a laboratory, the laboratory must be informed and the use of the preservative noted on the sample submission form.

A. **Formaldehyde:** 40% by volume, 36% by weight. Add 0.1 mL to each 30 mL of sample. Use this preservative *only* in samples tested for fat by chemical methods.[16]

B. **2-bromo-2-nitropropane-1, 3-diol (Bronopol®):** Use 1 tablet (containing 10 mg of active ingredient) or 0.05 mL (containing 20% active ingredient) per 50-mL sample. Samples must be transported and stored at 0° to 4.4°C.

Whereas the pure preservative does not interfere in analyses with infrared instruments, impurities or carrier materials may cause interference. Therefore, Bronopol® or similar products should be tested for absorption at the wavelengths used in the infrared testing being performed in the laboratory [chapter 15]. Samples should be tested for fat within 5 days of preservation and within 7 days for electronic somatic cell count (ESCC) methods only.

3.050 Sampling Raw Milk

3.051 *Precautions*[2,4,12,22,23]

1. Protect sampling instruments from exposure to contamination before and during use.
2. When using a dipper, remove it from the sanitizing solution, drain it completely, and rinse it at least twice in milk before transferring the sample.
3. Handle sample containers and caps aseptically. Do not drop, lay down, touch the inside of, or otherwise contaminate the containers or caps. If the container becomes contaminated or is suspect, discard it and use another.
4. Do not carry presterilized plastic bags or containers in pockets of clothing. Clipboards, covered containers, or boxes may be used carry empty single-service containers.
5. Precool multi-use sterile containers in the sample case as needed. If moisture is present, rinse containers with milk twice before filling with the portion to be tested.
6. Typically a single, universal sample is taken that will be analyzed for all components. If there is a need to collect separate microbiological, somatic cell and/or chemical samples, the microbiological sample must be taken first using aseptic technique. If separate samples are taken, they must be from the same source at the same time. Regulations often govern how samples may be taken and the handling of those samples.

3.052 *Farm Bulk Tanks*[23]

A. **Prepare to measure and sample:** Sanitize the outlet valve, connect milk transfer hose, connect power supply, wash and dry hands, and observe milk for any abnormality. If an abnormality is present, record on the report form and cease sampling.

B. **Measure milk**[23]

1. If the measuring stick is in the tank, dry the stick at milk level with a clean single-service paper towel, make the measurement, and record the result.
2. If the measuring stick is outside the tank, sanitize the stick with chemical sanitizer and dry it at the milk level with a clean single-service paper towel. Then make the measurement and record the result.

C. **Agitate milk adequately:** Agitate tank as specified in section 3.042.

D. **Check the temperature of the milk**[23]

1. Use a sanitized, standardized thermometer and record the result on the sample form.
2. Compare the accuracy of the bulk tank thermometer with the test thermometer monthly and record results [3.031].

E. **Collect sample by hand**[23]

1 Rinse dipper 2 times in the milk. Dip at least 15 to 20 cm (6 to 8 inches) to obtain a representative sample.
2. Do not hold the sample container over the milk while transferring the sample.
3. Fill sample containers not more than ¾ full (after closure) to permit proper mixing of the sample at the laboratory. Laboratories should not receive or test milk if sample containers are too full. Do not expel all the air when folding or "whirling" plastic bags. Leave ¼ of the volume of the bag as air space after the bag is closed and sealed.
4. Collect a 100-mL (3.4-oz.) representative sample from each producer's total milk supply. Sample all tanks individually and label each sample, including identifying each tank. If there is more than 1 bulk milk tank or split tanks on a farm, sample all tanks individually so the collector will have the same number of samples as tanks. These samples should not be composited. Submit the samples from multiple bulk tanks for separate analysis and reporting.
5. Provide a temperature control by collecting 2 samples at the first collection point (one sample to be used as the temperature control [TC], labeled as TC with time, date, temperature, and location identification).
6. Place the samples immediately in a sample case with a mixture of ice and water, or other refrigerant, to maintain 0° to 4.4°C and protect the sample from becoming submerged in water (unless inside a seal plastic bag).
7. Rinse the dipper in tap water immediately after use and return it to the sanitizing solution.
8. Prepare the sample report as outlined in section 3.041.
9. Transport the samples and sample data to the laboratory so that analysis may begin within 48 hours of collection. Ideally, the laboratory should receive samples within 24 hours of collection.

D. **Collect samples for compositional analysis with an automated sampler:** *Principle:* An automated device for sampling from bulk tanks is mounted on the intake line of the tank truck, preferably on the suction side. An electronically controlled peristaltic pump operates during the pumping cycle, removing a representative sample based on information set into the controller by the operator. This information consists of desired sample volume, volume of milk in the tank (in pounds), and speed of the truck's pump. Readers are referred to manufacturer's instructions for details and use.

3.053 *Milk Cans and Weigh Tanks*

A. **Agitate milk adequately:** See section 3.042.

B. **Check temperature of milk:** Use sanitized thermometer and record the result on a sampling form.

C. **Collect sample**

1. Hold the sample container away from the can or tank opening while filling.
2. Fill the sample immediately after the cans are emptied into the weigh tank. If the tank is not large enough for the producer's total volume of milk, collect proportionate amounts of milk from each filling into a single sample container.
3. Collect a temperature control.
4. Place the samples immediately into a mixture of ice and water and protect them from contamination.
5. Prepare sample report as outlined in section 3.041.
6. Transport the samples and sample data to the laboratory so that analysis may begin within 48 hours of collection. Ideally, the laboratory should receive samples within 24 hours of collection.

3.054 *Mobile Tank Trucks (Farm Pickup and Over-the-Road Tankers)*[23]

A. **Agitate the milk adequately:** See section 3.042.

B. **Check the temperature of the milk:** If milk is taken at location with a laboratory and the samples are taken directly to the laboratory and tested immediately (within 15 minutes), then the tank truck milk temperature serves as the laboratory receipt temperature. If the samples are going to be transported to another location, or if the samples will not be tested immediately, then a temperature control must be taken along with the samples.

C. **Collect the sample**

1. Collect a single sample from the farm pickup tanker. If tank is split, collect a separate sample from each compartment.
2. Collect duplicate samples from over-the-road tankers. The first sample is for the shipper; the second accompanies the tanker to its final destination. Collect two temperature controls, one each to accompany the two over-the-road tanker samples.
3. Place samples in a sample case with ice and immediately transfer to the laboratory.

3.055 *Dairy Plants*[22]

A. **Agitate the milk adequately:** Do not use hand agitators if tanks are large. Use an appropriate method to mix the tank. See section 3.042.

B. **Check the temperature of the milk.**

C. **Supply a temperature control:** Supply a temperature control from the first sampling location, label it as TC and with time, date, temperature, and location identification.

D. **Collect tank samples**

1. If used, sanitize the sampling cock. Use of sampling cocks may not give a representative microbiological sample, even after mixing.[12] The preferred method is to take the sample through a manhole.[22] If the sample must be taken using a sampling cock, discharge 2 liters of milk to flush the cock before taking the sample.
2. Sample the tanks individually, and collect a temperature control from each. If separate microbiological and chemical samples are taken, take microbiological samples first using aseptic technique. Label sample containers.
3. Place the samples in a sample case with ice, protect from contamination, and immediately transfer to the laboratory with sample data. Do not carry samples in-hand to the laboratory.

E. **Collect in-line samples**[22]

1. Sanitize the entry point.
2. Insert the needle of the syringe through the pipeline gasket or the closure of a stainless steel nipple clamped onto the line.
3. Transfer the sample from the syringe to a sample container. If separate microbiological and chemical samples are taken, take microbiological sample first using aseptic technique. Label sample containers.
4. Place the sample in a sample case with ice, protect from contamination and immediately transfer to the laboratory with sample data.

F. **Collect other commingled milk samples:** These samples may be collected from the weigh tank or the balance tank in the same manner.

3.056 *Milk Directly from the Udder (Cow Sample)*

1. Collect sample immediately before regular milking, working in a protected area.
2. Remove loose soil from the animals, and then wash the udder, especially under the teats, before allowing cows to enter the sample collection area.
3. Sanitize the teats and adjacent udder with warm disinfectant (e.g., 25 mg/L of iodophor).
4. Dry with clean, single-service towels.
5. Disinfect teat canal ends by opening the canal with finger pressure and swabbing with 70% alcohol. Alternatively, dip the teats in an iodophor teat dip, wait 10 seconds, and swab off excess with a cotton ball. Treat teats farthest from collector first.
6. Collect samples from the closest teats, removing 2 streams of milk into a separate vessel before collecting samples into sterile containers. Then collect samples from the farthest teats in the same way. Label sample containers.
7. Place the samples immediately in a sample case with ice and protect from contamination.

8. Deliver the samples and sample data to the laboratory within 12 hours. Cow samples typically are analyzed to provide information to a dairy farmer and/or veterinarian, usually to determine if a cow has mastitis or to determine if a cow treated with antibiotics has cleared. Caution is advised as cow samples may give unreliable results.

3.057 *Sediment Sampling*

A. **Mixed sample method:** For 18.92- to 37.85-L (5- to 10-gal.) cans and bulk storage tanks, a 500-mL, 120-mL, 60-mL, or 30-mL sample will be needed, depending on the diameter of the filter disc being used. Before mixing the sample, take a small strainer and transfer any floating or extraneous contaminants such as flies, hair, or debris to a separate disc and properly identify. Agitate contents of bulk storage tanks for at least 5 minutes, or according to manufacturer's recommendation, before removing test portions. Avoid contaminating the samples with foreign matter.

B. **Off-bottom method:** For 18.92- to 37.85-L cans, take a 500-mL sample with an off-bottom tester from an unstirred can of milk. Before withdrawing the sample, remove any floating or extraneous matter with a small strainer as directed above.

3.060 Sampling Pasteurized Products

3.061 *In-Line Samples*

Collect as stipulated in section 3.055 above.

3.062 *Packaged Retail Fluid Products*[4,12,22]

Randomly select representative samples of all products to be tested. On the form submitted to the laboratory, include the processing date (or the code date in the case of store-purchased samples). The reason for taking the sample is to determine where the sample came from and the age of the product taken.

When it is not practical to collect individual packages of a product (e.g., products packaged in large commercial packages), adequately mix the milk or milk product and aseptically transfer at least 100 mL of a representative sample to a sterile sample container.

Collect a temperature control. The TC must be at least half the size of the largest sample collected (e.g., if gallon size samples collected, TC must be ½ gallon or larger).

Identify the samples and immediately place them in a sample case with ice to maintain 0° to 4.4°C, protected from contamination (tops above refrigerant, or enclosed in leak-proof plastic bags, especially if being shipped), and deliver them to the laboratory with the sample data within 48 hours, preferably less.

3.063 *Dispenser Milk*

1. Collect a sample from the dispenser tube of a previously unopened container and place in a sample container without first flushing the milk through the tube. To determine the status of an in-use dispenser, collect a sample after drawing off about 500 mL of milk.

2. Collect a temperature control.
3. Identify the samples and immediately place them in a sample case with ice. Protect them from contamination and deliver them to the laboratory with the sample data within 48 hours, preferably less.

3.064 *Individual Coffee Creamers*

Because a single container usually provides an insufficient quantity for analytical procedures, randomly select 10 containers to satisfy testing requirements and to be representative of a lot. Containers should be delivered unopened to the laboratory (i.e., not combined in the field).

A. **Pasteurized and ultrapasteurized creamers:** Note codes, date, or lot numbers on the laboratory worksheet. Place containers in a plastic bag, seal the bag, and place it in the sample case with ice.

B. **Dried creamers:** Place packages of the dried product in a bag or box to avoid contamination and contact with moisture. Do not carry them in clothing. Hold and transport the samples at room temperature.

C. **Frozen creamers:** Follow general sampling procedures for ice cream [3.076]. Place the samples in a plastic bag or container to avoid contamination, and keep frozen (–18°C [0°F] or below) until analyzed. Frozen creamers are typically shipped with dry ice.

3.065 *Pressurized Containers*

A. **Retail containers**
   1. Select the necessary number of containers at random.
   2. Identify the samples and immediately place them in a sample case with ice, protect from contamination, and deliver to the laboratory with sample data.

B. **Commercial containers**
   1. Select the necessary number of containers at random.
   2. Mix the containers by inverting them 25 times, or thoroughly agitate for 30 seconds.
   3. Aseptically dispense a minimum of 100 mL of the contents of the containers into sample containers.
   4. Identify the samples and immediately place them in a sample case with ice, protect from contamination, and deliver to the laboratory with sample data.

3.066 *Closed Systems*[12]

When taking samples from a closed system (e.g., UHT system), the sample is taken using built-in sampling equipment. Use aseptic technique and take sample as specified by the manufacturer of the equipment.

3.070 Sampling Other Products

3.071 *Evaporated, Concentrated, and Condensed Milk*[4,12]

A. **Hermetically sealed retail containers**
   1. Select the required number of containers containing ≥100 g (3.4 oz.) at random.
   2. Identify all samples and transport unrefrigerated to the laboratory along with sample data.

B. **Bulk-tank and industrial-size containers**

1. Agitate the product in the container. Bulk tanks of concentrated product are difficult to mix and require longer agitation to become properly mixed. These products may require specially designed tanks and agitators or stirrers (with at least one edge conforming to the shape of the tank) to be adequately mixed. If it is too difficult to mix, it may be necessary to take several small samples and composite a representative sample. Also, it may be necessary to heat the product to 45°C for 30 minutes in order to adequately mix.
2. Aseptically transfer a representative portion (not less than 100 g) to a sterile sample container. Leave sufficient head space (about ¾ full) to allow proper mixing in the laboratory.
3. Identify the samples and immediately place them in a sample case with ice, protect from contamination, and deliver to the laboratory with sample data.

3.072 *Dry products*[4,12]

A. **Precautions**

1. Because dry products absorb moisture rapidly, make transfers quickly after opening the container to be sampled and seal the container immediately after sampling is completed.
2. If it is necessary to collect separate samples for microbiological and other analysis, aseptically collect the microbiological sample first. All samples must be collected from the same source and at the same time.
3. Place the sample into a clean and dry sample container that can be sealed air tight. Depending on the analysis, the sample container may also need to be opaque.[12]
4. Transport all dry samples to the laboratory unrefrigerated and protected from moisture.

B. **Retail containers**

1. When possible, collect intact containers (≥100 g).
2. If it is necessary to sample from large commercial containers, transfer 100 g or more of the product to a sterile, dry container with a dry, sterile spoon or spatula.
3. Label the samples and transfer them to the laboratory with sample data unrefrigerated and protected from moisture.

C. **Bulk containers**

1. With a dry, sterile tube or trier, aseptically transfer at least three plugs or columns from each container to a dry, sterile sample container. The total amount of sample transferred must be at least 100 g.
2. Label the samples and transfer them to the laboratory with sample data unrefrigerated and protected from moisture.

D. **Stitched bags**

1. Open bags carefully, avoiding contamination of the contents.
2. Use a dry, sterile tube, trier, spoon, or spatula, and aseptically transfer 100 g or more of the product to a dry, sterile sample container.
3. Label the samples and transfer them to the laboratory with sample data unrefrigerated and protected from moisture.

4. Reseal the bag to maintain product integrity.

3.073 *Butter, Margarine, and Related Products*[4,12]

Although butter is specifically mentioned in the following sections, the procedures also apply to margarine and other related products.

A. **Special equipment**

1. **Butter trier, sanitized:** Under commercial conditions, when numerous samples must be taken daily, a single, polished, stainless steel trier may be used for each sample if it is wiped thoroughly after each sample with clean tissue paper, dipped in 70% alcohol, ignited to remove excess alcohol, and tempered by being inserted twice into the butter to be sampled before the sample is removed. For composition or chemical examination, clean and dry the trier between each sample.
2. Sample jars or containers (preferably opaque), sterilized, size 240 mL (8 oz.) or larger.

B. **Procedure**

1. **Butter from churns:** Using a sanitized, stainless steel trier, remove three 120-g (4-oz.) portions of finished butter from the center and end locations of a batch of butter or from successive sampling points in the stream of butter from continuous churns. Identify the samples and immediately place them in a sample case with ice, protected from contamination, and transfer to a laboratory with sample data.
2. **Butter in boxes or bulk packages:** Remove at least 120 g of butter from 3 different corners of the container by inserting a stainless steel trier diagonally through the butter. Take plugs at least 75 mm (3 in.) long, including surface portions. With a sanitized spatula or spoon, transfer butter to a sterile sample container. Use a small portion of the sample to plug-seal the hole from which the plug was removed. (Note: A sample from the corner of the butter box, which includes the outside surface on three sides, is more effective for detecting surface mold contamination than a subsurface sample.) Identify the samples and immediately place them in a sample case with ice, protected from contamination, and transfer to a laboratory with sample data.
3. **Print butter:** Because of differences in the ratio between the surface area and weights of 113.5-g (4-oz.), 227-g (8-oz.), and 454-g (16-oz.) prints, it is preferable to remove samples from the print with a stainless steel trier to ensure uniformity in surface area per sample. Use a No. 8 sanitized cheese trier to take at least a 75-mm plug (about 120 g) from the end of the print and, with a sanitized spatula or spoon, transfer the plug (including surface portion) to the sample container. To sample a 113.5-g print, send the entire print to the laboratory. Identify the samples and immediately place them in a sample case with ice, protected from contamination, and transfer to a laboratory with sample data.

3.074 *Cottage Cheese and Similar Cultured Products*

1. Collect unopened containers (≥100 g) unless container size makes this impractical.

2. When collecting unopened containers is not practical, mix product and remove sample. If mixing is not practical, take representative subsamples and combine. Aseptically transfer 100 g or more of the product with a sterile instrument to a sample container.
3. Identify the samples and place them in a sample case with ice, protected from contamination.
4. To determine processing conditions in the manufacturing plant, the samples must be analyzed for *coliform* content within 24 hours of manufacture. In this case, the transport of the samples and sample data to the analyzing laboratory must be expedited.

3.075 *Cheese and Cheese Products*[4,12]

As these products are mostly sampled for compositional measurements, the sample container should be just large enough to hold the sample as to minimize compositional changes due to moisture migration.

A. **Small cheeses and retail packaged cheeses** *(≥100 g)***:** Collect the entire cheese or package of cheese.

B. **Blocks:** Using a stainless steel knife, make 2 cuts parallel to the sides, removing a piece of at least 100 g after discarding the surface layer.

C. **Large blocks** *(up to 640 lb.)***:** The sampling method depends on the cheese and the method of production. When possible, use a short stainless steel trier, wipe the surface of the block with 70% undenatured ethanol,[12] and take a 5- to 10-cm (2- to 4-inch) sample plug from the end of the block. Take a second from the center, and a third from halfway between the first and the second. Break off 2 to 2.5 cm from the outside edge of each plug, return it to the plug hole, and seal the plug hole over with a suitable sealing compound (e.g., a mixture of molten paraffin, beeswax, and white petrolatum [1:1:2], or one of white petrolatum and paraffin [1:1]). The remainder of the plug constitutes the sample.

Where only 1 plug can be taken, insert a long trier through a side-center sample hole and carefully withdraw the full plug. Break off 2 to 2.5 cm from the outer edge of the plug, return it to the plug hole, and seal as above. The remainder of the plug constitutes the sample.

D. **Barrel cheese**[1]

1. In a barrel container, the mass of cheese (225 to 250 kg, 500 to 550 lb.) cools slowly from the outside toward the center. By the time cooling is complete, a moisture pattern in the cheese is fixed with the highest moisture on the outside the lowest in the center, and the average somewhere in between.
2. The sampling procedure resulting from this study indicates that a trier with a 30.5-cm (12-inch) blade length should be inserted 7 cm (2.8 inches) from the edge of the cheese (near the periphery of the barrel), sloping toward the nearest outside edge of the barrel at a 11° angle from vertical. A trier guide fixed at the 11° angle is available and may be used as an aid. (For information on the guide, contact the National Cheese Institute [NCI], 1250 H Street, NW, Washington, DC 20005).
3. If the cheese barrel is full (that is, if there is no more than 2- to 3-cm headspace) it may be possible to draw a reliable sample through a

bung or sample port in the cover, which permits insertion of the trier at the 7-cm point. If the headspace is more than 3 cm, the cover should be removed. Otherwise, the point of the trier insertion will be distorted. In no instance should a barrel containing cheese from more than 1 vat be selected as a sample for moisture analysis.

4. For sample reliability, it is desirable that the trier be inserted to draw a full 27.9- to 30.5-cm (11- to 12-inch) plug from a full container. If a plug breaks short of 25.5 cm (10 inches), draw another plug from a different location 7 cm from the edge.
5. From a plug 25.5 to 30.5 cm long, remove the top 11.4 cm (4.5 inches) for sealing the plug hole.
6. Transfer the next 10.2-cm (4-inch) portion to the sample container. The remaining, bottom portion of the plug should be discarded.

E. **Crumbled, grated, dehydrated cheeses:** These types of cheeses are sampled by transferring at least 5 portions from a single lot of cheese to the sample container. Total amount transferred should not be less than 100 g.

F. **Surface samples:** Surface layers of cheese should be sampled only as required to establish the presence or absence of surface contamination, or to fulfill other special purposes. Therefore, specific sampling requirements depend on the analysis to be undertaken and should thus be determined in consultation with the analyzing laboratory.

3.076 *Ice Cream and Related Frozen and Semifrozen Products and Ingredients*[4,12]

A. **Shipment and storage:** Frozen product samples must be kept frozen (–18°C [–0°F] or below) during sampling and shipment to the analyzing laboratory. Dry ice is the refrigerant of choice. Samples of semifrozen products (mix, soft-serve) should be maintained at 0° to 4.4°C during sampling and shipment. Semifrozen samples must arrive at the laboratory so that microbiological analyses can begin within 48 hours of original collection. Samples of dry material may be transported without refrigeration. All samples must be sent to laboratories with sample data.

B. **Frozen products**

1. **Packaged:** Collect and submit samples in original, unopened containers (≥100 g).
2. **Bulk:** Aseptically transfer representative portions of at least 100 g to sterile sample containers for microbiological examination. If the bulk container has been opened previously, use sterile instruments to remove the surface portion to a depth of 2 cm around the area from which the sample is to be taken. With a second sterile instrument, aseptically transfer at least 100 g from the newly exposed surface to the sample container.

   If the object is to determine the care used by the retailer in vending operations, sample surface portions to a depth of 1 cm, collecting not less than 100 g. Sample individual servings of frozen dairy products as dipped by the retailer by taking representative portions of at least 100 g with a service dipper or other dispensing device, and treat such samples as regular bulk samples. If high bacterial counts have been previously observed on samples from the retailer's cabinet, take additional samples from unopened packages to determine whether responsibility for the high counts rests with the supplier or the retailer.

C. **Process samples:** When a particular part of the processing operation is being evaluated, take samples of unfrozen or partially frozen mixes either by passing a sterile sample container or dipper under properly sanitized orifices at certain intervals or by withdrawing samples with sterilized sampling instruments. Thoroughly agitate the contents of cans or vats before aseptically removing 100 g portions to sterile containers.

D. **Coloring and flavoring materials:** Mix individual solutions of coloring materials, extracts, flavors, etc., until they are homogeneous, and pour them directly and aseptically into a sample container; or transfer with a sterile sampling tube, syringe, or pipet, not less than 100 g from the original container. With a sterile spoon, aseptically transfer 100 g of well-mixed coloring powders, fruits, fruit preparations, nuts or nut preparations, cakes, pastries, or confections to a sample container. If cold-pack or frozen fruit is not thawed, use a high-speed electric drill with a sanitized auger, a hollow coring tube, or another suitably sharp, sanitized instrument to obtain enough material for the sample. Ensure a representative cross section of material from the outer edge to the center of the block.

E. **Stabilizers and emulsifiers:** With a sterile or sanitized trier, transfer at lest 3 plugs or columns (total not less than 120 g) from each container, or with a sterile or sanitized spoon or spatula, remove not less than 120 g of powder from various places. Transfer the samples to a sterile sample container, and immediately seal the sample container after the transfer is completed. If some portions of the package content are believed to be significantly different from the others, sample such portions separately.

F. **Sweetening agents:** Aseptically transfer at least 100 g of solid sweetener or 150 g of liquid sweetener to a sterile sample container.

G. **Eggs and egg products[4]:** Take samples from a representative number of containers in the lot. Determine the odor by smelling the sample after removing the microbiological sample.

   1. **Liquid eggs:** With a sterile tube or dipper, mix the contents of the container until homogeneous. With a sterile, long-handled dipper or ladle, aseptically transfer about 400 mL to a sterile sample container.
   2. **Frozen eggs:** Remove the top layer of the egg with a sterilized hatchet or chisel. Using a sterile auger or corer, take 3 cores from the top to the bottom of the container: first core in the center, second core midway between the center and the periphery, and third core near the edge. With a sterile spoon, transfer the cores to a sterile sample container.
   3. **Dried eggs:** For small packages, take the entire package as the sample. For boxes and barrels, remove the top layer with a sterile spoon or other sterile instrument, and with a sterile trier, remove at least 3 cores as described above. The sample should consist of about 400g. Aseptically transfer the core to a sample container with a sterile spoon or other suitable instrument.

3.077 *Aseptically Processed and Packaged Milk and Milk Products*

The routine sampling and testing of aseptically (ultrahigh temperature, UHT) processed and packaged milk and milk products are generally done at the processing location to meet low-acid, canned food regulations as described in the Code of Federal Regulations, Title 21, Part 113. Collect samples in original, unopened, hermetically sealed containers, and ship them and the sample data to a laboratory.

3.080 Sampling Product Containers, Closures, Packing Materials, Equipment, Water, and Air

3.081 *Paper Stock*[18]

Paper stock must be sampled before it enters into any converting operation. Partially converted items may also be sampled in intermediate stages of conversion. Sampling methods for these latter items, in general, comply with sampling methods for paper stock or finished products. Items fabricated from plastic, metal, or combinations of these materials are usually not sampled before conversion; therefore, sampling methods for only finished products are described below.

A. **Roll-stock sampling:** Either of the following 2 methods is acceptable.

1. Sample the roll stock as a butt roll with a minimum radial thickness of 2.54 cm (1 inch) of paper on the core and a minimum roll width of 30.48 cm (12 inch). With a lesser mill roll width, the full width of the roll would constitute the sample. If the width of the roll is more than 30.48 cm, the butt roll may be cut for convenience to a minimum of 30.48 cm by using a handsaw or a power band saw, taking care to minimize contamination. The cut web shall be firmly taped before the butt roll is removed from the roll stand. Wrap the roll-stock sample carefully in wrapping paper and seal with tape.
2. Cut samples form the roll of paper with a clean, sharp knife. Cut into the roll 2 laps deep and discard the first 2 layers. Then cut into the roll 6 laps deep to a size of approximately 20 × 25 cm, grasp the sample by the top and bottom sheets near the corners, and remove and tape in 3 or 4 places to keep the sheets aligned. This process protects the inner sheets for testing.

When samples are being cut from the roll of paper, 3 sides of the sample may be cut first, thus forming a flap. Staple or tape this flap to prevent undue exposure and riffling. Finally, cut the hinge side of the sample. Remove the assembled sample and place it in a clean paper envelope. Seal the envelope, and insert it into a stout manila or brown Kraft envelope. For sample protection, envelopes should be of a type that can be sealed, preferably with a pressure-sensitive adhesive rather than with envelopes that must be moistened.

B. **Sheeted-stock sampling:** Final samples must consist of a minimum of six sheets, each approximately 20 × 25 cm. Take sheeted paper selected for sampling from any portion of the stock except the bottom or top 1.5 cm. Reduce large sheets to a final sample size by using a guillotine-type cutter or equivalent tool that does not involve the direct handling of any sample sheets. Tape and package the stacks of cut sample sheets as described above. Top and bottom sheets constitute protective covers during sampling and shipping; discard them before testing.

3.082 *Cups, Lids, Hoods, etc.*[18]

Containers or closures to be examined for sanitary status shall be taken from lots consisting of at least 50 individual items. Containers or closures shall be taken from stock produced under normal operating procedures. Firm and flexible walled containers must be obtained after sanitization of the forming equipment but before the product is introduced to the package. A sample set from each filling or manufacturing line shall consist of a minimum of 4 50-cm^2 areas of surface when the swab test is used.

Single samples are defined as follows:

1. **Swab test:** Product contact area of 50 cm^2. If a single item has less than 50 cm^2 of contact surface, take sufficient individual items to provide at least 50 cm^2 (as in the case of containers of 100-mL [3.2-oz.] or less capacity).[24]
2. **Rinse test:** One container with greater than 100-mL capacity.[24]

3.083 *Fluid Product Packaging*

A. **Firm-walled uncapped items:** After sanitization, but before the product to be packaged is introduced, obtain from the line 4 paper, laminate, or plastic containers that are to be formed, filled, and sealed in a single-service device.

B. **Firm-walled capped items:** Randomly remove from the conveyor line 4 representative paper, laminate, or plastic containers that are formed, filled, and sealed in separate devices. Containers must be removed without their lips or interiors being touched just before they reach the filler valves. Insert the containers to be capped mechanically into the conveyor lines beyond the filler valves. Should an inspection show that the mechanical cappers are unsanitary, apply laboratory sterilized closures to 4 other containers that are taken from the conveyor before reaching the filler valves in addition to four that are mechanically capped. If unsanitary conditions are demonstrated, then take steps to sanitize the cappers.

C. **Flexible walled items**

1. Collect 4 bags used for dispensing or other, larger volume applications.
2. Deliver single-service milk and milk product containers promptly to the laboratory with sample data. *Do not* store or ship these containers in refrigerated cases or containers.[23]

3.084 *Equipment Cleanliness Sampling*

A. **Clean-in-place (CIP) equipment**[20]

1. The rinse solution method may be used on individual items of equipment or on systems designed for CIP. This method is not practical for other equipment because the volume of rinse solution required would be equivalent to the capacity of the entire unit and adequate agitation to flush surfaces thoroughly might not be possible.

2. The minimum amount of solution needed to flush the product contact surface of CIP items thoroughly is much greater than the amount that can be sterilized conveniently. Instead, determine the volume of water needed to fill the CIP system completely, sanitize the rinse solution by super-chlorination (25 mg of chlorine per liter) and hold for 10 minutes. Then neutralize the hypochlorite by adding an excess of sterile 10% sodium thiosulfate solution (2 mL/L of rinse solution). Tap water may also be sterilized by membrane filtration (pore size 0.45 µm), followed by the addition of sodium thiosulfate (1 mL of 10% solution per liter of water) to inactivate any residual chlorine.[17,20]
3. Introduce neutralized chlorine-treated water into the "ready for use" CIP unit. Start circulation and continue for 20 times the period required to move the same volume of water with the pump. Stop the pump and open the outlet valve at the lowest point in the system. Fill separate sterile sample containers at the beginning, middle, and end of the unit emptying step.
4. Use a sterile wide-mouthed container of sufficient size (at least 1 L) made of suitable plastic. Keep 1 L of the chlorine-treated water that has been neutralized, but not run through the CIP unit, for use as a control sample.

For large volumes of neutralized chlorine-treated rinses, the membrane filter method may be used to analyze both rinse and control samples.

B. **Ice cream freezers:** The sanitary condition of scrapers and of the interior surfaces of batch freezers may be determined by a modified rinse method. Prepare a sterile rinse solution in 100-mL quantities per 9.46-L capacity of batch freezer barrels to be tested. With the outlet valve of the barrel closed, pour sterile rinse into the inlet. Operate the scraper for 2 minutes and collect a sample through the outlet valve into a sterile sample container.

C. **Swab test procedure:** Use the swab test method to determine the sanitary condition of equipment and of large containers that cannot be tested by the rinse method. Open a sterile swab container, grasp the end of the stick (being careful not to touch any portion that might be inserted into the vial), and remove the swab aseptically. Open a vial of buffered rinse solution, moisten the swab head, and press out excess solution against the interior of the vial with a rotational motion. Hold onto the swab handle to make a 30° angle with the surface. Rub the moistened swab head slowly and thoroughly 3 times over approximately 50-cm^2 areas of surface of the item, as above; rinse the swab head in solution in the vial and then press out the excess moisture as above. Swab 4 more 50-cm^2 areas of surface of the item; rinse the swab in solution and remove excess solution after each swabbing. After the fifth area has been swabbed, position the swab head in the vial and bend and break the stick, leaving the head in the vial; alternatively, cut the stick with a pair of sterile scissors or other cutting device. Replace the screw cap, put the vial in a waterproof container, cool to 0° to 4.4°C and deliver to the laboratory to allow analysis within 48 hours of taking the sample. With calcium alginate swabs, after swabbing the fifth area and depositing the swab head in the rinse vial, add 0.5 mL of sterilized solubilizing solution.[24]

3.085 *Dairy Water Supply Sampling*[7,24]

Procedures and equipment for sampling water supplies are detailed in the current edition of *Standard Methods for the Examination of Water and Wastewater* or in the FDA *Milk Laboratory Evaluation Form—Dairy Waters (Coliform Group)*, FDA Form 2400k.

3.086 *Air Supply Sampling*

Sampling for airborne microorganisms in dairy plants involves collecting air samples in air pathways by which organisms may be introduced on the product or equipment. Samples may be taken 1) at openings in the equipment subject to potential contamination from organisms transported by air currents, 2) at selected points for testing the quality of room air (e.g., where the product is filled into containers), and 3) in areas where employees are concentrated. Because of air turbulence during operating hours, sampling by volumetric methods will be more effective and dependable than use of sedimentation technique.

Sampling time for all methods of collection usually is standardized at 15, 30, and 60 minutes, with the duration determined by experience or estimation. Samples may be taken monthly to detect specific microorganisms unless more frequent samples are necessitated by emergency conditions or suspected contamination.

3.090 Radionuclides in Milk and Dairy Products (Class 0)

Collect at least 3.78 L (1 gal.) of milk (raw or pasteurized), preserve with formaldehyde (10 mL of 40% formaldehyde per 3.78 L), and ship to the laboratory for analysis. Formaldehyde does not interfere with analysis of iodine 131 (^{131}I), barium 140, or cesium 137 by gamma spectroscopy, or of strontium 89 by ion exchange and/or by chemical methods. Addition of formaldehyde to raw milk does, however, cause transformation of ^{131}I to protein bound ^{131}I. In raw milk, the enzyme xanthine oxidase oxidizes formaldehyde (H_2CO) to hydrogen peroxide (H_2O_2) in the presence of oxygen, and H_2O_2 oxidizes ^{131}I to $^{131}I_2$, which binds protein. In pasteurized or dried milk, xanthine oxidase is inactive; consequently, addition of formaldehyde to processed milk has no effect on analyses of ^{131}I by ion-exchange methods. If raw milk is the sample of choice and ^{131}I is the only radionuclide of concern, no preservative should be added to the milk. Analysis can be simplified by passing milk through a column containing anion exchange resin at the sampling station and then shipping the column to the laboratory for further processing. This presupposes that all of the ^{131}I in the milk is in the inorganic form as iodide.

3.100 Cited References

1. BLATTNER, T.M.; OLSON, N.F.; WICHERN, D.W. Sampling barrel cheese for moisture analysis: comparison of methods. JAOAC **68**:718-721; 1985.
2. BRAZIS, A.R.; BLACK, L.A. Bacterial counts of bulk milk for interstate shipment: 1. effect of sampling procedures. J. Milk Food Technol. **25**:172-175; 1962.
3. CLAIBORNE, F.B.; COX, K.E. The direct microscopic count on preserved milk samples; an effective measure for uniform state-wide control. J. Milk Food Technol. **14**:105-108, 1951.
4. CUNNIFF, P.A., ED. *Official methods of analysis*, 16th ed. Washington, DC: AOAC; 1998.

5. DODGE, H.F.; ROMIG, H.G. *Sampling inspection tables*, 2nd ed. New York, NY: John Wiley and Sons; 1959.
6. FOOD AND DRUG ADMINISTRATION. *Bacteriological and analytical manual*, 8th ed. Gaithersburg, MD: AOAC Intl.; 1995.
7. GREENBERG, A.E.; CLESCERI, L.S.; EATON, A.D., eds. *Standard methods for the examination of water and wastewater*, 18th ed. Washington, DC: APHA; 1992.
8. INTERNATIONAL ASSOCIATION OF MILK, FOOD AND ENVIRONMENTAL SANITARIANS; U.S. PUBLIC HEALTH SERVICE; DAIRY INDUSTRY COMMITTEE. 3-A accepted practices for supplying air under pressure in contact with milk, milk products and product contact surfaces, serial #60403. J. Milk Food Technol. **35**:378-382; 1972.
9. INTERNATIONAL. ASSOCIATION OF MILK, FOOD AND ENVIRONMENTAL SANITARIANS; U.S. PUBLIC HEALTH SERVICE; DAIRY IINDUSTRY COMMITTEE. 3-A sanitary standards for storage tanks for milk and milk products, 01-06. J. Milk Food Technol. **37**:36-61; 1974.
10. INTERNATIONAL ASSOCIATION OF MILK, FOOD AND ENVIRONMENTAL SANITARIANS: U.S. PUBLIC HEALTH SERVICE; DAIRY INDUSTRY COMMITTEE. 3-A sanitary standards for farm milk cooling and holding tanks, no. 13-06. J. Milk Food Technol. **38**:646-653; 1975.
11. INTERNATIONAL COMMISSION ON MICROBIOLOGICAL SPECIFICATIONS FOR FOODS. *Microorganisms in Foods, 2nd ed. 2. Sampling for microbiological analysis: principles and specific applications*. Toronto, Canada: University of Toronto Press; 1986.
12. INTERNATIONAL DAIRY FEDERATION. *Milk and milk products—guidance on sampling*. Brussels, Belgium: IDF Standard 50C:1995.
13. INTERNATIONAL DAIRY FEDERATION. *Milk and milk products—sampling inspection by attributes*. Brussels, Belgium: IDF Standard 113A:1990.
14. INTERNATIONAL STANDARDS ORGANIZATION. *Sampling procedures and tables for inspection attributes*. Geneva, Switzerland: ISO 2859:1974.
15. INTERNATIONAL STANDARDS ORGANIZATION. *General information on sampling inspection, and guide to the use of ISO 2859 tables*. Geneva, Switzerland: ISO 2859:1974/ Addendum 1:1977.
16. LEVINE, B.S. *Effect of formaldehyde on the direct microscopic count of raw milk*. Pub. Health Rep. **65**:931-938; 1950.
17. MARSHALL, R.T.; APPEL, R. *Sanitary conditions in twelve fluid milk processing plants as determined by use of the rinse filter method*. J. Milk Food Technol. **36**:237-241; 1973.
18. PARROW, T. *Manual of recommended laboratory methods for sampling and microbiological testing of single service food packages and their components*. Syracuse, NY: Syracuse Research Corporation; 1978.
19. U.S. DEPARTMENT OF HEALTH AND HUMAN SERVICES. *Fabrication of single-service containers and closures for milk and milk products*. Washington, DC: U.S. Public Health Service, PHS/FDA: 1995.
20. U.S. DEPARTMENT OF HEALTH AND HUMAN SERVICES. *Grade A pasteurized milk ordinance*. Washington, DC: U.S. Government Printing Office; 1997.
21. U.S. DEPARTMENT OF HEALTH AND HUMAN SERVICES. *Evaluation of milk laboratories*. Washington, DC: U.S. Government Printing Office; 1995.
22. U.S. DEPARTMENT OF HEALTH AND HUMAN SERVICES. *Milk sample collector evaluation form: dairy plant sampling-raw and pasteurized milk*, FDA form 2399. Washington, DC: U.S. Government Printing Office; 1980.
23. U.S. DEPARTMENT OF HEALTH AND HUMAN SERVICES. *Bulk milk pickup tanker, hauler report and sampler evaluation form*, FDA form 2399a. Washington, DC: U.S. Government Printing Office; 1980.
24. U.S. DEPARTMENT OF HEALTH AND HUMAN SERVICES. *Milk laboratory evaluation forms*, FDA 2400 series. Washington, DC: U.S. Government Printing Office; 1995.

Chapter 4

Media and Dilution Water Preparation

G. L. Davis and P. J. Hickey
(M. Bulthaus, Tech. Comm.)

4.010 Introduction

Accuracy of microbial data obtained from testing dairy foods depends on which culture media are used and how these media are used in the laboratory. Media, reagents, and dilution water must be prepared and handled properly. Refer to chapter 2 for laboratory quality assurance procedures.

It is the responsibility of the individual analysts to know the properties of, and safety precautions for, the chemicals they use. For details, refer to manufacturers' material safety data sheets (MSDS).

Commercial dehydrated or prepared media are readily available for almost all methods and procedures given in this edition of *SMEDP* and should be used when available. For this reason, media formula or compositional information is not presented in this book. In those few exceptions where commercial media are not available, the formula of the media is given with the method. For commercial media, compositional information and directions for their preparation are on the label. If needed, information on standard methods agar (SMA) composition may be found in the 16th edition of *SMEDP*.[13]

4.020 Suitability of Water

Only water that has been treated to free it of traces of dissolved metals and bactericidal and inhibitory compounds should be used to prepare culture media, reagents, and dilution blanks. Inhibitor-free water is referred to as microbiologically suitable (MS) water. For routine use in microbiological analyses of dairy products it is the growth medium or dilution system prepared with the water that is of concern, and not the water itself. While culture media provide considerable protection from toxic agents present in the water,[16] it is still important that water used as a dilution fluid be free from substances toxic to microorganisms. A procedure to determine if dilution water may have a toxic effect is given in section 4.041, and water that passes the toxicity test is considered to be microbiologically suitable.

Guidelines for reagent-quality water have been published in *Standard Methods for the Examination of Water and Wastewater*,[4,5] the *Annual Book of ASTM Standards*,[1] *Preparation and Testing of Reagent Water in the Clinical Laboratory*,[14] and the *United States Pharmacopeia*[2] (*USP*). All of these publications recommend treatment of water to remove chemical and biological substances that may interfere with tests. Treatment should include one or more of the following: distillation, deionization, reverse osmosis, carbon adsorption, filtration, ultrafiltration, and ultraviolet oxidation. In general, MS water must be free of chemical contaminants such as chlorine and metals, exhibit low conductivity (high resistivity), and have low levels of heterotrophic organisms. Bottled water must meet *USP* requirements for purified water to be considered MS water. In addition, source water for treatment by filtration, ultrafiltration, UV oxidation, and/or reverse osmosis must be closely monitored because these types of treatments are incapable of removing all contaminants. For best results, water treatment should include distillation, mixed-bed deionization combined with activated carbon treatment and pre- and postfiltration, or reverse osmosis treatment with prefiltration and either distillation or mixed-bed deionization.

MS water should not be stored for long periods of time. Distilled water storage reservoirs must be drained and cleaned regularly. Open containers of *USP*-certified purified water should be protected from contamination. Point-of-use water purifiers must be maintained and tested according to the manufacturer's recommendations. Lengthy tubing and plumbing connections that are likely to permit the accumulation of bacteria must be avoided. MS water that is prepared from chlorinated source water must be tested regularly for residual chlorine. MS water must also be tested regularly for conductivity (or resistivity), metals, and heterotrophic bacteria.

4.030 Preparation of Dilution Water

Dilution blank preparations vary considerably in dairy and food laboratories around the world.[3,4,6,10,12,15,16] Janus[8] summarized the results of an IDF/ISO study involving 8 different diluents. The study group recommended quarter-strength Ringers solution as a reference standard, with peptone-salt diluent, peptone solution, and phosphate water as alternatives. The phosphate solution is retained in *SMEDP* because of its equivalence to other diluents[8] and the lack of sufficient evidence to dictate a change.[7,15] Distilled water performed as well as phosphated water (without magnesium chloride)[8,9] and would be usable where dilutions of milk and milk products are low. Use of a single diluent is essential, however, to ensure standardization.

4.031 *Stock Phosphate Solution*

Dissolve 34 g of potassium phosphate (monobasic) in 500 mL of MS water, adjust to pH 7.2 with sodium hydroxide, and make up to 1 L with MS water. Preferably, place in small vials. Sterilize at 121°C for 15 minutes. After sterilization, tightly seal the vials and store at 0° to 4.4°C.

4.032 *Stock Magnesium Chloride Solution*

Measure 38 g of anhydrous magnesium chloride into a 1-L volumetric flask and add MS water to make 1 L of solution. Dispense into suitable containers, sterilize, and store as described above [4.031].

4.033 *Phosphate Dilution Water (Class O)*

Add 1.25 mL of stock phosphate solution to MS water and make up to 1 L. Dispense in 99 ± 2-mL [2.045] or 9 ± 0.2-mL quantities, or in other volumes as required, and autoclave at 121°C for 15 minutes [4.091]. Bacteria should not be suspended in any dilution for more than 30 minutes at room temperature to minimize death or multiplication of the bacteria.

4.034 *Phosphate and Magnesium Chloride Dilution Water (Class O)*

Add 1.25 mL of stock phosphate solution and 5 mL of stock magnesium chloride solution to MS water and make up to 1 L. Dispense in 99 ± 2-mL [2.045], 9 ± 0.2-mL, or other quantities as required, and autoclave at 121°C for 15 minutes [4.091]. The addition of magnesium chloride may improve the recovery of microorganisms with metabolic injury induced by toxic substances in the dilution water.[6,11]

4.040 Water Toxicity Tests

4.041 *Dilution Water Toxicity Test (Class O)*

A screening test for dilution water toxicity can be conducted by preparing a dilution of the appropriate dairy food to provide 100 to 250 colonies per plate when 1 mL is plated. The diluted sample is then plated in duplicate after 0, 15, 30, and 45 minutes by the standard plate count (SPC) or equivalent procedure [chapter 6]. Distinct trends toward lower counts among successively plated samples suggest toxicity. Decreases of more than 20% in 45 minutes are indicative of dilution water toxicity.

4.042 *Water Quality Test (Class O)*

A detailed method is described in section 9020 B.3.C. of *Standard Methods for the Examination of Water and Wastewater*.[5]

4.050 Cleaning Glassware and Testing for Detergent Residues

Modern detergents are effective for cleaning laboratory glassware. Most of these detergents are of the anionic type, usually with alkaline substances such as phosphates, carbonates, or silicates. Some detergents, especially the cationic type with quaternary ammonium compounds, are highly inhibitory and great care must be exercised to ensure their removal. Detergents and soaps have an affinity for surfaces. They displace dirt and allow it to be washed away, but they themselves are difficult to remove completely.

4.051 *Cleaning Glassware*

Deposits of milk stone or calcium salts, which are resistant to ordinary detergents, are occasionally encountered. Remove salts by exposing glassware for several minutes to acid solutions and then rinsing thoroughly. Commercial dairy-acid cleaners, formulated to remove milk stone from milk-processing surfaces, can be used on laboratory glassware. Usage levels should be obtained from the label.

The detergent wash is best done with hot water after a preliminary rinsing with warm water to remove most of the soil. Soaking aids in the removal of stubborn residues. Six to 12 rinses with running tap water, followed by several rinses with MS water, are sometimes necessary to remove a detergent completely.

4.052 *Detergent Residues*

If glass petri dishes are used, laboratories should check for inhibitory residues whenever changing brands or lots of detergents. This procedure is described in chapter 2 [2.0412].

4.053 *Glassware pH Check*

Acid and alkaline residues can be detected on cleaned laboratory ware by adding and dispersing a few drops of aqueous 0.04% bromthymol blue (BTB) indicator. Localized blue (alkaline) or yellow (acid) zones in the pH indicator solution demonstrate the incomplete removal of cleaning solutions. Prepare the BTB solution by dissolving 0.1 g of BTB in 16 mL of 0.01N sodium hydroxide and diluting to 250 mL with MS water; the solution must be green.

4.060 Media

4.061 *Dehydrated Media*

Dehydrated media should be stored in tightly closed containers below 30°C and protected from light. If the environment is hot and humid, media may be stored in a refrigerator or freezer. Properly stored, most media remain stable until the manufacturer's expiration date; however, purchases should be planned to facilitate complete turnover within 1 year. Media should be dated upon receipt and when first opened.

After the seal has been broken, permitting entrance of air and moisture, the quality of a medium may depend on the storage environment. Use of a desiccator for storage of opened media will extend shelf life. If possible, media should be used or discarded within 6 months after breaking the seal. Suitable package sizes should be purchased to minimize the repeated use of a material from unsealed containers. Any medium that has absorbed moisture and become caked must be discarded. Contamination may take place if unclean spatulas are used to transfer material from containers.

4.062 *Prepared Media*

The life of any prepared medium, whether in tubes, bottles, or plates, depends on the storage conditions and type of medium. Prepared media should not be stored unless protected against water loss. This may be accomplished by using screw-capped tubes and bottles (with caps tightened after sterilization) instead of cotton-plugged or loosely covered containers. Prepared plates should be used within 1 week unless stored in moisture-proof containers such as plastic bags. Media in screw-capped tubes should be used within approximately 6 months.

Commercially prepared media should be used prior to the expiration date. If dehydration has occurred, media should be discarded.

4.070 Basic Steps in Media Preparation

Weigh carefully the proper amount of dehydrated medium.

Place the requisite amount of MS water into a suitable container (e.g., borosilicate glass; stainless steel or heat-resistant plastic such as polypropylene, polycarbonate, or polysulfone).

Add the weighed, dehydrated medium to part of the water. Mix with a stirring rod or magnetic stirrer. If necessary, adjust the medium pH with a suitable acid or alkali solution. Add the remaining water and mix again. [Note: Reconstituted media prepared from commercial dehydrates seldom require pH adjustment if made according to the manufacturer's directions. Errors in weighing dehydrated media and overheating may cause pH problems. Recheck medium preparation procedures if problems occur. If significant pH problems continue and medium preparation procedures are considered satisfactory, the commercial dehydrate should be replaced. See section 4.080 for information concerning pH adjustment.]

If necessary to effect complete solution, heat to boiling on wire gauze over a free flame or on a hot plate with a built-in magnetic stirrer. Stir often to prevent burning of the medium. A nonpressurized, free-flowing steam unit may be used. Media containing agar should be boiled 1 minute to ensure solution of the agar. Prolonged boiling may cause undesirable foaming. This can be reduced by holding the flask in cold water for a few seconds after the initial boiling has been accomplished. If necessary, restore water lost by evaporation. For example, weigh the container before and after heating. Add sufficient water to restore the original weight before distributing and sterilizing the rehydrated medium. A microwave oven may be used to dissolve dried medium if it is compatible with the container in use.

Distribute the medium into a suitable container. This can be most easily accomplished for a tubed liquid medium by using automatic pipeters. A hand-held adjustable pipeter is most suitable for small numbers of test tubes while an electrically operated dispensing apparatus is more satisfactory for large numbers [2.046]. In each instance, before use, the machine must be flushed with MS water followed by the medium until the water has been completely removed from the system. After use, the apparatus must be flushed with warm water, detergent solution, tap water, and MS water. If any residues accumulate, the apparatus should be disassembled and scrubbed. A small amount of water should be left in the syringe portion to prevent drying out and subsequent "freezing" of the plunger and barrel.

The amount of medium per container should be limited so that no part of the medium is more than 2.5 cm from the container wall or the surface of the agar. (This is to ensure rapid equilibration of temperature when the container is placed in a water bath.)

Sterilize at 121°C for 15 minutes [4.091] or according to recommended procedures for each medium. Checking of pH before use is recommended.

Melt and hold solid media at 44° to 46°C until ready for use, but not exceeding 3 hours. Hold inhibitory-substances media at 64°C [12.021, 12.022]. Solid media may be melted in boiling water, by flowing steam not under pressure, or in a microwave oven. The time to ensure complete solution will vary with the method and the volume in the container. Do not permit media to boil over in the microwave oven. If a precipitate forms, discard the media; do not remelt.

If it becomes necessary to formulate a dehydrated medium that is not commercially available, use only reagent-grade chemicals and ingredients approved by the *USP* and other components prepared by culture media suppliers. Follow the manufacturer's instructions for storing stock materials. Discontinue use of materials that show any evidence of contamination, decomposition, or dehydration.

4.080 Adjustment of pH

Prior to use, determine the hydrogen-ion concentration (pH) of culture media at 25°C electrometrically by using a potentiometer (pH meter). Determinations made at 45°C to take advantage of the fluid state of agar may be low! For example, SMA shows a pH of 7.04 at 25°C and a pH of 6.8 at 45°C.[17] Meters measure pH accurately only if samples and buffers are at the same temperature. Commercially prepared reference buffers should be used.

Prepare the pH meter as described in 2.0413. Macerate solid medium thoroughly with a glass rod before inserting electrodes. Be sure electrodes and sample are at 25°C. Alternatively, use flat surface electrodes that can test agar surfaces without prior mixing and breaking of the medium.

4.090 Sterilization

Before sterilization, bring the medium to boiling temperature while stirring frequently. Restore lost water if necessary [4.070] and autoclave. Because the pH of the medium may change during sterilization and because there may be potential browning reactions, it is important not to exceed the recommended temperature and time. Sugar broths should not be subjected to a sterilization cycle longer than 45 minutes. Reduce pressure with reasonable promptness to prevent boiling or undue changes in the nutritional properties of the medium. Remove from the autoclave when atmospheric pressure is attained. It is preferable to use flasks or bottles from which the melted medium may be poured into plates; however, if desired, test tubes containing 15- to 20-mL amounts may be used for pouring agar into plates.

4.091 *Steam Sterilization*

Sterilize media, water, and materials (such as rubber, cork, cotton, paper, and heat-labile plastic tubes and closures) that are likely to be charred in the dry-air sterilizer by autoclaving at 121°C for 15 minutes. Start timing after the temperature has reached 121°C. Autoclave media and dilution blanks within an hour of preparation. Slightly loosen stoppers to allow the passage of steam and air out of closed containers in the autoclave. Make certain the load is loosely packed. For efficient sterilization, separate containers by at least 1 cm in all directions. Before allowing steam pressure to rise, automatically or manually expel all air from the sterilizer through an exhaust valve. If manual means are used, make sure that all air has been exhausted and that only steam is being exhausted before pressurization begins. (If air remains in the chamber, a 15 pounds-per-square-inch gauge pressure can mean a temperature as low as 100°C!) Because the temperature obtained at a constant pressure of saturated steam will vary according to atmospheric pressure, rely on a properly operating and calibrated thermometer (not a pressure gauge) to ensure sterilization. Maintain and check autoclave as described in 2.041.

Carefully review label instructions before heat-treating any medium. For example, violet red bile agar (VRBA) requires boiling for 2 minutes rather than autoclaving.[9]

Avoid overloading autoclaves so that the rate of air exhaust or heating is not appreciably delayed. The volume of the load generally should not exceed 30% to 40% of the volume of the autoclave. The autoclave should reach 121°C slowly but within 15 minutes. The maximum time from applying the steam to unloading the autoclave should not exceed 45 minutes. A rapid come-up time does not necessarily result in more efficient autoclaving, since air is not replaced by steam when the steam enters the autoclave too rapidly. A steam flow that is too slow also results in decreased efficiency because air-steam mixtures form.

When nonliquid materials with slow heat conductance are to be sterilized, or where the packaged arrangement or volume of materials otherwise retards penetration of heat, allow extra time for materials to reach 121°C before beginning to time the sterilization period, and, if necessary, use longer sterilization periods to ensure sterility.

After sterilization, *gradually* reduce pressure within the autoclave (no less than 15 minutes is recommended) because liquids may be at temperatures above their boiling point at atmospheric pressure. Liquids can be lost through boiling when the pressure is lowered too rapidly. When dry materials such as sampling equipment or empty sample bottles are being sterilized, pressure may be released rapidly at the end of the 15-minute holding period at 121°C. This prevents collection of condensate and speeds up the drying of paper-wrapped equipment.

Used plates, pipets, tubes, etc., must be routinely decontaminated in microbiological laboratories. Dairy products, especially raw milk, may harbor potential pathogens such as staphylococci and streptococci. The same principles apply for loading the autoclave and sterilizing materials as for preparing media. Plastic petri dishes are most conveniently sterilized by placing them in heat-resistant, autoclavable bags, or other containers. When large quantities of used materials are autoclaved, the sterilization time shall be at least 30 minutes. Plastic dishes become amorphous when properly autoclaved. Sterilization tapes or other indicators can be applied to containers and placed in autoclaves to indicate that sterilization temperatures have been reached [2.041].

4.092 *Hot Air Sterilization*

Sterilize equipment with dry heat in hot-air sterilizers or ovens so that materials at the center of the load are heated to not less than 170°C for not less than 1 hour. (This usually requires exposure for about 2 hours at 170°C.) When the oven is loaded to capacity, use a longer period or a slightly higher temperature. Spore packs should be used to check sterilization efficiency.

4.100 Quality Control

General principles of quality control are covered in chapter 2. This chapter presents procedures that will provide minimal but adequate quality control in media production.

Whenever possible, use commercially dehydrated media.

Date the label of each bottle of dehydrated medium, indicating when it was received and when it was first opened.

A medium must be mixed completely to form a homogeneous solution in water before it can be sterilized and dispensed. Stirring that causes foaming should be avoided. Restore water lost by evaporation after ingredients are fully dissolved.

Autoclave performance should be monitored manually or with a continuous temperature-recording device. The bulb of the thermometer should be located properly on the exhaust line so as to measure minimum temperature within the sterilizing chamber. For each autoclave run, heat-indicating autoclave tape should be placed on each outer container. Records for sterilization runs should include the date, a brief listing of item(s) sterilized, temperature, and sterilization time. In addition, routine sterilization procedures should be checked periodically with a maximum-registering thermometer and either spore strips or suspensions.

Limit heating of the medium to the minimum necessary to ensure solution and sterilization. When the autoclave has reached atmospheric pressure following the recommended cycle, it should be opened immediately. Prolonged storage of melted media in a water bath should be avoided.

Check and document the final pH of each lot of medium at 25°C [4.080].

Aseptic technique must be followed strictly during dispensing of sterilized material. Hands should not touch any part of the dispensing surfaces that come in contact with sterile material. During interruptions in the cycle of a mechanical dispenser, the spout of the dispenser train should be placed inside a sterile container. A dispensing cycle should not be interrupted, however, except in an emergency.

Media containing dyes should be protected from light by storing them in the dark or a dark glass bottle, or by wrapping the container with brown paper or foil.

Each container of autoclaved medium should be labeled with the name of the medium and the autoclave run number.

Inclusive dates during which each lot and container of dehydrated medium were used should be recorded for future reference.

Before use, each lot of prepared medium should be inspected visually for volume, tightness of closure, clarity, consistency, and completeness of label. If possible, media should be tested with positive and negative microbial controls.

4.110 Cited References

1. AMERICAN SOCIETY FOR TESTING AND MATERIALS. *1994 annual book of ASTM standards*, Vol. 11.01, Designation D 1193-91, *Standard Specification for Reagent Water.* Philadelphia, PA: American Society for Testing and Materials; 1994.
2. ANONYMOUS. *United States pharmacopoeia*, 22nd ed. Easton, PA: Mack Printing Co.; 1989.

3. BUTTERFIELD, C.T. The selection of a dilution water for bacteriological examinations. J. Bacteriol. **23**:355-368; 1932.
4. CLESCERI, L.S.; GREENBERG, A.E.; EATON, A.D., EDS. *Standard methods for the examination of water and wastewater*, 20th ed. Washington, DC: APHA; 1998.
5. EATON, A.D.; CLESCERI, L.S.; GREENBERG, A.E., EDS. *Standard methods for the examination of water and wastewater*, 19th ed. Washington, DC: APHA; 1995.
6. HARTMAN, P.A. Modification of conventional methods for recovery of injured coliforms and salmonellae. J. Food Prot. **42**:356-361; 1979.
7. HUHTANEN, C.N.; BRAZIS, A.R.; ARLEDGE, W.L.; DONNELLY, C.B.; GINN, R.E.; RANDOLPH, H.E.; KOCH, E.J. A comparison of phosphate buffered and distilled water dilution blanks for the standard plate count of raw-milk bacteria. J. Milk Food Technol. **38**:264-268; 1975.
8. JANUS, J.A. Investigations into the bactericidal effect of diluents applied for the enumeration of *Enterobacteriaceae* in food products. Report of Group E 50. The Netherlands: International Dairy Federation; 1980. ISO/TC 34/SC 9.
9. JENSEN, J.P.; HAUSLER, W.J., JR. Productivity of boiled and autoclaved violet red bile agar. J. Milk Food Technol. **38**:279-280; 1975.
10. KING, W.L.; HURST, A. A note on the survival of some bacteria in different diluents. J. Appl. Bacteriol. **26**:504-506; 1963.
11. MACLEOD, R.A.; KUO, S.C.; GELINAS, R. Metabolic injury to bacteria: II. Metabolic injury induced by distilled water or Cu^{++} in the plating diluent. J. Bacteriol. **93**:961-969; 1967.
12. MALLETTE, M.F. A pH 7 buffer devoid of nitrogen, sulfur, and phosphorous for use in bacteriological systems. J. Bacteriol. **94**:283-290; 1967.
13. MARSHALL, R.T., ed. *Standard methods for the examination of dairy products*, 16th ed. Washington, DC: APHA; 1992.
14. NATIONAL COMMITTEE FOR CLINICAL LABORATORY STANDARDS. *Preparation and testing of reagent water in the clinical laboratory*, 2nd ed. Approved guideline. Villanova, PA: National Committee for Clinical Laboratory Standards; 1991. NCCLS Document C3-A2.
15. OBLINGER, J.L.; KENNEDY, J.E., JR. Evaluation of diluents used for total counts. J. Milk Food Technol. **39**:114-116; 1976.
16. RONALD, G.W.; MORRIS, R.L. The effect of copper on distilled water quality for use in milk and water laboratories. J. Milk Food Technol. **30**:305-309; 1967.
17. WALTER, W.G.; KUEHN, K.; BOUGHTON, A. Electrometric pH determinations of different agar media at 25° and 45°C. J. Milk Food Technol. **33**:343-345; 1970.

Chapter 5

Pathogens in Milk and Milk Products

D. R. Henning, R. Flowers, R. Reiser, and E. T. Ryser
(J. F. Frank, Tech. Comm.)

5.010 Introduction

Milk and milk products are no longer the cause of high morbidity and mortality rate that were prevalent in the U.S. prior to the advent of pasteurization.[13] Typhoid fever, scarlet fever, and tuberculosis were diseases common among raw milk consumers in the U.S. until the 1939 edition of the Milk Ordinance and Code highly recommended pasteurization. The work of industry sanitarians and public health officials has reduced the incidence of milkborne disease outbreaks and sporadic cases to low levels. However, milk and milk products occasionally are vehicles for disease. Summaries of foodborne disease outbreaks in the U.S. compiled from data voluntarily reported to the Centers for Disease Control and Prevention (CDC) indicate dairy products were vehicles for disease transmission in 1 to 2 percent of the foodborne disease outbreaks in the U.S. between 1988 and 1992.[12]

The sources of pathogenic organisms in raw milk are cows, workers involved with all milk handling operations from the farm to foodservice facilities, and the environments in which milk is handled. The cows can excrete pathogens through their udders or shed them from their skin or mucous membranes. Likewise workers may shed pathogens from their skin or mucous membranes or by handling products or product contact surfaces with unclean hands. The environmental source of contamination that most frequently introduces pathogens into raw milk is water.

Zoonoses, which have been transmitted to humans through unpasteurized milk, include brucellosis, infections by pathogenic strains of *Escherichia coli* (including *E. coli* O157:H7), leptospirosis, listeriosis, paratyphoid fever, salmonellosis, staphylococcal enterotoxic gastroenteritis, streptococcal infections, tuberculosis, foot and mouth disease, tickborne encephalitis, Q-fever, and toxoplasmosis.[44] In areas of the world where pasteurization or equivalent heat treatment of milk is routinely practiced, zoonotic diseases originating from contaminated milk are rare.

Pathogenic organisms that come from human sources and the environment are infrequently found in milk and milk products.[12] These organisms are inactivated by pasteurization, but postpasteurization contamination can occur.

Documented diseases resulting from the postpasteurization contamination of milk and milk products are: botulism, cholera, *Clostridium perfringens* infection, gastroenteritis, salmonellosis, staphylococcal enterotoxic gastroenteritis, streptococcal infections, tuberculosis, typhoid fever, infections with adenoviruses and enteroviruses, hepatitis A, amoebiasis, and giardiasis.[44]

The effective control of pathogenic microorganisms spread by milk integrates the "application of sanitation measures throughout the production, handling, pasteurization, and distribution of milk."[51] The Public Health Service recommended its first Standard Milk Ordinance in 1924 and has incorporated modifications and changes recommended through biennial conferences of the NCIMS since 1979.[65] The Pasteurized Milk Ordinance (PMO), with its appendixes, is recommended for legal adoption by states, counties, and municipalities to encourage a greater uniformity and a higher level of excellence in milk sanitation practices in the U.S. The PMO provides the time and temperature requirements that each particle of milk must attain to be legally pasteurized. Appendix I of the PMO provides the technical specifications for the pasteurization equipment, controls, and tests.[65]

Many heat treatments are used commercially for reducing the population of harmful microorganisms in milk and cream to a level at which they do not constitute a significant health hazard. The heat treatments defined are: 1) thermization, 2) pasteurization, 3) ultra high temperature treatment (UHT), and 4) sterilization.[15] These treatments have industrial and public health significance when applied to raw milk.

Pasteurization is intended to inactivate pathogenic vegetative cells.[65] The destruction of spoilage organisms is often another benefit of pasteurization, but is not the focus of milk safety programs. The coliform count is used as an index of postpasteurization contamination, but the absence of coliform organisms does not provide assurance that pathogenic organisms are also absent from the products. Enrichment and isolation procedures for the pathogens most likely to contaminate milk and milk products will be presented in this chapter, although it is recommended that this testing not be conducted in a production facility.

5.011 *Pathogens and Toxins of Significance in Milk and Milk Products*

This chapter will focus on 3 pathogenic bacterial pathogens, *Salmonella* species causing enteritis, *Listeria monocytogenes,* and enterotoxigenic *Staphylococcus aureus*. These pathogens have been causative agents in foodborne outbreaks in the recent past. Methodology for the isolation and identification of other pathogens infrequently associated with milkborne illnesses will not be discussed in detail. *Campylobacter* species, *Yersinia enterocolitica,* and *Escherichia coli* O157:H7 are organisms likely to be of concern to food microbiologists; methodology for their isolation and identification are available in other sources, including the *Bacteriological Analytical Manual* of the U.S. Food and Drug Administration.[61] A number of kits that employ genetic techniques (ribotyping, DNA probes, RNA probes, and polymerase chain reaction procedures such as random amplified polymorphic DNA and restriction fragment length polymorphism) and serological and immunological techniques (immunoblotting, magnetic immunocapture, ELISA, and electrophoresis) are available for detection of these pathogens. Many of these kits are "rapid" and can provide useful data if the false-positive and false-negative frequencies associated with the selected kit are acceptable. Several of these kits are described elsewhere in this chapter.

Salmonella species remain the most frequent foodborne pathogens associated with milk and milk products. There were 15 confirmed outbreaks in the 1988 to 1992 review by the CDC.[12] Ice cream is the vehicle most frequently implicated in salmonellosis. A multiple-antibiotic resistant *Salmonella* Thyphimurium was isolated from over 17,000 persons during an outbreak attributed to pasteurized milk from a Midwest dairy in 1985. Epidemiologists estimate that over 180,000 cases constituted this outbreak.[58] In another *Salmonella* outbreak in 1994, an estimated 224,000 consumers were sickened by *Salmonella* Enteritidis after eating ice cream from an upper Midwest manufacturer.[66]

Listeria monocytogenes is able to grow slowly at refrigerated temperatures.[28] There has not been an infective dose determined for the organism, so the presence of any viable *L. monocytogenes* is currently cause for a product recall.[54] The organism has been involved in a number of recalls of frozen desserts and high pH cheeses. An outbreak in the Los Angeles area in 1985 was attributed to a Mexican-style cheese, which had a pH above 5.4. There were 142 cases of listeriosis and 48 deaths.[51] Although most of the cases in the Mexican-style cheese outbreak were patients at high risk, an outbreak in Europe with a surface ripened cheese, Vauchrin Mont D'or, included non-pregnant adults who appeared to be normal, previously healthy individuals in more than 50% of the cases.[11]

Enterotoxigenic strains of *Staphylococcus aureus* produce toxins capable of causing nausea, vomiting, and diarrhea when consumed by humans.[13] These toxins can be formed in milk or milk products prior to pasteurization and still retain their toxic activity after pasteurization. The use of bulk tanks and other methods of rapid cooling of raw milk on the farm limits the growth of *S. aureus* strains, which contaminate the milk either from mastitis or the milking environment.[13] The presence of enterotoxigenic strains can become a problem if proper temperatures are not maintained prior to pasteurization. Cheddar, Monterey, and Kuminost cheese produced in a Missouri cheese factory in 1965 were the vehicles for a foodborne outbreak.[67] The cheese was made with pasteurized milk and postpasteurization contamination by a vacuumizing process prior to cheese making was suspected as the point of contamination. Slow and inactive starters did not produce sufficient lactic acid prior to milling to raise the lactic acid concentration above 0.35% in toxic vats. All nontoxic vats produced during the same time frame had lactic acid concentration above 0.40% at milling.

Also included in this chapter are cultural tests useful in diagnosing the microbial cause of inflammation in the mammary gland.

5.020 *Salmonella* Species Cultural Method (FDA-BAM, Class A1)

1. **Scope:** This method is applicable to all dairy products.
2. **References:** Chapter 2: Laboratory Quality Assurance and Safety.
   Chapter 3: Sampling Dairy and Related Products.
   Chapter 4: Preparation of Media, Dilution Water, and Sterilization.
   Chapter 9: Microbiological Methods for Dairy Products.
   Food and Drug Administration *Bacteriological Analytical Manual*: http://vm.cfsan.fda.gov/~ebam/bam-toc.html.
3. **Definition:** *Salmonella* are gram-negative rod-shaped enteric pathogens commonly isolated from fecal material and capable of extended survival in dry environments.
4. **Principle:** A milk or dairy product sample is introduced into a nutritious, nonselective medium to restore injured *Salmonella* cells to a stable physiological condition. Selective enrichment of the preenriched cultures increases the population of *Salmonella* relative to other microbial flora. Selective plating of the cultures on solid selective and differential media provides for isolation of pure colonies of suspect *Salmonella*. Biochemical tests are used to screen out most non-*Salmonella* isolates and serotyping is used to confirm the presence of the pathogen.
5. **Diluents, Culture Media, and Reagents:** For preparation of media and reagents refer to chapter 4.
   1. Lactose broth.
   2. Selenite cystine (SC) broth.
   3. Tetrathionate (TT) broth.
   4. Rappaport-Vassiliadis (RV) medium.
   5. Xylose lysine desoxycholate (XLD) agar.
   6. Hektoen enteric (HE) agar.
   7. Bismuth sulfite (BS) agar.
   8. Triple sugar iron agar (TSI).
   9. Tryptone (tryptophane) broth.
   10. Trypticase (tryptic) soy broth.
   11. Lauryl tryptose (LST) broth.
   12. Trypticase soy-tryptose broth (TSB).
   13. MR-VP broth.
   14. Simmons citrate agar.
   15. Urea broth.
   16. Urea broth (rapid).
   17. Malonate broth.
   18. Lysine iron agar (LIA) (Edwards and Fife).
   19. Lysine decarboxylase broth.
   20. Motility test medium (semisolid).
   21. Potassium cyanide (RCN) broth.
   22. Phenol red carbohydrate broth.
   23. Purple carbohydrate broth.
   24. MacConkey agar.
   25. Nutrient broth.
   26. Brain heart infusion (BHI) broth.
   27. Gelatinase solution: 5%.

28. Tryptose blood agar base.
29. Potassium sulfite powder, anhydrous.
30. Chlorine solution: 200 ppm, containing 0.1% sodium dodecyl sulfate.
31. Ethanol: 70%.
32. Kovacs' reagent.
33. Voges-Proskauer (VP) test reagents.
34. Creatine phosphate crystals.
35. Potassium hydroxide solution: 40%.
36. Sodium hydroxide solution: 1N.
37. Hydrochloric acid: 1N.
38. Brilliant green dye solution: 1%.
39. Bromcresol purple dye solution: 0.2%.
40. Methyl red indicator.
41. Sterile distilled water.
42. Tergitol Anionic 7.
43. Triton X-100.
44. Physiological saline solution: 0.85% (sterile).
45. Formalinized physiological saline solution.
46. *Salmonella* polyvalent somatic (O) antiserum.
47. *Salmonella* polyvalent flagellar (H) antiserum.
48. *Salmonella* somatic group (O) antisera: A, B, C_1 C_2, C_3, D_1, D_2, E_1, E_2, E_3, E_4, F, G, H, I, Vi, and other groups, as appropriate.
49. *Salmonella* Spicer-Edwards flagellar (H) antisera.

6. Apparatus and Glassware

1. Blender and sterile blender jars.
2. Sterile, 16-oz (500-mL) wide-mouth, screw-cap jars, sterile 500-mL Erlenmeyer flasks, sterile 250-mL beakers, sterile glass or paper funnels of appropriate size, and, optionally, containers of appropriate capacity to accommodate composited samples.
3. Sterile bent-glass or plastic spreader rods.
4. Balance with weights: 2000-g capacity, sensitivity of 0.1 g.
5. Balance with weights: 120-g capacity, sensitivity of 5 mg.
6. Incubator: 35° ± 1°C.
7. Refrigerated incubator or laboratory refrigerator: 4° ± 1°C.
8. Water bath: 48° to 50°C.
9. Water bath: 43° ± 0.2°C.
10. Water bath: 42° ± 0.2°C.
11. Sterile spoons or other appropriate instruments for transferring food samples.
12. Sterile culture dishes: 15 × 100 mm, glass or plastic.
13. Sterile pipets: 1 mL, with 0.01-mL graduations; 5 and 10 mL, with 0.1-mL graduations.
14. Inoculating needle and inoculating loop (about 3 mm id or 10 µL): nichrome, platinum-iridium, chromel wire, or sterile plastic.
15. Sterile test or culture tubes: 16 × 150 mm and 20 × 150 mm; serological tubes, 10 × 75 mm or 13 × 100 mm.
16. Test or culture tube racks.
17. Vortex mixer.

18. Sterile shears, large scissors, scalpel, and forceps.
19. Lamp (for observing serological reactions).
20. Fisher or Bunsen burner.
21. pH test paper (pH range 6 to 8): With maximum graduations of 0.4 pH units per color change.
22. pH meter.

7. Sampling and Pre-enrichment: The following methods are based on the analysis of a 25-g analytical unit at a 1:9 sample to broth ratio. With composited samples or other sample sizes, add enough broth to maintain a 1:9 ratio unless otherwise indicated.

A. **Liquid milk (skim milk, 2% fat milk, or whole and buttermilk) and frozen desserts:** Do not thaw frozen samples before analysis. If frozen samples must be tempered to obtain the analytical portion, thaw suitable portion as rapidly as possible to minimize increase in number of competing microflora and to reduce the potential of injuring *Salmonella* organisms. Thaw below 45° ± 1°C for 15 minutes with continuous agitation in a thermostatically controlled water bath, or thaw within 18 hours at 2° to 5°C. Aseptically weigh a 25-g sample into sterile, wide-mouth, screw-cap jar (500 mL) or other appropriate container and add 225 mL sterile lactose broth. Cap jar securely and let stand 60 minutes at room temperature. Mix well by swirling and determine pH with test paper. Adjust pH, if necessary, to 6.8 ± 0.2 with sterile 1 N NaOH or 1 N HCl. Cap jar securely and mix well before determining final pH. Loosen jar cap about ¼ turn and incubate 24 ± 2 hours at 35° ± 1°C. Continue as in 5.020.9 below.

B. **Nonfat dry milk**

1. **Instant:** Aseptically weigh 25-g sample into sterile beaker (250 mL) or other appropriate container. Using sterile glass or paper funnel (made with tape to withstand autoclaving), pour 25-g analytical units gently and slowly over surface of 225 mL brilliant green water contained in sterile 500-mL Erlenmeyer flask or other appropriate container. Alternatively, 25-g analytical units may be composited and poured over the surface of proportionately larger volumes of brilliant green water. Prepare brilliant green water by adding 2 mL 1% brilliant green dye solution per 1000 mL sterile distilled water and let stand undisturbed for 60 ± 5 minutes. Incubate loosely capped inoculated container, without mixing or pH adjustment, for 24 ± 2 hours at 35° ± 1°C. Continue as in 5.020.9.
2. **Noninstant:** Examine as described for instant nonfat dry milk, except that the 25-g analytical units may not be composited as described in 5.020.7.B1.
3. **Dry whole milk:** Aseptically weigh 25-g sample into sterile, wide-mouth, screw-cap jar (500 mL) or other appropriate container. Add 225 mL sterile distilled water and mix well by swirling. Cap jar securely and let stand 60 minutes at room temperature. Mix well by swirling and determine pH with test paper. Adjust pH, if necessary, to 6.8 ± 0.2. Cap jar securely and mix well before determining final pH. Add 0.45 mL 1% aqueous brilliant green dye solution

and mix well. Loosen jar cap ¼ turn and incubate jar 24 ± 2 h at 35° ± 1°C. Continue as in 5.020.9.

4. **Casein:** Aseptically weigh 25-g sample into sterile blender jar. Add 225 mL sterile lactose broth to sample and blend for 2 minutes. Aseptically transfer blended homogenate into sterile, wide-mouth, screw-cap jar (500 mL) or other appropriate container. Cap jar securely and let stand 60 minutes at room temperature. Mix well by shaking and determine pH with test paper. Adjust pH, if necessary, to 6.8 ± 0.2. Cap jar securely and mix well before determining final pH. Loosen jar cap ¼ turn and incubate jar 24 ± 2 hours at 35° ± 1°C. Continue as in 5.020.9.

8. **Preparation of Test Sample:** All samples should be aseptically mixed, stirred, blended, or otherwise prepared to make samples uniform.

9. **Procedure**

A. **Isolation of *Salmonella***

1. **Selective enrichment:** Tighten lid and gently shake incubated sample. Transfer 1-mL mixture to 10-mL selenite cystine (SC) broth and another 1-mL mixture to 10-mL tetrathionate (TT) broth. For highly contaminated samples, transfer 0.1-mL mixture to 10-mL Rappaport-Vassiliadis (RV) medium and another 1-mL mixture to 10-mL TT broth.
2. **Incubation of selective enrichment:** Incubate SC and TT broths 24 ± 2 hours at 35° ± 1°C. For highly contaminated samples, incubate RV medium 24 ± 2 hours at 42° ± 0.2°C (water bath). Incubate TT broth 24 ± 2 hours at 43° ± 0.2°C (water bath).
3. **Selective plating and incubation:** Mix (vortex, if tube) and streak 3-mm loopful (10 µL) incubated TT broth on bismuth sulfite (BS) agar, xylose lysine desoxycholate (XLD) agar, and Hektoen enteric (HE) agar. Prepare BS plates the day before streaking and store in dark at room temperature until streaked.

   Repeat with 3-mm loopful (10 µL) of RV medium (for samples that may be highly contaminated) and SC broth (for samples that may be highly contaminated).

   Reference AOAC[10] for option of refrigerating incubated sample preenrichments and incubated sample selective enrichments (SC and TT broths only). This option allows sample analyses to be initiated as late as Thursday while still avoiding weekend work.

   Incubate plates 24 ± 2 hours at 35° ± 1°C.
4. **Colony selection:** Examine selective agar plates for presence of colonies that may be *Salmonella.* Typical *Salmonella* colony morphology:

   a. Pick 2 or more colonies of *Salmonella* from each selective agar after 24 ± 2 hours incubation. Typical *Salmonella* colonies are as follows:

      (1) **Hektoen enteric (HE) agar:** Blue-green to blue colonies with or without black centers. Many cultures of *Salmonella* may produce colonies with large, glossy black centers or may appear as almost completely black colonies.

(2) **Xylose lysine desoxycholate (XLD) agar:** Pink colonies with or without black centers. Many cultures of *Salmonella* may produce colonies with large, glossy black centers or may appear as almost completely black colonies.

(3) **Bismuth sulfite (BS) agar:** Brown, gray, or black colonies; sometimes they have a metallic sheen. Surrounding medium is usually brown at first, but may turn black in time with increased incubation, producing the so-called halo effect.

b. If typical colonies are present on the BS agar after 24 ± 2 hours incubation, then pick 2 or more colonies. Irrespective of whether or not BS agar plates are picked at 24 ± 2 hours, reincubate BS agar plates an additional 24 ± 2 hours. After 48 ± 2 hours incubation, pick 2 or more typical colonies, if present, from the BS agar plates, only if colonies picked from the BS agar plates incubated for 24 ± 2 hours give atypical reactions in triple sugar iron agar (TSI) and lysine iron agar (LIA) that result in culture being discarded as not being *Salmonella*. See section 5.020.9A.4d below for details in interpreting TSI and LIA reactions.

c. Lightly touch the very center of the colony to be picked with sterile inoculating needle and inoculate TSI slant by streaking slant and stabbing butt. Without flaming, inoculate LIA slant by stabbing butt twice and then streaking slant. Since lysine decarboxylation reaction is strictly anaerobic, the LIA slants must have deep butt (4 cm). Store picked selective agar plates at 5° to 8°C.

d. Incubate TSI and LIA slants at 35° ± 1°C for 24 ± 2 hours. Cap tubes loosely to maintain aerobic conditions while incubating slants to prevent excessive H_2S production. *Salmonella* in culture typically produces alkaline (red) slant and acid (yellow) butt, with or without production of H_2S (blackening of agar) in TSI. In LIA *Salmonella* typically produces alkaline (purple) reaction in butt of tube. Consider only distinct yellow in butt of tube as acidic (negative) reaction. Do not eliminate cultures that produce discoloration in butt of tube solely on this basis. Most *Salmonella* cultures produce H_2S in LIA. Some non-*Salmonella* cultures produce a brick-red reaction in LIA slants.

All cultures that give an alkaline butt in LIA, regardless of TSI reaction, should be retained as potential *Salmonella* isolates and submitted for biochemical and serological tests. Cultures that give an acid butt in LIA and an alkaline slant and acid butt in TSI should also be considered potential *Salmonella* isolates and should be submitted for biochemical and serological tests. Cultures that give an acid butt in LIA and an acid slant and acid butt in TSI may be discarded as not being *Salmonella*. Test retained, presumed-positive TSI cultures as directed in 5.020.9B.2 and following to determine if they are *Salmonella* species including *S. arizonae*. If TSI cultures fail to give typical reactions for *Salmonella* (alkaline slant and acid butt) pick additional suspicious colonies from selective medium plate not giving presumed-positive culture and inoculate TSI and LIA slants as described above.

e. Apply biochemical and serological identification tests to

(1) Three presumptive TSI cultures recovered from set of plates streaked from SC broth (or RV medium for appropriate foods), if present, and 3 presumptive TSI agar cultures recovered from plates streaked from TT broth, if present.

(2) If 3 presumptive-positive TSI cultures are not isolated from one set of agar plates, test other presumptive-positive TSI agar cultures, if isolated, by biochemical and serological tests. Examine a minimum of 6 TSI cultures for each 25-g analytical unit.

5. **Atypical *Salmonella* colony morphology**

a. In the absence of typical or suspicious *Salmonella* colonies, search for atypical *Salmonella* colonies as follows:

(1) **HE and XLD agars:** Atypically a few *Salmonella* cultures produce yellow colonies with or without black centers on HE and XLD agars. In the absence of typical *Salmonella* colonies on HE or XLD agars after 24 ± 2 hours incubation, then pick 2 or more atypical *Salmonella* colonies.

(2) **BS agar:** Atypically some strains produce green colonies with little or no darkening of the surrounding medium. If typical or suspicious colonies are not present on BS agar after 24 ± 2 hours, then do not pick any colonies but reincubate an additional 24 ± 2 hours. If typical or suspicious colonies are not present after 48 ± 2 hours incubation, then pick 2 or more atypical colonies.

B. **Identification of *Salmonella***

1. **Mixed cultures:** Streak TSI agar cultures that appear to be mixed on MacConkey agar, HE agar, or XLD agar. Incubate plates 24 ± 2 hours at 35° ± 1°C. Examine plates for presence of colonies suspected to be *Salmonella* and proceed as in 5.020.9A.4.

a. **MacConkey agar:** Typical colonies appear transparent and colorless, sometimes with dark center. Colonies of *Salmonella* will clear areas of precipitated bile caused by other organisms sometimes present.

b. **Hektoen enteric (HE) agar:** See 5.020.9A.4a(1) (above).

c. **Xylose lysine desoxycholate (XLD) agar:** See section 5.020.9A.4a(2) (above).

2. **Pure cultures screening**

a. **Urease test (conventional):** With sterile needle, inoculate growth from each presumed-positive TSI slant culture into tubes of urea broth. Since occasional, uninoculated tubes of urea broth turn purple-red (positive test) on standing, include uninoculated tube of this broth as control. Incubate 24 ± 2 hours at 35° ± 1°C.

b. **Optional urease test (rapid):** Transfer two 3-mm loopfuls of growth from each presumed-positive TSI slant culture into tubes of rapid urea broth. Incubate 2 hours in 37° ± 0.5°C water bath. Discard all cultures giving positive test. Retain for further study all cultures that give negative test (no change in color of medium).

3. **Serological polyvalent flagellar (H) test**
   a. Test for polyvalent flagellar (H) at this point, or later (5.020.9B.4). Inoculate growth from each urease-negative TSI agar slant into either 1) BHI broth and incubate 4 to 6 hours at 35° ± 1°C until visible growth occurs (to test on same day); or 2) trypticase soy-tryptose broth and incubate 24 ± 2 hours at 35° ± 1°C (to test on following day). Add 2.5-mL formalinized physiological saline solution to 5 mL of either broth culture.
   b. Select 2 formalinized broth cultures and test with *Salmonella* polyvalent flagellar (H) antisera. Place 0.5 mL of appropriately diluted *Salmonella* polyvalent flagellar (H) antiserum in 10 × 75 mm or 13 × 100 mm serological test tube. Add 0.5 mL antigen to be tested. Prepare saline control by mixing 0.5 mL formalinized physiological saline solution with 0.5 mL formalinized antigen. Incubate mixtures in 48° to 50°C water bath. Observe at 15 minute intervals and read final results in 1 hour.
      (1) **Positive:** Agglutination in test mixture and no agglutination in control.
      (2) **Negative:** No agglutination in test mixture and no agglutination in control.
      (3) **Nonspecific:** Agglutination in both test mixture and control. Test the cultures giving such results with Spicer-Edwards antisera.
4. **Spicer-Edwards serological test**[26]: Use this test as an alternative to the polyvalent flagellar (H) test. It may also be used with cultures giving nonspecific agglutination in polyvalent flagellar (H) test (see 5.020.9B.3b(3) above). Perform additional biochemical tests [5.020.9B.7] on cultures giving positive flagellar test results. If both formalinized broth cultures are negative, perform serological tests on 4 additional broth cultures. If possible, obtain 2 positive cultures for additional biochemical testing. If all urease-negative TSI cultures from sample give negative serological flagellar (H) test results, perform additional tests [5.020.9B.5 (below)].
5. **Testing of urease-negative cultures**
   a. **Lysine decarboxylase broth:** If LIA test was typical, it need not be repeated. Use lysine decarboxylase broth for final determination of lysine decarboxylase if culture gives doubtful LIA reaction. Inoculate broth with small amount of growth from TSI slant suspicious for *Salmonella*. Replace cap tightly and incubate 48 ± 2 hours at 35° ± 1°C but examine at 24-hour intervals. *Salmonella* species cause alkaline reactions indicated by purple color throughout medium. Negative test is indicated by yellow color throughout medium. If medium appears discolored (neither purple nor yellow) add a few drops of 0.2% bromcresol purple dye and reread tube reactions.

b. **Phenol red dulcitol broth or purple broth base with 0.5% dulcitol:** Inoculate broth with small amount of growth from TSI culture. Replace cap loosely and incubate 48 ± 2 hours at 35° ± 1°C, but examine after 24 hours. Most *Salmonella* species give positive test, indicated by gas formation in inner fermentation vial and acid pH (yellow) of medium. Production of acid should be interpreted as a positive reaction. Negative test is indicated by no gas formation in inner fermentation vial and red (with phenol red as indicator) or purple (with bromcresol purple as indicator) color throughout medium.

c. **Tryptone (or tryptophane) broth:** Inoculate broth with small growth from TSI agar culture. Incubate 24 ± 2 hours at 35° ± 1°C and proceed as follows:

(1) **Potassium cyanide (KCN) broth:** Transfer 3-mm loopful of 24-hour tryptophane broth culture to KCN broth. Heat rim of tube so that good seal is formed when tube is stoppered with wax-coated cork. Incubate 48 ± 2 hours at 35° ± 1°C, but examine after 24 hours. Interpret growth (indicated by turbidity) as positive. Most *Salmonella* species do not grow in this medium, as indicated by lack of turbidity.

(2) **Malonate broth:** Transfer 3-mm loopful of 24-hour tryptone broth culture to malonate broth. Since occasional uninoculated tubes of malonate broth turn blue (positive test) on standing, include uninoculated tube of this broth as control. Incubate 48 ± 2 hours at 35° ± 1°C, but examine after 24 hours. Most *Salmonella* species cultures give negative test (green or unchanged color) in this broth.

(3) **Indole test:** Transfer 5 mL of 24-hour tryptophane broth culture to empty test tube. Add 0.2 to 0.3 mL Kovacs' reagent. Most *Salmonella* cultures give negative test (lack of deep red color at surface of broth). Record intermediate shades of orange and pink as ±.

(4) **Serological flagellar (H) tests for *Salmonella*:** If the polyvalent flagellar (H) test [5.020.9B.3] or the Spicer-Edwards flagellar (H) test tube test [5.020.9B.4] have not been performed, either test should be performed here.

Discard as not *Salmonella* any culture that shows either positive indole test and negative serological flagellar (H) test, or positive KCN test and negative lysine decarboxylase test.

6. **Serological somatic (O) tests for *Salmonella*:** Pretest all antisera with known cultures.

a. **Polyvalent somatic (O) test:** Using a wax pencil, mark off 2 sections about 1 × 2 cm each on inside of glass or plastic petri dish (15 × 100 mm). Commercially available sectioned slides may be used. Emulsify 3-mm loopful of culture from 24- to 48-hour TSI slant or, preferably, tryptose blood agar base (without blood) with 2 mL 0.85% saline. Add 1 drop of culture suspension to upper portion of each rectangular marked section. Add 1 drop of saline solution to lower part of 1 section only. Add 1 drop of *Salmonella* polyvalent somatic (O) antiserum to upper section only. With clean sterile transfer loop or needle, mix culture suspension with saline solution for 1 section and repeat for other section containing antiserum. Tilt mixtures in a back-and-forth motion for 1 minute and observe against dark background in good illumination. Consider any degree of agglutination a positive reaction. Classify polyvalent somatic (O) test results as follows:

(1) **Positive:** Agglutination in test mixture; no agglutination in saline control.

(2) **Negative:** No agglutination in test mixture; no agglutination in saline control.

(3) **Nonspecific:** Agglutination in test and in control mixtures. Perform further biochemical and serological tests as described in *Edwards and Ewing's Identification of Enterobacteriaceae*.[26]

b. **Somatic (O) group tests:** Test as above, using individual group somatic (O) antisera including V_i, if available, in place of *Salmonella* polyvalent somatic (O) antiserum. For special treatment of cultures giving positive V_i agglutination reaction, refer to AOAC.[10] Record cultures that give positive agglutination with individual somatic (O) antiserum as positive for that

Table 5.1. Biochemical and Serological Reactions of *Salmonella*

	Salmonella Species		
Test or Substrate	**Positive**	**Negative**	**Reaction[a]**
1. Glucose (TSI)	yellow butt	red butt	+
2. Lysine decarboxylase (LIA)	purple butt	yellow butt	+
3. H_2S (TSI and LIA)	blackening	no blackening	+
4. Urease	purple-red color	no color change	–
5. Lysine decarboxylase broth	purple color	yellow color	+
6. Phenol red dulcitol broth	yellow color and/or gas	no gas; no color change	+[b]
7. KCN broth	growth	no growth	–
8. Malonate broth	blue color	no color change	–[c]
9. Indole test	violet color at surface	yellow color at surface	–
10. Polyvalent flagellar test	agglutination	no agglutination	+
11. Polyvalent somatic test	agglutination	no agglutination	+
12. Phenol red lactose broth	yellow color and/or gas	no gas; no color change	–[c]
13. Phenol red sucrose broth	yellow color and/or gas	no gas; no color change	–
14. Voges-Proskauer test	pink-to-red color	no color change	–
15. Methyl red test	diffuse red color	diffuse yellow color	+
16. Simmons citrate	growth; blue color	no growth; no color change	v

[a]+, 90% or more positive in 1 or 2 days; –, 90% or more negative in 1 or 2 days; v, variable.
[b]Majority of *S. arizonae* cultures are negative.
[c]Majority of *S. arizonae* cultures are positive.

group. Record cultures that do not react with individual somatic (O) antiserum as negative for that group.

7. **Additional biochemical tests:** Classify as *Salmonella* those cultures that exhibit typical *Salmonella* reactions for tests 1–11, shown in Table 5.1. If 1 TSI culture from a 25-g analytical unit is classified as *Salmonella*, further testing of other TSI cultures from the same 25-g analytical unit is unnecessary. Cultures that contain demonstrable *Salmonella* antigens as shown by positive *Salmonella* flagellar (H) test but do not have biochemical characteristics of *Salmonella* should be purified and retested, beginning with 5.020.9A.4. Perform the following additional tests on cultures that do not give typical *Salmonella* reactions for tests 1–11 in Table 5.1 and that consequently do not classify as *Salmonella.*
   a. **Phenol red lactose broth or purple lactose broth:** Inoculate broth with small amount of growth from unclassified 24- to 48-hour TSI slant. Incubate 48 ± 2 hours at 35° ± 1°C, but examine after 24 hours.
      (1) **Positive:** Acid production (yellow) and gas production in inner fermentation vial. Consider production of acid with no gas as a positive reaction. Most cultures of *Salmonella* give negative test results, indicated by no gas formation in inner fermentation vial and red (with phenol red as indicator) or purple (with bromcresol purple as indicator) throughout medium. Discard as not *Salmonella* those cultures that give positive lactose tests, except cultures that give acid slants in TSI and positive reactions in LIA, or cultures that give positive malonate broth reactions. Perform further tests on these cultures to determine if they are *S. arizonae.*
   b. **Phenol red sucrose broth or purple sucrose broth:** Follow procedure described above. Discard as not *Salmonella* those cultures that give positive sucrose tests, except those that give acid slants in TSI and positive reactions in LIA.
   c. **MR-VP broth:** Inoculate medium with small amount of growth from each unclassified TSI slant suspected to contain *Salmonella.* Incubate 48 ± 2 hours at 35° ± 1°C.
      (1) **Perform Voges-Proskauer (VP) test at room temperature as follows:** Transfer 1 mL 48-hour culture to test tube and incubate remainder of MR-VP broth an additional 48 hours at 35° ±1°C. Add 0.6 mL alpha-naphthol and shake well. Add 0.2 mL 40% KOH solution and shake. To intensify and speed reaction, add a few crystals of creatine. Read results after 4 hours; development of pink-to-ruby red color throughout medium is positive test. Most cultures of *Salmonella* are VP-negative, indicated by absence of development of pink-to-red color throughout broth.
      (2) **Perform methyl red test as follows:** Transfer 5 mL of 96-hour MR-VP broth, add 5 to 6 drops of methyl red indicator. Read results immediately. Most *Salmonella* cultures give positive test, indicated by diffuse red color in medium. A dis-

Table 5.2. Criteria for Discarding Non-*Salmonella* Cultures

Test or Substrate	Results
1. Urease	positive (purple-red color)
2. Indole test	positive (violet color at surface)
Polyvalent flagellar (H) test or Spicer-Edwards flagellar test	negative (no agglutination)
3. Lysine decarboxylase	negative (yellow color)
KCN broth	positive (growth)
4. Phenol red lactose broth	positive (yellow color and/or gas)[a,b]
5. Phenol red sucrose broth	positive (yellow color and/or gas)[a]
6. KCN broth	positive (growth)
Voges-Proskauer test	positive (pink-to-red color)
Methyl red test	negative (diffuse yellow color)

[a]Test malonate broth positive cultures further to determine if they are *Salmonella arizonae.*

[b]Do not discard positive broth cultures if corresponding LIA cultures give typical *Salmonella* reactions; test further to determine if they are *Salmonella* species.

tinct yellow color is negative test. Discard as not *Salmonella* those cultures that give positive KCN and VP tests and negative methyl red test.

d. **Simmons citrate agar:** Inoculate this agar using a needle containing growth from unclassified TSI agar slant. Inoculate by streaking slant and stabbing butt. Incubate 96 ± 2 hours at 35° ± 1°C. Read results as follows:
   (1) **Positive:** Presence of growth, usually accompanied by color change from green to blue. Most cultures of *Salmonella* are citrate-positive.
   (2) **Negative:** No growth or very little growth and no color change.

8. **Classification of cultures:** Classify as *Salmonella* cultures that have reaction patterns comparable to those in Table 5.1. Discard as not *Salmonella* cultures that give results listed in any subdivision of Table 5.2. Perform additional tests described in *Edwards and Ewing's Identification of Enterobacteriaceae*[26] to classify any culture that is not clearly identified as *Salmonella* by classification scheme in Table 5.1, or not eliminated as not being *Salmonella* by test reactions in Table 5.2. If neither of 2 TSI cultures carried through biochemical tests confirms the isolate as *Salmonella,* perform biochemical tests beginning with those in 5.020.9B.5 on remaining urease-negative TSI cultures from same 25-g analytical unit.
   a. **Presumptive generic identification of *Salmonella*:** As alternative to conventional biochemical tube system, use any of 5 commercial biochemical systems (API 20E–Class B, Enterotube II–Class B, Enterobacteriaceae II–Class B, MICRO-ID–Class B, or Vitek GNI–Class B) for presumptive generic identification of foodborne *Salmonella*. Choose a commercial system based on a demonstration in the analyst's own laboratory of adequate correlation between commercial system and biochemical tube system delineated in this identification section. Commercial bio-

chemical kits should not be used as a substitute for serological tests. Assemble supplies and prepare reagents required for the kit. Inoculate each unit according to manufacturer's instructions and incubate for time and temperature specified. Add reagents, observe, and record results.

For presumptive identification, classify cultures as *Salmonella* or not *Salmonella*, according to reaction patterns in Table 5.1.

b. For confirmation of cultures presumptively identified as *Salmonella*, perform the *Salmonella* serological somatic (O) test [5.020.9B.6] or the Spicer-Edwards flagellar (H) test [5.020.9B.4], and classify cultures according to the following guidelines:
   (1) Report as *Salmonella* those cultures classified as presumptive *Salmonella* with commercial biochemical kits when the culture demonstrates positive *Salmonella* somatic (O) test and positive *Salmonella* (H) test.
   (2) Discard cultures presumptively classified as not *Salmonella* with commercial biochemical kits when cultures conform to Table 5.2 criteria for classifying cultures as not *Salmonella*.
   (3) Classify atypical cultures according to additional tests specified in 9.020.9A.5 or additional tests as specified by Ewing,[26] or send to a reference typing laboratory for definitive serotyping and identification.

9. **Treatment of cultures giving negative flagellar (H) test:** If biochemical reactions of certain flagellar (H)-negative culture strongly suggest that it is *Salmonella*, the negative flagellar agglutination may be the result of nonmotile organisms or insufficient development of flagellar antigen. Proceed as follows:
   a. Inoculate motility test medium in petri dish, using small amount of growth from TSI slant. Inoculate by stabbing medium once about 10 mm from edge of plate to depth of 2 to 3 mm. Do not stab to bottom of plate or inoculate any other portion.
   b. Incubate 24 hours at 35 ± 1°C. If organisms have migrated 40 mm or more, retest as follows:
      (1) Transfer 3-mm loopful of growth that migrated farthest to trypticase soy-tryptose broth.
      (2) Repeat either polyvalent flagellar (H) or Spicer-Edwards [5.020.9B.3, -B.4] serological tests. If cultures are not motile after the first 24 hours, incubate an additional 24 hours at 35° ± 1°C; if still not motile, incubate up to 5 days at 25° ± 1°C.
      (3) Classify culture as nonmotile if above tests are still negative.
10. **Suggested control cultures:** In addition to the positive control cultures (typical *Salmonella*), 3 additional *Salmonella* cultures are recommended to assist in the selection of atypical *Salmonella* colony morphology on selective agars. These cultures are a lactose-positive, H_2S-positive *S. arizonae* (ATCC 12325) and a lactose-negative, H_2S-negative *S abortus equi* (ATCC 9842); OR a lactose-positive, H_2S-negative *S diarizonae* (ATCC 29934). These cultures may be obtained from the American Type Culture Collection, 10801 University Boulevard, Manassas, VA 20110-2209.

10. **Expression of Results:** Express as the presence or absence of *Salmonella* in the test portion specifying the mass in grams or the volume in milliliters of sample tested.

11. **Precision:** See chapter 1: Precision Parameters.

12. **Test Report:** The test report shall identify the method used and results obtained. The report will also identify any variation in the test not specified in this method as well as problems that may have impacted the test result. Each sample will be described in such a manner as to ensure traceability as to its origin.

5.030 Rapid Screening Tests for *Salmonella*

5.031 *Introduction*

Rapid screening methods are acceptable alternatives to conventional culture methods for detection of *Salmonella* in foods based on comparative studies that establish that they are equivalent to the standard culture methods.[1] Because of the public health, regulatory, and potential legal significance of *Salmonella* in foods, validation of method performance by a widely accepted protocol is desirable. Numerous rapid methods have been proposed for detection of *Salmonella* in foods that employ a variety of technologies ranging from relatively simple rapid biochemical screening to sophisticated nucleic acid amplification and detection systems. The objective of this section is to present rapid methods that have been validated against a standard method using a widely recognized and accepted protocol.

The most widely recognized and accepted method validation schemes are the ISO and AOAC International's Official Methods of Analysis (AOAC-OMA) program. The AOAC Research Institute (AOAC-RI) performance tested program was developed to specifically address the validation of rapid test kits containing proprietary components. Several rapid methods for *Salmonella* have been evaluated via the AOAC-OMA and AOAC-RI programs. A number of rapid test kits have also been evaluated against the ISO *Salmonella* method. These evaluations have employed various validation schemes that are accepted in specific countries but not on an international basis. Therefore, the methods described below are limited to those validated by AOAC-OMA and AOAC-RI.

These 2 validation schemes differ principally in that the AOAC-OMA program requires that a collaborative study be performed involving several laboratories. The AOAC-RI program requires independent laboratory verification of selected claims made by the manufacturer of the test kit. Both programs require that the manufacturer of the kit supply an extensive amount of data to verify performance parameters (e.g., sensitivity, specificity, range of application to products) inclusively with regard to *Salmonella* and exclusivity to competing organisms. The AOAC-RI program also includes verification of the manufacturers' quality systems for production, shelf life of the kit, and ruggedness testing of the method across a range of conditions that might be encountered in routine use.

The validated rapid methods are most often screening tests that require confirmation. If the screening methods are more productive than the standard culture method, positive assays may be obtained with the rapid method that cannot be confirmed culturally. These reactions are considered false-positives, but may in fact represent "true-positives" that cannot be confirmed because of failure of the confirmation procedure. In other cases, the rapid method may be as sensitive in detection of salmonellae as the cultural method, but not produce identical results (i.e., neither method provides 100% detection, but false-negative rates are similar). In comparing data, consider that the basis for detection of *Salmonella* by the rapid methods is normally different from that for isolation by culture methods, but both usually rely on pre- and selective enrichment steps.

Positive results by culture methods require that 3 cultural conditions be met. First, *Salmonella* must grow to the level necessary to ensure that cells are transferred into selective enrichments. Second, a sufficient number of salmonellae must be present in at least one of the selective enrichment cultures to ensure that one *Salmonella* cell is streaked onto a selective plate. Third, the relative proportion of salmonellae to other organisms capable of growth on the selective/differential isolation media must be such that at least one isolated colony of *Salmonella* can be obtained. The basis for obtaining positive results by culture is primarily selectivity and the importance of preenrichment for resuscitation of injured cells cannot be minimized.

Rapid screening methods require that a sufficient number of salmonellae/mL be present to allow detection by DNA hybridization or serological or biochemical tests. High numbers of competitors might inhibit growth of salmonellae to the level necessary for detection by the rapid methods as well as prevent isolation by standard culture conditions. However, under certain conditions sufficient numbers of salmonellae could develop to produce positive results by the rapid assays, but not by the culture procedure because of large populations of competitive flora (e.g., swarming *Proteus*). Additionally, other conditions could allow cultural isolation of *Salmonella* present at levels below the threshold sensitivity of rapid methods.

It is probably unrealistic to expect 100% agreement between conventional culture and rapid assay results due to the differences in detection methods. The high sensitivity of standard cultural methods for *Salmonella* will ensure a high agreement between approved rapid and conventional culture methods.[1] Rapid methods that have been evaluated by AOAC and/or AOAC-RI are discussed briefly, but not in the detail needed to perform the test. The published method (AOAC-OMA) and the package insert for the kit (AOAC-RI) should be consulted for performance of the methods.

5.032 *Fluorescent Antibody Method—Class O*[45]

Many of the rapid methods proposed for detection of salmonellae are based on immunological reactions. The fluorescent-antibody (FA) technique was the first immunological method applied to the detection of salmonellae. Thomason et al.[60] reported that the 0, V_i and H antigens of *Salmonella typhi* could be stained with fluorescent-labeled antibodies and observed by fluorescence microscopy. With the advent of antisera of greater sensitivity and specificity, a protocol was developed for detection of salmonellae in foods.

A historical summary of the development of the FA–Class O procedure has been published.[59] The AOAC-approved method employs a 24-hour preenrichment (for all foods but raw meat samples, which are placed directly in selective enrichment), and a 24-hour selective enrichment followed by a 4-hour postenrichment.[27] Portions of the postenrichment are then stained and examined for fluorescent cells. The presence of fluorescent cells morphologically typical of salmonellae constitutes a presumptive-positive result that must be confirmed by cultural methods. Negative results are generally available 1 day earlier than with conventional culture methods.

Thomason et al.[60] compiled data from 3 studies and indicated a 97.6% agreement between standard culture methods and FA, and a false-negative and false-positive rate of 0.1% and 2.3%, respectively. However, some laboratories observed much higher false-positive rates, especially with certain products.[59] Staining and reading of stained slides is both laborious and subjective, requiring a high degree of technical training and experience.

5.033 *Hydrophobic Grid Membrane Filtration (HGMF)—Class A1*

This method uses a membrane filter impregnated with hydrophobic material in a grid pattern of 1,600 compartments.[2,55] The hydrophobic material acts as a barrier, preventing the spread of growth units between adjacent compartments. An appropriate dilution of an enriched sample is filtered. The HGMF filter is then placed on a plate of appropriate agar. Colonies are isolated within the grid following incubation.

A HGMF–Class A1 method for *Salmonella* has been approved by the AOAC for the analysis of 6 foods—nonfat dry milk, powdered eggs, cheese powders, pepper, chocolate, and raw poultry.[3,25] The test sample is incubated in the appropriate preenrichment medium for 18 to 24 hours at 35° ± 1°C. A 0.1-mL volume of the preenriched test sample is subcultured in 10 mL of tetrathionate brilliant green (TBG) broth. After 6 to 8 hours of incubation, a 1-mL portion of diluted (raw poultry) or undiluted (the other 5 foods) selective TBG enrichment is filtered through the HGMF. The filters are then placed on plates. Following incubation of the selective lysine agar (SLA) at 43° ± 1°C and the hektoen enteric (HE) agar plates at 35° ± 1°C for 24 hours, the filters are examined for *Salmonella*. Suspect colonies, if present, are confirmed by the conventional AOAC culture method.[14] Since the original collaborative study of the HGMF method, the method has been modified and SLA and HE plates replaced by a single EF-18 agar plate.[14]

Use of the HGMF–Class A1 method has limitations. Its performance beyond the analysis of the 6 foods previously mentioned has not been fully assessed. Further, the use of a single selective enrichment and a single selective plating agar may preclude the detection of strains that are more readily recovered by other selective enrichment broths and/or selective agars.

5.034 *Immunodiffusion–Class A1*[10,37]

Detection of *Salmonella* in the self-contained and disposable unit, *Salmonella* 1-2 TEST–Class A1 (BioControl Systems, Inc., Bothell, WA), is based on the formation of an opaque zone or band when *Salmonella* bacteria are immobilized by polyvalent H (flagellar) antibodies in a semisolid motility medium. The clear, plastic device consists of 2 interconnected chambers: a motility chamber containing L-serine and a peptone-based, nonselective motility medium and an inoculation chamber containing L-serine and tetrathionate broth with brilliant green dye (TBG).

Most food samples are preenriched for 24 ± 2 hours at 35° ± 1°C as described in the cultural reference method. The preenrichment culture is then seeded into the inoculation chamber of the 1-2 TEST system. Raw milk and products with potential for being highly contaminated are enriched and then transferred to TBG and incubated 6-8 hours at 42° ± 0.5°C.[22,29] Enrichment cultures of raw milk and other highly contaminated products are then added to the inoculation chamber of the 1-2 TEST system.[29] Preparation of the 1-2 unit involves 3 steps. First, the TBG in the inoculation chamber is activated by the addition of 1 drop of iodine-iodide solution. Then 1 drop of a *Salmonella* antibody solution is added to the motility chamber. The blue-colored antibody preparation facilitates reading of the immobilization reaction.

Following removal of the chamber plug that seals the opening between the motility chamber and the inoculation chamber, a 0.1-mL portion of preenrichment (processed food), or selective enrichment (highly contaminated products) culture is added to the inoculation chamber. The 1-2 unit is incubated for a minimum 14 hours at 35° ± 1°C. Motile *Salmonella* organisms, if present, migrate from the inoculation chamber into the motility chamber. A visible band of precipitation occurs where motile *Salmonella* and diffusing antibody interface. Such presumptive-positive reactions are then confirmed by streaking a loopful of TBG from the inoculation chamber onto selective plating media as described by the method.[4] Isolates are then confirmed using the reference method.

In addition to yielding presumptive-positive results for processed foods and raw milk samples 1 day earlier than with the conventional culture method, the *Salmonella* 1-2 TEST offers other advantages. It is easy to use, requires no specialized training or sophisticated equipment, and is readily adaptable for use in laboratories that handle small or large numbers of test samples. Because the detection of *Salmonella* by the 1-2 TEST is based on immunosuppression of motility, nonmotile serovars such as *S. gallinarum* and *S. pullorum* and other variants will not be detected.

In 1986, DeSmedt et al.[23] developed a motility enrichment technique based on the use of a semisolid selective medium. The analytical procedure consisted of preenrichment for 20 hours, followed by motility enrichment for 24 hours and serological tests on the migrated cultures. Since then, the method has undergone collaborative study in which it has been compared with the method of the International Office of Cocoa, Chocolate and Sugar Confectionery (IOCCC) for detecting *Salmonella* in cocoa and chocolate products.[46] The rapid immunodiffusion method has been found to be at least as sensitive as the IOCCC method and in some cases it has provided superior detection of lactose fermenting *Salmonella*. This method was subsequently compared to the AOAC reference method and a collaborative study performance.[22,38] The method was approved by AOAC in 1992 for detection of *Salmonella* in cocoa and chocolate products.

5.035 *Enzyme Immunoassays*

A. ***Salmonella*-Tek™–Class A1:** The *Salmonella*-Tek™–Class A1 employs 2 *Salmonella*-specific antibodies, MOPC 467 and 6H4. Preenrichment is in nonselective medium for 24 ± 2 hours at 35° ± 1°C, selective enrichment is in tetrathionate brilliant green broth (TBG) and selenite cystine (SC) for 18 to 24 hours, and postenrichment is in M broth for 6 hours (35° ± 1°C). A centrifugation and heating step is performed prior to the EIA procedure. After boiling, portions of the cooled M broth cultures are dispensed into the wells of the microelisa strips and incubated with agitation to allow capture of *Salmonella* antigens. The wells are then washed, and peroxidase-labeled conjugate binds to the captured *Salmonella* antigen (if present) to form an antibody-antigen antibody-peroxidase complex. Unbound conjugate is removed from the wells by washing, and enzyme substrate is added. If a blue color develops, the sample is presumptive-positive for *Salmonella*. The reaction is stopped with an acid solution that turns the blue color to an intense yellow. The plates are read on an EIA reader, all presumptive-positives must be confirmed culturally.

Five other EIA techniques, including enrichment protocols similar to *Salmonella*-Tek™–Class A1, have undergone comparative and collaborative studies.

B. **TECRA™–Class A1:** The TECRA™ EIA (Bioenterprises Pty. Ltd., Roseville, N.S.W., Australia), in contrast to *Salmonella*-Tek™, uses polyclonal rather than monoclonal antibodies. The assay is performed in microtiter plates or strip wells and can be read visually or spectrophotometrically. The TECRA™ EIA (AOAC[7,35,37]) method has no requirement for sophisticated instrumentation. Wash steps can be performed manually and assay results can be readily obtained visually, eliminating the need for an EIA spectrophotometer.

C. **Q-TROL™–Class A1:** The Q-TROL™–Class A1 *Salmonella* assay (Dynatech Laboratories, Inc., Chantilly, VA) uses monoclonal antibodies and a fluorogenic reagent. More than 1,700 food samples were analyzed by the Q-TROL™ culture method (AOAC[6]). A colorimetric enzyme assay using the substrate phenolphthalein monophosphate (PMP) and the enzyme alkaline phosphatase was also developed and compared with the fluorogenic assay. The results indicated that the colorimetric assay was at least as sensitive as the previously approved fluorogenic assay.[27,39]

D. **VIDAS SLM–Class A1:** The VIDAS SLM–Class A1 method for detection of *Salmonella* is an automated qualitative enzyme-linked fluorescent immunoassay. The VIDAS SLM method (AOAC[19]), including cultural enrichment steps and assay, requires 48 hours for completion. The enrichment sequence is similar to other EIA methods discussed above but has the advantage that the assay is fully automated.

E. **ASSURANCE EIA–Class A1:** (BioControl Systems, Inc., Bothell, WA) This is a polyclonal enzyme immonoassay using microwell plates. Results are read as optical density using a microplate reader. This test is readily automated.

F. **LOCATE EIA–Class A1:** Recently the LOCATE EIA–Class A1 method for *Salmonella* (Rhone-Poulenc Diagnostics, Ltd.) received AOAC approval.[42] This is a microactive assay similar to the *Salmonella*-Tek™–Class A1, TECRA™–Class A1, and the Assurance EIA–Class A1 assays and incorporates similar enrichment steps.

The extensive evaluations of the EIA methods clearly indicate that this technology is an attractive alternative to conventional culture methods for detection of salmonellae in foods. This analytical approach provides detection of salmonellae one day earlier than by conventional cultural methods, with low numbers of both false-negative and false-positive results for most processed products. Relatively high false-positive rates have been reported for some raw products.[20,21,24,35] Advantages of the methods include automation and a definitive endpoint that contrasts with the subjective interpretation associated with culture methods.

G. **DNA Hybridization–Class A4:** Genetic relatedness among related bacteria can be measured by a DNA hybridization (DNAH) technique that probes for unique nucleotide sequences in target organisms. The performance of a DNA probe hybridization assay for *Salmonella* in foods (GENE-TRAK Systems, Framingham, MA) was compared to the AOAC culture method.[40] The results showed that the sensitivity of the DNAH method compared favorably with the culture method under all test conditions and, in some cases, DNAH method appeared to provide superior detection.

A collaborative study compared the sensitivity of the DNAH procedure to the standard culture method for detection of *Salmonella* in 6 artificially contaminated foods: ground pepper, soy flour, dry whole egg, milk chocolate, nonfat dry milk, and raw deboned turkey.[36] The results of this collaborative study and earlier comparative studies led to an AOAC approval of the DNAH method.[5,34,36] The isotopic DNAH method includes preenrichment (18 to 24 hours), 6-hour selective enrichment in tetrathionate brilliant green broth (TBG) and selenite cystine broth (SC), and a 12 to 16 hour postenrichment in GN broth for processed foods. After inoculation of the postenrichment GN broth with 0.1 mL of each of the TBG and SC cultures, both selective enrichments are incubated for 12 to 16 hours. A portion of the GN enrichment culture is then filtered and the DNAH assay performed on the filters.

Positive reactions are reported when counts for the test filter are >500 cpm above the average of 3 negative control filters. The assay itself requires about 4 hours to perform and the culture steps required a minimum of 42 hours. Thus, the total time required for the DNAH method is 46 hours. The DNAH assay is a screening method and positive results are confirmed by culture methods. Both postenrichment and reincubated selective enrichment cultures are streaked to selective agar media for confirmation of positive DNAH assays.

Subsequent to approval of the isotopic DNAH method, a nonisotopic, colorimetric DNAH method was developed.[1,7] The colorimetric assay employed DNA probes different from those used in the isotopic method. The target for the colorimetric assay probes is ribosomal RNA (i.e., the assay is based on hybridization of the DNA probes to target rRNA). The assay, which is carried out in an aqueous environment, involves hybridization between rRNA and *Salmonella*-specific oligonucleotide probes, capture of rRNA target:DNA probe hybrids onto a solid support, and a colorimetric endpoint detection.

Following preenrichment, selective enrichment, and postenrichment of test samples as described above for the DNAH assay, bacteria are lysed and *Salmonella*-specific fluorescent-labeled detection and poly-deoxyadenylic acid (poly dA) capture probes are added. The mixture is then incubated to allow hybridization of both probes to target rRNA, if present. A polydeoxythymidylic acid (poly dT) coated plastic dipstick solid phase is then introduced into the hybridization solution. Base pairing between the poly dA tail sequence of the capture probe and the poly dT on the dipstick facilitates capture of the DNA probe:rRNA target hybrids onto the dipstick. Unbound labeled probe is removed by washing the dipstick, followed by incubation in a solution containing antifluorescent antibody (Ab) conjugated to horseradish peroxidase (HRP). The peroxidase conjugate binds to the fluorescent label on the hybridized detector probe. Unbound conjugate is washed away, and the dipstick is incubated in a substrate-chromogen solution. Reaction of HRP with substrate-chromagen results in development of a blue color. The enzyme/substrate reaction is stopped by addition of acid with a concomitant change in color from blue to yellow. Absorbance at 450 nm in excess of threshold value indicates the presence of *Salmonella* in the test samples.

The colorimetric DNAH assay can be completed in 2.5 hours following approximately 44 hours of culture enrichments. Chan et al.[14] compared the productivity of the colorimetric DNAH method with the AOAC culture method. An AOAC collaborative study was performed by Curiale et al.[17] and no significant difference appeared in the ability of the methods to detect salmonellae in any of the 6 artificially contaminated foods examined in this study. The method subsequently received AOAC approval.[18]

Table 5.3. AOAC-RI Performance Tested Methods for Detection of *Salmonella* in Foods and Environmental Samples (All methods are Class A4)

Test Kit	Manufacturer	License No.	Matrixes
Path-Stik	Lumac B.V.	941001	food
Reveal	Neogen	960801	food
Bioline ELISA	Bioline	961001	food
Salmonella Screen *Salmonella* Verify	Vicam L.P.	961002	food
Oxoid Rapid Test for *Salmonella* Samples	Oxoid Ltd.	960902	food, environmental
Salmonella DLP Assay	Gene-Trak Systems Corp.	961101	food, environmental
Dynabeads Anti-*Salmonella* Kit	Dynal S.A.	970401	food
BIND *Salmonella* Rapid Assay Kit	Idexx Laboratories, Inc.	970501	food
Bax for *Screening Salmonella*	Qualicon	970801	food
TECRA Unique *Salmonella*	TECRA Diagnostic	971001	food, environmental

5.036 *AOAC-RI Performance Tested Methods—Class A4*

Ten test kit methods for rapid detection of *Salmonella* species in foods have been certified as Performance Tested [Table 5.3]. Prior to 1998, AOAC-RI did not require that the data on which the certification was based be published. Therefore, the validation data for the approval of methods listed are not readily available in the scientific literature. Information on the methods and their performance should be requested directly from the manufacturers.

5.037 *Immunological-Based Tests*

A. ***Salmonella* Screen/*Salmonella* Verify–Class A4** *(Vicam L.P.):* This kit employs antibody coated magnetic beads to capture salmonellae from enrichment broths permitting competing microflora and food residues to be removed by washing. The captured *Salmonella* can then be plated directly to selective/differential agar media for isolation and identification. The Vicam *Salmonella* Verify kit includes a step where colonies developing from the beads can be quickly screened by a latex agglutination technique to determine if they are perspective *Salmonella* species.

B. **Dynabeads Anti-*Salmonella* Kit–Class A4:** *(Dynal, Inc.):* This kit employs anti-*Salmonella* magnetic labeled beads to capture salmonellae from enrichment broths and remove competing microflora and food residue. The captured *Salmonella* can then be plated directly to selective/differential agar media for isolation and identification.

C. **TECRA Unique *Salmonella*–Class A4** *(TECRA Diagnostics):* A 22-hour dipstick test that includes a 16-hour enrichment step followed by capture, wash, replication (4 to 5 hours at 35° to 37°C), conjugate binding, wash, and color development steps within a disposable device composed of a series of tubes containing the appropriate reagents.

D. **Bioline ELISA–Class A4 method** *(Bioline):* A 36-hour microtitre strip assay.

E. **Reveal dipstick–Class A4 method** *(Neogen Corp.):* An immunological dipstick method that has received AOAC-RI approval for food testing. This method includes preenrichment and selective enrichment steps followed by the dipstick assay.

F. **Path-Stik–Class A4 method** *(Celsis-Lumac Ltd):* An immunological dipstick method that has received AOAC-RI approval for food testing. This methods includes preenrichment and selective enrichment steps followed by the dipstick assay.

G. ***Salmonella* DLP Assay–Class A4:** Gene-Trak Systems Corp. has received Performance Tested certification for the food dipstick assay modification of its AOAC-OMA method.

H. **BAX–Class A4** *(Qualicon):* This is a one-day *Salmonella* detection method, BAX for screening *Salmonella*, based on polymerase chain reaction (PCR) amplification of *Salmonella*-specific nucleic acid. After preenrichment (20 hours) and a short (3 hours) secondary enrichment step, cells are lysed and added to PCR tubes, which contain the reagents, required to perform the amplification. *Salmonella*-specific PCR gene product is detected using a gel electrophoresis procedure. The BAX–Class A4 *Salmonella* method requires approximately 28 hours including enrichment, amplification, and assay steps.

I. **Oxoid *Salmonella* Rapid Test–Class A4** *(Unipath):* This is a biochemical screening method. Samples are preenriched (18 to 24 hours) in appropriate media and then aliquots transferred to a disposable culture vessel containing an elective medium and 2 tubes. Each tube contains a selective medium in the lower portion of the tube and an indicator medium in the upper portion separated by a porous partition. *Salmonella* grow in the elective enrichment and migrate into the tubes through the lower selective media to the upper indicator media where their presence is indicated by a color change. After a 24-hour incubation of the enrichment/screening system, tubes are examined for the possible presence of *Salmonella*. Tubes producing positive results are screened using the Oxoid *Salmonella* Latex Test, and positive reactors reported as presumptively containing *Salmonella*.

J. **Bind *Salmonella* Assay–Class A4** *(Idexx Laboratories):* This is a bacterial ice nucleation detection method. It is a one-day (22-hour) *Salmonella* screening method that includes preenrichment followed by a simple assay system based on bacteriophage infection of *Salmonella* resulting in expression of ice nucleation proteins that lead to ice crystal formation, which can be detected with a colorimetric assay.

5.040 *Listeria Monocytogenes* Cultural Method—(FDA-BAM, Class A1)

1. **Scope:** This method is applicable for the isolation of *Listeria* from raw milk, fluid dairy products, ice cream, dried dairy products, a variety of cheeses, and environmental test samples.
2. **References:** Chapter 2: Laboratory Quality Assurance and Safety.
   Chapter 3: Sampling Dairy and Related Products.
   Chapter 4: Preparation of Media, Dilution Water, and Sterilization.
   Chapter 9: Microbiological Methods for Dairy Products.
   Food and Drug Administration *Bacteriological Analytical Manual*:
   http://vm.cfsan.fda.gov/~ebam/bam-toc.html.
3. **Definition:** *Listeria monocytogenes* is a gram-positive, catalase positive, nonsporeforming rod that produces lactic acid from glucose and other fermentable sugars. It causes enteric and systemic infections in animals and man.
4. **Principle:** Milk, dairy product, or environmental samples are introduced into a nutritious, nonselective medium to restore injured *Listeria* cells to a stable physiological condition. Selective agents are added to the preenrichment culture to increase population of *Listeria* in relation to competing microflora. Plating of enrichment culture on solid selective and differential media is used to obtain isolated colonies of *Listeria*. Biochemical screening of isolated colonies, along with hemolytic response on sheep blood agar, provide identification of *L. monocytogenes* cultures.
5. **Diluents, Culture Media, and Reagents:** For preparation of media and reagents refer to AOAC.[8]
   1. Acriflavin HCl: 0.5% (w/v) filter-sterilized stock solution in distilled water.

2. Agar (Difco).
3. Blood agar base No. 2 (Unipath).
4. Cycloheximide: 1.0% (w/v) filter-sterilized stock solution in 40% (v/v) solution of ethanol in water.
5. Sheep blood: Defibrinated, sheep blood agar.
6. Ethanol: Absolute.
7. Glycine anhydride.
8. Gram stain kit.
9. Hydrogen peroxide solution: 3% for catalase test.
10. Lithium chloride-phenylethanol-moxalactam (LPM) agar; LPM + esculin/Fe^{3+}.
11. Nalidixic acid (sodium salt): 0.5% (w/v) filter-sterilized stock solution in distilled water.
12. Nutrient broth.
13. Physiological saline solution: 0.85%.
14. Carbohydrate fermentation broth containing 1 mL of a 0.5% (w/v) solution of dextrose, esculin, maltose, rhamnose, mannitol or xylose per 9 mL of purple carbohydrate fermentation broth base.
15. SIM medium or motility test medium (MTM).
16. Trypticase soy agar with 0.6% yeast extract (TSAYE).
17. Trypticase soy broth with 0.6% yeast extract (TSBYE).
18. Tryptose broth and agar.
19. Oxford medium (OXA).
20. Enrichment broth, pH 7.3 (EB).
21. PALCAM agar.

6. **Apparatus and Glassware**
   1. Balance: Gram-range.
   2. Coverslips: Glass.
   3. Erlenmeyer flask: 500 mL.
   4. Fermentation tubes (Durham).
   5. Grease pencil or magic marker.
   6. Incubators: 30° and 35° ± 1°C.
   7. Immersion oil.
   8. Inoculating loop.
   9. Inoculating needle.
   10. Microscope slides.
   11. Phase contrast microscope with oil immersion phase objective (100×).
   12. Petri plates.
   13. Pipets: 25, 10, and 1 mL.
   14. Test tubes: 16 × 124 mm or other appropriate sizes, screw cap.
   15. Blender and jars or stomacher and stomacher bags.
   16. Dissecting or low-power microscope with illuminator.

7. **Preparation of Test Sample:** All samples should be aseptically mixed, stirred, blended, or otherwise prepared to make samples uniform.

8. **Sample Preparation and Pre-enrichment:** The following method is based on the analysis of a 25-g analytical unit at a 1:9 sample/broth ratio. Products to be transported to the laboratory should be kept frozen if they were frozen when taken from the sampling site. If they were at any other

temperature they should be refrigerated at 4° ± 1°C until analyzed. In the laboratory the test sample, either liquid or solid, is added to the enrichment broth, pH 7.3 (EB) and macerated and blended by the stomacher. Blend or stomach as required for thorough mixing. Keep the EB culture in the blender jar or stomacher bag or alternatively, transfer to a sterile 500-mL Erlenmeyer flask. Incubate the EB culture 4 hours at 30° ± 1°C.

9. **Procedure for Isolation of *Listeria***

A. **Enrichment:** Add 0.455 mL acriflavin, 1.8 mL nalidixic acid, and 1.15 mL cycloheximide to the preenrichment culture and reincubate for 44 hours for a total of 48 hours (preenrichment and enrichment incubation time) at 30° ± 1°C.

B. **Isolation procedure**

1. After 24 and 48 hours of incubation, streak the EB culture to Oxford agar (OXA) and either lithium chloride-phenylethanol-moxalactam agar (LPM) (with or without esculin/Fe^{3+}) or PALCAM agar.
2. Incubate OXA and PALCAM plates at 35°C for 24 to 48 hours, and LPM plates at 30° ± 1°C for 24 to 48 hours.
3. Examine OXA and PALCAM for black colonies surrounded by black haloes, indicative of esculin hydrolysis. Examine LPM plates using a strong beam of white light that strikes the bottom of the plate at a 45° angle (Figure 5.1). When examined either directly or via a low-power or dissecting microscope (with the mirror detached) from an eye position directly above the plate (i.e., at 90° to the plate), suspect *Listeria* colonies appear sparkling blue (like bluish crushed glass) or white.
4. Transfer 5 or more typical colonies from OXA, PALCAM, and/or LPM to trypticase soy agar plus yeast extract (TSAYE) and streak for isolation.
5. Incubate TSAYE plates at 30° ± 1°C for 24 to 48 hours until growth is satisfactory.

C. **Identification procedure:** Examine the TSAYE plates for typical colonies using the modified Henry lighting arrangement. See Figure 5.1.

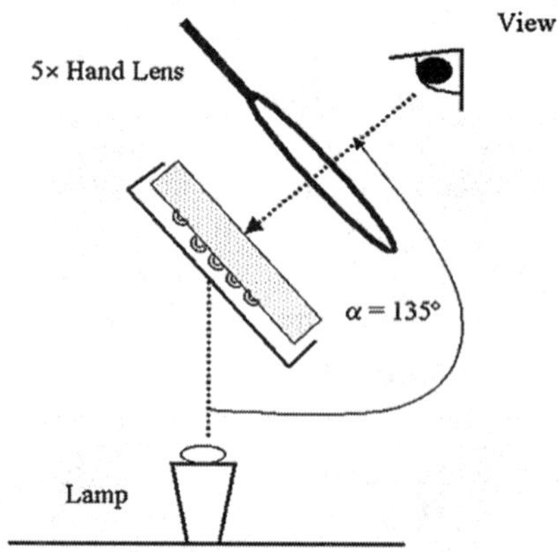

Figure 5.1. Modified Henry technique for observing bluish-green hue of *Listeria* colonies. Angle of transillumination (α = 135°).

1. Pick a typical colony and prepare a wet mount using 0.85% saline for the suspending medium. Be sure to choose a colony with sufficient growth to prepare a reasonably heavy suspension and emulsify thoroughly. If the suspension is too light, the few cells present will adhere to the glass and appear nonmotile. When viewed through the oil-immersion objective of a phase-contrast microscope, *Listeria* appears as a slim, short rod with slight rotating or tumbling motility. Always use a known culture for comparison. Cocci, large rods, or rods with rapid swimming motility are not *Listeria*.
2. Test a typical colony for catalase activity. All *Listeria* spp. are catalase-positive. Gram stain a 16- to 24-hour culture. All *Listeria* spp. are short, gram-positive rods with older cultures showing variable reactions and shorter coccoidal-like cells.
3. Transfer a typical colony into a tube of trypticase soy broth plus yeast extract (TSBYE) and incubate at 35°C for 24 hours. This culture, which can be kept at 4° ± 1°C for several days, will be used as the inoculum for various biochemical tests.
4. Draw a grid of 20 to 25 spaces on the backside of a heavily poured and well-dried (check for moisture before using) plate of sheep blood agar.
5. From the TSAYE plate, heavily stab 1 colony per grid space, reserving 3 grid spaces for 2 positive controls (*L. monocytogenes* and *Listeria ivanovii*) and 1 negative control (*Listeria innocua*).
6. Incubate the blood agar plate for 48 hours at 35° ± 1°C.
7. Examine the blood agar plate containing the culture stabs with a bright light. *L. monocytogenes* and *Listeria seeligeri* will produce zones of weak clearing around the stab. *L. innocua* produces no zone of hemolysis, whereas *L. ivanovii* produces a well-defined zone of clearing around the stab. Do not try to speciate the isolate at this point, but note the extent of hemolytic activity.
8. Inoculate SIM motility medium or motility test medium (MTM) from the TSBYE culture.
9. Observe daily during 7 days of incubation at room temperature (20° to 25°C). All *Listeria* are motile and produce a typical umbrella-like growth pattern.

Table 5.4. Differentiation of *Listeria* Species

Species	Hemolytic (beta)	Use Mannitol	Rhamnose	Sheep Xylose	Blood Stab
L. monocytogenes	+	–	+	–	+
L. ivanovii	+	–	–	+	+
L. innocua	–	–	V[a]	–	–
L. welshimeri	–	–	V[a]	+	–
L. seeligeri	+	–	–	+	+
L. grayi	–	+	–	–	–

[a] V = variable

10. From the TSBYE culture, inoculate the purple carbohydrate fermentation broth tubes containing dextrose, esculin, maltose, rhamnose, mannitol, and xylose (use of durham tubes is optional).
11. Incubate up to 7 days at 35° ± 1°C. Positive-reacting *Listeria* spp. produce acid without gas. All *Listeria* spp. should be positive for dextrose, esculin, and maltose, whereas all *Listeria* spp. except *Listeria grayi* should be negative for mannitol. [Note: The esculin test can be omitted if pigmentation of the isolate on OXA, PALCAM, or LPM plus esculin/Fe3+ is unequivocal.] Xylose-Rhamnose reactions for all six *Listeria* spp. are shown in Table 5.4.

D. **CAMP test:** The Christie-Atkins-Munch-Peterson (CAMP) test is useful for speciating *Listeria*, particularly when results from blood agar stabs are questionable. To perform the test, streak a *beta*-hemolytic strain of *Staphylococcus aureus* (ATCC 49444 or ATCC 25923) and a culture of *Rhodococcus equi* (ATCC 6939) (both available from the American Type Culture Collection, Manassas, VA) in parallel and diametrically opposed to each other on a plate of sheep blood agar. Separate these horizontal streaks so that the *Listeria* strains to be tested along with a positive control (*L. monocytogenes*) and negative control (*L. innocua*), which are to be streaked at a right angle to the horizontal streaks, are close to but not touching the horizontal streaks. After 24 to 48 hours of incubation at 35° ± 1° C, examine plates for enhanced hemolysis in the zone of influence near the horizontal streaks. Figure 5.2 shows the arrangement of the streaked cultures on a CAMP plate. Hemolytic activity of *L. monocytogenes* and *L. seeligeri* is enhanced near the *S. aureus* streak, whereas the hemolysis produced by *L. ivanovii* is stronger near the *R. equi* streak. The remaining *Listeria* spp. are non-hemolytic and do not react in this test. The CAMP test differentiates *L. ivanovii* from *L. seeligeri* and can differentiate a weakly hemolytic *L. seeligeri* from *L. welshimeri*. Isolates giving typical reactions for *L. monocytogenes* except for hemolysin production should be CAMP tested before being identified as non-hemolytic *L. innocua*.

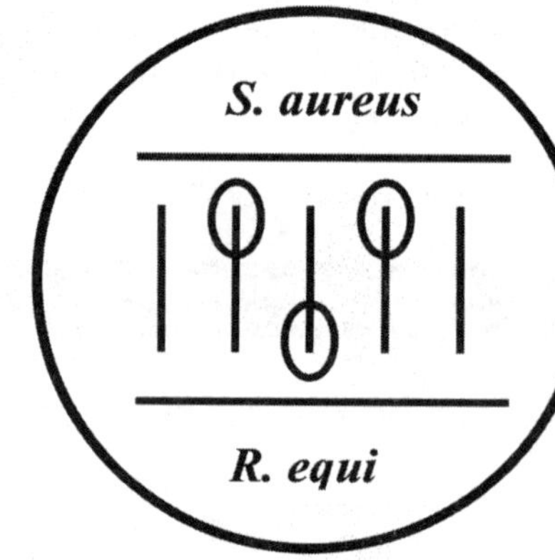

Figure 5.2. CAMP test on sheep blood agar plate. Horizontal streaks of *Staphylococcus aureus* (*S.aureus*) and *Rhodococcus equi* (*R. equi*). Typical hemolytic patterns for five species of *Listeria* streaked vertically are diagrammed. (L-R) *Listeria welshimeri, Listeria monocytogenes, Listeria ivanovii, Listeria seeligeri, Listeria innocua.*

E. **Speciation of *Listeria*:** All *Listeria* species are small, catalase-positive, gram-positive rods that are motile in wet mounts and exhibit an umbrella-like growth pattern in semi-solid motility media. Dextrose, esculin, and maltose are used by all *Listeria* with some species also using mannitol, rhamnose, and xylose with production of acid. *L. grayi* produces acid from mannitol. Since *L. monocytogenes*, *L. ivanovii*, and *L. seeligeri* hemolyze sheep blood, all 3 species yield a positive CAMP reaction. Of these 3, only *L. monocytogenes* fails to use xylose and is positive for rhamnose. Difficulties in differentiating *L. ivanovii* and *L. seeligeri* can be overcome using the CAMP test. Hemolytic activity of *L. seeligeri* is enhanced near the *S. aureus* streak whereas *L. ivanovii* shows particularly strong hemolysis near the *R. equi* streak. Among the nonhemolytic species, *L. innocua* may yield the same rhamnose-xylose reactions as *L. monocytogenes* but is negative in the CAMP test. Occasional isolates of *L. innocua* are unable to use both rhamnose and xylose. *L. welshimeri*, which is rhamnose positive, may be confused with a weakly hemolytic *L. seeligeri* unless resolved by the CAMP test.

10. **Expression of Results:** The results are expressed by presence or absence of *Listeria* in the test portion, specifying the mass in grams, or the volume in milliliters of sample tested.

11. **Precision:** There are no precision parameters for this test.

12. **Test Report:** The test report shall identify the method used and results obtained. The report will also identify any variation in the test not specified in this method as well as problems that may have impacted the test result. Each sample will be described in such a manner as to ensure traceability as to its origin.

5.041 *Cold Enrichment—Class O*

Isolation of *L. monocytogenes* from dairy products often proves to be challenging and regardless of the method used, *Listeria* must be isolated in pure culture and identified using the aforementioned biochemical tests. Early workers found that refrigerated storage of the specimen in a nonselective medium such as tryptose broth for 1 week to 6 months before plating on blood agar enhanced recovery of *Listeria*. This technique, known as cold enrichment, relies on the ability of *Listeria* to outcompete other microorganisms during cold storage and has been successfully used to recover *Listeria* from many foods.[43,62] However, the time-consuming nature of cold enrichment now precludes its routine use in food microbiology testing laboratories.

5.042 *International Dairy Federation (IDF) Method—Class A1*

The IDF method, which closely resembles the FDA method [5.050], is widely used in Europe for recovering *Listeria* spp. from dairy products.[8] Major differences between this method and the FDA method include: 1) use of the same enrichment broth with the same selective agents but without 4 hours of nonselective enrichment; 2) adjustment of the selective enrichment broth to pH 7.3 when testing acidic dairy products; and 3) use of Oxford agar as the only selective plating medium with the plates incubated for 48 hours at 37° ± 1°C rather than 35° ± 1°C. The IDF protocol for identifying suspected *Listeria* isolates is essentially identical to that used in the FDA method. AOAC International has adopted the IDF procedure as an official first action method for examining dairy products.[62]

5.043 *Rapid Methods*

Purified isolates can be rapidly identified (additional tests may be required to speciate completely) using any of the following biochemically based commercially available test kits: 20 S™–Class B or API-ZYM–Class B (Analytical Products)[62]; Vitek automicrobic gram-positive and gram-negative identification cards–Class A2 (BioMerieux Vitek)[8,32]; or API Listeria–Class B (BioMerieux Vitek).[32] The Micro-ID™ kit–Class A2 (Organon Teknika Corp.) allows speciation of *Listeria* provided the CAMP reaction is known.[8,32]

A variety of nonconventional rapid methods based on 1) detection of specific antigens in enzyme-linked immunosorbant assays (ELISA) by polyclonal or monoclonal antibodies, or 2) hybridization of *Listeria* DNA with a specifically labeled DNA probe has been developed for identifying *Listeria* to the genus and species level. These methods can be used to screen enrichment cultures and can greatly accelerate identification of *Listeria*-positive samples.[8,32] Commercially available AOAC approved ELISA test kits for identifying *Listeria* to the genus level include *Listeria*-Tek–Class A4 (Organon-Teknika), Assurance *Listeria*–Class B (BioControl Systems, Inc.),[8,30] and the TECRA Listeria Visual Immunoassay–Class A4 (Bioenterprises Pty. Ltd.).[32,49] VIP–Class A4, a visual immunoprecipitae assay (BioControl Systems, Inc.) for detecting *L. monocytogenes* and related species also has received AOAC approval.[54] Other genus-specific immunoassays include the fully automated VIDAS *Listeria* assay (Class A4, BioMerieux Vitek) and Listertest (Class A4, VICAM),[32] which uses immunomagnetic beads. The fully automated VIDAS *L. monocytogenes* assay is one of very few ELISA assays that is specific for *L. monocytogenes*.

Several nonradioactive DNA probe test kits are commercially available for identifying *Listeria* isolates to the genus or species level. The AOAC approved Gene-Trak Colorimetric Listeria assay–Class A2 (Gene-Trak Systems) is specific for the genus *Listeria*.[32] A similar *L. monocytogenes*-specific assay is also available from the same manufacturer and is awaiting AOAC approval. AccuProbe™–Class B, a chemilluminescent genus-specific assay (Gen-Probe), is suitable for identifying colonies from isolation or purification agar or in pure broth cultures.[32,62] Finally, Qualicon has recently developed two additional DNA-based *Listeria* identification systems: 1) the automated Riboprinter Microbial Characterization System–Class B, which will identify all pure *Listeria* cultures to the species level based on ribotype analysis, and 2) a PCR-based amplification method (Class B) for specific detection of *L. monocytogenes* in enrichment cultures.

5.050 *Staphylococcus Aureus* Direct Plate Count[9] (FDA-BAM, Class A1)

1. **Scope:** This method is suitable for the analysis of foods in which more than 100 *Staphylococcus aureus* cells per gram may be present.

2. **References:** Chapter 2: Laboratory Quality Assurance and Safety.
   Chapter 3: Sampling Dairy and Related Products.
   Chapter 4: Preparation of Media, Dilution Water, and Sterilization.
   Chapter 9: Microbiological Methods for Dairy Products.
   Food and Drug Administration *Bacteriological Analytical Manual*:
   http://vm.cfsan.fda.gov/~ebam/bam-toc.html.
3. **Definition:** *Staphylococcus aureus* are gram-positive, catalase-positive cocci that grow in grape-like clusters and produce a strongly positive coagulase reaction. They cause a variety of disease syndromes including gastroenteritis resulting from consumption of enterotoxin.
4. **Principle:** Serial dilutions of product are plated on a selective and differential agar medium to yield colonies typical of *S. aureus*. Colonies are confirmed by coagulase reaction. Numbers of *S. aureus* per gram of sample is calculated based on the proportion of coagulase positive colonies.
5. **Diluents, Culture Media, and Reagents:** For preparation of media and reagents refer to AOAC.[9]
   1. Baird-Parker medium (BP).
   2. Trypticase (tryptic) soy agar (TSA).
   3. Brain heart infusion (BHI) broth.
   4. Coagulase plasma (rabbit) with EDTA.
   5. Lysostaphin.
   6. Tryptone yeast extract agar.
   7. Paraffin oil: sterile.
   8. 0.02 M phosphate saline buffer, containing 1% NaCl.
   9. Hydrogen peroxide for catalase test: 3%.
6. **Apparatus and Glassware**
   1. Drying cabinet or incubator for drying surface of agar plates.
   2. Sterile streaking rods with an angled spreading surface 45 to 55 mm long.
   3. Same basic equipment as for conventional plate count.
7. **Sampling and Pre-enrichment:** If samples can not be examined immediately, samples should be frozen and stored at –20°C or lower until examined. Unfrozen samples should be refrigerated at 0° to 4°C until examined, but in no case should examination start after 36 hours of storage. Nonperishable, canned, or low-moisture food can be stored at room temperature until analysis is initiated.

   Liquid or solid milk or dairy foods are to be shaken or mixed thoroughly to ensure an even distribution of microorganisms in the sample. Preenrichment should not be used for the direct plate count procedure.
8. **Preparation of Test Sample:** Fifty grams of sample and 450 mL of Butterfield's phosphate-buffered dilution water are blended or stomached for 2 minutes. This is a 1:9 food to diluent ratio.

   Serial decimal dilutions are prepared and shaken vigorously 25 times in a 30-cm arc in 7 seconds.

   Not more that 15 minutes should elapse from the time sample is blended until all dilutions are plated on the selective-differential medium.

9. Procedure

A. **Plating:** For each dilution to be plated, aseptically transfer 1 mL sample suspension to 3 plates of BP agar medium, distributing the 1 mL of inoculum equally onto 3 plates. Spread inoculum over surface of agar plate using sterile spreading devices. Retain plates in upright position until inoculum is absorbed by agar medium (about 10 minutes on properly dried plates). If inoculum is not readily absorbed by medium, place plates upright in incubator for about 1 hour. Invert plates and incubate 45 to 48 hours at 35° ± 1°C. Select plates containing 20 to 200 colonies, unless only plates at lower dilutions (>200 colonies) have colonies with typical appearance of *S. aureus*. Colonies of *S. aureus* are typically circular, smooth, convex, moist, 2 to 3 mm in diameter on uncrowded plates, gray to jet-black, frequently with light-colored (off-white) margin, surrounded by opaque zone and frequently with an outer clear zone. Colonies have buttery to gummy consistency when touched with inoculating needle. Occasionally, nonlipolytic strains of similar appearance may be encountered, except that surrounding opaque and clear zones are absent. Strains isolated from frozen or desiccated foods that have been stored for extended periods frequently develop less black coloration than typical colonies and may have rough appearance and dry texture.

If several types of colonies that appear to be *S. aureus* are present, count the number of colonies of each type. Use plates of the lowest dilution plated, which contain <20 colonies. If plates containing >200 colonies of typical *S. aureus* appearance and plates of higher dilution have no typical colonies, use these plates to enumerate *S. aureus*. Select more than 1 colony of each type counted and test for coagulase production. Add number of colonies on set of triplicate plates represented by colonies giving positive coagulase test and multiply by sample dilution factor.

B. **Coagulase testing:** Transfer suspect *S. aureus* colonies into small tubes containing 0.2 to 0.3 mL BHI broth and emulsify thoroughly. Inoculate agar slant of suitable maintenance medium (e.g., TSA with loopful of BHI suspension). Incubate BHI culture suspension and slants 18 to 24 hours at 35° ± 1°C. Retain slant cultures at room temperature for ancillary or repeat tests in case coagulase test results are questionable. Add 0.5 mL reconstituted coagulase plasma with EDTA to BHI culture and mix thoroughly. Incubate at 35° ± 1°C and examine periodically over 6-hour period for clot formation. Only firm and complete clots that stay in place when tube is tilted or inverted are considered positive for *S. aureus*. Partial clotting must be tested further. Test known positive and negative cultures simultaneously with suspect cultures of unknown coagulase activity. Make gram stains of all suspect cultures and observe microscopically.

C. **Expression of result:** Use confirmed counts from all plates having up to 200 colonies. In cases where a proportion of the colonies selected for confirmation are confirmed as *S. aureus*, calculate the number of *S. aureus* colonies for the plate as the appropriate percentage of the presumptive count.

The number of *S. aureus* per gram or milliliter is equal to the confirmed colonies multiplied by the sample dilution factor. The result is expressed as a number between 1.0 and 9.9 multiplied by 10^x, with x being the appropriate power of 10.

If the confirmed count is less than 10, report the number of *S. aureus* per gram as an estimate count of 10 x d, with d being the reciprocal of the dilution factor of the dilution from which the highest counts were obtained.

If the confirmed count is greater than 200, calculate an estimated count from dishes having a count nearest 200 colonies and multiply by the reciprocal of the dilution factor. Report as the estimated number of *S. aureus* per gram.

10. **Precision:** See chapter 1: Precision Parameters [1.110].

11. **Test report:** The test report shall identify the method used and results obtained. The report will also identify any variation in the test not specified in this method as well as problems that may have impacted the test result. Each sample will be described in such a manner as to ensure traceability as to its origin.

5.060 Ancillary Tests for *Staphylococcus Aureus*

Isolates that produce a weak coagulase test are subjected to the thermonuclease test in order to confirm identity. The isolates obtained by these methods can be used for the determination of their ability to produce staphylococcal enterotoxins.[41]

1. **Scope:** These tests are used to confirm colonies obtained by direct plating as *S. aureus* should the coagulase test produce questionable or inconclusive results.[16,33,63]

2. **References:** Chapter 2: Laboratory Quality Assurance and Safety.
   Chapter 4: Preparation of Media, Dilution Water, and Sterilization.

3. **Definition:** See 5.060.

4. **Principle:** Selected colonies are tested for characteristics other than coagulase production that allow differentiation of *S. aureus* from other staphylococci and other competing microflora. *S. aureus* produces catalase, which distinguishes it from lactic acid bacteria and many other gram-positive microorganisms.

   Under anaerobic conditions most *S. aureus* isolates have the ability to reduce both glucose and mannitol to lactic acid, while most *Staphylococcus epidermidis* can reduce glucose to lactic acid but cannot reduce mannitol. Micrococci can not reduce either glucose or mannitol to lactic acid. While the reduction of mannitol to lactic acid is not definitive, coupled with the other ancillary test, it can be of assistance in the confirmation of *S. aureus.*

   Several species of staphylococci produce an enzyme that specifically lyses the cell wall of *Staphylococcus aureus* in the presence of lysostaphin, which causes a suspension of cells to clear over a period of 2 hours.

   S. aureus produces a characteristic heat stable nuclease that is at least as indicative of the species as is coagulase. The enzyme, which digests

DNA and RNA, survives boiling for 20 minutes. After heat treatment, if the solution is still capable of digesting DNA, the test organism that produced the thermonuclease can be considered a *S. aureus* isolate.

5. **Apparatus and Glassware**
   1. Incubator: 37° ± 1°C.
   2. Water bath: Capable of operating at 50° ± 1°C.
   3. Drying cabinet: Ventilated capable of being controlled at 50° ± 1°C, or 37° ± 1°C.
   4. Petri plates.
   5. Test tubes: 10 mm × 75 mm.
   6. Test tubes: 13 mm × 100 mm.
   7. Pipets: 1.0 mL with 0.1-mL divisions.
   8. Glass or plastic spreaders for spread plating.
   9. Glass slide.

6. **Diluents, Culture Media, and Reagents**
   1. Phosphate-buffered saline: (PBS) 0.85% saline with 1.0 mL of phosphate buffer solution (42.5 g KH_2PO_4 in 1 L water, pH 7.2 ± 0.1).
   2. Hydrogen peroxide: 3%.
   3. Lysostaphin (Sigma).
   4. Paraffin oil: sterile.
   5. Purple broth base containing 0.5% glucose.
   6. Purple broth base containing 0.5% mannitol.
   7. Tween 80 solution: 1%.
   8. Brain heart infusion broth.
   9. Toluidine blue-deoxyribonucleic agar.

7. **Sampling:** Culture slants on trypticase soy agar (TSA) are retained from the questionable coagulase test. The slants are maintained at room temperature.

8. **Procedure**

   A. **Catalase test**
      1. Scrape of a loop across the growth on an agar slant (or several colonies from a Baird-Parker plate) and emulsify in a 13- × 100-mm culture tube containing 0.5 mL of a 1% Tween-80 solution.
      2. Add 0.5 mL of 3% hydrogen peroxide and loosely cover the tube (culture tube cap). Do not perform this assay on an open slide since the effervescence can create aerosols of pathogenic organisms.
      3. Effervescence is an indication of a positive test.

   B. **Anaerobic utilization of glucose and mannitol**
      1. Heavily inoculate a tube of purple broth containing 0.5% glucose and a tube containing 0.5% mannitol with the isolate to be tested. Layer enough sterile mineral oil over the surface of the broth to create a height of a least 25 mm. Positive, negative, and blank media controls should be run simultaneously.
      2. Incubate the test samples for 5 days at 37° ± 1°C.
      3. After 5 days a positive result is indicated by a color change from purple to yellow.

C. **Lysostaphin sensitivity**
   1. Transfer a colony or a loopful of cells to 100 μL of PBS in a culture tube (13 × 100 mm). Using a vortex mixer suspend the cells in the buffer.
   2. Transfer 50 μL of the suspension to a second tube containing 100 μL of PBS; this serves as the negative control.
   3. Add 100 μL of lysostaphin solution containing 25 μg of lysostaphin per mL to the first tube of cells and incubate the tubes at 37° ± 1°C for 2 hours.

      The test is considered positive if clearing of the suspension occurs within 2 hours. If it does not clear, the test is considered negative. Most *S. aureus* are lysed by lysostaphin.

D. **Thermostable nuclease production[50]:** Inoculate 15 to 20 mL of brain heart infusion broth from the maintenance slant of the suspect culture prepared prior to the coagulase test. Incubate for 18 hours at 35° ± 1°C. Pour broth into a centrifuge tube and adjust pH to 5.5. The tube is capped and placed into a boiling water bath for 20 minutes, followed by chilling in an ice bath before centrifugation for 45 minutes at 7,000 × G. Use a Pasteur pipet to transfer drops of the supernatant fluid to wells cut in the deoxyribonuclease medium. Plates are incubated for 1 hour at 50° ± 1°C and flooded with 4 N HCl. Clear zones indicating nuclease activity within a ring of precipitate are immediately visible against a black background if heat-stable nuclease is present.

   Agar medium plates for the nuclease assay are prepared by adding the following to 100 mL of water: 0.6 g of trizma base, 0.045 g of deoxyribonucleic acid, 1.25 g of agar, 1 g of NaCl, and 0.2 mL of a 0.01 M $CaCl_2$ solution. The pH is adjusted to 9.0 with 1 N HCl and boiled for 20 minutes before pouring into 60- × 15-mm petri dishes. Immediately before use, wells are punched in the agar about 1 cm apart with a No. 2 cork borer, and the plugs removed by aspiration.

9. **Expression of Results:** The individual ancillary test is negative or positive per the criteria listed for the test. Table 5.5 is consulted to determine if the additional characteristics can resolve the questionable coagulase test result in regard to the culture's identity.

Table 5.5. Typical Characteristics of *Staphylococcus aureus*, *Staphylococcus epidermidis*, and Micrococci[a]

Characteristic	*S. aureus*	*S. epidermidis*	micrococci
Catalase activity	+	+	+
Coagulase production	+	–	–
Thermostable nuclease production	+	–	–
Lysostaphin sensitivity	+	+	–
Anaerobic utilization of			
Glucose	+	+	–
Mannitol	+	–	–

[a]+, Most (90% or more) strains positive; –, most (90% or more) strains negative.

10. **Test Results:** The test report shall identify the ancillary tests used and the results obtained. The report will also identify any variation in the test not specified in these ancillary methods as well as problems that may have impacted the test results. Each sample will be described in such a manner as to ensure traceability as to its origin.

5.070 Enterotoxin Production and Isolate Analysis

Isolates of *Staphylococcus aureus* may or may not produce enterotoxins. If an isolate is capable of producing toxins, more toxin will be produced by the organism in culture systems than will be produced in the food from which it was isolated. Because of the sensitivity of current ELISA test kits (sensitivity to equal to or less than 1.0 ng/mL), elaborate culture systems such as the membrane over agar or semisolid agar techniques are no longer necessary. Shallow standing cultures of toxin producing isolates of *S. aureus* will produce enough toxin to be detected by the various kits.

The colonies of *S. aureus* isolated by procedure 5.060 are suitable for testing for the production of staphylococcal enterotoxins. Transfer 4 to 8 typical colonies to a tube containing 5.0 mL of sterile PBS. Mix the tube thoroughly and transfer 100 µL of the suspension to a 5.00-mL of sterile brain heart infusion in a 250-mL Erlenmeyer flask.

Incubate the flask statically or with gentle shaking for 18 to 24 hours.

Centrifuge the culture and save the supernatant for toxin analysis. If not tested the same day, freeze the supernatant until testing.

In order to reduce the possibility of staphylococcal protein A interference with the test, add 20 µL of normal rabbit sera (NRS) per mL of culture supernatant. The NRS must be prescreened for the absence of antibodies to the enterotoxins. This reagent is available from Toxin Technology, Inc., Sarasota, Florida, USA.

The treated culture supernatant can be tested as a substitute for the sample extract in any of the commercial kits listed in 5.100. It may be necessary to make dilutions of the supernatant if quantization of the toxin is desirable. Most often if toxin is produced, it is produced in quantities greater than the minimal detectable amount (1.0 ng/mL).

It is necessary to select multiple colonies at the onset of this procedure in order to be certain that any one of the colonies is a toxin producer. Alternately, 4 to 8 colonies from the suspect food can be individually tested; however, this will add significantly to the time and cost of the assay.

5.080 Screening for Staphylococcal Enterotoxins[64]–(Class B)

1. **Scope:** This method applies to fluid milk, dried milk, cheeses, and solid dairy products.
2. **References:** Chapter 2: Laboratory Quality Assurance and Safety.
   Chapter 3: Sampling Dairy and Related Products.
   Chapter 4: Preparation of Media, Dilution Water, and Sterilization.
3. **Definition:** The staphylococcal enterotoxins (SE) are a group of closely related but serologically distinct proteins made by some isolates of *Staphylococcus aureus*, which when ingested may cause the symptoms of staphylococcal food poisoning. There are now 9 enterotoxins: A, B, C, D, E, G, H, I, and J.[47] At this time, test kits and reagents are only available for

toxins A to E. There are at least 8 subtypes of staphylococcal enterotoxin C (SEC); however, they all cross react with polyvalent antisera.[52] Therefore, for the purposes of detection in food products, they can be referred to as SEC.

4. **Principle:** The TECRA kit® (Class B) is an antibody-based enzyme-linked immunoabsorbent assay (ELISA). It is a sandwich ELISA, which uses a mixture of highly specific antibodies to capture the SE's and a mixture of horseradish peroxidase, conjugated second antibody for detecting the presence of staphylococcal enterotoxins. As set up, the kit can not distinguish among the 5 enterotoxin serotypes (A to E). If the presence of enterotoxins is indicated by the results from this test, confirmation of its presence is required.

5. **Diluents, Culture Media, and Reagents**
   1. Tris buffer: 0.25 M, pH 8.0.
   2. Sodium hydroxide: 1 M.
   3. Hydrochloric acid solution: 0.1 M.
   4. Sodium hypochlorite solution (household bleach).
   5. Distilled or deionized water.
   6. Reagents supplied with the TECRA® kit.
   7. Antibody-coated Removawell strips (48 coated wells).
   8. Concentrated wash solution.
   9. Sample additive solution.
   10. Positive control.
   11. Negative control.
   12. Conjugate diluent.
   13. Conjugate.
   14. Substrate diluent.
   15. Substrate.
   16. Stop solution.

6. **Apparatus and Glassware**
   1. Centrifuge.
   2. Incubator: 35° to 37°C.
   3. pH paper: 0 to 14, pH meter optional.
   4. Blender: Waring or Stomacher.
   5. Pipeters: Adjustable; 50 to 200 µL; 5 to 50 µL.
   6. Pipet tips.
   7. Syringes: Disposable, approximately 25 mL.
   8. Absorbent cotton.
   9. Centrifuge tubes: 15 mL, polypropylene
   10. Wash bottle: Plastic, 500-mL.
   11. Plastic wrap (e.g., Saran Wrap®).
   12. Microtiter plate shaker, optional.
   13. Microtiter plate reader: 414-mm range recommended.

7. **Sampling:** See chapter 3.

8. **Sample Preparation**
   A. **Fluid milk products:** The pH should be in the 7 to 8 range, adjust with the appropriate sodium hydroxide or hydrochloric acid solutions.

Add 50 µL of the sample additive solution to 5 mL of the test sample and mix thoroughly. A 200-µL portion of the mixture can be tested directly in the ELISA.

B. **Dried milk products:** Reconstitute the dried product to the solids concentration that would be normal for use. To 5 mL of the reconstituted milk add 50 µL of sample additive solution. This mixture can be tested directly in the ELISA.

C. **Cheese and other solid dairy products:** Weigh 10 g of sample and add 20 mL of water and blend thoroughly. Adjust pH to 4 with hydrochloric acid solution—use care to maintain pH above 3 since enterotoxins are denatured below pH 3. Centrifuge at 1,000 to 3,000 × g for 10 minutes. Filter the supernatant through a cotton plugged syringe and save the filtrate. (Prepare the cotton filter as follows: Insert enough cotton into a 25-mL syringe barrel to make a plug approximately 0.5 cm thick. Force about 5 mL of water through the cotton to pack the filter.) Adjust the pH of the filtrate to 7 to 8 with the sodium hydroxide solution. To 5 mL of the pH-adjusted filtrate add 50 µL of sample additive solution and mix thoroughly. Use 200 µL of this mixture to test in the ELISA.

9. **Procedure:** The short incubation times and the presence of thimerosal in most reagents allow the assay to be conducted using nonsterile conditions.

Mix all reagents thoroughly prior to use, but do not over agitate. The kits are manufactured on a lot-by-lot basis and the reagents are balanced for each lot; therefore, reagents from one kit should not be used with any other kit. The kits are assigned an expiration date. Expired kits should be discarded. The reagents in the kit are temperature sensitive. The assay is performed at room temperature (20° to 25°C); however, the kit and all diluted reagents should be stored under refrigeration (2° to 8°C). Unused wells should be stored in the sealed pouch provided in the presence of silica gel desiccant. At the time of testing, secure the necessary number of wells in the 96-well frame provided. After the test, the spent wells should be removed from the frame and discarded. As much as possible, use the aseptic technique; do not touch the rim of the wells with fingers or pipet tips during the various manipulations. Be careful not to cross contaminate wells—working with multiple samples and wells can be confusing.

A. **Enterotoxin assay**

1. Remove enough wells from the well pack to perform the assay. One well is needed for each sample plus 1 well for the positive control and 1 well for the negative control. Secure the necessary number of wells in the frame provided.
2. Activate the wells by completely filling the wells with wash solution. Incubate the wells at room temperature for at least 10 minutes before adding the 200 µL of test sample or controls.
3. After incubation, empty wells by tipping the frame. Tap the inverted plate on a paper towel several times to shake out any residual wash buffer.

4. To individual wells add 200 µL of the test samples and the controls. Wrap the frame in plastic wrap and place in a 35° to 37°C incubator for 2 hours.
5. After incubation, invert the plate over a trough or beaker containing 2% sodium hypochlorite solution. Tap the inverted frame on paper towels as before. Fill the wells with wash solution, and empty and tap. Repeat this wash step 3 times.
6. Add 200 µL of conjugate to each well. Cover and incubate at room temperature for 1 hour.
7. After incubation, empty the plate and wash 5 times with wash buffer as above.
8. To each empty wells add 20 µL of reconstituted substrate. Incubate the well for 30 minutes at room temperature. After 30 minutes, gently tap the side of the frame to distribute the color and observe over a white background. Looking directly into the wells, compare the colors to the color chart provided. Observe the system periodically until the color of the positive control is about equal to that of number 4 on the color chart (30 to 45 minutes total time).
9. Stop the reaction by adding 20 µL of the stop solution to each well. Tap the side of the frame to ensure mixing.
10. Record the results either visually or use a microplate reader.
11. *Interpretation of results using the color chart by visual observation:* Compare the colors of the individual wells with the color chart and use a white background. The positive control is the primary reference. Allowing the color to develop to the same intensity as the control (4) on the chart ensures maximum sensitivity and reproducibility. Color must develop in the positive control; if it does not, the test should be repeated using fresh reagents. If the color of the negative control is darker than the reference (2), the wells may not have been properly washed and the test should be repeated. The test sample is considered positive if the color development is at least as intense as reference (3) and the negative control is no darker than reference (2).
12. *Interpretation of results using a microplate reader:* Although using a plate reader is not mandatory, it is highly recommended. A single, dual, or variable wave length plate reader can be used as long as it can read an absorbance at 414 ± 10 mm. The instrument should be zeroed with the wash buffer and the absorbance of the positive control should be equal to or greater than 1.0 to ensure that all reagents are working properly. The absorbance of the negative control should be equal to or less than 0.2. If it is greater than 0.2, the test should be repeated. The test sample would be considered positive if the absorbance is greater than 0.2. However, if the absorbance is slightly greater than 0.2, the test should be repeated.
13. Positive TECRA®–Class B kit results must be confirmed.
14. Confirmation of TECRA®–Class B results with the microslide gel double diffusion test.

    The TECRA® kit results should be confirmed using the microslide gel double diffusion assay detailed by AOAC. Briefly, a template for reagents is placed over a thin layer of agar on a microscope slide. Specific antisera for the various toxins are placed in the center wells of the test system. Peripheral wells are used for the controls and the test samples. The test samples, controls, and sera diffuse from the wells and, if the test is positive, a line of immunoprecipitate forms between the sample or control wells and the sera well. Because this test system has limited sensitivity, an elaborate extraction concentration procedure is required to recover the enterotoxin from a suspect food sample. The reagents, sera, and toxin controls as well as the templates are available from Toxin Technology, Inc., Sarasota, Florida. The microslide technique as described appears straightforward; however, it is laborious and time consuming and requires considerable practice to perform successfully. This test should not be attempted by the typical dairy laboratory.

10. **Expression of Results:** An absorbance of more than 0.2 indicates a presumptive positive. When confirmed by the microslide gel double diffusion test, the sample can be reported as positive for one or more of the staphylococcal enterotoxin A through E. Confirmation with a specific staphylococcal enterotoxin antiserum by the microslide double gel diffusion assay permits reporting that the specific enterotoxin was present in the culture.

11. **Precision:** There are no precision parameters for this test. The test has a sensitivity of 0.5 µg/mL.

12. **Test Report:** The test report shall identify the method used and results obtained. The report will also identify any variation in the test not specified in this method as well as problems that may have impacted the test result. Each sample will be described in such a manner as to ensure traceability as to its origin.

5.090 Other Kits for Staphylococcal Enterotoxin Detection in Foods–Class B

A. Other kits for detection of staphylococcal enterotoxin in foods include:

1. Ridascreen®–Class B, R-Biopharm GmbH, Darmstadt, Germany. U.S. supplier: Biotek Instruments, Winouski, Vermont.
2. Transia®–Class B, Transia-Diffchamb S.A., Lyon, France.
3. SET-RPLA®–Class B, Unipath, 800 Proctor Ave., Ogdensburg, New York.
4. VIDAS®–Class B, BioMerieux Vitek, Inc., Hazelwood, Missouri.

5.091 *Comments on Test Kits*

All these kits are capable of detecting the SEs at or below the 1 ng/g level in food. SET-EIA is the most sensitive at 0.1 ng/mL of food extract. Most of the kits have undergone some type of collaborative testing or review, but not the extensive AOAC collaborative studies. The extracts as prepared for the TECRA® procedure could be used in most test kits. Su and Lee-Wong have published an excellent review of these procedures.[56] Two of the kits are able to differentiate enterotoxin types and may be useful for confirmation of the

TECRA® in lieu of the microslide analysis. Therefore, if there is a problem with the conjugate in one kit, the problem should be avoided by the use of the other. Although the Transia kit and the SET-RPLA kit do not have *Staphylococcus Enterotoxin Examination* (SEE) specific antibodies incorporated in the capture and conjugated antibodies, the anti SEA used in them cross reacts with SEE. Therefore, should there be SEE present in the test sample, in all likelihood it would be detected as SEA.

5.092 *Recommendation*

Although the various test kits now make the detection of enterotoxins relatively easy, all the test kits have their own quirks and drawbacks. In addition, all the kits are quite expensive and have expiration dates. Unless the testing laboratory makes the detection of staphylococcal enterotoxins a routine procedure, there are many drawbacks. For instance, the TECRA® and Ridascreen kits are both peroxidase based; therefore, foods that contain natural peroxidases (radishes, pickles, peppers, etc.) can and do cause false positives unless the peroxidase is inactivated before testing. The Transia kit does not provide a negative control; therefore, all positive results are suspect and must be confirmed. The SET-RPLA kit is subject to false-positive agglutination, and the Vidas B kit, although the least expensive to run (per test), requires a high capital outlay for equipment.[1] Because high *S. aureus* counts are a relatively rare occurrence and staphylococcal enterotoxin analysis is complex, it is recommended that enterotoxin analyses not be added to routine laboratory procedures, but performed by a reference laboratory.

5.100 Mastitis Culture Tests

1. **Scope:** This method is used to diagnose the cause of inflammation of the mammary gland in dairy animals.
2. **References:** Chapter 3: Sampling Dairy and Related Products.
   Chapter 4: Preparation of Media, Dilution Water, and Sterilization.
3. **Definition:** Common bacterial mastitis pathogens include streptococci, enterococci, staphylococci, and gram-negative and gram-positive bacilli.
4. **Principle:** Aseptically collected samples from individual mammary glands, composites from a single cow, or commingled from multiple cows are spread onto the surface of bovine blood agar, which are incubated to produce colonies that are identified by appearance, hemolytic pattern, and biochemical and/or microscopic tests.
5. **Diluents, Culture Media, and Reagents**
   1. Ethanol: 70% or isopropanol.
   2. Iodophor disinfectant: 1%.
   3. Water: Potable.
   4. Blood agar with esculin: Prepare with typticase soy agar II (blood agar base) or tryptose blood agar base. Add 0.1 g esculin per 100 mL agar prior to autoclaving, cool to 45° to 48°C, and add 5 mL sterile whole bovine or ovine blood (defibrinated or containing an anticoagulant). Test each lot of blood for antihemolysins by streaking a prepared plate with a culture of cultures of *Staphylococcus aureus* capable of producing a clear zone of alpha hemolysis and an incomplete zone

of beta hemolysis (4 to 6 mm wide). Washed red blood cells may be used instead of whole blood, in which case no test for antihemolysins is needed.

5. Purple broth base containing 0.5% lactose and 6.5% NaCl.
6. Hydrogen peroxide: 3%.
7. Coagulase plasma (rabbit) with EDTA.
8. Staphylococcal hemolysin, or a culture of *Staphylococcus aureus* capable of producing a broad zone of incomplete hemolysis.

6. Apparatus and Glassware

1. Sample containers with rack: sterile glass or plastic tubes with screw caps or push-on type lids or 4-oz. sterile plastic sample bags. Identify with waterproof marker.
2. Ice chest: Should contain a rack for placing containers to keep them upright and tops out of cracked ice.
3. Cotton gauze sponge or absorbent cotton.
4. Single-service paper towels.
5. Brush: Suitable for removing adhering bedding or other materials for udder.
6. Transfer loops: 0.01 mL for transfer of individual quarter sample or 0.05 mL for transfer of composite sample; platinum-rhodium wire or disposable plastic are satisfactory.
7. Cotton swabs (sterile): For transfer of large volumes of sample.
8. Petri dishes: 100 mm or larger.
9. Incubator: 37° ± 1°C; humidity kept high to avoid desiccation of agar.
10. Bent-glass rod spreader or sterile plastic spreader.

7. Sampling: If teats and udder are clean, proceed to section C.

A. Brush particles of bedding and dry soil from the udder with a dry paper towel or brush.

B. Wash dirty teats with a disinfectant-saturate clean paper towel. Dry with a second dry towel. Dip teat in 1% iodophor and wipe dry with a clean paper towel after 30 seconds.

C. Remove and discard 2 streams of milk from each teat to be sampled to reduce the number of potentially contaminating bacteria in the teat canal.

D. Swab vigorously the end of each teat with a cotton pledget or gauze sponge saturated with 70% ethanol or isopropanol. Use a separate swab for each teat. If the renewed surface of the swab does not remain clean, apply another sponge. Treat teats on the far side of the udder first, then those on the near side.

1. Remove samples from the near-side teats first. Avoid touching any surface of the sample container that milk will ultimately touch. Hold the tube cap with the inner surface down and the container as nearly horizontal as possible to minimize opportunity for falling material to enter. Turn the teat to near horizontal position and direct streams of milk into the container. Do not allow the container to touch the teat.
2. Collect 3 to 5 mL. Close the container as quickly as possible and place on ice.

E. Store samples at 4° ± 1°C and preferably culture within 24 hours.

8. **Preparation of the Sample:** To resuspend milk fat and bacteria within sample, warm to approximately 25° ± 1°C by placement with tops clearly above waterline in a 37° ± 1°C water bath for 15 seconds. Mix and allow foam to subside before plating.

9. **Procedure**

A. Streak 0.01-mL samples from individual quarters onto separate quadrants of a single plate. Streak or spread samples of 0.05 mL onto ½ plate and 0.1 mL onto a full plate. Use a bent rod to spread inoculum from composite samples over at least ½ plate to provide isolated colonies. Begin spreading from the outside of the plate, lightly streaking numerous trails toward the center. Take care to avoid overlapping streaks of samples on the same plate. Permitting a small amount of milk to remain at the beginning of the streak will enhance growth of *Corynebacterium bovis*. [Note: Some bacteria are inhibited when they reside within the heavy concentration of abnormal milk. This is particularly noted among staphylococci that grow at the edge of a layer of such milk. The portion of the colony outside the streak is larger than the portion within the milk.]

B. Incubate plates 24 hours at 37° ± 1°C and examine for fast growing organisms. Return plates to incubators that have no typical colonies to permit a visualization of slow growing bacteria. If abnormal samples continually yield no colonies, incubation under anaerobic or partial CO_2 environments and for extended periods may be necessary. Microscopic examination of a smear of precipitate from a centrifuged sample may provide clues for special methods of isolation.

C. **Identification of mastitis pathogens**

1. **Presumptive identification:** Analysts should be experienced in recognizing probable identities based on size, color, and shape of colonies plus hemolytic and esculin reactions.
2. **Streptococci and enterococci:** Commonly encountered streptococci and enterococci are *Streptococcus agalactiae, Streptococcus uberis, Streptococcus dysgalactiae, Streptococcus bovis, Enterococcus faecium,* and *Enterococcus faecalis*. On esculin-blood agar these bacteria form translucent, convex colonies 1 to 3 mm in diameter, usually surrounded by a zone of greening (α-hemolysis) or clearing (β-hemolysis) of the red blood cells. These bacteria are catalase-negative, gram-positive cocci that divide in 1 plane only, like rods. They can

Table 5.6. CAMP-Esculin Reactions of Several *Streptococcus* Species Encountered in the Bovine Mammary Glands

Species	CAMP Test	Esculin Hydrolysis
S. agalactiae	+	–
S. uberis	+ or –	+
S. dysgalactiae	–	–

be further differentiated by the CAMP-esculin test. This test is performed on blood agar containing 0.1% esculin and 0.01% ferric citrate that is added before sterilization. A culture or sterile filtrate of *S. aureus* capable of producing a broad zone of incomplete hemolysis is streaked across the center of this plate. Alternately, streak *S. aureus* hemolysin onto the plate. The presumptive streptococci or enterococci colonies are streaked at right angles and within 2 mm of the line of staphylococcal inoculum or over the zone containing the hemolysin. Examine plates after aerobic incubation at 37° ± 1°C for 18 to 24 hours. Cultures that are CAMP-positive produce zones of complete clearing in semicircular or arrowhead shapes with the zone of incomplete hemolysis produced by the *Staphylococcus.* Browning of the medium around streptococcal colonies indicates hydrolysis of esculin. Interpret reactions according to Table 5.6.

Enterococci can be differentiated from the streptococci by their ability to grow and produce acid in lactose broth containing 6.5% NaCl and brom cresol purple indicator. Differentiation of this entire group of bacteria is facilitated by use of miniaturized rapid identification systems.

3. **Stapholococci and micrococci:** Staphylococci and micrococci are gram-positive, catalase-positive cocci that divide in multiple planes. They produce opaque white to cream-colored colonies that are 2 to 3 mm in diameter on uncrowded areas of blood agar. Micrococci produce little or no hemolysis and generally occur in small numbers because they get into samples from their habitat around the teat orifice. Colonies of *Staphylococcus aureus,* the most common cause of bovine mastitis in many dairy herds, are usually surrounded by zones of hemolysis. This hemolysis typically consists of a broad zone of incomplete hemolysis that is often accompanied by a narrow zone of complete hemolysis at the edge of the colony. Some strains of *S. aureus* produce only zones of complete hemolysis, while a few produce no hemolysis. Generally, presence of a pure culture of numerous colonies typical in appearance of this group of bacteria is strong evidence of causation of bovine mastitis. High-somatic cell counts add confidence to this diagnosis. The catalase test is performed by applying a drop of 3% hydrogen peroxide to a portion of a colony on a glass slide. Avoid removal of blood cells because they may contain catalase. Appearance of bubbles (oxygen) on the slide is a positive test. The coagulase test is useful in confirmation of *S. aureus* although a few strains of this species produce a negative reaction and a few non-aureus strains of staphylococci give positive reactions. The test is performed by mixing in a tube 0.5 mL each of the coagulase plasma (rabbit) and an 18-hour broth culture of the suspect bacterium. The tube incubated at 37° ± 1°C in a water bath is examined for clotting (positive) at 1, 2, and 4 hours. For further test of identity of staphylococci, see 5.060.

4. **Gram-negative bacilli:** The commonly encountered gram-negative mastitis bacteria are in the genera *Escherichia, Klebsiella, Enterobacter* (coliform bacteria), and *Pseudomonas*. These bacteria produce large, moist, translucent colonies on blood agar. Many of them are potential contaminants of samples, but their presence in pure culture is evidence of intramammary infection. Colonies of *Ps. aeruginosa* are generally highly hemolytic, spread readily over the agar surface, and produce both a green, water-soluble pigment and a strong apple odor. They are easily differentiated from the coliforms by their inability to ferment lactose and positive oxidase reaction. Coliforms produce acid and gas in triple sugar iron (TSI) agar, whereas *Ps. aeruginosa* fails to change the color of TSI agar, or turns it more alkaline. Coliform bacteria can be differentiated with a rapid test kit. *Escherichia coli* generally produces a green sheen on eosin methylene blue (EMB) agar whereas *Enterobacter* and *Klebsiella* produce moist, large colonies with dark centers. It is seldom necessary to proceed beyond this stage in identification in diagnosing the cause of mastitis. If more information is desired, consult the reference given in the bibliography.[52] Other gram-negative bacteria that have been associated with bovine mastitis include *Citrobacter freundii*, an oxidase-negative lactose fermenter and H_2S producer; *Proteus vulgaris*, an oxidase-negative, urease-positive, lactose nonfermenter; and *Serratia* spp., which are oxidase-negative, urease-negative, lactose nonfermenters.
5. **Gram-positive bacilli:** Small numbers of cases of bovine mastitis have been reportedly caused by the following bacteria.
   a. **Corynebacterium bovis:** Slow growing, very small, white to creamy, nonhemolytic colonies that have rough, dull surface. Growth is enhanced by oleic acid found in milkfat and by 0.1% Tween-80. Nonsporing cells are irregular in shape and stain with granular appearance. Catalase is produced.
   b. **Actinomyces pyogenes:** Convex, smooth and glistening, hemolytic colonies 0.5 to 1.5 mm in diameter form on incubation for 48 hours. Gram-stained cells are similar to those of *C. bovis*.
   c. **Bacillus cereus:** Gram-positive, aerobic, spore-forming cells that produce large, hemolytic colonies that often have a green-gray color and a ground-glass appearance.
6. **Mycobacteria, *nocardia*, and mycoplasmas:** These bacteria are slow-growing and unusual in appearance. They are easily missed in culture tests or mistaken in identity.
   a. **Mycobacteria:** Acid-fast rods that may appear as beaded and filamentous with a tendency to branch.
   b. ***Nocardia* spp.:** Extremely dangerous to humans and should be handled under a biohazard hood. After 48-hour incubation the colonies may resemble staphylococci, but continued incubation produces pigmented, rough, powdery-like surfaces resulting from growth of aerial hyphae. Cells are gram-positive, branched, slender filaments accompanied by short rods and cocci.

c. **Mycoplasma:** Require a special PPLO medium for growth and an atmosphere of 10% CO_2. Colonies formed are so small they may require a stereoscope (25×) to identify them. Larger colonies have a fried egg appearance caused by a light periphery surrounding a dark center.

5.110 Cited References

1. ANDREWS, W.H. A review of culture methods and their relation to rapid methods for the detection of *Salmonella* in foods. Food Technol. **39:**77; 1985.
2. ASSOCIATION OF OFFICIAL ANALYTICAL CHEMISTS. Changes in methods. *Salmonella* detection in foods: Hydrophobic grid membrane filter method. JAOAC **68:**405; 1985.
3. ASSOCIATION OF OFFICIAL ANALYTICAL CHEMISTS. Changes in methods. *Salmonella* in foods: Enzyme immunoassay screening method. JAOAC **69:**381; 1986.
4. ASSOCIATION OF OFFICIAL ANALYTICAL CHEMISTS. Changes in methods. *Salmonella* detection in foods: enzyme immunoassay screening method. JAOAC **69:**405; 1986.
5. ASSOCIATION OF OFFICIAL ANALYTICAL CHEMISTS. Changes in methods. *Salmonella* in foods: DNA hybridization method. JAOAC **70:**394; 1987
6. ASSOCIATION OF OFFICIAL ANALYTICAL CHEMISTS. Changes in official methods. *Salmonella* in foods: Fluorogenic monoclonal EIA screening method. JAOAC **72:**203; 1989.
7. ASSOCIATION OF OFFICIAL ANALYTICAL CHEMISTS. Changes in official methods. *Salmonella* in foods: Colorimetric polyclonal EIA screening method. JAOAC **72:**210; 1989.
8. ASSOCIATION OF OFFICIAL ANALYTICAL CHEMISTS. *Listeria*, 16th ed. Gaithersburg, MD: Official Methods of Analysis of AOAC International, 1995: 94A-106B.
9. ASSOCIATION OF OFFICIAL ANALYTICAL CHEMISTS. *Official Methods of Analysis of AOAC International,* 16th ed. Gaithersburg, MD: AOAC International; 1995.
10. ASSOCIATION OF OFFICIAL ANALYTICAL CHEMISTS. *Official Methods of Analysis*, 16th ed. (Supplements 1996, 1997 and 1998) Gaithersburg, MD: AOAC; 1995.
11. BANNISTER, B.A. *Listeria monocytogenes* meningitis associated with eating soft cheese. J. Infect. Dis. **15:**165-168; 1987.
12. BEAN, N.H.; GOULDING, J.S.; DANIELS, M.T.; ANGULO, F.J. Surveillance for foodborne disease outbreaks—United States, 1988–1992. J. Food Protect. **60:**1265-1286; 1997.
13. BRYAN, F.L. Epidemiology of milk-borne diseases. J. Food Prot. **46:**637-649; 1983.
14. CHAN, S.W.; WILSON, S.G.; JOHNSON, A.; WHIPPLE, K.; SHAH, A.; WILBY, A.; OTTAVIANI, M.; VERA-GARCIA, M.; MOZOLA, M.; HOBERT, D. Comparative study of a colorimetric DNA hybridization assay and the conventional culture procedure for the detection of *Salmonella* in foods. JAOAC **73:**419; 1990.
15. CODEX COMMITTEE ON MILK AND MILK PRODUCTS. *Heat Treatment Definitions*. CXMMP 98/8. Rome: Codex alimentarius commission; 1998:1-10.
16. COLLINS, C.H.; LYNNE, P.M. *Microbiological methods*. London, England: Buttersworth; 1984.
17. CURIALE, M.S.; KLATT, M.J.; MOZOLA, M.A. Colorimetric deoxyribonucleic acid hybridization for rapid screening of *Salmonella* in foods. JAOAC **73:**248; 1990.
18. CURIALE, M.S.; KLATT, M.J.; GEHLE, W.E.; CHANDONNET, H. Colorimetric and fluorometric substrate immunoassays for the detection of *Salmonella* in all foods: A comparative study. JAOAC **73:**961; 1990.
19. CURIALE, M.S.; GANGAR, V.; GRAVENS, C. Vidas enzyme-linked fluorescent immunoassay for detection of *Salmonella* in food: Collaborative study. JAOAC Int. **80:**491; 1997.
20. D'AOUST, J.-Y.; SEWELL, A.M. Detection of *Salmonella* by the enzyme immunoassay (EIA) technique. J. Food Sci. **51:**484; 1986.
21. D'AOUST, J.-Y.; SEWELL, A.M. Detection of *Salmonella* with the BioEnzaBead™ enzyme immunoassay technique. J. Food Prot. **51:**538; 1988.

22. D'AOUST, J.-Y.; SEWELL, A.M. Reliability of the immunodiffusion 1-2 Test™ system for detection of *Salmonella* in foods. J. Food Prot. **51:**853; 1988.
23. DE SMEDT, J.M.; BOLDERDIJK, R.F. Dynamics of *Salmonella* isolation with modified semisolid Rappaport-Vassiliadis medium. J. Food Prot. **50:**658; 1987.
24. ECKNER, K.F.; FLOWERS. R.S.; ROBISON, B.J.; MATTINGLY, J.A.; GABIS, D.A.; SILLIKER, J.H. Comparison of *Salmonella* BioEnzaBead™ immunoassay method and conventional culture procedure for detection of *Salmonella* in foods. J. Food Prot. **50:**379; 1987.
25. ENTIS, P.; BRODSKY, M.H.; SHARP, A.N.; JARVIS, G.A. Rapid detection of *Salmonella* spp. in food by use of the ISO-GRID hydrophobic grid membrane filter. Appl. Environ. Microbiol. **43:**261; 1982.
26. EWING, W.H. *Edwards and Ewing's Identification of Enterobacteriaceae*, 4th ed. New York: Elsevier Science Publishing Co.; 1986.
27. FANTASIA, L.D.; SCHRADE, J.P.; YOGER, J.F.; DEBLER, D. Fluorescent antibody method for the detection of *Salmonella*: Development, evaluation, and collaborative study. JAOAC **58:**828; 1975.
28. FARBER, J.M.; LOSOS, J.Z. *Listeria monocytogenes*: a foodborne pathogen. Can. Med. Assoc. J. **138:**413-418; 1988.
29. FELDSINE, P.T.; FALBO-NELSON, M.T.; HUSTEAD, D.L.; FLOWERS, R.S.; FLOWERS, M.J. Comparative and multilaboratory studies of two immunodiffusion method enrichment protocol and the AOAC/Bacteriological Analytical Manual culture method for the detection of *Salmonella* in all foods. JAOAC Int. **78:**987; 1995.
30. FELDSINE, P.T.; LIENAU, A.H.; FORGEY, R.L.; CALHOON, R.D. Assurance polyclonal enzyme immunoassay for detection of *Listeria monocytogenes* and related *Listeria* species in selected foods: collaborative study. JAOAC **80:**775-790; 1997.
31. FELDSINE, P.T.; LIENAU, A.H.; FORGEY, R.L.; CALHOON, R.D. Visual immunoprecipitate assay (VIP) for *Listeria monocytogenes* and related *Listeria* species detection in selected foods: collaborative study. JAOAC **80:**791-805; 1997.
32. FENG, P.; U.S. FOOD AND DRUG ADMINISTRATION. *Bacteriological analytical manual*, 8th ed., Appendix 1. Rapid methods for detecting foodborne pathogens. Gaithersburg, MD: AOAC International; 1995.
33. FLOWERS, R.S.; ANDREWS, W.; DONNELLY, C.W.; KNOWING, E. *Pathogens in milk and milk products.* In: MARSHALL, R.T., ed. *Standard Methods for the Examination of Dairy Products*, 16th ed. Washington, DC: APHA; 1992: 103-212.
34. FLOWERS, R.S.; ECKNER, K.F.; GABIS, D.A.; ROBISON, B.J.; MATTINGLY, J.A.; SILLIKER, J.H. Microbiological Methods. Enzyme immunoassay for detection of *Salmonella* in foods: Collaborative study. JAOAC **69:**786; 1986.
35. FLOWERS, R.S.; KLATT, M.J. Evaluation of a visual immunoassay for detection of *Salmonella* in foods. Annual Meeting of IFT; 1987. Abstract 122.
36. FLOWERS, R.S.; KLATT, M.J.; ROBISON, B.J.; MATTINGLY, J.A.; GABIS, D.A.; SILLIKER, J.H. Enzyme immunoassay for detection of *Salmonella* in low-moisture foods: Collaborative study. JAOAC **70:**530; 1987.
37. FLOWERS, R.S.; KLATT, M.J.; KEELAN, S.L. Visual immunoassay for detection of *Salmonella* in foods: collaborative study. JAOAC **71:**973; 1988.
38. FLOWERS, R.S.; KLATT, M.J. Immunodiffusion screening method for detection of motile *Salmonella* in foods: collaborative study. JAOAC **72:**303; 1989.
39. FLOWERS, R.S.; KLATT, M.J.; KEELAN, S.L.; SWAMINATHAN, B.; GEHLE, W.D.; CHANDONNET, H.E. Fluorescent enzyme immunoassay for rapid screening of *Salmonella* in foods. JAOAC **72:**318; 1989.
40. FLOWERS, R.S.; MOZOLA, M.A.; CURIALE, M.S.; GABIS, D.A.; SILLIKER, J.H. Comparative study of a DNA hybridization method and the conventional culture procedure for detection of *Salmonella* in foods. J. Food Sci. **52:**781; 1987.
41. FREED, R.C.; EVENSON, M.L.; REISER, R.F.; BERGDOLL, M.S. Enzyme linked immunosorbent assay for detection of staphylococcal enterotoxins in foods. Appl. Environ. Microbial. **44:**1349-1355; 1982.
42. GANGAR, V.; CURIALE, M.S.; D'ONORIA, A.; DONNELLY, C.; DUNNIGAN, P. LOCAATE enzyme-linked immunosorbent assay for detection of *Salmonella* in food. JAOAC **81:**419; 1988.

43. GRAY, M.L.; STAFSETH, H.; THORP, F., Jr.; SHOLL, L.B.; RILEY, W.F., Jr. A new technique for isolating listerellae from the bovine brain. J. Bacteriol. **55:**471-476; 1948.

44. HEESCHEN, W.H. Introduction. In: GEHRIGER, G., ed. *The significance of pathogenic microorganisms in raw milk.* Brussels: International Dairy Federation; 1994:8-11.

45. INSALATA, N.F.; CHORDASH, R.A. Fluorescent antibody detection of salmonellae. In: *Compendium of Methods for the Microbiological Examination of Foods,* 2nd. ed. Washington, DC: APHA; 1984.

46. INTERNATIONAL COMMISSION ON MICROBIOLOGICAL SPECIFICATIONS FOR FOOD. *Microorganisms in Foods. 2. Sampling for Microbiological Analysis: Principles and Specific Applications,* 2nd ed. Intern. Comm. On Microbiology. Spec. for Foods. Toronto, Ontario: Univ. of Toronto Press; 1986.

47. JARRAUD, S.; et al. *egc,* A highly preventive operon of enterotoxin gene, forms a putative nursery of superantigens in *Staphylococcus aureus.* J. Immunol. **166:**669-677; 2001. An erratum to this paper was published in J. Immunol. **166:**4259.

48. JOHNSON, J.L. *Isolation and identification of* Listeria monocytogenes *from meat, poultry and egg products.* Chapter 8 in *USDA-FSIS Microbiology Laboratory Guidebook,* 3rd ed., vol. 1., Washington, DC: U.S. Govt. Print. Off.; 1998.

49. KNIGHT, M.T.; NEWMAN, M.C.; BENZINGER, M.J., Jr.; AGIN, J.R. TECRA *Listeria* visual immunoassay (TLVIA) for detection of *Listeria* in foods: Collaborative study. JAOAC. **79:**1083-1094; 1996.

50. KOUPAL, A.; DEIBEL, R.H. Rapid qualitative method for detecting staphylococcal nuclease in foods. Appl. Environ. Microbiol. **35:**1193; 1978.

51. LINNAN, M.J.; MASCOLA, L.; LOU, X.D.; GOULET, V.; MAY, S.; SALMINEN, C.; HIRD, D.; YONEKURA, M.L.; HAYES, P.; WEAVER, R.; AUDURIER, A.; PLIKAYTIS, B.D.; FANNIN, S.L.; KLEKS, A.; BROOME, C.V. Epidemic listeriosis associated with Mexican-style cheese. N Engl. J Med. **319:**823-828; 1989.

52. MARR, J.C.; LYON, J.D.; ROBERTSON, J.R.; LUPHER, M.; DAVIS, W.C.; BOBACH, G.A. Characterization of novel type C staphylococcal enterotoxins: biological and evolutionary implications. Infect. Immun. **61:**4254-4262;1993.

53. NATIONAL MASTITIS COUNCIL. *Laboratory Handbook on Bovine Mastitis.* Arlington, VA: National Mastitis Council, Inc.; 1999.

54. RYSER, E.T.; MARTH, E.H. Listeria, *listeriosis and food safety,* 1st ed. New York: Marcel Dekker; 1991.

55. SHARPE, S.N.; MICHAUD, G.L. Hydrophobic grid-membrane filters: New approach to microbiological enumeration. App. Microbiol. **28:**223; 1974.

56. SU, Y.-C., LEE-WONG, A.C. Current Perspectives on detection of staphylococcal enterotoxins. J. Food Prot. **60:** 196-202; 1997.

57. TAPPERO, J.W.; SCHUCHAT, A.; DEAVER, K.A.; MASCOLA, L.; WENGER, J.D. Reduction in the incidence of human listeriosis in the United States: effectiveness of prevention efforts? JAMA. **273**:1118-1123; 1995.

58. TAUXE, R.V. *Salmonella*: A postmodern pathogen. J. Food Prot. **54:**563-568; 1991.

59. THOMASON, B.M. Current status of immunofluorescent methodology for salmonellae. J. Food Prot. **44:**381; 1981.

60. THOMASON, B.M.; CHERRY, W.B.; MOODY, M.D. Staining bacterial smears with fluorescent antibody. III. Antigenic analysis of *Salmonella typhosa* by means of fluorescent antibody and agglutination reactions. J. Bacteriol. **74:**525; 1957.

61. U.S. FOOD AND DRUG ADMINISTRATION. *Bacteriological Analytical Manual.* 8th ed. McLean, VA: AOAC; 1995.

62. U.S. FOOD AND DRUG ADMINISTRATION. *Bacteriological analytical manual,* 8th ed., Chapter 10: *Listeria.* Arlington, VA: AOAC International; 1995, 10.01-10.13.

63. U.S. FOOD AND DRUG ADMINISTRATION. *Bacteriological Analytical Manual,* 8th ed., Chapter 13. *Staphylococcus aureus.* Arlington, VA: AOAC International; 1995.

64. U.S. FOOD AND DRUG ADMINISTRATION. *Bacteriological Analytical Manual,* 8th ed. *Staphylococcus aureus.* Staphylococcal enterotoxins: visual ELISA: Polyvalent (Types A-E) screening for determining enterotoxigenicity and identifying staphylococcal enterotoxins in foods. Arlington, VA: AOAC; 1995.

65. U.S. PUBLIC HEALTH SERVICE. *Grade "A" Pasteurized milk ordinance, Item 16p, 1995 Revision. Pasteurization—Aseptic processing,* Publication No. 229. Washington, DC: U.S. Department of Health and Human Services; 1995.
66. VOUGHT, K.J.; TATINI, S.R. *Salmonella enteritidis* contamination of ice cream associated with a 1994 multistate outbreak. J. Food Prot. **61**:5-10; 1998.
67. ZEHREN, V.L.; ZEHREN, V.F. Relation of acid development during cheesemaking to development of staphylococcal enterotoxin A. J. Dairy Sci. **51**:645-649; 1967.

5.120 Other References

ASSOCIATION OF OFFICIAL ANALYTICAL CHEMISTS. *Official Methods of Analysis,* 14th ed. (Supplements, 1986, 1987). Arlington, VA: AOAC; 1984.

INTERNATIONAL DAIRY FEDERATION. *Annual momento, Commission A.* Brussels: IDF; 1990.

WARBURTON, D.W.; FELDSTINE, P.T.; FALBO-NELSON, M.T. Modified immunodiffusion method for detection of *Salmonella* in raw, flesh and highly contaminated foods: Collaborative study. JAOAC **78:** 59; 1995

Chapter 6

Microbiological Count Methods

D. T. Laird, S. A. Gambrel-Lenarz, F. M. Scher, T. E. Graham, and R. Reddy
(L. J. Maturin, Tech. Comm.)

6.010 Introduction

Microbiological count methods are the accepted laboratory methods used to estimate the microbial population of a tested substance. These procedures are used throughout the dairy industry and regulatory enforcement agencies for the determination of quality and detection of microbial contamination in raw and processed milk. This is accomplished by the testing of producer samples, inline samples, and retail samples. Cultured dairy products (e.g., cultured buttermilk, fermented acidophilus, etc.), dairy products to which bacterial cultures are added, and acidified products are not ordinarily tested for total microbial content for spoilage.

The most commonly used microbiological count method is the standard plate count (SPC) agar method. This method is used by the dairy industry for estimating the microbial populations in most types of dairy products and samples and for determining quality and sources of contamination at successive stages of processing. The SPC, which is the reference method recognized by the NCIMS and specified in the Grade A Pasteurized Milk Ordinance,[35] estimates the microbial population (primarily mesophilic, aerobic, and facultative bacteria) of raw and pasteurized milk and milk products.

Although SPC is a time-consuming method, it is relatively accurate for determining viable bacteria in dairy products. The direct microscopic count (DMC) used by some plants to estimate the microbial content of raw milk is not sufficiently accurate for quality or regulatory purposes. In the present environment, there is interest in rapid and/or less costly tests that provide results comparable to SPC. Therefore, other alternative tests have been developed to supplement SPC. Alternative methods are compared to the reference SPC method by individual analysts using the alternate procedure. This validation determines an analyst's ability to perform the alternate method to produce results comparable to the official or reference SPC method. The recommended protocol to evaluate the performance of an individual analyst against the standard method is located in section 6.020.10H.

Although standardization of equipment, materials, and incubation in SPC has been of considerable value, questions continue to be raised concerning the ability of this procedure to completely reflect the sanitary practices used in the production and handling of milk. Therefore, additional information about the microbial quality of a sample may be gained by the preliminary incubation (PI) of milk in conjunction with determining the SPC.[4,6,10,22,23,32,38] A more complete picture of the microbial content of dairy products (e.g., lactic acid bacteria, psychrotrophic, thermoduric and thermophilic bacteria, and yeast and mold counts) may also be obtained by using other media at other temperatures for various periods of time [chapter 8].

The plate loop count (PLC) procedure is specifically used to examine raw milk based on a single dilution [6.030]. It is satisfactorily precise with countable media plates in the range of 25 to 250 colonies. Limitations of the PLC method occur when the raw milk counts exceed 200,000 per milliliter.[39] The PLC has limited value for raw milk with <25,000 cfu/mL. This method has been observed to yield 10% to 20% lower results than the SPC method.[29]

The Petrifilm™ aerobic count (PAC) plate method is a ready-made plating procedure that uses a dehydrated cold water soluble gelling agent [6.040]. PAC plates are applicable for the enumeration of bacteria in raw milk,[4,15,30,36] pasteurized milk,[6,13,34,35] and other dairy products.[8] The PAC method has been collaboratively studied with milk[14,30] and dairy products[8] and has not been found to be significantly different from the SPC method.

The Redigel™ aerobic count pectin (ACP) gel medium uses pectin as the gelling agent so that all operations are carried out at room temperature [6.050]. The Redigel™ ACP method is applicable in matrices similar to the SPC. It has been collaboratively studied with milk, cream, and cultured products[30]; however, it is not at the present recognized by the NCIMS.

The spiral plate count (SPLC) method is applicable to raw milk, pasteurized milk, and milk products [6.060].[9] It has been collaboratively tested with milk[13,27] and found not to be significantly different from the SPC method. SPLC is a mechanical method that requires less analyst involvement than does the SPC method. It is recognized by the NCIMS for raw milk only.

6.020 Standard Plate Count Method (Class O)

1. **Scope:** The standard plate count (SPC) method is applicable to raw and processed liquid and dry dairy products. SPC has limited applicability to nonheat-treated cultured products.

2. **References:** Chapter 1: Standard Methods.
   Chapter 2: Laboratory Quality Assurance and Safety.
   Chapter 3: Sampling Dairy and Related Products.
   Chapter 4: Preparation of Media, Dilution Water, and Sterilization.
   Chapter 8: Tests for Groups of Microorganisms.

Chapter 9: Microbiological Methods for Dairy Products.

3. **Definition:** The standard plate count: Total colony-forming units (CFU) of bacteria, yeasts, and molds per milliliter or gram under stated conditions of the method.
4. **Principle:** Measured aliquots of milk and milk products are introduced directly or diluted into or onto standard methods agar (SMA) using specific techniques. Plates are incubated aerobically at 32° ± 1°C for 48 ± 3 hours. Determination of the number of microorganisms per mL/gm of a sample is obtained by selecting plates containing 25 to 250 cfu/mL or gm or selecting plates with counts closest to this range.
5. **Diluents, Culture Media, and Reagents:** See chapter 4: Preparation of Media, Dilution Water, and Sterilization.
   A. Buffer, stock phosphate, or stock $MgCl_2$ solution (optional).
   B. Dilution blanks, phosphate buffer[5]: Fill dilution bottles with phosphate buffer so that each bottle contains 99 ± 2 mL after sterilization. Autoclave the filled bottles at 120° ± 1°C for 15 minutes. When autoclave conditions restrict heat penetration, 20 to 30 minute sterilization periods may be required.

      After dilution buffer blanks have been sterilized and allowed to cool to room temperature, check entire lot for bottles obviously containing less than or more than 99 ± 2 mL. Discard these bottles. Of the remaining dilution blanks, randomly select 1 blank for every 25 remaining. In general, for 2 to 25 blanks select 1 to check for volume; for 26 to 50, check 2; for 51 to 75, check 3; etc. Use a class "A" graduate cylinder or equivalent to determine if the volume is 99 ± 2 mL. If all blanks that are checked are within specification then the lot of blanks may be used. If 1 or more are out of specification then the *entire* lot may not be used.

      When less than 99-mL amounts are needed, use 9 ± 0.2 mL and 90 ± 2 mL dilution blanks. Use of a properly calibrated automatic measuring devices is optional.

      When bulk sterilized buffer is used, measure the diluent directly into sterile dilution bottles. Use these prepared dilution blanks on the same day that the bulk buffer is made and sterilized.

      Ready-to-use plastic, single-service dilution blanks are commercially available. Volume [see above] and toxicity [chapter 4] checks on commercially prepared dilution blanks are performed as described for laboratory prepared dilution blanks.
   C. Dilution buffer blanks, 2% sodium citrate: Fill and autoclave dilution bottles as in section 6.020.5.A.
   D. Sodium citrate: ACS.
   E. Standard methods agar (SMA): Dehydrated.
   F. Ethyl alcohol: 70%.
6. **Apparatus and Glassware:** See chapter 2: Laboratory Quality Assurance and Safety.
   1. Autoclave: Capable of raising to temperature within 15 minutes (preferably within 5 minutes) of starting air exhaust and capable of maintaining 120° ± 1°C. Total time in autoclave for SMA must be less

than 1 hour. Exposure of media to excessive heat or to heat for prolonged periods will cause degradation of the media components and may result in reduced microbial growth.

2. Balance: Sensitive to at least 0.1 g.
3. Weights: Certified class S or S1 or equivalent ASTM 1, 2, or 3 weights.
4. Colony counter: Quebec dark field model or equivalent with grid plate.
5. Dilution bottles: Capacity 150 mL with indelible mark at 99 ± 1 mL.
6. Hand tally.
7. Incubator: 32° ± 1°C.
8. Media storage bottles: Allow for a 1-inch (2.5-cm) airspace at the top.
9. pH meter: Electronic readable to 0.1 pH units (preferably with double juncture reference electrodes). Printer optional.
10. Microwave oven (optional).
11. Petri dishes: Glass or plastic, flat bottom, 80 mm inside diameter and 12 mm deep.
12. Pipets or pipeters that conform to APHA standards.
13. Pipet containers: Nontoxic.
14. Refrigerator: Range capable from 0° to 4.4°C.
15. Shaker, mechanical dilution bottle: See *SMEDP*, 11th edition.
16. Sterilizing oven: Hot air 170°C to 220°C.
17. Stomacher or blender with corresponding sterile stomacher bags or autoclaveable blender jars (optional).
18. Thermometer: NIST certified or equivalent, graduation level not more than 0.5°C between 0° and 100°C; otherwise not more than 1.0°C covering all other laboratory temperatures ranges.
19. Thermometers: ± 1°C accurate compared to NIST thermometer, mercury in glass (plastic laminated preferred), alcohol/spirit or digital.
20. Media water bath: 45° ± 1°C, circulating, appropriate water level, and adequate size for workload.

7. Sampling: See chapter 3: Sampling Dairy and Related Products.

8. Preparation of Test Sample

A. **Raw and pasteurized fluid milk and liquid milk products:** Maintain samples at 0° to 4.4°C with refrigeration or iced water from collection to completion of analysis.

Begin analysis within 48 hours (preferably within 24 hours) of collecting the sample(s). Time begins at the initial collection from the source and not from when samples are picked up from an intermediate site to be transported to the laboratory by another person. Picking up samples that someone else has previously collected is not considered sample collection but sample pick up.

When the sample arrives at the laboratory, determine the temperature of each set of samples by inserting a precooled thermometer into a separate pilot container (temperature control [TC]) treated exactly the same as the samples in the set, and record the temperature. Do not insert thermometer into any sample intended for microbiological examination before the microbial test portion has been removed. Fluid milk samples that have been frozen should not be tested microbiologically since freezing causes significant changes in the viable microbial count in milk.[31]

Unless otherwise specified, mix liquid samples by shaking 25 times in 7 seconds with a 1-foot (30-cm) movement.[19] A mechanical shaker may be used to shake the dilution blanks uniformly for 15 seconds [6.020.6].

Liquid samples in sealed containers such as retail containers should be completely inverted 25 times or until contents are homogeneous.

To ensure a homogeneous sample when no air space is present, aseptically open the container and pour the product from the filled containers back and forth into a sterile container 3 times.

The interval between the completion of mixing and removing the test portion must not exceed 3 minutes.

Before opening a sample container, remove all obvious materials that may contaminate the sample from the closure. If necessary, wipe the tops of unopened sample containers with a sterile cloth/paper towel saturated with 70% ethyl alcohol.

Depending on the expected count, make appropriate serial dilutions by aseptically pipeting 1 or 11 mL of sample into 99 mL-phosphate buffer dilution blanks to yield a final dilution that is expected to yield plates with 25 to 250 cfu. Raw milk is normally diluted to 1:100 and 1:1000 while processed milk is normally diluted to 1:10 and 1:100 prior to plating.

B. **Butter, margarine, and related products:** Melt samples by rotating containers filled to not more than 50% of capacity with butter or a similar product in a water bath set at not more than 40° ± 1°C (for less than 15 minutes) until the product is fluid enough to pipet.

Using pipets and dilution blanks that have been prewarmed to 40° to 45°C, prewet an 11 mL wide mouth pipet with warm sterile dilution buffer (drawing liquid into pipet and discharging back into the same dilution blank).

With a minimum of product adhering to the outside (insert pipet tip no more than 2.5 cm into the sample) of the 11-mL pipet, immediately transfer 11 grams of uniformly mixed and melted fat serum mixture into 99 mL of a prewarmed phosphate buffer dilution blank. Shake the sample 25 times in 7 seconds with a 1 foot (30 cm) movement.

Depending on expected count, make appropriate serial dilutions by aseptically pipeting diluted sample into warmed diluent to yield plates with 25 to 250 cfu.

C. **Dry dairy products:** All samples are to be aseptically mixed, stirred, ground, blended, or otherwise prepared in order to make the sample uniform.

Weigh portions with a sterile weighing scoop (or equivalent) onto sterilized squares of hardsurface paper or aluminum foil, or directly into a dilution blank.

For initial dilutions, temper phosphate buffer dilution blanks to 40° to 45°C. Aseptically transfer a 1-g portion directly into a tempered dilution blank or into sterile, dry, wide-mouth, screw-capped dilution bottle and add warmed diluent.

Optionally, transfer 11 g of dry product directly into 99 mL of dilution water or to an empty sterile bottle and then add warmed diluent.

Disperse the sample completely in initial dilution blanks before making any further dilutions [6.020.8].

For samples with low solubility, dissolve weighed sample in sterile buffer containing 2% sodium citrate and having a pH below 8.0. Do not use this buffer with Petrifilm™ aerobic count plates [6.040.8].

Allow any incompletely dispersed samples to soak for 2 minutes, shake the diluted sample, and proceed with making appropriate serial dilutions by aseptically pipeting diluted sample into phosphate buffered dilution buffer to yield plates with 25 to 250 cfu.

D. **Cheese and other cultured and culture-added products:** All samples are to be aseptically mixed, stirred, ground, blended, or otherwise prepared in order to make the sample uniform.

Aseptically transfer 11 g of cheese to a sterile blender warmed to 40° to 45°C and add 99 mL of 2% sodium citrate dilution buffer warmed to 40° to 45°C. Blend for 2 minutes at a speed sufficient to *emulsify* the sample thoroughly. Invert the container to rinse particles from the interior walls and remix for approximately 10 seconds. Do not allow the temperature of the blended sample to exceed 40°C. If heating is unavoidable, mixing for less than 2 minutes may be used provided that complete emulsification is obtained.

Alternatively add 11 g of sample and 99 mL of 2% sodium citrate dilution buffer at 40° to 45°C to an 18 × 30 cm polyethylene bag. Place and lock the bag into a stomacher (as per manufacturer's instructions) and mix for 2 minutes. Avoid foam when pipeting the sample.

Make appropriate serial dilutions by aseptically pipeting mixed sample into phosphate buffer to yield plates with 25 to 250 cfu.

E. **Ice cream and related food products:** Thaw frozen samples at a temperature up to 40°C for no more than 15 minutes. Stir or mix to make homogeneous before weighing.

For initial dilutions, aseptically transfer an 11 g portion into a sterile, dry, wide-mouth dilution blank and add diluent. Optionally, transfer 11 g of product directly into 99 mL of dilution buffer. Make appropriate serial dilutions by aseptically pipeting mixed sample into phosphate buffer to yield plates with 25 to 250 cfu.

F. **Other dairy or related food products:** See chapter 9: Microbiological Methods for Dairy Products for additional preparation instructions.

9. Procedure

A. **Use of pipet aids and pipeters:** Pipet aids and pipeters are necessary to fill pipets. *Mouth pipeting is not permitted.* The type of pipet aid used must not alter the characteristics of APHA milk pipets in terms of the techniques involved in filling and adjusting to volume and emptying, including the blowout of the last drop of milk sample and the touch-off of the last drop of diluted sample.

B. **Dilution of samples:** Identify each plate with the sample number, dilution, and other desired sample or laboratory information prior to shaking samples and making dilutions.

Make appropriate serial dilutions by aseptically pipeting the mixed sample into phosphate buffer.

When the SPC is expected to yield a count between 25,000 and 250,000 cfu/mL or gm, prepare plates containing 10^{-2} and 10^{-3} dilutions and normal dilutions for raw milk. When low counts (< 25,000) are expected, plate the samples at 10^{-1} and 10^{-2} dilutions and normal dilutions for finished products. In certain circumstances the sample may need to be plated without dilution (10°).

Dilution schemes have always presented problems on how the dilution factor is determined even when 1 mL/11 mL are put into a 99-mL dilution blank. The following is an example calculation for dilutions:

Sample volume put in blank/Total volume (sample plus diluent) in blank = dilution fraction

(Reciprocal of dilution fraction = dilution factor)

11/11+99 = 11/110 = **1/10** (also 10^{-1} or 0.1)

(dilution factor = 10/1 or 10)

1/1+99 = **1/100** (also 10^{-2} or 0.01)

(dilution factor = 100/1 or 100)

C. **Handling of pipets:** Use sterile pipets for the initial transfer and for each subsequent transfer from the same container. If the pipet becomes contaminated before the transfer is completed, discard and replace it with another sterile pipet. Do not flame to decontaminate pipets. Use a separate sterile pipet for transfers from each different dilution. Add test portions of milk to room temperature dilution blanks. Do not prepare dilutions in direct sunlight.

Aseptically adjust pipets in containers or bags so that about 2 to 3 inches of the ends of the pipets are exposed.

When removing sterile pipets from a pipet container, do not drag the pipet tip over any exposed exteriors of the pipets remaining in the container as the exposed ends of the pipets are subject to contamination. Remove pipets by placing the bottom of a finger on the end of a pipet and pulling it outward from the container or bag about 6 inches. Tilt the end of pipet down in order to lift the tip up. Lift the pipet and remove the pipet so that the tip is not dragged across the exposed ends of pipets left in the container or bag.

D. **Measuring sample portions:** Without coming in contact with any outer surface of the sample container or dilution blank, insert the tip of the pipet into the sample or dilution. Do not insert the pipet more than 2.5 cm below the surface of the sample or dilution or through foam unless unavoidable. It may be necessary to wait (within the 3 minutes allowed) for the foam to settle or to manipulate or tilt the sample container in order for the foam to break or to force the foam to another location in the container to expose a foam-free area on the sample surface.

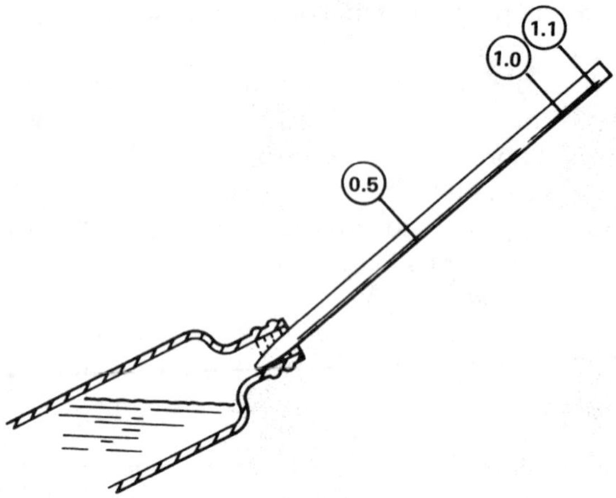

Figure 6.1. Measuring diluted sample.
Lower side of pipet touches the inside surface of the container.

Draw test portions above the desired pipet graduation mark and raise the pipet tip above the surface of the sample. Bring the pipet tip in contact with the inside of the sample container (above the surface of the sample remaining in the container) or in contact with the dilution blank neck (or in the case of commercial dilution blanks with no necks, above the level of the dilution) to ensure drainage is complete and excess liquid does not adhere when the pipet is removed from the sample or dilution bottle.[7] Adjust the level of the sample in the pipet down to the desired graduation mark. Figure 6.1 demonstrates the proper pipet placement for a dilution blank. Angles and surface contact are similar for sample containers and commercial dilution blanks without necks.

When measuring a dairy products with a viscosity similar to that of whole milk or dairy products that are less viscous, complete each transfer by holding the pipet at an angle of about 45°. The bottom of the pipet tip must touch the inside bottom of a petri dish or the inside neck of a dilution bottle (or for commercial dilution blanks without necks on a dry area above the dilution). Let the sample column drain from the desired graduation mark to the pipet tip rest point for 2 to 4 seconds. Move the tip to a dry spot and promptly and gently blow the last drop out with pipet or pipeting device (avoid making bubbles). Do not blow out by mouth. Dilution and plating schemes are shown in Figure 6.2.

E. **Mechanical and electronic pipeters:** In addition to standard pipets, fixed-volume mechanical and electronic pipeters may be used to measure and transfer milk and milk product samples. The procedures above generally apply; however, operators should check the manufacturer's instructions.

F. **Concentrated and cultured dairy products:** Where the solids content or sample viscosity appreciably exceeds that of whole milk, prepare an initial 10^{-1} or 10^{-2} dilution by weighing a test portion into a warmed (40° to 45°C), buffered dilution blank. Weigh 11 g (or 1 g) aseptically into dilution bottles containing 99 mL of sterile, warmed buffer. The viscosity of these dairy products differs at different temperatures. Differences in specific gravity depend on the sample's composition. Furthermore, the amount of trapped air will vary, even in properly agitated samples.

G. **Delivering dilutions with a milk pipet:** When delivering a diluted sample of a dairy product, hold the pipet at an angle of about 45° with the lower part of the pipet tip touching the inside bottom of a petri dish or the inside neck of a dilution bottle (or for commercial dilution blanks without necks on a dry area above the dilution). Lift the cover of the petri dish just high enough to insert the pipet. Deposit the sample on the inside of the dilution blank neck or away from the center of the petri dish to aid in mixing the sample in the SMA. Allow 2 to 4 seconds for the diluted milk or milk product to drain from the graduation mark to the pipet tip. Raise the pipet to a vertical position and touch the pipet tip once against a dry spot on the petri dish or on the inside of the dilution bottle neck. *Do not blow out.* When 0.1-mL quantities are measured with a 1.1 mL-pipet, hold the pipet as directed and let the diluted sample drain to the proper graduation point but *do not retouch* the pipet to the plate. After depositing the test portions in each series of plates, promptly pour the SMA.

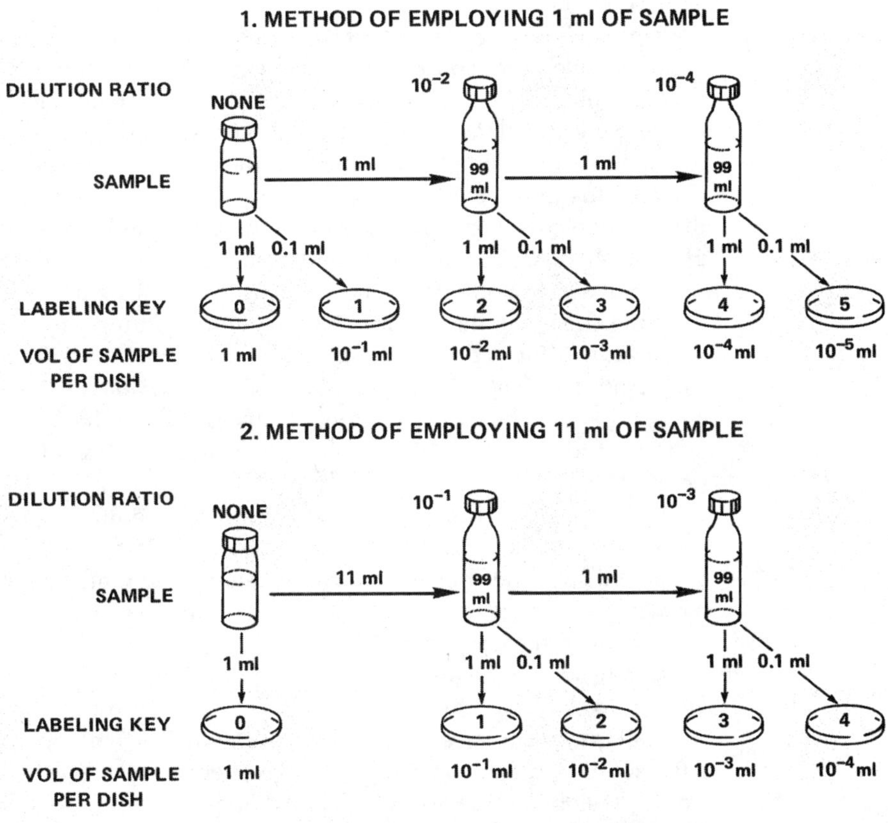

Figure 6.2. Examples for preparing dilutions.

H. **Plating of samples**

1. **Melting of sterile medium:** Melt the required amount of sterile SMA in boiling water, in a microwave oven, or by exposing it to flowing steam (not under pressure) in a partially closed container. Avoid prolonged exposure to unnecessarily high temperatures during and after melting. If the medium is melted in 2 or more batches, use all of each batch in its order of melting, provided that the contents of separate containers remain fully melted. Discard medium that develops atypical characteristics such as precipitate or clumps. Do not melt more medium than will be used in 3 hours. Do not resterilize the medium. Freshly sterilized medium, after it has been tempered to 45° ± 1°C, may also be used for up to 3 hours after tempering.
2. **Tempering medium:** Cool the melted medium promptly to approximately 45° ± 1°C and hold in a circulating water bath at a temperature between 44° and 46°C.[20] Place the bulb of a thermometer in the medium in a separate temperature control (TC) container identical to and with the same volume of medium as the first container. This TC medium must have been exposed to the same heating and cooling as the test medium. Do not depend on the sense of touch or time to indicate the proper temperature of the medium before pouring agar. Each batch of media must have its own TC container.
3. **Pouring and mixing agar:** Select the number of samples to be plated in any one series so that not more than 20 minutes (preferably only 10 minutes) elapse between diluting the first sample and pouring the last plate in the series.[3,17,18] Should a continuous plating operation be done by a team, plan the work so that the time between the initial measurement of a test portion into diluent or directly into a dish and the pouring of the last plate for that sample is less than 20 minutes. Do not pour plates in direct sunlight.

   Remove agar bottle from the water bath and wipe any water from the outside of the medium bottles before pouring.

   Introduce 10 to 12 mL of liquefied medium at 44° to 46°C into each plate by gently lifting the cover of the petri dish just high enough to pour the medium. Carefully avoid spilling the medium on the outside of the container or on the inside of the plate lid when pouring.

   As each plate is poured,[24] thoroughly mix the medium with the test portions in the petri dish by rotating the dish first in one direction and then in the opposite direction, rotating and tilting the dish by hand or using mechanical rotators. Take care not to splash the mixture over the edge or on the lid.

   Having spread the mixture evenly over the bottom of the plate, allow it to solidify (within 10 minutes) on a level surface. Poured dry milk product plates must be overlaid with 3 to 5 mL of SMA. After solidification, invert the plates to prevent spreading colonies from developing due to accumulated moisture and place the plates in the incubator within 10 minutes.

I. **Sterility controls of medium, dilutions, and equipment:** Check the sterility of dilution buffer, medium, pipets, pipeter tips, and petri dishes by pouring control plates for each lot used. In addition, prepare air quality control plates for morning and afternoon platings.

Prior to mixing and pipeting the first sample, pick a dilution blank from the lot(s) to be used and pour approximately 1.0 mL directly into a sterile petri plate. From this same dilution blank, pipet 1.0 mL of buffer into sterile petri plates, one for each pipet or pipeter tip volume/size to be used. Pour about 10 to 12 mL of SMA agar into each of these plates. In addition, pour 10 to 12 mL of SMA into 2 sterile petri plates. One is to be covered immediately and serves as the medium control. Immediately remove the cover of the second plate and leave exposed for 15 minutes (use a timer) in the area where the plating will be done. This is the air quality control plate. At this point, begin mixing and pipeting the test samples. After the 15 minutes have elapsed, replace the cover on the air quality control plate. Place all of the control plates into the incubator along with the first set of test plates that have solidified. Control plates are acceptable if no growth is observed, except for the air quality plate. The air quality plate is acceptable if ≤15 colonies are observed. If more than 15 colonies are observed, take steps to improve air quality.

J. **Incubation:** Incubate plates at 32° ± 1°C for 48 ± 3 hours.[2,40] For dry products, incubate plates at 32° ± 1°C for 72 ± 3 hours. Plates must reach the temperature of incubation within 2 hours. Stack plates no more than 6 plates high with at least one inch between each stack.

Control excessive humidity in the incubator by adjusting vents and/or airflow. Excessive humidity may promote spreader formation. Low humidity may suppress growth on test sample plates by causing excessive drying of the media. To increase humidity, place pans of water in the incubator. For static type incubators, place the pan on the bottom near the heat source. For forced air incubators, place the pans near where the air is blowing. Some incubators have built-in humidity controls, in which case the manufacturer's instructions should be followed to control the humidity.

Agar in plates should not lose more than 15% of its weight due to moisture loss during 48 hours of incubation [chapter 2].

K. **Counting colonies on plates:** Count colonies on plates promptly after the incubation period. Record the dilutions used and the number of colonies counted or estimated on each plate. If impossible to count at once after the required incubation, store the plates at 0° to 4.4°C for not more than 24 hours,[12] but *avoid* making this a routine practice. When counting colonies on plates, proceed according to the directions given below. For each grouping of samples, record the results of sterility tests on materials (dilution blanks, agar, etc.) used when pouring plates and the incubation temperature used.

1. **Visual counting of plates:** Count colonies with the aid of magnification under uniform and properly controlled artificial illumination. Plates should be examined in subdued light. Routinely use a colony counter equipped with a guide plate ruled in square cen-

timeters.[1] Avoid mistaking particles of undissolved medium, debris, sample, or precipitated matter in plates, for pinpoint colonies. Examine doubtful objects carefully, using higher magnification (e.g., dissecting scope) when required, to distinguish colonies from foreign matter. Arrange schedules of laboratory analysts to prevent eye fatigue and the inaccuracies that result from eyestrain or fatigue.

a. **Normal plates** *(25 to 250 or less than 25 colonies):* Select spreader-free plate(s). Count all colonies, including those of pinpoint size, on selected plate(s). Record the dilution(s) used and the total number of colonies counted.

b. **Crowded plates** *(more than 250 colonies):* When both dilutions have counts >250 cfu, do not record counts from the highest dilution as too numerous to count (TNTC) unless estimated counts can not be made. If the number of colonies per plate exceeds 250, count colonies in those portions of the plate that are representative of colony distribution and calculate an estimated standard plate count (ESPC) from these counts. If there are fewer than 10 colonies per square centimeter, count colonies in 12 squares. Select, if representative, 6 consecutive squares horizontally across the plate and 6 squares at right angles, being careful not to count a square more than once. When there are more than 10 colonies per square centimeter, count colonies in 4 representative squares. In both instances, multiply the average number of colonies found per square centimeter by the area of the plate used to determine the estimated number of colonies per plate. Each laboratory must determine the area ($\Pi \times r^2$) in square centimeters of the plates in use.

c. **Spreaders:** Spreading colonies are usually of 3 distinct types. The first type is a chain of colonies, not too distinctly separated, that appears to be caused by the disintegration of a bacterial clump. The second type develops in the film of water between the agar and the bottom of the dish. The third type forms in the film of water at the edge or on the surface of the agar. If plates prepared from a sample have spreader growth such that: 1) the area covered by the spreader or the area covered by the spreader plus the repressed area exceeds 25% of the plate area, or 2) the area of repressed growth caused by the spreaders exceeds 25% of the plate area, report the plate as spreader (SPR). When it is necessary to count colonies on plates containing spreaders not eliminated by either condition cited above, count each distinct spreader as one source. If one or more chains appear to originate from separates sources, count each source as one colony. Do not count each individual growth in such chains as a separate colony. The second and third types usually result in distinct colonies and are counted as such. Combine the spreader count and the colony count to compute the plate count.

d. **Laboratory accidents or bacterial growth inhibitors:** When a plate from a sample is known to be contaminated, abused, or is otherwise unsatisfactory due to laboratory handling, record the plate as a laboratory accident (LA). When unsatisfactory samples are received, indicate why they are unsatisfactory but do not report as an LA. If the test for inhibitory substances is positive for a sample, record the SPC (also coliform count) as a growth inhibitor (GI). Analysts may be inclined to suspect the presence of inhibitory substances in a sample when plates have no growth or have proportionally less growth in lower dilutions. Such developments should not be cited as evidence of inhibition until the presence of inhibitory substances has been confirmed.

2. **Automated counting (Class B):** Automated colony counters (Class B), when validated in individual laboratories to yield counts that 90% of the time are within 10% of those obtained manually, may be used for counting plates for nonregulatory purposes. When using colony-counting instruments, exercise the following precautions:
   a. Align the petri dish carefully on the colony-counter stage.
   b. Avoid "counting" the stacking ribs or legs of plastic petri dishes.
   c. Do not count plates having unsmooth (rippled) agar surfaces.
   d. Avoid plates having food particles or air bubbles in the agar.
   e. Do not count plates having spreaders or extremely large surface colonies.
   f. Avoid scratched plates.
   g. Wipe fingerprints and films off the petri dish bottom before counting.

10. Expression of Results

A. **Computing and recording counts[21,26]:** When computing the SPC (plate in countable range of 25 to 250 cfu/mL or gm), report only the first 2 significant digits to avoid creating a fictitious impression of precision and accuracy. When making this conversion, round off to 2 significant figures by raising the second digit to the next highest number when the third digit is 6, 7, 8, or 9 and by rounding down when the third digit is 1, 2, 3, or 4. When the third digit is 5, round up if the second digit is odd and round down when the second digit is even. Use zeroes for each successive digit toward the right from the second digit. In other words, round to the nearest even 2 digit number along with the appropriate number of zeros.

Examples

Actual Count	Reported Count
12,700	13,000
12,400	12,000
15,500	16,000
14,500	14,000

B. **Sequential plates with 25 to 250 colonies:** Calculate the SPC as follows: $N = \Sigma C/[(1 \times n_1) + (0.1 \times n_2)]d$, where:

N = number of colonies per milliliter or gram of product.
ΣC = sum of all colonies on all plates counted.
n_1 = number of plates in lower dilution counted.
n_2 = number of plates in next higher dilution counted.
d = dilution from which the first counts were obtained.

Examples

1:10	1:100
232	33

$$\begin{aligned} N &= (232 + 33)/[(1 \times 1) + (0.1 \times 1)]10^{-1} \\ &= 265/0.11 \\ &= 2{,}449 \\ &= 2{,}400 \end{aligned}$$

1:100	1:1000
232	33

$$\begin{aligned} N &= (232 + 33)/[(1 \times 1) + (0.1 \times 1)]10^{-2} \\ &= 265/0.011 \\ &= 24{,}490 \\ &= 24{,}000 \end{aligned}$$

C. **Both plates with fewer than 25 colonies:** When plates from both dilutions yield fewer than 25 colonies each, record the count as less than 25 times is the reciprocal of the dilution, called the dilution factor [6.020.9].

Example

1:100	1:1000	SPC/mL (g)
18	2	<2,500 ESPC
0	0	<2,500 ESPC

D. **All plates with more than 250 colonies:** When plates from both dilutions yield more than 250 colonies each (but fewer than 100 per square centimeter), estimate counts form the plates nearest 250 and multiply by the reciprocal of the *d/l* or dilution factor.

Example

1:100	1:1000	SPC/mL (g)
TNTC	640	640,000 ESPC

E. **All plates with more than an average of 100 colonies per square cm:** Estimate the SPC as greater than 100 times the highest dilution plated times the area of the plate (Πr^2, where r = radius or ½ diameter, (Π=3.1416). The examples below have an average count of 110 per square centimeter.

Example

1:100	1:1000	SPC/mL (g)
TNTC	7,150*	>6,500,000*ESPC
TNTC	6,490**	>5,700,000**ESPC
TNTC	2,200***	>2,000,000***ESPC

* based on a plate area of 65 cm^2 (9 cm inside diameter)
** based on a plate area of 57 cm^2 (8.5 cm inside diameter)
*** based on a plate area of 20 cm^2 (5 cm inside diameter)

Report all counts as the SPC or the ESPC per milliliter or gram, as applicable. When instrumental colony counters (I) are used, report counts as SPC (I) or ESPC (I).

F. **All plates with spreaders, demonstrated growth inhibitors, or laboratory accidents:** Report as SPR, GI, or LA, respectively.

G. **Interpreting counts:** The matter of interpreting counts is beyond the scope of this book. Consult local regulations and the latest edition of the Grade A Pasteurized Milk Ordinance.[35]

H. **Avoiding personnel errors and determination of count agreement between analysts:** Avoid inaccuracies in counting caused by carelessness, impaired vision, or failure to recognize colonies. Laboratory workers should duplicate their own counts on the same plate within 8% and the counts of other analysts within 10% on 90% of samples.[28]

The following procedure is used to determine if the counts obtained from one plate by *3 or more analysts* are in agreement based on the expected counting error.[11,28]

1. Rank counts from high to low and convert each to its logarithm:

Rank	Analyst	Count	Logarithm
1	D	108	2.0334
2	F	101	2.0043
3	A	97	1.9868
4	E	95	1.9777
5	C	93	1.9685
6	B	81	1.9085

2. **Determine the differences among counts:** Determine the differences between counts by subtracting from the largest logarithm the next largest logarithm in turn (e.g., when comparing the first and second logarithms 2.0334 to 2.0043, use P = 2, 0.0554 from Table 6.1; when comparing the first and third logarithm, 2.0334 to 1.9868, use P = 3, 0.0584 from Table 6.1). If the difference exceeds the value listed in Table 6.1 for $R_p \times S_m$ (R_p = significant studentized range at α = .05, and S_m = standard error of the mean based on previous estimates of analyst performance), the difference is significant.

Table 6.1. Least Significant Differences (α = .05) for Comparing Counts Reported by Analysts on the Same Plate[a]

Plate (P)[b]	$R_p \times S_m$[c]
2	.0554
3	.0584
4	.0604
5	.0618
6	.0630
7	.0638
8	.0646
9	.0652
10	.0658

[a] Assuming S_m = 0.0200 with *df* = α.

[b] The critical value ($R_p \times S_m$) chosen to compare counts depends on the rank order. If the counts being compared are consecutive, use P = 2. When the counts are separated by two other counts, use P = 4, etc.

[c] R_p = significant studentized range at α = .05; S_m = the standard error of the mean.

Rank	Analyst	Count	Logarithm	Difference	$R_p \times S_m$
1	D	108	2.0334		
2	F	101	2.0043	0.0291	0.0554
3	A	97	1.9868	0.0466	0.0584
4	E	95	1.9777	0.0557	0.0604
5	C	93	1.9685	0.0649	0.0618
6	B	81	1.9085	0.1249	0.0630

Analysts C and B are significantly different from analyst D.

3. **Repeat after dropping the highest count:** When the process is repeated (dropping analyst D's count) starting with analyst F, who was previously ranked second, it is apparent that analyst B is again significantly low.

Rank	Analyst	Count	Logarithm	Difference	$R_p \times S_m$
2	F	101	2.0043		
3	A	97	1.9868	0.0175	0.0554
4	E	95	1.9777	0.0266	0.0584
5	C	93	1.9685	0.0358	0.0604
6	B	81	1.9085	0.1249	0.0630

4. **Repeat after dropping the third highest count:** The steps above are repeated continuing with the count of analyst A (rank 3) until no significant difference is observed.

   The data are summarized below:

Rank	Analyst	Count
1	D	108[a]
2	F	101[a,b]
3	A	97[a,b]
4	E	95[a,b]
5	C	93[b]
6	B	81[c]

[a,b,c]Counts with the same letter do not differ from one another at the $\alpha = .05$ level.

5. **Summary of interpretation of counts:** Analyst B is counting significantly lower than all other analysts and needs training. Analysts C and D differ from one another and need to discover the cause. Attention should be focused on an analyst (high or low) who differs from the majority of the other analysts. In general, problems with colony recognition or, occasionally, visual acuity are the primary causes of differences.

11. **Precision:** See chapter 1: Standard Methods.

12. **Test Report:** The test report must identify the method used and results obtained. The report is to identify any variation in the test not specified in this method as well as problems that may have impacted the test result. Each sample will be described in such a manner as to ensure traceability as to its origin.

6.030 Plate Loop Count (PLC) Method (Class O)

1. **Scope:** This alternate method of the SPC is applicable only to the examination of raw milk, and results are valid within the plated range of 25 to 250 colonies.

2. **References:** Chapter 1: Standard Methods.
   Chapter 2: Laboratory Quality Assurance and Safety.
   Chapter 3: Sampling Dairy and Related Products.
   Chapter 4: Preparation of Media, Dilution Water, and Sterilization.
   Chapter 8: Tests for Groups of Microorganisms.
   Chapter 9: Microbiological Methods for Dairy Products.
3. **Definition:** The plate loop count: Total cfu/mL of bacteria, yeasts and molds under procedures and conditions of the method as stated.
4. **Principle:** A 0.001-mL aliquot of a raw milk sample is introduced into SMA using the plate loop count device. Plates inoculated with the PLC device are incubated and counted in the same manner as the SPC. Determination of the number of microorganisms per mL of a raw milk sample is based on a single dilution.
5. **Diluents, Culture Media, and Reagents:** See 6.020.5.
   See also chapter 4: Preparation of Media, Dilution Water, and Sterilization.
6. **Apparatus and Glassware**
   1. Loop: Welded true circle, ID 1.45 ± 0.06 mm calibrated to contain 0.001 mL of raw milk, made of B & S gauge No. 26 platinum-rhodium (3.5%) or platinum-iridium (15%) wire, attached to a 75-mm-length wire, 30° bend about 3 to 4 mm from the loop with the loop opening toward hub, loop fits over a No. 54 drill bit but not over a No. 53 drill bit.
   2. Luer-Lok hypodermic 13-gauge needle: Sawed off 24 to 36 mm from where the barrel enters the hub.
   3. Cornwall continuous pipeting outfit: Becton, Dickinson & Co., No. 1251, consisting of metal pipeting holder, a Cornwall Luer-Lok syringe, filling outfit, 2-mL capacity calibrated to deliver 1 mL.
   4. Rubber tubing: Attached to the syringe and extending into a capped buffer dilution blank of sufficient length to facilitate sampling process.
   5. Cover: Glass tube (or equivalent) to protect loop during sterilization and handling.
   6. Template: Showing wire angle and lengths. (See Figure 6.3.)
   7. Drill bits: Sizes No. 53 and No. 54.
7. **Sampling:** See chapter 3: Preparation of Media, Dilution Water, and Sterilization.
8. **Preparation of Test Sample:** See 6.020.8.

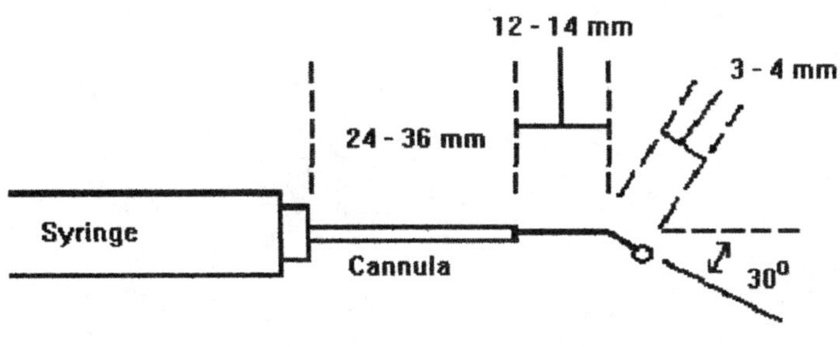

Figure 6.3. Plate loop count template.

Table 6.2. Example of Alternate Method Validation

Sample Number	SPC	Log_{10} PLC	Log Diff.	Sq. Log Diff.	PLC	Log_{10} SPC	Log Diff.	Sq. Log Diff.
1a	32,000	4.50515	0.04275	0.00183	28,000	4.44716	0.05799	0.00336
1b	29,000	4.46240			32,000	4.50515		
2a	140,000	5.14613	0.08432	0.00711	130,000	5.11394	0.06215	0.00386
2b	170,000	5.23045			150,000	5.17609		
3a	96,000	4.98227	0.13167	0.01734	130,000	5.11394	0.03218	0.00104
3b	130,000	5.11394			140,000	5.14613		
4a	30,000	4,47712	0.11394	0.01298	31,000	4.49136	0.08842	0.00782
4b	39,000	4.59106			38,000	4,57978		
5a	32,000	4.50515	0.09691	0.00939	31,000	4.49136	0.04420	0.00195
5b	40,000	4.60206			28,000	4.44716		
6a	100,000	5.00000	0.02228	0.00050	95,000	4.97772	0.02228	0.00050
6b	95,000	4.97772			100,000	5.00000		
7a	240,000	5.38021	0.03779	0.00143	230,000	5.36173	0.06070	0.00368
7b	220,000	5.34242			200,000	5.30103		
8a	50,000	4.69897	0.02531	0.00064	45,000	4.65321	0.07106	0.00505
8b	53,000	4.72428			53,000	4.72428		
9a	36,000	4.55630	0.02482	0.00062	38,000	4.57978	0.06127	0.00375
9b	34,000	4.53148			33,000	4.51851		
10a	84,000	4.92428	0.02020	0.00041	83,000	4.91908	0.02145	0.00046
10b	88,000	4.94448			79,000	4.89763		
11a	61,000	4.78533	0.02758	0.00076	63,000	4.79934	0.01401	0.00020
11b	65,000	4.81291			61,000	4.78533		
12a	88,000	4.94448	0.00491	0.00002	84,000	4.92428	0.01579	0.00025
12b	89,000	4.94939			81,000	4.90849		

13a	87,000	4.93952	0.00496	0.00002	82,000	4.91381	0.02172	0.00047
13b	88,000	4.94448			78,000	4.89209		
14a	61,000	4.78533	0.04074	0.00166	62,000	4.79239	0.04646	0.00216
14b	67,000	4.82607			69,000	4.83885		
15a	54,000	4.73239	0.09893	0.00979	45,000	4.65321	0.05115	0.00262
15b	43,000	4.63347			40,000	4.60206		
16a	140,000	5.14613	0.08432	0.00711	160,000	5.20412	0.02633	0.00069
16b	170,000	5.23045			170,000	5.23045		
17a	29,000	4.46240	0.04742	0.00225	36,000	4.55630	0.09390	0.00882
17b	26,000	4.41497			29,000	4.46240		
18a	87,000	4.93952	0.00496	0.00002	89,000	4.94939	0.04630	0.00214
18b	88,000	4.94448			80,000	4.90309		
19a	59,000	4.77085	0.04658	0.00217	56,000	4.74819	0.03218	0.00104
19b	53,000	4.72428			52,000	4.71600		
20a	30,000	4.47712	0.11394	0.01298	30,000	4.47712	0.07918	0.00627
20b	39,000	4.59106			36,000	4.55630		
21a	130,000	5.11394	0.06215	0.00386	120,000	5.07918	0.07918	0.00627
21b	150,000	5.17609			100,000	5.00000		
22a	59,000	4.77085	0.04658	0.00217	65,000	4.81291	0.03476	0.00121
22b	53,000	4.72428			60,000	4.77815		
23a	110,000	5.04139	0.16273	0.02648	120,000	5.07918	0.03476	0.00121
23b	160,000	5.20412			130,000	5.11394		
24a	41,000	4.61278	0.06872	0.00472	38,000	4.57978	0.01158	0.00013
24b	35,000	4.54407			37,000	4.56820		
25a	200,000	5.30103	0.04576	0.00209	170,000	5.23045	0.02633	0.00069
25b	180,000	5.25527			160,000	5.20412		

Sum 242.494 0.12836 241.804 0.06564 Sum/50 4.84989 0.00257 4.83608 0.00131 |Sum/50 SPC – Sum/50 PLC| = |4.84989 – 4.83608| = 0.01381 (satisfactory as is < 0.036).

Sum/50 SPC = 0.00257 (satisfactory as is < 0.005).

Sum/50 PLC = 0.00131 (satisfactory as is < 0.005).

9. **Procedure**

A. **Analyst validation of the plate loop count method:** As with any alternate method, PLC must be determined to produce comparable results to the SPC prior to use in a laboratory. Each analyst that will be performing this method needs to compare his or her performance using both PLC and SPC. These comparisons must be satisfactory, and records of the comparisons must be maintained.

PLC and SPC must be done on the same milk samples. Samples are plated in duplicate using both methods. This process is continued until 25 samples have been plated that have counts in the 25 to 250 cfu/mL range. While all plating does not have to be done on the same day, all preparations from any one sample must be done at the same time with both procedures.

B. **Validation of alternate methods:** Each analyst performing an alternate method is to satisfactorily validate that method. Duplicate counts of the alternate method (e.g., PLC) and the standard method (e.g., SPC) are converted to $\log_{10}$ counts. The difference between the $\log_{10}$ counts for the duplicate counts are squared and the squared values are summed for all samples for each method. The sum of the $\log_{10}$ counts are divided by 50 to obtain the mean $\log_{10}$ count for the alternate and standard methods.

The mean $\log_{10}$ count for the 50 alternate method observations must not differ from the mean $\log_{10}$ count of the standard method by more than 0.036. In addition, the sum of the squared $\log_{10}$ differences for each method divided by 50 can not be greater than 0.005. An example of a validation is shown in Table 6.2.

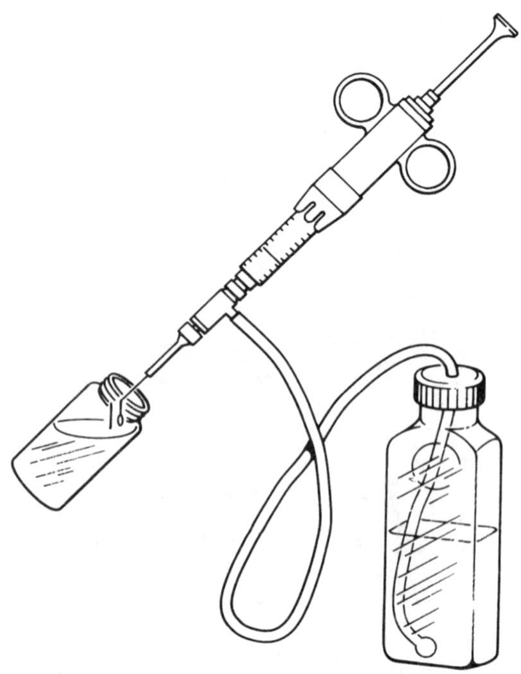

Figure 6.4. Plate loop count device.

This statistical protocol is designed to determine that an analyst is proficient with the 2 methods in use. It is NOT designed for comparing the precision and accuracy of any 2 methods that is required as a part of a collaborative study for method acceptance.[13]

C. **Procedure**

1. Kink the end of the wire loop. Insert the kinked end into the shank of the sawed-off needle such that from the start of the 30° bend is about 12 to 14 mm from the end of the barrel (Figure 6.3).
2. Attach the needle to the pipeting outfit and cover the loop and needle with glass tube (or equivalent).
3. Sterilize assembled outfit wrapped in Kraft paper (or equivalent) or in a closed container by autoclaving at 120° ± 1°C for 15 minutes. Allow to cool to room temperature prior to use.
4. Check device wire angle and length with template.
5. Place tubing into sterile buffer and prime PLC device. (See Figure 6.4.)
6. Identify plates: Samples and controls (air quality, buffer, SMA, initial rinse, loop rinses after each 20 samples and final rinse).
7. Flame loop before use for 15 seconds and allow to cool.
8. Discharge several 1-mL discharges to waste.
9. Shake samples and wait for foam to settle.
10. Tilt sample containers to allow foam to recede and expose surface of milk sample.
11. Dip loop into each sample (avoiding foam) to the bend in shank and withdraw vertically from sample surface 3 times in 3 seconds with a 2.5-cm uniform movement.
12. Raise petri plate cover, insert loop, and carefully depress syringe plunger. The sterile buffer must flow across sample filled loop to wash the 0.001 mL sample onto the petri plate.
13. Pour plates using 12 to 15 mL of tempered SMA.
14. Incubate as with SPC.

10. Expression of Results: See 6.020.9 and 6.020.10.

1. Record plate counts for each sample tested on bench sheets.
2. Calculation of results is based on a single dilution of 1:1000 of the sample.
3. Plates having 25 to 250 cfu are multiplied by the dilution faction of 1000 and reported as plate loop count per mL (PLC/mL).
4. Plates having <25 cfu are reported as <25,000 estimated plate loop count per mL (EPLC/mL).
5. Plates having >250 cfu are reported as the estimated count [6.020.10] multiplied by 1000. Report as EPLC/mL.
6. Spreader growth report as SPR.
7. Growth inhibitor report as GI.
8. Laboratory accident report as LA.

11. Precision: See chapter 1: Standard Methods.

12. Test Report: The test report should identify the method used and results obtained. The report is to identify any variation in the test not specified in this method as well as problems that may have impacted the test result. Each sample will be described in such a manner as to ensure traceability as to its origin.

6.040 Petrifilm™ Aerobic Plate Count (PAC) Method (Class A1)

1. **Scope:** The Petrifilm™ aerobic plate count method is applicable to all dairy products including raw milk and liquid milk products, dried milk products, cheese, processed cheese, butter, margarine, frozen milk products, custard, desserts, and cream.

   Do not use PAC plates for laboratory pasteurized counts (LPC). As with the SPC method, in cases when looking specifically for lactic acid bacteria an alternate method should be considered [chapter 8].

2. **References:** Chapter 1: Standard Methods.
   Chapter 2: Laboratory Quality Assurance and Safety.
   Chapter 3: Sampling Dairy and Related Products.
   Chapter 4: Preparation of Media, Dilution Water, and Sterilization.
   Chapter 8: Tests for Groups of Microorganisms.
   Chapter 9: Microbiological Methods for Dairy Products.

3. **Definition:** See 6.020.3.

4. **Principle:** The Petrifilm™ aerobic count plate (PAC) method is a ready-made culture medium system that consists of 2 plastic films coated with adhesive, powdered standard-methods nutrients, and a dehydrated cold water-soluble gelling agent. An indicator dye, triphenyltetrazolium chloride (TTC), is included to help visualize the colonies when counting. This microbial method uses premade media. The medium is inoculated by peeling back the top film and pipeting 1 mL of the test sample directly onto the bottom film. Pipets, plate loop continuous pipeting syringes, or automatic pipeters may be used to add the 1 mL of sample. The top film is dropped and the inoculum is distributed evenly over the circular plating surface with a plastic spreading device. Plates are incubated aerobically at 32° ± 1°C for 48 ± 3 hours.

5. **Diluents, Culture Media, and Reagents:** See chapter 4: Preparation of Media, Dilution Water, and Sterilization.

   See also 6.020.5.

   See manufacturer's instructions (3M Co., 3M Center, Bldg. 275-5W-05, St. Paul, MN 55144-1000).

   A. **Appropriate sterile diluents:** Butterfield's phosphate buffer (IDF phosphate buffer, 0.0425 g/L KH_2PO_4, adjusted to pH 7.2). *Do not use buffers containing citrate, bisulfite, or thiosulfate* with Petrifilm™ plates as they may inhibit growth.
      1. **NaOH, 1.0 *N* sterile solution:** For pH adjustment of diluted acidic products.
      2. **HCl, 1.0 *N* sterile solution:** For pH adjustment of diluted alkaline products.

   B. **Storage and disposal:** Store unopened Petrifilm™ plate pouches at temperatures 0.5° to 8°C. Just prior to use, allow pouches to come to room temperature before opening and record date opened on the package. Return any unused plates to pouch. To prevent exposure to moisture, *do not refrigerate or freeze opened pouches*. Seal opened pouches by folding the end of the pouch over and taping or clipping shut. Store resealed pouches in a cool, dry location for no longer than one month. Exposure of Petrifilm™ plates to temperatures >25°C (77°F) and/or relative humidity >50% can affect the performance of the plates.

As with other microbial detection systems, inoculated PAC plates may contain viable bacteria that may be a biohazard. Follow current industry standards for disposal.

Expiration date and lot number are noted on each package of Petrifilm™ plates. The lot number is also noted on individual plates.

6. **Apparatus and Glassware:** See 6.020.6.
   1. Petrifilm™ aerobic count spreader.
   2. Refrigerator: Capable of 0.0° to 4.4°C.
   3. Incubator: Capable of 32° ± 1°C.
   4. Thermometer: ± 1°C accuracy.
   5. Colony counter or other illuminated magnifier.
   6. Hand tally.
   7. Balance: Sensitive to 0.1 gram.
   8. Dilution bottles: Capacity 150 mL with indelible mark at 99 ± 1 mL.
   9. Pipets, pipeters, or plate loop device: Conforms to APHA standards.
   10. Stomacher with corresponding sterile stomacher bags.
   11. Blender with autoclaveable blender jars.
7. **Sampling:** See chapter 3: Sampling Dairy and Related Products.
8. **Preparation of Test Sample**

   A. **Raw and pasteurized fluid milk and liquid milk products:** See 6.020.8.

   B. **Butter, margarine, and related products:** See 6.020.8.

   C. **Dry dairy products**
   1. See 6.028.
   2. Low solubility samples, dissolve in warmed (40° to 45°C), sterile, phosphate buffer dilution blank. *Do not use buffers containing citrate with Petrifilm™ plates.*
   3. Acidic products, adjust pH of the diluted sample to 6.6 to 7.2 with 1.0 *N* NaOH. For alkaline products, adjust pH with 1.0 *N* HCl.

   D. **Cheese and other cultured and culture-added products**
   1. See 6.020.8.
   2. Do not use buffers containing citrate with Petrifilm™ plates. If the procedure indicates citrate buffer, substitute warmed (40° to 45°C), sterile, buffered phosphate dilution buffer.
   3. For acidic products, adjust pH of the diluted sample to 6.6 to 7.2 with 1.0 *N* NaOH.

   E. **Ice cream and related food products:** See 6.020.8.

   F. **Other dairy or related food products:** See 6.020.8.
9. **Procedure**

   A. **Plating samples**
   1. Prepare controls as in 6.020.9. The buffer, pipet and pipet tip, and media controls are combined into a single control for the PAC procedure. For the air quality plate, dispense 1 mL of sterile buffer

onto the plate and spread as described below. Allow this plate to sit for 1 minute and then completely open the plate to completely expose both wet surfaces. Set a timer for 15 minutes and then start preparing the test samples. After 15 minutes replace the top film and incubate the plate with the other controls and samples. The combined control is acceptable if no colonies are observed. The air quality plate is acceptable if ≤10 colonies are observed.

2. Make appropriate serial dilutions by aseptically pipeting mixed sample into phosphate buffer dilution blank to yield a dilution expected to give 25 to 250 colony forming units per mL of diluted sample.
3. Place PAC plates on a flat, level surface.
4. Lift the top film and carefully inoculate 1 mL of undiluted or diluted sample by pipet, pipeter, or plate loop continuous pipeting syringe.
5. Replace the top film by dropping.

B. **Spread sample:** Distribute the sample evenly by placing the plastic spreader ridge side down over the sample. Apply steady downward pressure on the center of the plastic spreader. Do not slide the spreader across the film when spreading or removing the spreader. Leave plate undisturbed for at least 1 minute to permit solidification of the gel.

C. **Incubation**

1. Incubate plates in a horizontal position with the clear side up in stacks not exceeding 20 units, at 32° ± 1°C for 48 ± 3 hours.
2. Avoid excessive humidity in the incubator, but prevent excessive drying of the medium by controlling ventilation and air circulation. Petrifilm™ AC plates should not lose more than 15% of their weight during 48 hours of incubation [chapter 2].

D. **Counting colonies:** Count the colonies on plates promptly after incubation period. Record the dilutions used and the number of colonies counted or estimated for each plate. If impossible to count at once, after the required incubation, plates may be stored in a sealed plastic container at 0.0° to 4.4°C for no longer than 24 hours, but avoid making this a routine practice. When counting colonies on plates, proceed according to the directions given below. For each lot of samples, record the results of sterility tests on materials (dilution buffer/pipet/tips, media [combined control], air quality, etc.).

E. **Manual counting of plates**

1. Use a standard colony counter or other magnified light source to enumerate all red colonies regardless of size or intensity.
2. The circular growth area is approximately 20 cm^2. Estimates can be made on plates containing greater than 250 colonies by counting the number of colonies in one or more representative squares and determining the average number per square. Multiply the average number per square by 20 to determine the estimated count per plate and report as estimated Petrifilm™ aerobic count (EPAC).
3. Some organisms can liquefy the gel, allowing them to spread out

and obscure the presence of other colonies. If liquefied gel interferes with the counting, estimate the count by counting the squares in unaffected areas. See above.

4. High concentrations of colonies on the plates will cause the entire growth area to become red or pink. Occasionally, on overcrowded plates, the center may appear to lack visible colonies, but many small colonies may be seen on the edges. If this occurs, dilute the sample further to obtain a more accurate count. The history of a sample is important, since it indicates when further dilution is necessary.

F. **Laboratory accidents or bacterial growth inhibitors:** When a plate from a sample is known to be contaminated, abused, or otherwise unsatisfactory due to laboratory handling, record the plate as a laboratory accident (LA). When unsatisfactory samples are received, indicate why they are unsatisfactory, but do not report as LA. If the test for inhibitory substances is positive for a sample, record the SPC (also coliform count) as growth inhibitor (GI). The analyst may be inclined to suspect the presence of inhibitory substances in a sample when plates have no growth or have proportionally less growth in lower dilutions. Such developments should not be cited as evidence of inhibition, until the presence of inhibitory substances has been confirmed.

G. **Automated counting of plates**

1. **Petrifilm™ information management system (PIMS):** PIMS has been validated through the NCIMS Laboratory Methods Committee to be an equivalent enumeration device for use with the Petrifilm™ AC plates.

   Refer to manufacturer's instructions for set-up and operational information.

2. **Control cards**
   a. Store control cards in a clean, dry, closed container.
   b. Scan and record control card result prior to the start of and at the end of each operation period.
   c. Scan and record control card result at a minimum of once per each hour of operation.
   d. If a control card scan yields a result <92 or >108, preset audible and message alarms will alert the operator of a failure.
   e. Inspect control card for defects. If permanent defects are observed, replace control card.
   f. Scan and report new control card result.
   g. Maintain records of control card scans.

H. **Personal errors:** For one analyst, the count is to be ±10% between visual and PIMS results.

If 2 or more analysts use R_pS_m method, compare the results. Include PIMS results as an analyst [6.020.10 and Table 6.1].

10. Expression of Results: Computing and recording counts [6.020.10].

11. Precision: See chapter 1: Standard Methods.

12. Test Report: The test report must identify the method used and results obtained. The report is to identify any variation in the procedure not specified in this method as well as problems that may have impacted the test result. Each sample will be described in such a manner as to ensure traceability as to its origin.

13 **Bibliography**

6.050 Pectin Gel Method (Redigel™) (Class A1)

1. **Scope:** The pectin gel method using Redigel™ aerobic count medium is applicable to all raw and processed liquid and dry dairy products. The method has limited applicability to cultured products not having received heat processing after culturing.

2. **References:** Chapter 1: Standard Methods.
   Chapter 2: Laboratory Quality Assurance and Safety.
   Chapter 3: Sampling Dairy and Related Products.
   Chapter 4: Preparation of Media, Dilution Water, and Sterilization.
   Chapter 8: Tests for Groups of Microorganisms.
   Chapter 9: Microbiological Methods for Dairy Products.

3. **Definition:** See 6.020.3.

4. **Principle:** An aliquot of a liquid or diluted solid sample is introduced into or onto the Redigel™ aerobic pectin gel medium and pretreated Redigel™ dish. Plates are incubated as with SPC. Determination of the number of microorganisms per mL or gm of product is obtained by selecting plates chosen at dilution levels that will result in a significant result.

5. **Diluents, Culture Media, and Reagents:** See chapter 4: Preparation of Media, Dilution Water, and Sterilization.

   See also 6.020.5.

   Refer to manufacturer's instructions (3M Co., 3M Center, Bldg. 275-5W-05, St. Paul, MN 55144-1000).

   A. **Storage and disposal**
      1. *Media bottles:* ≤25°C (77°F).
      2. *Pretreated Redigel™ dishes:* Closed packages at room temperature (15° to 30°C or 59° to 86°F)

   B. **Shelf life**
      1. *Media bottles and dishes:* Expiration date and lot number are noted on individual bottle or box.
      2. As with other microbial detection systems, inoculated Redigel™ PGPC plates may contain viable bacteria that may be a biohazard. Follow current industry standards for disposal.

6. **Apparatus and Glassware:** See 6.020.6.

7. **Sampling:** See chapter 3: Sampling Dairy and Related Products.

8. **Preparation**

   A. Raw and pasteurized fluid milk and liquid milk products: See 6.020.8.
   B. Butter, margarine, and related products: See 6.020.8.
   C. Dry dairy products: See 6.020.8.
   D. Cheese and other cultured and culture-added products: See 6.020.8.
   F. Ice cream and related food products: See 6.020.8.
   G. Other dairy or related food products: See 6.020.8.

9. **Procedure:** Allow Redigel™ media to warm to room temperature before use.
   A. **One-dish or 10-dish bottle**
      1. Lift the lid of a pretreated Redigel™ dish and pour the liquid pectin gel [~10 mL] into the dish.
      2. Replace the lid and swirl the dish to cover the bottom with pectin gel.
      3. The sample must be added within 5 minutes after the liquid pectin gel is added. Add the sample or sample inoculum to the liquid pectin gel in the dish (0.1-1 mL depending on the desired dilution).
      4. Immediately swirl several times to thoroughly mix the sample with the pectin gel.
      5. Place the dish on a level surface and allow the medium to solidify for approximately 40 minutes and then incubate.
   B. **Incubation:** See 6.020.9.
   C. **Manual counting of colonies:** See 6.020.9.
10. **Expression of Results:** For computing and recording counts see section 6.020.10.
11. **Precision:** See chapter 1: Standard Methods.
12. **Test Report:** The test report must identify the method used and results obtained. The report is to identify any variation in the procedure not specified in this method as well as problems that may have impacted the test result. Each sample will be described in such a manner as to ensure traceability as to its origin.

6.060 Spiral Plate Count (SPLC) Method (Class A2)

1. **Scope:** The spiral plate count method is applicable to the examination of raw milk with valid results within the range of 400 to 400,000 cfu/mL.
   Note: The prior method described in *SMEDP* 16th edition for use with Model C and D platers (no longer manufactured) is still valid.
2. **References:** Chapter 1: Standard Methods.
   Chapter 2: Laboratory Quality Assurance and Safety.
   Chapter 3: Sampling Dairy and Related Products.
   Chapter 4: Preparation of Media, Dilution Water, and Sterilization.
   Chapter 8: Tests for Groups of Microorganisms.
   Chapter 9: Microbiological Methods for Dairy Products.
3. **Definition:** See 6.020.3.
4. **Principle:** The spiral plater (SPLC) aspirates a liquid sample by syringe and deposits it onto the surface of a prepared SMA agar plate in an Archimedes spiral pattern, with more sample in the center and less toward the plate edge. A total of 50 µL is deposited in default mode. This reduction in liquid deposited creates a 3-log dilution effect, allowing samples containing between 400 and 400,000 cfu/mL to be deposited and counted without prior dilution. The sample volume deposited on any portion of the plate is known. After proper incubation, colonies appear along the spiral track and are counted on a special grid [Figure 6.5] that associates a calibrated volume with each area. The number of bacteria in

the sample is estimated by dividing the number of colonies in a defined area by the volume contained in the same area.

The spiral plating method is AOAC approved[13] and studies have shown that the method is proficient not only with raw milk analysis,[9,27,37] but also with other samples and applications.[16,25,27,33,37]

5. **Diluents, Culture Media, and Reagents:** See chapter 4: Preparation of Media, Dilution Water, and Sterilization.

   See also 6.020.5.

   A. **Counting grid**
      1. The counting grid [Figure 6.5] is divided into 4 equal quadrants; each quadrant is divided by 6 arcs (segments) labeled 8–13.
      2. **High-count plates:** The grid is divided into 8 circumferential sectors labeled a, b, c, d, e, f, g, and h.

         A segment is the area between 2 arc lines within a quadrant. The grid is used to relate colonies in areas on a spiral plate to the volume in which they were deposited. The sample volume becomes greater as the counting proceeds from the outside edge of the plate toward the center.

   B. **Bacterial suspension:** 10^3 to 10^6 cfu/mL.

   C. Crystal violet solution.

   D. Bleach solution.

6. **Apparatus and Glassware**
   1. Autoplate 4000®: (Spiral Biotech, Inc., 2 Technology Way, Norwood, MA 02062, http://www.spiralbiotech.com). The Autoplate 4000® is a microprocessor-controlled spiral plater with an automated controlled-depletion system for cleaning and a stepper-motor driven syringe for uptake and plating of samples.

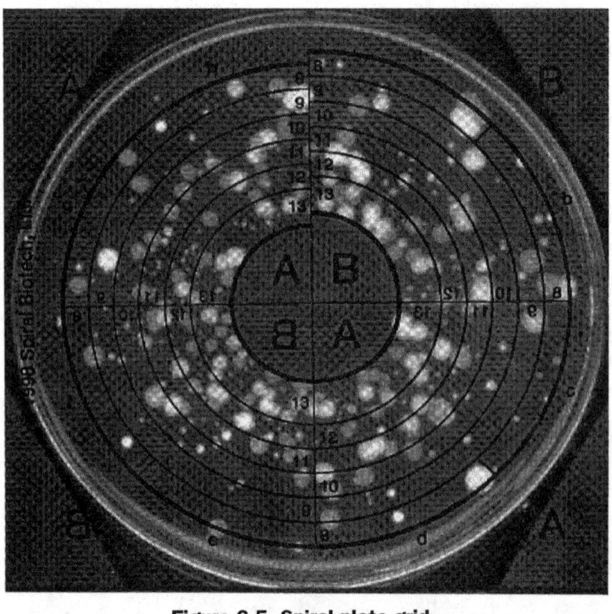

Reprinted with permission.

Figure 6.5. Spiral plate grid.

2. Spiral counting grid: For relating deposited sample volumes to specific portions of the petri dishes.
3. Vacuum source: 50 to 60 cm Hg and a 1-liter vacuum flask or bottle for trapping liquids.
4. Disposable micro beakers: 5 mL or equivalent.
5. Petri dishes: 100 × 15 mm/polyethylene bags about 30 × 20 × 40 cm.
6. Sodium hypochlorite solution: About 5% (equivalent to full strength commercial bleach solution) or equivalent.
7. Dye solution: Crystal violet 0.7% (w/v) solution.
8. Polypropylene reservoirs: 3 with a 75-mL capacity.

7. **Sampling:** See chapter 3: Sampling Dairy and Related Products.

8. **Preparation of Test Sample:** Prepare fresh SMA agar or melt premade SMA agar, avoiding prolonged exposure to high temperatures [6.020.8]. Pipet 15 to 20 mL of sterile SMA agar tempered to 60° to 70°C (TC required) into each petri dish, either by hand or calibrated automated dispenser. Allow agar to solidify on a sanitized, level surface, preferably under a laminar flow hood. After solidification, examine plates for uniformity of agar depth (no more than 2-mm difference), invert and allow to cool to room temperature. Place the solidified agar plates in polyethylene bags, close with ties or a heat sealer, and store inverted at 0° to 4.4°C for no longer than 2 weeks. Bring the prepared plates to room temperature and allow to dry for 12 to 24 hours before inoculation. Observe for any visible imperfections in the agar such as surface colonies (discard batch) or bubbles (do not use).

9. **Procedure**

A. **Calibration**

1. Before using the grid for the first time, the volume of the sample represented by each part of the grid must be determined by running a calibration. Maintain records of this calibration.
2. Make consecutive 1:2 dilutions of a bacterial suspension from 10^3 to 10^6 cfu/mL, resulting in 11 bacterial concentrations.
3. Plate all dilutions in duplicate by both the SPC method [6.020] and the SPLC method using the same medium and incubator.
4. After incubation, count and calculate the SPC per mL for each dilution. Count the spiral plates over the grid surface; use the counting rule of 20 to record the number of colonies counted and the grid area over which they were counted.
5. Each of the SPLC colony counts for a particular grid area (SPLC per area), divided by the SPC per mL for the corresponding bacterial concentration, will indicate how much volume was deposited on that particular grid area.

(SPLC per area) / (SPC per mL) = volume (mL) for the grid area.

B. **Procedure:** Since this is an alternate procedure, analysts must validate the SPLC to the SPC using the protocol in section 6.030.5.

1. Turn on vacuum source and Autoplate 4000®. Make sure that settings are for 50-µL deposition, 100-mm dish size, and "min" fill (for one plate per sample) or "max" fill (for multiple replicates when comparing to the SPC method).

2. Check stylus alignment daily according to manufacturer's directions and adjust if necessary.
3. Fill sterile cleaning reservoirs (autoclaved at 120° ± 1°C for 15 minutes) with sterile water or disinfectant to the top of their tolerance bands, as indicated, and place in position on the Autoplate 4000®.
4. Label the plate with sample information and make a vertical mark on the side of the plate bottom to indicate the start of sample deposition.
5. Shake samples and plate within 3 minutes.
6. Pour or pipet 3 to 4 mL of sample into a sterile 5-mL beaker and place it in position on the Autoplate 4000®.
7. Expose a plate to air for 15 minutes next to spiral plater at beginning during plating.
8. Remove the agar plate cover and place the plate on the turntable so that the vertical mark aligns with the radial scribed line on the turntable.
9. Press "all" to initiate a cycle of cleaning, filling, and plating.
10. After plating (inoculation) occurs, remove plate and replace lid.
11. If performing multiple replicate plates, as required when comparing to the SPC method, press "plate" to inoculate a replicate plate.
12. After absorption of liquid, invert the plate(s) and incubate as SPC.

C. **Controls**

1. **Dye plate control:** Prior to plating samples, run a crystal violet dye plate and examine the plate for a good distribution pattern.
   a. Conduct rinse controls before plating, after every 20 samples, and when sampling is complete.
   b. Check that bleach solution is rinsing free with no residual chlorine.
   c. Run a known sample after the last sample and before the final rinse control and maintain record.
   d. Check accuracy of instrument dispensing by running a validation routine with the validation test fixture quarterly; refer to the manufacturer's instructions.

D. **Counting and reporting spiral plate counts:** Count plates promptly after incubation. When it is impossible to count the plates at once, store the plates at 0° to 4.4°C for no longer than 24 hours, but avoid making this a routine practice.

E. **Counting rule of 20**

1. After incubation, center the spiral plate against the spiral grid with the vertical mark on the side of the plate aligned with 12 o'clock on the grid.
2. Choose any quadrant and count the colonies beginning in the outer segment No. 8 toward the center until 20 colonies have been counted, then finish counting the segment in which the 20th colony occurred. Similarly, count the same segment in the opposite quadrant.
3. Record the sum of the counts from the 2 segments. Record the number of the innermost segment counted.
4. If the number of colonies in segment No. 8 in 1 quadrant exceeds

75, recount plate by counting the circumferentially adjacent sectors (single spirals) in ⅛ increments (marked "a" to "h" on the grid) until at least 50 colonies have been counted. Record count and last sector counted.

5. Determine the number of cfu/mL by dividing count obtained by the volume contained in all the segments or sectors counted.

10. **Expression of Results:** Report count as SPLC/mL using only the first 1 left-hand digit [6.020].

(Segment count + Opposite segment count)/volume = SPLC count/mL

If there are not at least 20 colonies in the 6 segments of the quadrant, all of the colonies on the whole plate must be counted.

If a spreader covers no more than half of a plate, count well-distributed colonies in the spreader-free portion of the plate.

If plates show excessive colonies and cannot be counted, record as TNTC for highest dilutions factor and report as >400,000 ESPLC/mL.

If fewer than 20 colonies are counted on a total plate, report as <400 ESPLC/mL.

If plates show no colonies, record plate count as 0.

Do not count:

1. If spreaders interfere with the counting of the plate.
2. If the presence of a growth inhibitor is detected. Report the results as growth inhibitor (GI).
3. With irregular distributions of colonies caused by dispensing errors. Report the results as a laboratory accident (LA).

11. **Precision:** See chapter 1: Standard Methods.

12. **Test Report:** The test report must identify the method used and results obtained. The report is to identify any variation in the procedure not specified in this method as well as problems that may have impacted the test result. Each sample will be described in such a manner as to ensure traceability as to its origin.

6.070 Cited References

1. ARCHAMBAULT, J.; CUROT, J.; McCRADY, M.H. The need of uniformity of conditions for counting plates with suggestions for a standard colony counter. Am. J. Public Health **27**:809-812; 1937.
2. BABEL, F.J.; COLLINS, E.B.; OSLON, J.C.; PETERS, I.I.; WATROUS, G.H.; SPECK, M.L. The standard plate count of milk as affected by the temperature of incubation. J. Dairy Sci. **38**:499-503; 1955.
3. BERRY, J.M.; McNEILL, D.A.; WITTER, L.D. Effect of delays in pour plating on bacterial counts. J. Dairy Sci. **52**:1456-1457; 1969.
4. BISHOP, J.R. Jr., JUAN, J.Y. Improved methods for quality assessment of raw milk. J Food Prot. **51**:955-957; 1988.
5. BUTTERFIELD, C.T. Experimental studies of natural purification in polluted waters: VII. the selection of a dilution water for bacteriological examinations. J. Bacteriol. **23**:355-368; 1932.
6. BYRNE, R.D.; BISHOP, J.R. Jr., BOLING, J.W. Estimation of potential shelf-life of pasteurized fluid milk utilizing a selective preliminary incubation. J Food Prot. **54**:308-309; 1989.
7. COURTNEY, J.L. The relationship of average standard plate count ratios to employee proficiency in plating dairy products. J. Milk Food Technol. **19**:336-344; 1956.
8. CURIALE, M.S.; FAHEY, P.; FOX, T.L.; McALLISTER, J.S. Dry rehydratable films for

enumeration of coliforms and aerobic bacteria in dairy products: collaborative study. JAOAC **72:**312-318; 1989.

9. DONNELLY, C.B.; GILCHRIST, J.E.; PEELER, J.T.; CAMPBELL, J.E. Spiral plate count method for the examination of raw and pasteurized milk. Appl. Environ. Microbiol. **32:**21-27; 1976.
10. DRUCE, R.G.; THOMAS, S.B. Preliminary incubation of milk and cream prior to bacteriological examination: a review. Dairy Sci. Abstr. **30:**291-307; 1968.
11. DUNCAN, D.B. Multiple range and multiple F tests. Biometrics **11:**1-42; 1955.
12. FOWLER, J. L.; CLARK, W.S., Jr.; FOSTER, J.F.; HOPKINS, A. Analyst variation in doing the standard plate count as described in *Standard methods for the examination of dairy products*. J. Food Prot. **41:**4-7; 1978.
13. GILCHRIST, J.E.; DONNELLY, C.B.; PEELER, J.T.; CAMPBELL, J.E. Collaborative study comparing the spiral plate and aerobic plate count methods. JAOAC **60:**807-812; 1977.
14. GINN, R.E.; PACKARD, V.S.; FOX, T.L. Enumeration of total bacteria and coliforms in milk by dry rehydratable film methods; a collaborative study. JAOAC **69:**527-531; 1986.
15. GINN, R.E.; PACKARD, V.S.; FOX, T.L. Evaluation of the 3M dry medium culture plate (Petrifilm™ SM) method for determining numbers of bacteria in raw milk. J. Food Prot. **47:**753-755; 1984.
16. GREENWOOD, M.H.; COETZEE, E.F.C.; FORD, B.M.; GILL, P.; HOOPER, W.L.; MATTHEWS, S.C.W.; PATRICK, S.; PETHERS, J.V.S.; SCOTT, R.J.D. The microbiology of selected retail food products with an evaluation of viable counting methods. J. Hygiene. **92:** 67-78; 1984.
17. HARTMAN, P.A.; WEBER, J.A. Holding times of raw milk dilutions: a reassessment. J. Milk Food Technol. **35:**713-714; 1972.
18. HUHTANEN, C.N.; BRAZIS, A.R.; ARLEDGE, W.L.; COOK, E.W.; DONNELLY, C.B.; GINN, R.E.; JEZESKI, J.J.; PUSCH, D.; RANDOLPH, H.E.; SING, E.L. Effects of time of holding dilutions on counts of bacteria from raw milk. J. Milk Food Technol. **35:**126-130; 1972.
19. HUHTANEN, C.N.; BRAZIS, A.R.; ARLEDGE, W.L.; COOK, E.W.; DONNELLY, C.B.; GINN, R.E.; MURPHY, J.N.; RANDOLPH, H.E.; SING, E.L.; THOMPSON, D.I. Effect of dilution bottle mixing methods on plate counts of raw-milk bacteria. J. Milk Food Technol. **33:**269-273; 1970.
20. HUHTANEN, C.N.; BRAZIS, A.R.; ARLEDGE, W.L.; COOK, E.W.; DONNELLY, C.B.; GINN, R.E.; MURPHY, J.N.; RANDOLPH, H.E.; KOCH, E.J. Temperature equilibration times of plate count agar and a comparison of 50° versus 45°C for recovery of raw-milk bacteria. J. Milk Food Technol. **33:**319-322; 1975.
21. INTERNATIONAL DAIRY FEDERATION. *Milk and milk products: enumeration of microorganisms—colony count at 30°C. provisional IDF standard 100A*. Brussels, Belgium: Intern. Dairy Fed.; 1987.
22. JOHNS, C.K. Preliminary incubation for raw milk samples. J. Milk Food Technol. **23:**137-141; 1960.
23. JOHNS, C.K. Use of counts after preliminary incubation to improve raw milk quality for a Denver plant. J. Milk Food Technol. **38:**481-482; 1975.
24. KOBURGER, J.A. Stack-pouring of petri plates: a potential source of error. J. Food Prot. **43:**561-562; 1980.
25. MANNINEN, M.T., FUNG, D.Y.C., HART, R.A. Spiral system and laser colony scanner for enumeration of microorganisms. J. Food Safety. **11:**177-187; 1991.
26. NIEMELA, S. *Statistical evaluation of results from quantitative microbiological examinations.* Report no. 1, 2nd ed. Uppsala, Sweden: Nordic Committee in Food Analysis; 1983.
27. PEELER, J.T.; GILCHRIST, J.E.; DONNELLY, C.B.; CAMPBELL, J.E. A collaborative study of the spiral plate method for examining milk samples. J. Food Prot. **40:**462-464; 1977.
28. PEELER, J.T.; LESLIE, J.E.; DANIELSON, J.W.; MESSER, J.W. Replicate counting errors by analysts and bacterial colony counters. J. Food Prot. **45:**238-240, 1982.
29. PEELER, J.T.; MESSER, J.W.; SANDERS, R.L.; BACHELOR, H.K. A comparison of pre-

liminary incubation counts and standard plate counts of grade A bulk tank milk from eleven states. Dairy, Food and Environ. Sanitat. **9:**494-497, 1989.

30. PITON, C.; GRAPPIN, R. A model for statistical evaluation of precision parameters of microbiological methods: application to dry rehydratable film methods and IDF reference methods for enumeration of total aerobic mesophilic flora and coliforms in raw milk. JAOAC **74:**92-103; 1991.
31. READ, R.B., JR.; BRADSHAW, J.G.; FRANCIS, D.W. Effect of freezing raw milk on standard plate count. J. Dairy Sci. **52:**1720-1723, 1969.
32. REINBOLD, G.W.; JOHNS, C.K.; CLARK, W.S., JR. Modification of the preliminary incubation treatment for raw milk samples. J. Milk Food Technol. **32:**42-43; 1969.
33. SCHALKOWSKY, S. Plating Systems. In: Pierson, M.D. *Foodborne microorganisms and their toxins; developing methodology*. Stern, NJ: EDS P; 1986:107-127.
34. SUHREN, G. Enumeration of total and coliform bacteria in pure cultures, raw and pasteurized milk by dry rehydratable film and standard methods. Milchwissenschaft. **45:**139-144; 1990.
35. U.S. DEPARTMENT OF HEALTH AND HUMAN SERVICES. *Grade A pasteurized milk ordinance: Recommendations of the Public Health Service*, Publication No. 229, Washington, DC: U.S. Govt. Print. Off.; 1989 Rev.
36. VAN HEDDEGHEM, A.; REYBROECK, W. Determination of the total bacteria and the coliform bacteria in raw milk with the Petrifilm method. Landbouwtijdschrift. **43:**839-848; 1990.
37. WEXLER, H.M.; MOLITORIS, E.; MURRAY, P.R.; WASHINGTON, J.; ZABRANSKY, R. J.; EDELSTEIN, P.H.; FINEGOLD, S. M. Comparison of spiral gradient endpoint and agar dilution methods for susceptibility testing of anaerobic bacteria; multi-laboratory collaborative evaluation. J. Clinical Microbiol. **34:**170-174; 1996.
38. WHITE, C.H. Rapid methods for estimation and prediction of shelf-life of milk and diary products. J. Dairy Science **76:**3126-3132; 1993.
39. WRIGHT, E.O.; REINBOLD, G.W.; BURMEISTER, L.; MELLON, J. Prediction of standard plate count of manufacturing-grade raw milk from the plate loop count. J. Milk Food Technol. **33:**168-170; 1970.
40. YALE, M.W.; PEDERSON, C.S. Optimum temperature of incubation for standard methods of milk analysis as influenced by the medium. Amer. J. Public Health and the Nation's Health **26:**344-349; 1936.

6.080 Other References

BETTS, G.D.; BETTS, R.P.; TAYLOR, R. Evaluation of 3M Petrifilm™ for aerobic plate count, yeast and mould count and *Escherichia coli* count. Campden Food and Drink Research Association. Technical Memorandum No. 703; 1994.

CHAMBAULT, J.; CUROT, J.; McCRADY, M.H. The need of uniformity of conditions for counting plates with suggestions for a standard colony counter. Am. J. Public Health **27:**809-812; 1937.

CHAIN, V.S.; FUNG, D.Y.C. Comparison of Redigel, Petrifilm™, spiral plate system, isogrid, and aerobic plate count for determining the numbers of aerobic bacteria in selected foods. J. Food Prot. **54:**208-211; 1991.

CUNNIFF, P., ED. *Official methods of analysis of AOAC INTERNATIONAL*, 16th ed., 4th rev. Washington, DC: AOAC; 1998: 10.

CURIALE, M.S.; SONS, T.; McALLISTER, J.S.; HALSEY, B.; FOX, T.L. Dry rehydratable film for enumeration of total aerobic bacteria in foods: collaborative study. JAOAC **73:**242-248; 1990.

FOOD AND DRUG ADMINISTRATION. *Form 2400a—standard plate count, coliform, and simplified count methods.* Washington, DC: U.S. Govt. Print. Off.; 1999.

FUNG, D.Y.C.; CHAIN, V.S. Comparative analysis of Redigel and aerobic plate count methods for viable cell counts of selected foods. Food Micro. **8:**299-301; 1991.

HUGHES, D.; SUTHERLAND, P.S. Evaluation of Petrifilm SM for determining bacteriological counts on raw milk by comparison with the standard plate count and micropipette count techniques. Australian J Dairy Technology 42:59-61; 1987.

MARSHALL, R.T., ed. *Standard methods for the examination of dairy products*, 16th ed. Washington, DC: APHA; 1992.

MOSTELLER, T.M.; BISHOP, J.R., Jr. Sanitizer efficacy against attached bacteria in a milk biofilm. J. Food Prot. **56:**34-41; 1993.

OTTAVIANI, F.; ARVATI, G. Evaluation of new rapid systems for the determination of the total load and of the total coliforms in milk and milk products. II Latte. **13:**299-303; 1988.

PETERZ, M.; NILSSON, A.C. Determination of counts, number of aerobic bacteria and coliforms in foods by petrifilm method and agar plating—comparative study. Var Foeda. **43:**386-389; 1991.

ROTH, J.N. A temperature-independent pectin gel method for aerobic plate count in dairy and nondairy food products: collaborative study. JAOAC **71:**343-349; 1988.

SMITH, L.B.; ZOTTOLA, E.A.; FOX, T.L.; CHAUSSE, K. Use of Petrifilm to evaluate the microflora of frozen dessert mixes. J Food Prot. **52:**549-551; 1989.

TERAMOTO, T. Assessment of simple culturing Petrifilm for measuring numbers of colon bacillus and bacteria. Pharm. Tech Japan. **2:**1-5; 1986.

THOMPSON, D.I.; DONNELLY, C.B.; BLACK, L.A. A plate loop method for determining viable counts of raw milk. J. Milk Food Technol. **23:**167-171; 1960.

YNDESTAD, M. Petrifilm™—An alternative to traditional agar plates for culture of bacteria and moulds. Norsk Veterinae Rtidsskrift. **104:**411-414; 1992.

YOSHIDA, K.; MIZUOCHI, S.; HARTUA, M.; SIMIZU, Y. ; MORICHI, T. Evaluation of the Petrifilm™ method for the determination of viable bacterial counts in raw milk. Food Hygiene. **28:**483-486; 1987.

Chapter 7

Coliform and Other Indicator Bacteria

P. M. Davidson, L. A. Roth, and S. A. Gambrel-Lenarz
[J. Bruhn, Tech. Comm.]

7.010 Introduction

The coliform group of bacteria comprises all aerobic and facultatively anaerobic, gram-negative, nonspore-forming rods that are able to ferment lactose with the production of acid and gas at 32° or 35°C within 48 hours. (The temperature of incubation should be specified when reporting results.) One source of these organisms is the intestinal tract of warm-blooded animals. Certain bacteria of nonfecal origin are also members of this group. Typically, these organisms are classified in the genera *Escherichia*, *Enterobacter*, and *Klebsiella*. A few lactose-fermenting species of other genera are also included in the coliform group. In proportion to the numbers present, the existence of any of these types in dairy products is suggestive of unsanitary conditions or practices during production, processing, or storage.

Application of the test for coliforms is not intended to detect fecal pollution, but to measure the quality of the practices used to ensure proper processing and to minimize bacterial contamination of processed dairy products.[8,27]

Results of tests on raw samples are to be interpreted differently from those obtained when testing pasteurized milk.[29,34] Coliforms in small numbers may enter raw milk and cream under normal conditions of production and handling.[2] Some laboratories perform coliform estimates on raw milk to determine the degree of contamination during milk production. However, for raw and pasteurized samples, in the absence of a storage interval and temperature records for milk and cream before testing, it is impossible to conclude from positive tests alone to what degree bacterial growth following initial contamination may have contributed to test results. For cultured products, some limitations on the sample's age before testing seem necessary because of the rapid and marked reductions encountered in coliform counts within 24 hours of processing.[16] Coliforms isolated from pasteurized products suggest improper pasteurization and/or postpasteurization contamination, indicating the presence of defective equipment or a need for improved plant sanitation. Coliform tests are conducted following pasteurization primarily to detect bacterial recontamination of milk, cream, and other processed dairy products.[38]

The choice of method will largely depend on limits for the number of coliforms in which the analyst is interested. Other considerations are the materials required, laboratory facilities, and labor available to process the required volume of work conveniently.

In preliminary surveys of pasteurized dairy products, 1 or 2 plates, each containing 1 mL of sample, are sufficient. Well-operated pasteurization plants normally achieve coliform counts of fewer than 5 colonies per milliliter on processed samples. For increased sensitivity on such samples, a larger sample should be used: 4-mL portions in plates poured with 15 to 20 mL of medium are satisfactory.[20]

The multiple-tube or MPN procedure is one alternative if examination of a larger sample is desired. The multiple-tube method results in a most probable number that is an estimate of the bacteria present in a sample within limitations of the procedure.[28]

Some dairy foods may contain injured cells that will not grow on violet red bile agar (VRBA) when the specified colony count procedures without resuscitation are used. To obtain more accurate counts in instances where samples might contain injured coliforms, the coliform test may be modified when using a solid medium. This entails using a resuscitation step with the pour-plate technique, in which the sample is first plated with approximately 10 mL of tryptic soy agar.[18,19,33]

Escherichia coli is currently the best known fecal indicator, and its recovery from dairy products suggests that other organisms of fecal origin, including pathogens, may be present.

A fluorogenic assay for detection of *Escherichia coli* is based on the nearly exclusive presence of the enzyme β-glucuronidase in *E. coli*. A microbiological medium containing the substrate 4-methylumbelliferyl-β-D- glucuronide (MUG) is employed. *E. coli* growing in the medium produces the enzyme that cleaves MUG and results in fluorescence under long-wavelength UV light (366 nm). Only a few microorganisms produce gas in lauryl sulfate tryptose (LST) broth as well as act upon MUG. Ninety-six percent of *E. coli* strains produce the enzyme β-glucuronidase.[13]

The Petrifilm™ dry rehydratable methods are sample-ready plating procedures that use a dehydrated cold water-soluble gelling agent, selective nutrients, and a tetrazolium indicator that facilitates colony enumeration. These microbial methods use premade films that do not involve media preparation. Incubation space and waste management are optimized since a stack of 15 1-mL Petrifilm™ plates occupy approximately the same space as 1 standard petri dish.

Petrifilm™ coliform count (PCC) plates are applicable for the enumeration of coliform in raw milk,[4(17.3.02),6,30] pasteurized milk,[4(17.3.02),5,21] and dairy products.[4(17.3.03)] The PCC method has been collaboratively studied with milk[4(17.3.02,-.03)]and dairy products[4(17.3.03)] and was found to be not significantly different from the VRB method. The Petrifilm™ high-sensitivity coliform count (PHSCC) plates are applicable for the enumeration of low levels of coliforms in dairy products. A 5-mL sample is plated onto one PHSCC plate. The PHSCC method has been collaboratively studied with milk and dairy products and was found to be not significantly different from the VRB method.[4(17.3.03A),6] Petrifilm™ rapid coliform count (PRCC) plates are applicable for the presumptive indication of coliforms in 6 to 14 hours and confirmed coliforms in 8 to 24 hours. The AOAC collaborative study found the PRCC method to be an acceptable alternative for early detection and confirmation of coliforms in raw milk, pasteurized milk, and dairy products. The Petrifilm™ *E. coli*/coliform count plate (PEC) is useful in the enumeration of coliforms and *E. coli* in dairy products.[4(17.3.04),5,7,15] The PEC method has been collaboratively studied for *E. coli* and total coliforms with cheese and was found to be not significantly different from the MPN method.[4(17.3.04)]

The Redigel™ methods use pectin as the gelling agent so that all operations are carried out at room temperature. The Redigel™ VRB test (RVRB) method is useful for coliform enumeration and is applicable in matrices similar to the VRB agar method. It has been collaboratively studied with milk, cream, and cultured products.[4(17.3.01)] The Redigel™ colichrome 2 (RCC2) test method is applicable for the enumeration of coliforms and *E. coli*. The AOAC precollaborative study found the RCC2 method to be an acceptable alternative for the detection of coliforms and *E. coli* in raw and pasteurized milk, cheese, cottage cheese, and yogurt.

The hydrophobic grid membrane filter (HGMF) method uses a membrane filter imprinted with hydrophobic material in a grid pattern.[12] Hydrophobic lines divide the membrane filter surface into separate compartments of equal and known size and act as barriers to the spread of colonies. The number of squares occupied by colonies is enumerated and converted to the MPN value of organisms by using the formula. To enumerate *E. coli*, a fluorogenic agent (4-methylumbelliferyl-β-D-glucuronide) has been incorporated into one of the media used in the HGMF analysis to determine the presence of the enzyme β-glucuronidase.

For additional information concerning coliforms in other dairy products, refer to discussions of concentrated [9.030] and dry milk products [9.050]; butter, margarine, and related products [9.060]; cheese and other cultured products [9.070]; and ice cream and related products [9.080].

7.020 Colony Count Technique (without resuscitation) (Class O)

1. **Scope:** The method is applicable to milk and fluid milk products.

2. **References:** Chapter 2: Laboratory Quality Assurance and Safety.
   Chapter 3: Sampling Dairy and Related Products.
   Chapter 4: Preparation of Media, Dilution Water, and Sterilization.
   Chapter 6: Microbiological Count Methods.
   Chapter 9: Microbiological Methods for Dairy Products.

3. **Definitions**
   A. **Coliform group positive presumptive test:** Typical dark red colonies (normally measuring at least 0.5 mm in diameter on uncrowded

plates) appearing within 24 ± 2 hours of incubation at 32°± 1°C on VRBA.[1,14,24,40]

B. **Confirmed test:** A *confirmed test* should be made of atypical colonies from VRBA plates by transferring each of 5 colonies (if available) to tubes of 2% brilliant green bile (BGB) broth and incubating at 32° or 35°C. BGB broth tubes showing gas after 48 ± 3 hours of incubation at 35° ± 1°C represent confirmed coliforms.

4. **Principle:** Sample is decimally diluted in diluent and plated with VRBA into petri dishes for enumeration of coliform bacteria as coliform colony-forming units per milliliter. Plates are incubated at 24 ± 2 hours of incubation at 32°± 1°C.

5. **Diluents, Culture Media, and Reagents**

   A. **General:** See chapter 6 for standard equipment and supplies.

   B. **Diluent:** See chapter 6.

   C. Culture medium.

   D. **VRBA:** See chapter 4. Use commercially available dehydrated media and prepare according to the manufacturer's instructions.

   E. **Brilliant green bile (BGB) broth, 2%:** See chapter 4. Use commercially available dehydrated media and prepare according to the manufacturer's instructions. Dispense medium in quantities of 10 mL into culture tubes containing Durham tubes and sterilize according to manufacturer's instructions. The Durham tubes should not contain air bubbles following sterilization.

6. **Apparatus and Glassware:** See chapter 6.
   Incubator capable of 32° ± 1°C.

7. **Sampling:** See chapter 3.

8. **Procedure**

   A. **Colony count method procedure:** Transfer 1 mL of each sample or a decimal dilution thereof onto a sterile plate. Add to each plate 10 to 15 mL of VRBA tempered to 44° to 46°C. Pour an agar control [chapter 6] for each flask of medium used. Select the number of samples to be plated in any one series so there is not more than a 20-minute time lapse between diluting the first sample and pouring the last plate in the series.

   To facilitate mixing of the sample and the agar medium when plating viscous products such as cream, ice cream, and buttermilk, prepare initial dilutions of the sample of 1:2 or 1:10 in warmed (about 40° to 45°C) dilution blanks and distribute 10 mL into 3 dishes using 15 to 20 mL of medium per dish.

   Mix the contents of the plates thoroughly using conventional mixing procedures. Allow the mixtures to solidify (5 to 10 minutes) on a level surface; then distribute an additional 3 to 4 mL of the plating medium as an overlay, completely covering the surface of the solidified medium to inhibit surface colony formation. Invert and incubate the plates for 24 ± 2 hours at 32° ± 1°C.

   It is preferable to record results from only those plates that contain *between 15 and 150* coliform colonies. Count the dark red colonies measuring 0.5 mm or more in diameter on uncrowded plates, and record results. When fermentable substances other than lactose are present in samples, confirm the presence of lactose fermenters by appropriate transfers of either dark red colonies on VRBA or broth from tubes showing gas to 2% BGB.

On crowded plates (more than 150 colonies), coliform colonies may show atypical characteristics and may measure less than 0.5 mm in diameter. Furthermore, on crowded plates, strains of some noncoliforms and yeasts may produce colonies comparable in color and size to colonies of coliforms.[28] In such instances, pick representative colonies, and confirm the presence of lactose fermenters.

Results from plates having excessive numbers of colonies may be unreliable. Avoid crowded plates, if possible, by plating a sufficient number of dilutions with selected volumes of the sample. Plates from serial dilutions that do not demonstrate a proportionate change in the numbers of colonies corresponding to the dilutions plated indicate the possibility of an injured coliform population.[36] In these instances it may be necessary to use the multiple-tube fermentation technique [7.030] or a modified VRBA procedure [7.040] to obtain the most accurate assessment of the coliform population.

B. **Confirmed test with colonies from a solid medium (Class O):** If it is necessary to confirm coliform colonies on VRBA, transfer typical and/or atypical colonies to tubes of BGB broth and incubate for 48 ± 3 hours at 32°or 35° ± 1°C. The presence of gas in the inverted Durham tube or effervescence after gentle agitation indicates a positive confirmed test. Failure to show gas production within 48 hours indicates the absence of coliforms. If growth on a solid medium is without clearly isolated colonies, streak the growth on the surface of solidified VRBA plates for isolation, incubate for 24 ± 2 hours at 32° ± 1°C, and transfer isolated colonies to BGB broth. Confirm the presence of coliform bacteria as indicated above.

9. Calculation and Expression of Results

A. **Calculation:** Calculate *N*, the number of colony-forming units of coliforms per milliliter or gram of sample using the following:

$$N = \Sigma c / (n_1 + 0.1\, n_2)d$$

Where:

Σc = Sum of all colonies on all plates counted.
n_1 = Number of plates in first dilution counted.
n_2 = Number of plates in second dilution counted.
d = Dilution from which the first counts were obtained.

B. **All plates with fewer than 15 colonies:** When plates from both dilutions yield fewer than 15 colonies each, record the count as less than 15 times d/L, where d/L is the reciprocal of the dilution factor [chapter 6].

C. **All plates with more than 150 colonies:** If *more than 150* colonies develop on the highest-dilution plate, estimate counts from plates nearest 150 and multiply by the reciprocal of the dilution.

D. **All plates with spreaders, demonstrated growth inhibitors, or laboratory accident:** See chapter 6.

10. **Precision:** When 5 or more coliform colonies appear on single plates, counts are usually more precise than those obtained using 5 fermentation tubes.[25] When fewer than 15 coliform colonies routinely develop on the plate(s) from diluted sample(s), lower dilutions should be plated. Keep in mind that precision decreases as the number of colonies per plate decreases.[3] If fewer than 5 coliform colonies routinely develop on the plate(s) from undiluted sample(s),[26] multiple-tube procedures, Petrifilm™ HSCC, or hydrophobic grid membrane filtration should be considered.

    Caution should be exercised before drawing conclusions from the results of a single examination by either the tube or the plate method.[26,27] The precision of results obtainable is low when 1) few positive tubes appear among several inoculated with one or more sample volume(s), or 2) a very low colony count is obtained from several plates.[22]

11. **Test Report and Interpretation:** Use only 2 significant figures followed by zeros. Record the method of choice when reporting results. It is important to determine that the chosen test meets with regulatory as well as customers' and suppliers' requirements. The estimate of coliform numbers will vary with the method and the media used. Likewise, while modification of a method might be desirable, interpretation of the test may be changed with variance from the published procedure. An example is the extension of incubation times that can result in increased population estimates.[35] In addition, external factors such as sampling methods, testing protocols, preparation time, and handling may influence recovery and results for enumeration.

    Because organisms giving positive coliform tests are practically nonexistent in properly pasteurized milk collected directly from pasteurizers, the presence of such organisms is usually indicative of contamination introduced by equipment and/or processing downstream from the pasteurizer.

7.030 Most Probable Number Technique (Class O)

To provide a more sensitive test for estimating low (e.g., < 5 CFU/g) coliform populations or to estimate coliforms that may have been injured, the fermentation tube technique has historically been used. The multiple-tube or MPN procedure is one alternative for enumerating coliforms in a larger sample than is possible with the plating procedure. Because of the irregular distribution of bacteria, even when coliforms average 1 per milliliter, the probabilities are that 37% of the 1-mL portions of a sample will contain no coliforms; however, if each test is made with 5 portions of 1 mL apiece, completely negative results may be expected less than 1% of the time.

Processed products may contain bacterial cells that have been stressed during processing or storage, resulting in injured coliforms that may be unable to grow in solid or liquid selective media. Thus, counts on some manufactured milk products may be erroneously low and may not indicate the true population of viable coliforms present. Environmental stresses such as heat, chemicals, freezing, dehydration, or acid pH of the food matrix (e.g., yogurt, buttermilk, or juices) may injure coliforms, thus adversely affecting the quantitative recovery of the organisms in selective media.[31] This has been found to be true for fluid milk, cheese, and acidified or frozen dairy products.[13,23,33] In such instances, modified procedures using solid media are available to facilitate the recovery of injured coliforms [7.040].[11,18,19,32,32] However, liquid media have better potential than solid media for estimating the viable populations of heat-injured coliform bacteria.[36,37] Although the multiple-tube fermentation technique using LST broth is not as precise in estimating coliform populations as solid media methods, it is the most sensitive in detecting injured cells.

1. **Scope:** This procedure specifies methods for the enumeration of presumptive coliform species of bacteria by means of the culture technique involving a liquid medium and calculation of the number of presumptive coliform species of bacteria per gram or milliliter by the most probable number (MPN) technique after incubation at 35°C.

   The method is applicable to milk and liquid milk products, dried milk, sweet whey, dried buttermilk, lactose, acid, lactic acid and rennet casein, caseinate and dried acid whey, cheese and processed cheeses, butter, frozen milk products, dairy custards, and creams.

2. **References:** Chapter 2: Laboratory Quality Assurance and Safety.
   Chapter 3: Sampling Dairy and Related Products.
   Chapter 4: Preparation of Media, Dilution Water, and Sterilization.
   Chapter 6: Microbiological Count Methods.
   Chapter 9: Microbiological Methods for Dairy Products.

3. **Definitions**
   A. **Positive presumptive test:** A *positive presumptive test* for members of the coliform group is indicated when fermentation tubes containing lauryl sulfate tryptose (LST) broth show gas formation within 48 ± 3 hours of incubation at 35° ± 1°C
   B. **Confirmed test:** A *confirmed test* should be made of positive LST broth tubes by transferring 1 loopful to a tube of BGB broth. BGB broth tubes showing gas after 48 ± 3 hours of incubation at 35° ± 1°C represent confirmed coliforms.

4. **Principle:** Three consecutive dilutions of a sample are placed into 3 sets of 3, 5, or 10 culture tubes containing lauryl sulfate tryptone broth and Durham tubes. Tubes are incubated at 24 ± 2 hours of incubation at 35°± 1°C with the resultant fermentation of the media. Tubes are scored as either positive (presence of gas only) or negative (no gas). Coliform count for the sample is determined by consulting the MPN table.

5. **Diluents, Culture Media, and Reagents**
   A. **General:** See chapter 6 for standard equipment and supplies.
   B. **Diluent:** See chapter 6.
   C. **Culture Media.**
   D. **LST broth:** See chapter 4. Use commercially available dehydrated media and prepare according to manufacturer's instructions.
   E. **BGB broth, 2%:** See chapter 4. Use commercially available dehydrated media and prepare according to manufacturer's instructions.

6. **Apparatus and Glassware**

A. **Apparatus:** Inoculation loop (3 mm) and needle.

B. **Glassware**

1. Culture tubes of sufficient capacity to contain 10 times the sample volume and that allow head space for adequate mixing.
2. Durham tubes of appropriate dimensions for use with the test tubes.

7. **Sampling:** See chapter 3.

8. **Procedure**

A. **Dilution of samples:** Dilute (if necessary) samples according to chapter 6.

B. **Inoculation and incubation of tubes:** Transfer 1-mL portions of the sample and/or a decimal dilution for 3 consecutive dilutions to each of 3 or 5 tubes of LST broth. (Five tubes are recommended if low numbers of coliforms are expected.) Incubate the tubes for 24 ± 2 hours at 35° ± 1°C and examine for gas production either in the inverted Durham tube or by effervescence when the tube is gently shaken. Record results and, if required, begin a confirmed test for all gas-positive tubes. Positive LST broth tubes should be confirmed by transfer to 2% BGB broth. Incubate the gas-negative tubes for an additional 24 ± 2 hours, examine for additional gas-positive tubes, and begin the confirmed test for any additional gas-positive tubes detected. Record all LST tubes showing gas within 48 ± 3 hours, and calculate the presumptive MPN of coliform bacteria per gram or milliliter.

Note: Avoid introducing air into the inverted tubes. If small bubbles of gas appear in Durham tubes during storage, steaming the tubes will drive off the gas. *Do not* use such tubes if they show turbidity.

C. **Confirmed test for coliform bacteria:** Gently agitate the positive LST tubes and transfer 1 loopful from each tube (avoid transferring the pellicle) to a tube of BGB broth. Incubate the BGB tubes for 48 ± 3 hours at 35° ± 1°C. Record all BGB tubes showing gas, and report the confirmed MPN of coliform bacteria per gram or milliliter [7.030.9.C].

9. **Expression of Results**

A. **MPN tables:** The inherent complexity of computing MPNs and confidence limits means that most laboratory workers must use published tables to determine the MPN. Tables 7.1 and 7.2 show the MPNs of microorganisms corresponding to the frequency of positive tubes obtained from 3 1:10 dilution series. Results for both 3 tubes [Table 7.1] and 5 tubes [Table 7.2] per dilution are given along with the 95% confidence limits. Tables 7.1 and 7.2 provide combinations of positive results that occur often enough to be statistically significant; the less likely combinations—those that occur less than 1% of the time—have been omitted. Should further insight into these tabular differences or the methods used to compute the values be needed, the original work should be reviewed.[9,10] In the rare situation where the appropriate combination of positive results is not found within these tables, it is generally recommended that the analysis be repeated.

Tables 7.3 and 7.4 give examples for determining MPN estimates for a 3-tube and 5-tube MPN series, respectively. Note that the tabular

Table 7.1. Selected Most Probable Number (MPN) Estimates and 95% Confidence Limits[2] of Estimates for Fermentation Tube Tests When Three Tubes with 0.1-g, 0.01-g, and 0.001-g (or -mL) Amounts Are Used

Number of Positive Tubes Out of Three				95% Confidence Limits	
0.1 g	0.01 g	0.001 g	MPN/g or mL[a]	Lower	Upper
0	0	0	<3	–	–
0	1	0	3+	<1	17
1	0	0	4	<1	21
1	0	1	7+	2	27
1	1	0	7	2	28
1	2	0	11+	4	35
2	0	0	9	2	38
2	0	1	14+	5	48
2	1	0	15	5	50
2	1	1	20+	7	60
2	2	0	21	8	62
3	0	0	23	9	130
3	0	1	39	10	180
3	1	0	43	10	210
3	1	1	75	20	280
3	2	0	93	30	380
3	2	1	150	50	500
3	2	2	210+	80	640
3	3	0	240	90	1400
3	3	1	460	100	2400
3	3	2	1100	300	4800
3	3	3	>1100	–	–

Note: All figures under "MPN/g or mL" in this table may be multiplied by 100 for reporting "MPN/100 g or mL."

[a] Normal results, obtained in 95% of tests, are *not* followed by a plus. Less likely results, obtained in only 4% of tests, *are* followed by a plus. Combinations of positive tubes not shown in the table occur in less than 1% of tests, and their frequent occurrence is an indication that technique is faulty or that assumptions underlying the MPN estimate are not being fulfilled. MPN estimates for combinations that are not shown in the table may be obtained by extrapolating to the next highest combination shown in the table; for example, a result of 2/0/2 would have an MPN of approximately 20, which is the MPN for a more likely result of 2/1/1.

values are treated in terms of the actual sample volumes planted in these dilutions.

When more than 3 dilutions of a sample are prepared, the results from only 3 consecutive dilutions are used in determining the MPN. First, for all dilutions having all tubes positive, select the highest dilution (i.e., the smallest sample volume) [example "e" of Tables 7.3 and 7.4]. Second, use the next 2 higher dilutions (smaller volumes) [examples "a" and "b" of Tables 7.3 and 7.4]. When none of the tested dilutions yields all tubes positive, select, if possible, the first 3 consecutive dilutions for which the middle dilution contains the positive result [example "c" of Tables 7.3 and 7.4]. If a positive result occurs in a higher dilution (smaller sample volume) than in the 3 selected, add the number of positive tubes in this dilution to the highest dilution (smallest sample volume) of the 3 selected [example "d" of Tables 7.3 and 7.4].

Table 7.2. Selected Most Probable Number (MPN) Estimates and 95% Confidence Limits[2] of Estimates for Fermentation Tube Tests When Five Tubes with 0.1-g, 0.01-g, and 0.001-g (or -mL) Amounts Are Used[a]

Number of Positive Tubes Out of Five				95% Confidence Limits	
0.1 g	0.01 g	0.001 g	MPN/g or mL[a]	Lower	Upper
0	0	0	<2	–	–
0	0	1	2+	<1	10
0	1	0	2	<1	10
1	0	0	2	<1	11
1	0	1	4+	1	15
1	1	0	4	1	15
1	2	0	6+	2	18
2	0	0	4	1	17
2	0	1	7+	2	20
2	1	0	7	2	21
2	1	1	9+	3	25
2	2	0	9	3	25
3	0	0	8	3	24
3	0	1	11	4	29
3	1	0	11	4	30
3	1	1	14+	6	35
3	2	0	14	6	35
3	2	1	17+	7	40
3	3	0	17+	7	41
4	0	0	13	5	38
4	0	1	17	7	45
4	1	0	17	7	46
4	1	1	21	9	55
4	2	0	22	9	56
4	2	1	26+	12	65
4	3	0	27	12	67
4	3	1	33+	15	77
4	4	0	34+	16	80
5	0	0	23	9	68
5	0	1	31	13	110
5	1	0	33	14	120
5	1	1	46	20	150
5	1	2	63+	22	180
5	2	0	49	21	170
5	2	1	70	30	210
5	2	2	94+	40	250
5	3	0	79	30	250
5	3	1	110	40	300
5	3	2	140	60	360
5	4	0	130	50	390
5	4	1	170	70	480
5	4	2	220	100	580
5	4	3	280+	120	690
5	4	4	350+	160	820
5	5	0	240	100	940
5	5	1	350	100	1300

continued

Table 7.2. *Continued*

Number of Positive Tubes Out of Five				95% Confidence Limits	
0.1 g	0.01 g	0.001 g	MPN/g or mL[a]	Lower	Upper
5	5	2	540	220	2000
5	5	3	920	300	2900
5	5	4	1600	600	5300
5	5	5	>1600	–	–

Note: All figures under "MPN/g or mL" in this table may be multiplied by 100 for reporting "MPN/100 g or mL."

[a] Normal results, obtained in 95% of tests, are *not* followed by a plus. Less likely results, obtained in only 4% of tests, *are* followed by a plus. Combinations of positive tubes not shown in the table occur in less than 1% of tests, and their frequent occurrence is an indication that technique is faulty or that assumptions underlying the MPN estimate are not being fulfilled. MPN estimates for combinations that are not shown in the table may be obtained by extrapolating to the next highest combination shown in the table; for example, a result of 4/0/2 would have an MPN of approximately 21, which is the MPN for a more likely result of 4/1/1.

Table 7.3. Examples of Determining Most Probable Number (MPN) Estimates: Three-Tube Series

	Sample Amount (g or mL)					Reported Positive	MPN
Example	0.1	0.01	0.001	0.0001	0.00001	Values	Estimate/g or mL
a	3/3[a]	3/3	2/3	0/3	0/3	3-2-0	930
b	3/3	3/3	3/3	2/3	0/3	3-2-0	9300
c	0/3	0/3	1/3	0/3	0/3	0-1-0	30
d	3/3	3/3	2/3	1/3	1/3	3-2-2	2100
e	3/3	3/3	3/3	3/3	3/3	3-3-3	>110,000

Note: All figures under "MPN/g or mL" in this table may be multiplied by 100 for reporting "MPN/100 g or mL."

[a] Number of positive tubes/Number of tubes inoculated.

Table 7.4. Examples of Determining Most Probable Number (MPN) Estimates: Five-Tube Series

	Sample Amount (g or mL)					Reported Positive	MPN
Example	0.1	0.01	0.001	0.0001	0.00001	Values	Estimate/g or mL
a	5/5[a]	5/5	2/5	0/5	0/5	5-2-0	490
b	5/5	5/5	5/5	2/5	0/5	5-2-0	4900
c	0/5	0/5	1/5	0/5	0/5	0-1-0	20
d	5/5	5/5	3/5	1/5	1/5	5-3-2	1400
e	5/5	5/5	5/5	5/5	5/5	5-5-5	>160,000

Note: All figures under "MPN/g or mL" in this table may be multiplied by 100 for reporting "MPN/100 g or mL."

[a] Number of positive tubes/Number of tubes inoculated.

Often it is necessary to calculate the MPN from initial sample amounts other than those listed in Tables 7.1 and 7.2. If the largest (greatest) sample used for the table reference is 0.01 g, multiply the MPN index listed in the table by 10. Thus, results of a 5-tube MPN determination showing 3 positive 0.01-g portions, 2 positive 0.001-g portions, and 1 positive 0.0001-g portion (3-2-1) are read from Table 7.2 as 17 and multiplied by 10 to arrive at 170 as the actual MPN per gram for the sample. Similarly, if the greatest portion used for the table reference is 1 g rather than 0.1 g, divide the MPN derived from the table by 10. Thus, the results of a 3-tube MPN determination for coliforms showing 3 positive 1-g portions, 1 positive 0.1-g portion, and no positive 0.01-g portions (3-1-0) are read from Table 7.1 as 43 and divided by 10 to arrive at 4.3 as the presumptive MPN per gram for the sample.

B. **MPN formula:** An alternative approach to obtain the MPN per gram uses the following formula[33]:

$$MPN/g = ((MPN/g)_{Table} \div 100) \times \text{middle-tube dilution factor}$$

To obtain an MPN per 100 g, multiple by 100.

C. **Reporting results:** Results should be recorded as "number of microorganisms per quantity (gram or milliliter) of sample by the MPN method" (e.g., coliform MPN per gram = 11). With the report of microbiological counts by the MPN method, include the number of tubes used in each dilution (i.e., the 5-tube MPN or the 3-tube MPN).

10. **Precision:** Given that the tabulated numbers are correctly computed, the next consideration should be an appreciation of the confidence limit surrounding a given value in each table. That is, the tabular MPN estimate represents a range and not an absolute value: MPN estimates are often credited with unfounded precision. Tables 7.1 and 7.2 include 95% confidence limits for the tabular MPN estimates. The strict interpretation of these limits is that, if the analyst assumes that the true number of organisms lies between these limits, the assumption will be correct 95% of the time. Woodward[39] published tables of confidence limits for 3- and 5-tube multiple dilution assays and pointed out that, for a 3-tube test, the 95% confidence limits cover a 33-fold range from approximately 14% to 458% of the actual tabular MPN estimate; for a 5-tube multiple-dilution test, the 95% confidence limits cover a 13-fold range from approximately 24% to 324% of the MPN.

    Caution should be exercised before drawing conclusions from the results of a single examination by either the tube or the plate method.[26,27] The precision of results obtainable is low when 1) few positive tubes appear among several inoculated with one or more sample volume(s), or 2) a very low colony count is obtained from several plates.[22]

11. **Test Report:** Record the method of choice when reporting results. It is important to determine that the chosen test meets with regulatory as well as customers' and suppliers' requirements. The estimate of coliform numbers will vary with the method and the media used. Likewise, while variations in a method might be desirable, they may impact on the results. An example is the extension of incubation times which can result

in increased population estimates.[35] In addition, external factors such as sampling methods, testing protocols, preparation time, and handling may influence recovery and results for enumeration.

7.040 Modified VRBA Procedures (Class B)

Processed products may contain bacterial cells that have been stressed during processing or storage, resulting in injured coliforms that may be unable to grow in solid or liquid selective media. Thus, counts on some manufactured milk products may be erroneously low and may not indicate the true population of viable coliforms present. Environmental stresses such as heat, chemicals, freezing, dehydration, or acid pH of the food matrix (e.g., yogurt, buttermilk, or juices) may injure coliforms, thus adversely affecting the quantitative recovery of the organisms in selective media.[31] This has been found to be true for fluid milk, cheese, and acidified or frozen dairy products.[17,23,33] In such instances, modified procedures using solid media are available to facilitate the recovery of injured coliforms.[11,18,19,32,33]

1. **Scope:** This procedure specifies a method that can be used to enumerate coliform species of bacteria that may be injured in fluid milks, cheeses, and acidified and frozen dairy desserts.
2. **References:** Chapter 2: Laboratory Quality Assurance and Safety.
   Chapter 3: Sampling Dairy and Related Products.
   Chapter 4: Preparation of Media, Dilution Water, and Sterilization.
   Chapter 6: Microbiological Count Methods.
   Chapter 9: Microbiological Methods for Dairy Products.
3. **Diluents, Culture Media, and Reagents:** See chapter 6 for standard equipment and supplies.
   Violet red bile agar-2 (VRBA-2).
   Tryptic soy agar, TSA: see chapter 4.
4. **Sampling:** See chapter 3.
5. **Procedure:** Plates are incubated at 32° ± 1°C for 2 ± 0.5 hours. After the preliminary incubation, the inoculated base medium is overlaid with about 10 mL of VRBA-2 (VRBA with double the usual concentrations of bile salts No. 3, neutral red, and crystal violet). After solidification, the plates are incubated at 32° ± 1°C for 24 ± 2 hours and counted.
6. **Expression of Results:** The procedures described in 7.040.5 are not normally used for control purposes. They do, however, provide information that may be useful to the dairy food processor. The fact that VRBA-2 was used should be included in the report of results.
7. **Precision:** Precision parameters have not been determined for this test.
8. **Test Report:** The test report specifies the method used and the results obtained, indicating clearly the method of expression used and the repeatability if calculated. Any exceptions to operating details of the method must be specified.

7.050 Confirmed Test for *Escherichia coli* (Class O)

Information for verifying *Escherichia coli* is provided for testing laboratories that have a specific need for determining numbers of *E. coli.*

Isolates suspected of being *E. coli* have traditionally been confirmed based on their IMViC pattern. However, this profile alone is not enough to identify the species because at least 7 species may have the same pattern as typical and atypical *E. coli*. Care must be taken to avoid misidentifying the isolate, especially if it was obtained by direct streaking or from less selective enrichment media. Isolates that are presumed to be *E. coli* must conform to the coliform definition prior to being tested by the methods described in this section (i.e., produce gas from lactose and produce typical colonies on L-EMB plates).

1. **Scope:** This method can be used on coliform cultures isolated from dairy foods previously analyzed.
2. **References:** Chapter 2: Laboratory Quality Assurance and Safety.
   Chapter 3: Sampling Dairy and Related Products.
   Chapter 4: Preparation of Media, Dilution Water, and Sterilization.
   Chapter 6: Microbiological Count Methods.
   Chapter 9: Microbiological Methods for Dairy Products.
3. **Definition:** *E. coli*: In a pure culture, a microorganism that ferments lactose with the production of gas within 48 hours at 35°C; that appears as a gram-negative, with nonspore-forming rods or cocci; and that gives IMViC patterns + + – – (biotype 1) or – + – – (biotype 2).
4. **Principle**
   A. Cultures that are suspect as being coliforms are purified and then determined if they are gram-negative rods or cocci that ferment lactose in 48 hours to gas.
   B. Confirmed coliform cultures have 10 examined for their biochemical characteristics using the IMViC test procedure
5. **Diluents, Culture Media, and Reagents:** See chapter 6 for standard equipment and supplies.
   1. L-EMB agar.
   2. LST broth.
   3. EC broth.
   4. Methyl red-Voges-Proskauer (MR-VP) medium.
   5. Tryptone broth: 1%.
   6. Koser's citrate broth.
   7. Kovacs' indole reagent: p-dimethylaminobenzaldehyde, 5 g; amyl alcohol, 75 mL; and hydrochloric acid (concentrated), 25 mL. Dissolve p-dimethylaminobenzaldehyde in the amyl alcohol and slowly add the hydrochloric acid. Store at 4°C. (Discard if color is darker than light straw.)
   8. Methyl red indicator: Methyl red, 0.19 g; ethanol, 95%, 300 mL. Dissolve methyl red in ethanol and make up to 500 mL with distilled water.
   9. α-naphthol solution: 5% in absolute ethanol.
   10. 40% aqueous potassium hydroxide.
   11. Creatine crystals.
6. **Apparatus and Glassware:** The apparatus required for the preparation of the test sample, dilutions, and plating in liquid and solid media.

7. **Sampling:** See chapter 3.
8. **Procedure:** Gently agitate the positive LST tubes, and transfer 1 loopful from each tube (avoid transferring the pellicle) to a tube of EC broth. When coliform populations are being estimated using solid media (e.g., VRBA), colonies may be tested for *E. coli* identity.
   A. Transfer the colonies to EC broth and follow the same procedure as for tubes inoculated from LST.
   B. Incubate the EC tubes for 48 ± 2 hours at 45.5° ± 0.2°C. To achieve the required temperature control, use a water bath or water-jacketed air incubator. Subculture all EC tubes showing gas within 48 ± 2 hours by streaking on L-EMB agar and incubating for 24 ± 2 hours at 35° ± 1°C.
   C. Examine the plates for typical nucleated, dark-centered colonies with or without a metallic sheen. Pick 2 typical colonies and transfer them to SMA slants. If no typical colonies are present on the L-EMB plates, pick 2 or more colonies considered likely to be *E. coli* and transfer them to SMA slants.
   D. Incubate the SMA slants for 18 to 24 hours at 35° ± 1°C. Perform a gram stain, and submit all cultures appearing as gram-negative short rods or cocci to the following biochemical tests (IMViC test):
      1. **Indole production:** Inoculate a tube of tryptone broth and incubate for 24 ± 2 hours at 35° ± 1°C. Test for indole by adding 0.2 to 0.3 mL of Kovacs' reagent. Do not shake the tube after adding the reagent. A distinct red color in the upper layer represents a positive test.
      2. **Voges-Proskauer test:** Inoculate a tube of MR-VP broth and incubate for 48 ± 2 hours at 35° ± 1°C. Aseptically transfer 1 mL to a 13- × 100-mm tube to test for acetylmethylcarbinol. Add 0.6 mL of α-naphthol solution and 0.2 mL of 40% potassium hydroxide and mix. Add a few crystals of creatine. Shake and let stand for 2 hours. The test is positive if an eosin pink color develops.
      3. **Methyl red test:** Incubate the remainder of the MR-VP culture for an additional 48 ± 2 hours, and add 5 drops methyl red solution to each tube. The test is positive if the culture turns red, negative if yellow or orange.
      4. **Citrate utilization:** Lightly inoculate a tube of Koser's citrate broth and incubate for 96 ± 2 hours at 35° ± 1°C. Growth resulting in distinct turbidity represents a positive test.
      5. **Production of gas from lactose:** Inoculate a tube of LST broth and incubate for 48 ± 2 hours at 35° ± 1°C. Gas in the Durham tube or effervescence after gentle agitation is a positive reaction.

      All cultures that ferment lactose with the production of gas within 48 hours at 35°C; that appear as gram-negative, non-spore-forming rods or cocci; and that give IMViC patterns + + – – (biotype 1) or – + – – (biotype 2) are considered to be *E. coli*. As an alternative to the IMViC tests, commercially available microidentification kits may be used to identify *E. coli*.
9. **Expression of Results:** Results expressed on the basis of the most probable number of *E. coli* in the sample. Calculate the MPN of *E. coli* based on

the number of EC tubes that have been shown to contain *E. coli* in 3 successive dilutions.

10. **Precision:** No precision parameters are reported for this method.
11. **Test Report:** The test report identifies the method used and the results obtained, indicating clearly the method of expression used and the repeatability if calculated. Any exceptions to operating details of the method must be specified.

7.060 Fluorogenic Assay (MUG Test) for Detection of *Escherichia coli* in Solid Media[13] (Class B)

This method specifies a procedure for the enumeration of coliform species of bacteria by means of a cultural technique involving a medium containing MUG and calculating the number of coliforms after incubation.

1. **Scope:** This method is applicable to milk and milk products, frozen dairy desserts, cheeses and processed cheeses, butter, and dried products.
2. **References:** Chapter 2: Laboratory Quality Assurance and Safety.
   Chapter 3: Sampling Dairy and Related Products.
   Chapter 4: Preparation of Media, Dilution Water, and Sterilization.
   Chapter 6: Microbiological Count Methods.
   Chapter 9: Microbiological Methods for Dairy Products.
3. **Definition**
   Coliform species of bacteria are those that at 32°C have 0.5 mm of larger colony size on the MUG agar. *Escherichia coli* are indicated by colonies producing a blue fluorescence when the plates are exposed to the longwave UV light.
4. **Principle**
   A. Prepare samples and conduct plating on VRBA with MUG in place of VRBA.
   B. Resuscitation of potentially injured cells if desired following the procedures in 7.040 using TSA and VRBA to which 100 µg/mL MUG has been added to both media.[13]
   C. Count coliforms and *E. coli* colonies using the longwave UV light.
5. **Diluents, Culture Media, and Reagents:** See chapter 6 for standard equipment and supplies.
   VRBA containing 100 µg/mL of MUG (LST-MUG) (Sigma Chemical Co., St. Louis, MO; Hach Co., Ames, IA).
6. **Apparatus and Glassware:** Longwave ultraviolet light source (366 nm), 4 to 6 watts (UV Products Inc., San Gabriel, CA; American Scientific Products, McGaw Park, IL).
7. **Sampling:** See chapter 3.
8. **Preparation of Test Sample:** See chapter 6.
9. **Procedure**
   A. Prepare samples and conduct plating as described in section 7.020 using VRBA with MUG in place of VRBA.
   B. If resuscitation of potentially injured cells is desired, follow the procedure in 7.040 using TSA and VRBA to which 100 µg/mL MUG has been added to both media.

C. Total coliforms are represented as dark red colonies larger than 0.5 mm in diameter. *Escherichia coli* colonies produce a blue fluorescence when the plates are exposed to the longwave UV light.

10. **Expression of Results:** The results are expressed as coliforms per gm or mL and *E. coli* per gm or mL.

11. **Precision:** No precision parameters are known for this method

12. **Test Report:** The test report should specify the methods of sampling and analysis plus the results obtained, indicating clearly the method of expression used and the repeatability if calculated. Any exceptions to operating details of the method must be specified.

7.070 Petrifilm™ Dry Rehydratable Film Methods

7.071 *Petrifilm™ Coliform Count (PCC) Plate method (Class A1)*

1. **Scope:** This method is applicable to dairy products including raw milk and liquid milk products; chocolate milk, evaporated milk, and dried milk products; cheese and processed cheese; butter and margarine; frozen milk products; and cream.

2. **References:** Chapter 2: Laboratory Quality Assurance and Safety.
   Chapter 3: Sampling Dairy and Related Products.
   Chapter 4: Preparation of Media, Dilution Water, and Sterilization.
   Chapter 6: Microbiological Count Methods.
   Chapter 9: Microbiological Methods for Dairy Products.

3. **Definition:** The Petrifilm™ coliform count plate (PCC) method is a sample-ready culture medium system that consists of 2 plastic films coated with modified violet red bile (VRB) nutrients, a dehydrated cold water-soluble gelling agent, and a tetrazolium indicator that facilitates colony enumeration. The countable range of the plate is 15 to 150 colonies. Estimates can be made on plates containing less than 15 or greater than 150 colonies.

4. **Principle:** This method allows for the enumeration of coliforms as colony-forming units per milliliter or gram under conditions of the method as stated. The PCC plate is inoculated with 1 mL of sample. The sample is spread over approximately a 20 cm^2 growth area. The gelling agent is allowed to solidify, the plates are incubated and then enumerated. Coliform colonies growing on the PCC plate produce acid, which causes the pH indicator to deepen the gel color. Gas associated with red colonies differentiates coliforms from other gram-negative organisms.

   The PCC plate is suitable for enumeration of total coliforms when incubated at 30°C to 37°C. Enumeration of thermotolerant (fecal) coliforms is achieved by incubation at 41°C to 45°C.

5. **Diluents, Culture Media, and Reagents:** See manufacturer's instructions for use (3M Microbiology Products, 3M Center, Bldg. 275-5W-05, St. Paul, MN 55144-1000).

   A. **Storage and disposal:** Store unopened Petrifilm™ plate pouches at temperatures ≤8°C (46°F). Just prior to use, allow pouches to come to room temperature before opening. Return unused plates to pouch. To prevent exposure to moisture, do not refrigerate or freeze opened pouches. Seal opened pouches by folding the end of the pouch over and taping shut. Store resealed pouches in a cool, dry place for no longer than 1 month. Exposure of Petrifilm™ plates to temperatures >25°C (77°F) and/or relative humidity >50% can affect the performance of the plates.

As with other microbial detection systems, used PCC plates may contain viable bacteria that may be a biohazard. Follow current industry standards for disposal.

Expiration date and lot number are noted on each package of Petrifilm™ plates. The lot number is also noted on individual plates.

B. **Sterile diluent:** Butterfield's phosphate buffer (IDF phosphate buffer, 0.0425 g/L KH_2PO_4, adjusted to pH 7.2). Do not use buffers containing citrate, bisulfite, or thiosulfate with Petrifilm™ plates; they can inhibit growth.

C. **Reagents**
   1. NaOH solution (1.0 *N*) for pH adjustment of diluted acidic products.
   2. HCl solution (1.0 *N*) for pH adjustment of diluted alkaline products.
   3. Ethyl alcohol, 70%, for sample container decontamination.

6. Apparatus and Glassware
   1. PCC spreader.
   2. Refrigerator: Capable of ≤8°C (46°F).
   3. Incubator: Capable of 32 ± 1°C.
   4. Thermometer: ± 1°C accuracy.
   5. Colony counter or other illuminated magnifier.
   6. Hand tally.
   7. Balance: Sensitive to 0.01 gram.
   8. Dilution bottles: Capacity 150 mL with indelible mark at 99 ± 1 mL.
   9. Pipets: 1 mL or pipeters that conform to APHA standards.
   10. Stomacher blender with corresponding sterile stomacher bags or autoclaveable blender jars.
   11. pH meter or pH paper.

7. Sampling: See chapter 3: Sampling Dairy and Related Products.

8. Preparation: See chapter 6: Microbiological Count Methods for sample preparations.

A. **Pasteurized whole and reduced fat milks and raw milk:** [6.020.8.A, 6.020.9]

Depending on expected count, inoculate 1 mL directly or make appropriate serial dilutions by aseptically pipeting diluted sample into diluent to yield a dilution that gives 15 to150 colony forming units per mL of diluted sample plated. One mL of a direct yields a 1-coliform-per-gram sensitivity.

B. **Cream, half-and-half, condensed milk, egg nog, cottage cheese, butter, margarine, and related products:** Make 1:5 dilution (24.75 g/99 mL sterile diluent). Mix well and plate 1 mL on each of 2 plates. Multiply total of counts on 2 plates by 2.5 to obtain count/g.

C. **Alternative for butter and margarine:** Homogenization may be facilitated by use of prewarmed (40°C to 45°C) phosphate buffer dilution blank. Alternative [7.072.8.C].

D. **Chocolate milk:** Make a 1:10 minimum dilution (11 g/99 mL sterile diluent). Mix well and plate 1 mL on each of 2 plates. Multiply total of counts on 2 plates by 5 to obtain count/g. Alternative [7.072.8.B].

E. **Sour cream, dips, yogurt, and buttermilk:** Proceed as in [7.071.8.A] except after dilution preparation, adjust pH to 6.6 to 7.2 with 0.1*N* NaOH (approximately 0.1 mL/g of sample). Alternative [7.072.8.E].

F. **Ice cream and related products:** [6.020.8.E, 6.020.9].
Prepare a 1:5 dilution. Proceed as in [6.020.5].

Alternative [7.072.8.B].

Alternative: Hydrate PCC plates with 1 mL of sterile diluent and allow at least 1 hour for gel to solidify. Lift the top film of the prehydrated PCC plate (gel will adhere to top film) and dispense 0.5 mL of a 2:3 homogenate (10 g/5 mL of sterile diluent) onto the bottom film of each of 3 plates. Replace the top film gently over sample. Add the coliform count from the 3 plates to obtain the count/g.

Alternative: Proceed as in [7.071.A] except plate 1 plate and multiply result by 3 to obtain the count/g.

G. **Cheese:** [6.020.8.D, 6.020.9].
Proceed as in [7.071.8.A]. Do not use citrate buffer to homogenize sample.

Alternative [7.072.8.E].

H. **Other dairy or related food products:** See chapter 9: Microbiological Methods for Dairy Products for additional preparation instructions.

9. Procedure

A. **Method**

1. Make appropriate serial dilutions by aseptically pipeting mixed sample into phosphate buffer dilution blank to yield a dilution that gives 15 to150 colony forming units (CFU) per mL of diluted sample.
2. Place the PCC plate on a flat level surface.
3. Lift the top film and carefully inoculate 1 mL of undiluted or diluted sample by pipet or pipeter.
4. Roll the top film down onto the sample to prevent trapping air bubbles.
5. Place the plastic spreader smooth side down on the center of the plate and press gently on the center of the spreader to distribute the sample evenly. Spread the inoculum over the entire Petrifilm™ growth area before gel is formed. Do not slide the spreader across the film.
6. Remove the spreader and leave the plate undisturbed for at least one minute to permit the gel to solidify.

B. **Incubation:** Incubate plates with the clear side up in stacks not exceeding 20 units at 32°C ± 1°C for 24 hours ± 2 hours. Alternative incubation temperatures may be used depending on the method and information desired.

C. **Counting colonies:** Count plates promptly after incubation period. Record the dilutions used and the number of colonies counted or estimated for each plate. If impossible to count at once, after the required incubation, plates may be stored frozen for later enumeration at temperatures ≤ –15°C for no longer than a week. Avoid making this a routine practice. When counting colonies on plates, proceed according to the directions given below. For each lot of samples, record the results of sterility tests on materials (dilution blanks, pipet/tips, air, etc.) used when pouring plates and the incubation temperature used.

D. **Manual counting of plates:** PCC plates can be counted on a standard colony counter or other illuminated magnifier. Coliform colonies are red and associated with entrapped gas. Colonies not associated with gas (greater than one colony diameter from gas bubble) are not counted as coliforms. Do not count colonies on the foam dam since they are removed from the selective influence of the medium. Do not count artifact bubbles that may be present.

The circular growth area is approximately 20 cm^2. Estimates can be made on plates containing greater than 150 colonies by counting the number of colonies in 1 or more representative squares and determining the average number per square. Multiply the average number per square by 20 to determine the estimated count per plate.

Gas produced by a coliform may disrupt the colony so that the colony outlines the bubble. This should be counted as a single coliform.

PCC plates with colonies that are too numerous to count (TNTC) have 1 or more of the following characteristics: 1) many small colonies, 2) many gas bubbles, and 3) deepening of the gel color due to acid production. When any of these characteristics occur, dilute the sample further to obtain a more accurate count.

E. **Laboratory accidents or bacterial growth inhibitors:** When a plate from a sample is known to be contaminated or is otherwise unsatisfactory, record the plate as a laboratory accident (LA).

10. **Expression of Results:** Computing and recording counts same as 7.020.9.

11. **Precision:** See chapter 1: Precision Parameters.

12. **Test Report:** The test report identifies the method used and results obtained. The report will also identify any variation in the test not specified in this method as well as problems that may have impacted the test result. Each sample will be described in such a manner as to ensure traceability as to its origin.

7.072 *3M™ Petrifilm™ High-Sensitivity Coliform Count (PHSCC) Plate Method (Class A2)*

1. **Scope:** This method is applicable to dairy products including raw milk, liquid milk products, chocolate milk, evaporated milk, dried milk products, cheese and processed cheese, butter and margarine, frozen milk products, frozen yogurt, and cream.

2. **References:** Chapter 2: Laboratory Quality Assurance and Safety.
   Chapter 3: Sampling Dairy and Related Products.
   Chapter 4: Preparation of Media, Dilution Water, and Sterilization.
   Chapter 6: Microbiological Count Methods.
   Chapter 9: Microbiological Methods for Dairy Products.
3. **Definition:** This method allows for the enumeration of coliforms as colony-forming units per milliliter or gram under conditions of the method as stated. The countable range of the plate is 15 to 150 colonies. Estimates can be made on plates containing less than 15 or greater than 150 colonies
4. **Principle:** The Petrifilm™ high-sensitivity coliform count plate (PHSCC) method is a sample-ready culture medium system that consists of 2 plastic films coated with modified VRB nutrients, a dehydrated cold water-soluble gelling agent, and a tetrazolium indicator that facilitates colony enumeration. The PHSCC plate is useful for the enumeration of low levels of coliform bacteria. A 5-mL sample is plated onto 1 plate. This allows a 1-coliform-per-gram sensitivity if a 1:5 dilution of product is made. A 2-per-gram sensitivity if achieved if a 1:10 dilution is used. The sample is spread over approximately a 60-cm^2 growth area. The gelling agent is allowed to solidify, the plates are incubated, and then enumerated. Coliform colonies growing on the PHSCC plate produce acid, which causes the pH indicator to deepen the gel color. Gas associated with red colonies differentiates coliforms from other gram-negative organisms.

   The PHSCC plate is suitable for enumeration of total coliforms when incubated at 30°C to 37°C.
5. **Diluents, Culture Media, and Reagents:** See manufacturer's instructions for use (3M Microbiology Products, 3M Center, Bldg. 275-5W-05, St. Paul, MN 55144-1000).
6. **Apparatus and Glassware**
   1. PHSCC spreader.
   2. Pipets: Minimum capacity of 5 mL or pipeters that conform to APHA standards.
   3. Refrigerator: Capable of ≤8°C (46°F).
   4. Incubator: Capable of 32° ± 1°C.
   5. Thermometer: ± 1°C accuracy.
   6. Colony counter or other illuminated magnifier.
   7. Hand tally.
   8. Balance: Sensitive to 0.01 gram.
   9. Dilution bottles: Capacity 150 mL with indelible mark at 99 ± 1 mL.
   10. Stomacher blender with corresponding sterile stomacher bags or autoclaveable blender jars.
   11. pH meter or pH paper.
7. **Sampling:** See chapter 3: Sampling Dairy and Related Products.
8. **Preparation**
   A. **Pasteurized whole and reduced fat milks and raw milk:** [6.020.8.A, 6.020.9]. Depending on expected count, inoculate 5 mL directly or make appropriate serial dilutions by aseptically pipeting diluted sam-

ple into diluent to yield a dilution that gives 15 to 150 colony forming units per mL of diluted sample plated.

B. **Chocolate milk, cream, ice cream, or sweetened condensed milk:** [6.020.8.A, 6.020.8.E, 6.020.9]. Prepare a 1:5 minimum dilution (24.75 g/99 mL sterile diluent). Mix well and plate 5 mL on 1 plate. Five mL of a 1:5 mL dilution yields a 1-coliform-per-gram sensitivity.

C. **Butter, margarine, and related products:** [6.020.8.B, 6.020.9]. Prepare a 1:5 minimum dilution in 40° to 45°C prewarmed sterile dilution bottles. Mix well and plate 5 mL on 1 plate. Five mL of a 1:5 dilution yields a 1-coliform-per-gram sensitivity.

D. **Dry dairy products:** [6.020.8.C, 6.020.9]. Prepare a 1:10 minimum dilution (11 g/99 mL sterile diluent). Five mL of a 1:10 yields a 2-coliform-per-gram sensitivity. Alternative: Ten mL of a 1:10 dilution plated onto 2 PHSCC plates yields a 1-coliform-per-gram sensitivity.

Do not use buffers containing citrate with Petrifilm™ plates.

Adjust pH of the diluted sample to 6.5 to 7.5. For acidic products, adjust pH with 1.0*N* NaOH. For alkaline products, adjust pH with 1.0*N* HCl. [6.020.8.C, 6.020.9]

E. **Cheese and other cultured and culture-added products:** [6.020.8.D, 6.020.9]. Prepare a minimum 1:10 dilution. Do not use buffers containing citrate with Petrifilm™ plates. If the procedure indicates citrate buffer, substitute warmed (40° to 45°C), sterile, buffered phosphate dilution water. [7.071.5.B]

Adjust pH of the diluted sample to 6.5 to 7.5.

F. **Other dairy or related food products:** See chapter 9: Microbiological Methods for Dairy Products for additional preparation instructions.

9. Procedure

A. **Method**

1. Make appropriate serial dilutions by aseptically pipeting mixed sample into phosphate buffer dilution blank to yield a dilution that gives 15 to 150 colony forming units per mL of diluted sample.
2. Place the PHSCC plate on a flat level surface.
3. Lift the top film and carefully inoculate 5 mL of undiluted or diluted sample by pipet or pipeter.
4. Roll the top film down onto the sample gently to prevent pushing sample off the film.
5. Place the plastic spreader smooth side down on the center of the plate and press gently on the center of the spreader to distribute the sample evenly. Do not slide the spreader across the film.
6. Remove the spreader and leave the plate undisturbed for 2 to 5 minutes to permit the gel to solidify.

B. **Incubation:** Incubate plates with the clear side up in stacks not exceeding 10 units at 32°C ± 1°C for 24 hours ± 2 hours.

C. **Counting colonies:** Count plates promptly after incubation period. Record the dilutions used and the number of colonies counted or estimated for each plate. If impossible to count at once, after the required incubation, plates may be stored frozen for later enumeration at temperatures ≤ –15°C for no longer than a week. Avoid making this a routine practice. When counting colonies on plates, proceed according to the directions given below. For each lot of samples, record the results of sterility tests on materials (dilution blanks, pipet/tips, air, etc.) used when pouring plates and the incubation temperature used.

D. **Manual counting of plates:** PHSCC plates can be counted on a standard colony counter or other illuminated magnifier. Coliform colonies are red and associated with entrapped gas. Colonies not associated with gas (greater than one colony diameter from gas bubble) are not counted as coliforms. Do not count artifact bubbles that may be present.

The circular growth area is approximately 60 cm^2. Estimates can be made on plates containing greater than 150 colonies by counting the number of colonies in one or more representative squares and determining the average number per square. Multiply the average number per square by 60 to determine the estimated count per plate.

Gas produced by a coliform may disrupt the colony so that the colony outlines the bubble. This should be counted as a single coliform.

PHSCC plates with colonies that are too numerous to count (TNTC) have 1 or more of the following characteristics: 1) many small colonies, 2) many gas bubbles, and 3) deepening of the gel color due to acid production. When any of these characteristics occur, dilute the sample further to obtain a more accurate count.

E. **Laboratory accidents or bacterial growth inhibitors:** When a plate from a sample is known to be contaminated or is otherwise unsatisfactory, record the plate as a laboratory accident (LA).

10. **Expression of Results:** Computing and recording counts same as 7.020.9.
11. **Precision:** See chapter 1: Precision Parameters.
12. **Test Report:** The test report identifies the method used and results obtained. The report will also identify any variation in the test not specified in this method as well as problems that may have impacted the test result. Each sample will be described in such a manner as to ensure traceability as to its origin.

7.073 *3M™ Petrifilm™ Rapid Coliform Count (PRCC) Plate Method (Class A3)*

1. **Scope:** This method is applicable to dairy products including raw milk; pasteurized fluid milks; chocolate milk; evaporated milk; dried milk products; cultured products (including cheese and processed cheese, cottage cheese, sour cream and yogurt); butter and margarine; frozen milk products (including ice cream, ice mix, and frozen yogurt); and cream.
2. **References:** Chapter 2: Laboratory Quality Assurance and Safety.
   Chapter 3: Sampling Dairy and Related Products.
   Chapter 4: Preparation of Media, Dilution Water, and Sterilization.
   Chapter 6: Microbiological Count Methods.
   Chapter 9: Microbiological Methods for Dairy Products.

3. **Definition:** This method allows for the enumeration of coliforms as colony-forming units per milliliter or gram under conditions of the method as stated. The countable range of the plate is 15 to 150 colonies. Estimates can be made on plates containing less than 15 or greater than 150 colonies

4. **Principle:** The Petrifilm™ rapid coliform count plate (PRCC) method is a sample-ready culture medium system that consists of 2 plastic films coated with modified VRBA nutrients, a dehydrated cold water-soluble gelling agent, a pH indicator to detect acid, and a tetrazolium indicator that facilitates colony enumeration. The PRCC plate is inoculated with 1 mL of sample. The sample is spread over approximately a 20-cm^2 growth area. The gelling agent is allowed to solidify and the plates are incubated and then enumerated. As colonies grow on the PRCC plate and produce acid, the pH indicator in the plate changes from red-orange to yellow, providing presumptive indication of coliforms. Gas trapped around coliform colonies indicates confirmed coliforms.

5. **Diluents, Culture Media, and Reagents:** See manufacturer's instructions for use (3M Microbiology Products, 3M Center, Bldg. 275- 5W-05, St. Paul, MN 55144-1000).

6. **Apparatus and Glassware**
   1. PRCC spreader.
   2. Refrigerator: Capable of ≤8°C (46°F).
   3. Incubator: Capable of 32° ± 1°C.
   4. Thermometer: ± 1°C accuracy.
   5. Colony counter or other illuminated magnifier.
   6. Hand tally.
   7. Balance: Sensitive to 0.01 gram.
   8. Dilution bottles: Capacity 150 mL with indelible mark at 99 ± 1 mL.
   9. Pipets: 1 mL or pipeters that conform to APHA standards.
   10. Stomacher blender with corresponding sterile stomacher bags or autoclaveable blender jars.
   11. pH meter or pH paper

7. **Sampling:** See chapter 3: Sampling Dairy and Related Products.

8. **Preparation**

   A. **Pasteurized whole and reduced fat milks and raw milk:** [6.020.8.A, 6.020.9]. Depending on expected count, inoculate 1 mL direct or make appropriate serial dilutions by aseptically pipeting diluted sample into diluent to yield a dilution that gives 15 to 150 colony forming units per mL of diluted sample plated. One mL of a direct yields a 1-coliform-per-gram sensitivity.

   B. **Butter, margarine, and related products:** [6.020.8.B, 6.020.9]. Make a 1:10 minimum dilution (11 g/99 mL sterile diluent). Mix well and plate 1 mL on each of 2 plates. Multiply total of counts on 2 plates by 5 to obtain count/g.

   Alternative for butter and margarine: Homogenization may be facilitated by use of prewarmed (40°C to 45°C) phosphate buffer dilution blank. Alternative [7.072.8.C].

C. **Dry dairy products:** [6.020.8.C, 6.020.9]. Same as 7.072.8.D.

Adjust pH of the diluted sample to 6.5 to 7.5. For acidic products, adjust pH with 1.0*N* NaOH. For alkaline products, adjust pH with 1.0*N* HCl.

D. **Cheese and other cultured and culture-added products:** [6.020.8.D, 6.020.9]. Same as 7.072.8.E. Do not use buffers containing citrate with Petrifilm™ plates. If the procedure indicates citrate buffer, substitute warmed (40°C to 45°C) sterile, buffered phosphate dilution water.

Adjust pH of the diluted sample to 6.5 to 7.5. For acidic products adjust pH with 1.0*N* NaOH.

E. **Ice cream and related food products:** [6.020.8.A, 6.020.8.E, 6.020.9]. Same as 7.072.8.B.

F. **Other dairy or related food products:** See chapter 9: Microbiological Methods for Dairy Products for additional preparation instructions.

9. Procedure

A. **Method:** Make appropriate serial dilutions by aseptically pipeting a mixed sample into phosphate buffer dilution blank to yield a dilution that gives 15 to150 colony forming units per mL of diluted sample. Same as 7.072.9.A.

B. **Incubation**

1. Incubate plates with the clear side up in stacks not exceeding 20 units at 35°C ± 1°C for 24 hours ± 2 hours.
2. Examine plates for coliform growth at any time during the 24 ± 2 hour incubation interval depending on the desired information and method being followed. Because coliform growth is affected by temperature, time out of the incubator should be minimized to avoid extending the detection time.

C. **Counting colonies:** Record the dilutions used and the number of colonies counted or estimated for each plate. When counting colonies on plates, proceed according to the directions given below. For each lot of samples, record the results of sterility tests on materials (dilution blanks, pipet/tips, air, etc.) used when pouring plates and the incubation temperature used.

D. **Manual counting of plates:** The early result (6 to 14 hours) or presumptive coliform count is based on acid production indicated by yellow halos with or without red centers indicating CFUs. Indirect back lighting may enhance early detection of yellow acid zones on PRCC plates. Coliform colonies may begin to appear at 6 hours of incubation as discrete yellow zones.

Continue incubating plates to detect additional acid zones and/or red colonies associated with acid.

Some coliforms produce large amounts of acid. For these organisms, fusion of the yellow acid zones could occur at about 20 colonies per plate. The circular growth area is approximately 20 cm^2. Estimates can be made on plates containing greater than 50 acid zones by counting the number of acid zones in 1 or more representative squares and determining the average number per square. Multiply the average number by 20 to determine total count per plate.

PRCC plates can be counted on a standard colony counter or other illuminated magnifier. Do not count colonies on the foam dam since they are removed from the selective influence of the medium. Do not count artifact bubbles that may be present.

Estimates can be made on plates containing greater than 150 colonies by counting the number of colonies in 1 or more representative squares and determining the average number per square. Multiply the average number per square by 20 (growth area is approximately 20 cm^2) to determine the estimated count per plate.

The confirmed coliform count is characterized by gas associated with red CFUs.

Too numerous to count (TNTC) coliform count (>4 hours). High concentrations of coliforms (>1000 CFUs/plate) may cause the entire growth area to turn yellow after 4 hours of incubation. When this occurs, the plate is TNTC for coliforms and further dilution of the sample is required to obtain a more accurate count.

E. **Laboratory accidents or bacterial growth inhibitors:** When a plate from a sample is known to be contaminated or is otherwise unsatisfactory, record the plate as a laboratory accident (LA).

10. **Expression of Results:** Computing and recording counts same as 7.020.9.

11. **Precision:** See chapter 1: Precision Parameters.

12. **Test Report:** The test report identifies the method used and results obtained. The report will also identify any variation in the test not specified in this method as well as problems that may have impacted the test result. Each sample will be described in such a manner as to ensure traceability as to its origin.

7.074 *3M™ Petrifilm™* E. Coli/Coliform Count (PEC) Plate Method *(Class A1)*

1. **Scope:** This method is applicable to dairy products including raw milk, liquid milk products, cheese, frozen milk products, and cream for the detection of *Escherichia coli* and other coliforms.

   Do not use this plate alone for the detection of *E. coli* O157:H7. As with most other *E. coli*/coliform media, this plate will not specifically indicate whether any *E. coli* O157:H7 strain is present. Because most O157 strains are atypical *E. coli*, they will appear as non-*E. coli* coliforms (red with gas).

2. **References:** Chapter 2: Laboratory Quality Assurance and Safety.
   Chapter 3: Sampling Dairy and Related Products.
   Chapter 4: Preparation of Media, Dilution Water, and Sterilization.
   Chapter 6: Microbiological Count Methods.
   Chapter 9: Microbiological Methods for Dairy Products.

3. **Definition:** This method allows for the enumeration of *E. coli* and other coliform as colony forming units per milliliter or gram under conditions of the method as stated.

4. **Principle:** The Petrifilm™ *E. coli*/coliform count plate (PEC) method is a sample-ready culture medium system that consists of 2 plastic films coat-

ed with modified VRBA nutrients, a dehydrated cold water-soluble gelling agent, an indicator of glucuronidase activity (5-bromo-4-chloro-3-indolyl-β-D-glucuronide) (BCIG) and a tetrazolium indicator that facilitates colony enumeration. The PEC plate is inoculated with 1 mL of sample. The sample is spread over approximately a 20-cm^2 growth area. The gelling agent is allowed to solidify and the plates are incubated and then enumerated. In general, *E. coli* colonies are blue to red-blue and closely associated (approximately one colony diameter) with entrapped gas. Coliform colonies are bright red and closely associated with entrapped gas.

5. **Diluents, Culture Media, and Reagents:** See manufacturer's instructions for use (3M Microbiology Products, 3M Center, Bldg. 275-5W-05, St. Paul, MN 55144-1000).

6. **Apparatus and Glassware**
   1. PEC spreader.
   2. Refrigerator: Capable of ≤8°C (46°F).
   3. Incubator: Capable of 32° ± 1°C.
   4. Thermometer: ± 1°C accuracy.
   5. Colony counter or other illuminated magnifier.
   6. Hand tally.
   7. Balance: Sensitive to 0.01 gram.
   8. Dilution bottles: Capacity 150 mL with indelible mark at 99 ± 1 mL.
   9. Pipets: 1 mL or pipeters that conform to APHA standards.
   10. Stomacher blender with corresponding sterile stomacher bags or autoclaveable blender jars.
   11. pH meter or pH paper.

7. **Sampling:** See chapter 3: Sampling Dairy and Related Products.

8. **Preparation**

   A. **Raw and pasteurized fluid milk and liquid milk products:** [6.020.8.A, 6.020.9]. Depending on expected count, inoculate 1 mL directly or make appropriate serial dilutions by aseptically pipeting diluted sample into diluent to yield a dilution that gives 15 to 150 colony-forming units per mL of diluted sample plated. One mL of a direct yields a 1-coliform-per-gram sensitivity.

   B. **Cheese:** [6.020.8.D, 6.020.9]. Make a 1:10 minimum dilution (11 g/99 mL sterile diluent). Do not use buffers containing citrate with Petrifilm™ plates. If the procedure indicates citrate buffer, substitute warmed (40°C to 45°C), sterile, buffered phosphate dilution water.

   For optimal bacterial growth or recovery adjust pH of the sample or diluted sample to 6.6 to 7.2. For acidic products, adjust pH with 1.0*N* NaOH. For alkaline products, adjust pH with 1.0*N* HCl.

   Mix well and plate 1 mL on each of 2 plates. Multiply total of counts on 2 plates by 5 to obtain count/g.

   C. **Ice cream and related food products:** [6.020.8.A, 6.020.8.E, 6.020.9]. Make a 1:10 minimum dilution (11 g/99 mL sterile diluent). Mix well and plate 1 mL on each of 2 plates. Multiply total of counts on 2 plates by 5 to obtain count/g.

   D. **Other dairy or related food products:** See chapter 9: Microbiological Methods for Dairy Products for additional preparation instructions.

9. **Procedure:** Same as 7.071.9.

   A. **Incubation:** Incubate plates with the clear side up in stacks not exceeding 20 units at 35°C ± 1°C. Alternative incubation temperatures may be used depending on the method and information desired. For total coliform results incubate plates for 24 hours ± 2 hours. For total *E. coli* incubate plates for 48 hours ± 2 hours. Regardless of incubation time, whenever a blue colony associated with gas is observed, it is a confirmed *E. coli.*

   B. **Counting colonies:** Count plates promptly after incubation period. Record the dilutions used and the number of colonies counted or estimated for each plate. If impossible to count at once, after the required incubation, plates may be stored frozen for later enumeration at temperatures ≥ –15°C for no longer than a week. Avoid making this a routine practice. When counting colonies on plates, proceed according to the directions given below. For each lot of samples, record the results of sterility tests on materials (dilution blanks, pipet/tips, air, etc.) used when pouring plates and the incubation temperature used.

   C. **Manual counting of plates:** PEC plates can be counted on a standard colony counter or other illuminated magnifier. Do not count colonies on the foam dam since they are removed from the selective influence of the medium. Do not count artifact bubbles that may be present.

   Enumerate blue to red-blue colonies associated with entrapped gas, regardless of size or intensity of color, as confirmed *E. coli*. Other coliform colonies will be red and associated with entrapped gas. Colonies not associated with gas (greater than one colony diameter from gas bubble) are not counted as coliforms. The total coliform count consists of both the red and blue colonies associated with gas at 24 hours. Reincubate plates an additional 24 ± 2 hours to detect any additional *E. coli* growth. Regardless of incubation time, whenever a blue colony associated with gas is observed, it is a confirmed *E. coli.*

   The circular growth area is approximately 20 cm^2. Estimates can be made on plates containing greater than 150 colonies by counting the number of colonies in 1 or more representative squares and determining the average number per square. Multiply the average number per square by 20 to determine the estimated count per plate.

   Gas produced by a coliform or *E. coli* may disrupt the colony so that the colony outlines the bubble. This should be counted as a single CFU.

   PEC plates with colonies that are too numerous to count (TNTC) have 1 or more of the following characteristics: 1) many small colonies, 2) many gas bubbles, and 3) deepening of the gel color. High concentrations of *E. coli* will cause the growth area to turn blue, while high concentrations of coliforms (non-*E. coli*) will cause the area to turn dark red. When any of these characteristics occur, dilute the sample further to obtain a more accurate count.

   D. **Laboratory accidents or bacterial growth inhibitors:** When a plate from a sample is known to be contaminated or is otherwise unsatisfactory, record the plate as a laboratory accident (LA).

10. **Expression of Results:** The results are expressed as coliforms per gm or mL and *E. coli* per gm or mL.
11. **Precision:** See chapter 1: Precision Parameters.
12. **Test Report:** The test report identifies the method used and results obtained. The report will also identify any variation in the test not specified in this method as well as problems that may have impacted the test result. Each sample will be described in such a manner as to ensure traceability as to its origin.

7.080 Pectin Gel Method

7.081 *3M™ Redigel™ VRB Test (RVRB) Method (Class A1)*

1. **Scope:** This method is applicable to raw and processed milk and cream, cultured dairy products including cheese, cottage cheese, sour cream and yogurt, and dry dairy products.
2. **References:** Chapter 2: Laboratory Quality Assurance and Safety.
   Chapter 3: Sampling Dairy and Related Products.
   Chapter 4: Preparation of Media, Dilution Water, and Sterilization
   Chapter 6: Microbiological Count Methods.
   Chapter 9: Microbiological Methods for Dairy Products.
3. **Definition:** This method provides a nutrient base for growth of coliforms and other gram-negative organisms and allows for the enumeration of coliforms as colony forming units per mL or gm under conditions of the method as stated.
4. **Principle:** A specified aliquot of a liquid or diluted solid sample is introduced into or onto the Redigel™ aerobic pectin gel medium and pretreated Redigel™ dish. Plates are incubated aerobically at 32°C ± 1°C for 24 hours ± 2 hours. Determination of the number of coliform per mL or gm of product is obtained by selection of plates chosen at dilution levels that will result in a significant result.
5. **Diluents, Culture Media, and Reagents:** See manufacturer's instructions for use (3M Co., 3M Center, Bldg. 275-5W-05, St. Paul, MN 55144-1000).
   A. **Storage and disposal**
      1. **Bottles:** ≤25°C (77°F).
      2. **Pretreated Redigel™ dishes:** Closed packages at room temperature (15° to 30°C or 59° to 86°F). As with other microbial detection systems, Redigel™ PGVRB plates may contain viable bacteria that may be a biohazard. Follow current industry standards for disposal.

   B. **Shelf life**
      1. **Bottles:** Expiration date and lot number are noted on individual bottle or box.
      2. **Dishes:** Expiration date and lot number are noted on individual dish, package and box.
      3. **Sterile diluent:** Butterfield's phosphate buffer (IDF phosphate buffer, 0.0425 g/L KH_2PO_4, adjusted to pH 7.2).
      4. **Ethyl alcohol:** 70%, for sample container decontamination, if desired.

6. **Apparatus and Glassware**
   1. Incubator: Capable to 32° ± 1°C.
   2. Thermometer: ± 1°C accuracy.
   3. Colony counter or other illuminated magnifier.
   4. Hand tally.
   5. Balance: Sensitive to 0.01 gm.
   6. Dilution bottles: Capacity 150 mL with indelible mark at 99 ± 1 mL.
   7. Pipets, pipeters, or plate loop device that conforms to APHA standards.
   8. Stomacher or blender with corresponding sterile stomacher bags or autoclaveable blender jars.
7. **Sampling:** See chapter 3: Sampling Dairy and Related Products.
8. **Preparation**

   A. **Pasteurized whole and reduced fat milks and raw milk:** [6.020.8.A, 6.020.9]. Depending on expected count, inoculate 1 mL direct or make appropriate serial dilutions by aseptically pipeting diluted sample into diluent to yield a dilution that gives 15 to 150 colony-forming units per mL of diluted sample plated. One mL of a direct yields a 1-coliform-per-gram sensitivity.

   B. **Butter, margarine, and related products:** Make 1:5 dilution (24.75 g/99 mL sterile diluent). Mix well and plate 1 mL on each of 2 plates. Multiply total of counts on 2 plates by 2.5 to obtain count/g.

   Alternative for butter and margarine: Homogenization may be facilitated by use of prewarmed (40°C to 45°C) phosphate buffer dilution blank.

   C. **Dry dairy products:** [6.020.8.C, 6.020.9]. Make a 1:10 minimum dilution (11 g/99 mL sterile diluent). Mix well and plate 1 mL on each of 2 plates. Multiply total of counts on 2 plates by 5 to obtain count/g.

   D. **Cheese and other cultured and culture-added products:** [6.020.8.D, 6.020.9]. Make a 1:10 dilution (11 g of cheese / 99 mL 2% sodium citrate diluent).

   E. **Ice cream and related food products:** [6.020.8.E, 6.020.9]. Same as 7.071.8.F.

   F. **Other dairy or related food products:** See chapter 9: Microbiological Methods for Dairy Products for additional preparation instructions.
9. **Procedure:** Redigel™ media is preferred to be at room temperature before use.

   A. **One-dish or 10-dish bottle**
   1. Lift the lid of a pretreated Redigel™ dish and pour the liquid pectin gel from a 1-dish bottle into the dish. Alternatively, pour or pipet 10 to 12 mL from a 10-dish bottle into the dish or dishes.
   2. Replace the lid and swirl the dish to cover the bottom with pectin gel. The sample must be added within 5 minutes after the liquid pectin gel is added. Add the sample or sample inoculum to the liquid pectin gel in the dish (0.1 to 1 mL depending on the desired dilution).
   3. Immediately swirl several times to thoroughly mix the sample with the pectin gel.

4. Place the dish on a level surface and allow the medium to solidify for approximately 40 minutes and then incubate.

B. **Incubation:** Incubate plates at 32° ± 1°C for 24 ± 2 hours for the total coliform count. Plates must reach the temperature of incubation within 2 hours.

C. **Counting colonies on plates:** Count plates promptly after the incubation period. Record the dilutions used and the number of colonies counted or estimated on each plate. If impossible to count at once, after the required incubation, store the plates at 0° to 4.4°C for not more than 24 hours; avoid making this a routine practice. When counting colonies on plates, proceed according to the directions given below. For each lot of samples, record the results of sterility tests on materials (dilution blanks, agar, etc.) used when pouring plates and the incubation temperature used.

D. **Manual counting of plates:** Count colonies with the aid of magnification under uniform and properly controlled artificial illumination. Plates should be examined in subdued light. Routinely use a colony counter equipped with a guide plate ruled in square centimeters.[4(17.3.01)] Examine doubtful objects carefully, using higher magnification when required to distinguish colonies from foreign matter. Arrange schedules of laboratory analysts to prevent eye fatigue and the inaccuracies that result from eyestrain.

1. **Normal plates** *(15 to 150 or less than 15 colonies):* Count all colonies, including those of pinpoint size, on selected plate(s). Record the dilution(s) used and the total number of colonies counted.
2. **Crowded plates** *(more than 150 colonies):* Do not record counts on crowded plates from the highest dilution as too numerous to count (TNTC). If the number of colonies per plate exceeds 250, count colonies in those portions of the plate that are representative of colony distribution, and calculate an estimated RVRB (ERVRB) from these counts. If there are fewer than 10 colonies per square centimeter, count colonies in 12 squares; select, if representative, 6 consecutive squares horizontally across the plate and 6 squares at right angles, being careful not to count a square more than once. When there are more than 10 colonies per square centimeter, count colonies in four such representative portions. In both instances, multiply the average number of colonies found per square centimeter by the area of the plate used to determine the estimated number of colonies per plate. Each laboratory must determine the area in square centimeters of the plates in use.

E. **Laboratory accidents or bacterial growth inhibitors:** When a plate from a sample is known to be contaminated or is otherwise unsatisfactory, record the plate as a laboratory accident (LA).

10. Expression of Results: Computing and recording counts is same as 7.020.9.

11. Precision: See chapter 1: Precision Parameters.

12. Test Report: The test report identifies the method used and results obtained. The report will also identify any variation in the test not specified in this method as well as problems that may have impacted the test result. Each sample will be described in such a manner as to ensure traceability as to its origin.

7.082 *3M™ Redigel™ Colichrome2 Test (RCC2) Method (Class A3)*

1. **Scope:** This method is applicable to all raw and processed milk and cream as well as cultured dairy products including cheese, cottage cheese, sour cream, and yogurt.
2. **References:** Chapter 2: Laboratory Quality Assurance and Safety.
   Chapter 3: Sampling Dairy and Related Products.
   Chapter 4: Preparation of Media, Dilution Water, and Sterilization.
   Chapter 6: Microbiological Count Methods.
   Chapter 9: Microbiological Methods for Dairy Products.
3. **Definition:** The RCC2 test provides a nutrient base for growth of *E. coli* and other coliforms. RCC2 medium contains chromogenic galactoside and glucuronide in the medium to differentiate *E. coli* and other coliforms from noncoliform bacteria. Most noncoliform bacteria hydrolyze neither substrate and appear as white or cream colonies. Coliforms hydrolyze the galactoside and are pink to red. However, coliforms that are *E. coli* hydrolyze the glucuronide in addition to the galactoside and are purple. Gram-positive bacteria are inhibited by bile salts in the medium. This medium is pectin-based and gels at room temperature when poured into a Redigel™ pretreated dish and allows for the enumeration of coliforms as colony forming units per mL or gm under conditions of the method as stated.

   Do not use this plate alone for the detection of *E. coli* O157:H7. As with most other *E. coli*/coliform media, this plate will not specifically indicate whether any *E. coli* O157:H7 strain is present. Because most O157 strains are atypical *E. coli*, they will appear as non-*E. coli* coliforms (pink to red in color).
4. **Principle:** A specified aliquot of a liquid or diluted solid sample is introduced into or onto the RCC2 pectin gel medium and pretreated Redigel™ dish. Plates are incubated aerobically at 32°C ± 1°C for 24 ± 2 hours. Determination of the number of coliform per mL or gm of product is obtained by selection of plates chosen at dilutions levels that will result in a significant result.
5. **Diluents, Culture Media, and Reagents:** See manufacturer's instructions for use (3M Co., 3M Center, Bldg. 275-5W-05, St. Paul, MN 55144-1000).

   A. **Storage and disposal**
      1. **Bottles:** ≤25°C (77°F).
      2. **Pretreated Redigel™ dishes:** Closed packages at room temperature (15° to 30°C or 59° to 86°F). As with other microbial detection systems, RCC2 plates may contain viable bacteria that may be a biohazard. Follow current industry standards for disposal.

   B. **Shelf life**
      1. **Bottles:** Expiration date and lot number are noted on individual bottle or box.

2. **Dishes:** Expiration date and lot number are noted on individual dish, package, and box.
3. **Sterile diluent:** Butterfield's phosphate buffer (IDF phosphate buffer, 0.0425 g/L KH_2PO_4, adjusted to pH 7.2).
4. **Ethyl alcohol:** 70% for sample container decontamination, if desired.

6. **Apparatus and Glassware**
   1. Incubator: Capable to 32° ± 1°C.
   2. Thermometer: ± 1°C accuracy.
   3. Colony counter or other illuminated magnifier.
   4. Hand tally.
   5. Balance: Sensitive to 0.01 gm.
   6. Dilution bottles: Capacity 150 mL with indelible mark at 99 ± 1 mL.
   7. Pipets, pipeters, or plate loop device that conform to APHA standards.
   8. Stomacher or blender with corresponding sterile stomacher bags or autoclaveable blender jars.
7. **Sampling:** See chapter 3: Sampling Dairy and Related Products.
8. **Preparation**

   A. **Pasteurized whole and reduced fat milks and raw milk:** [6.020.8.A, 6.020.9]. Depending on expected count, inoculate 1 mL direct or make appropriate serial dilutions by aseptically pipeting diluted sample into diluent to yield a dilution that gives 15 to 150 colony forming units per mL of diluted sample plated. One mL of a direct yields a 1-coliform-per-gram sensitivity.

   B. **Butter, margarine, and related products:** Make 1:5 dilution (24.75 g/99 mL sterile diluent). Mix well and plate 1 mL on each of 2 plates. Multiply total of counts on 2 plates by 2.5 to obtain count/g.

   Alternative for butter and margarine: Homogenization may be facilitated by use of prewarmed (40°C to 45°C) phosphate buffer dilution blank.

   C. **Dry dairy products:** [6.020.8.C, 6.020.9]. Make a 1:10 minimum dilution (11 g/99 mL sterile diluent). Mix well and plate 1 mL on each of 2 plates. Multiply total of counts on 2 plates by 5 to obtain count/g.

   D. **Cheese and other cultured and culture-added products:** [6.020.8.D, 6.020.9]. Same as in 7.071.8.G.

   E. **Ice cream and related food products:** [6.020.8.E, 6.020.9]. Same as in 7.071.8.

   F. **Other dairy or related food products:** See chapter 9: Microbiological Methods for Dairy Products for additional preparation instructions.

9. **Procedure:** Redigel™ media is preferred to be at room temperature before use.

   A. **One-dish or 10-dish bottle**
      1. Lift the lid of a pretreated Redigel™ dish and pour the liquid pectin gel from a 1-dish bottle into the dish. Alternatively, pour or pipet 10 to 12 mL from a 10-dish bottle into the dish or dishes.
      2. Replace the lid and swirl the dish to cover the bottom with pectin gel. The sample must be added within 5 minutes after the liquid

pectin gel is added. Add the sample or sample inoculum to the liquid pectin gel in the dish (0.1 to 1 mL depending on the desired dilution).

3. Immediately swirl several times to thoroughly mix the sample with the pectin gel.
4. Place the dish on a level surface and allow the medium to solidify for approximately 40 minutes and then incubate.

B. **Incubation:** Incubate plates at 32° ± 1°C for 24 ± 2 hours for the total coliform count. Plates must reach the temperature of incubation within 2 hours.

C. **Counting colonies on plates:** Count plates promptly after the incubation period. Record the dilutions used and the number of colonies counted or estimated on each plate. If impossible to count at once after the required incubation, store the plates at 0° to 4.4°C for not more than 24 hours; avoid making this a routine practice. When counting colonies on plates, proceed according to the directions given below. For each lot of samples, record the results of sterility tests on materials (dilution blanks, agar, etc.) used when pouring plates and the incubation temperature used.

D. **Manual counting of plates:** Count colonies with the aid of magnification under uniform and properly controlled artificial illumination. Plates should be examined in subdued light. Routinely use a colony counter equipped with a guide plate ruled in square centimeters.[41] Examine doubtful objects carefully, using higher magnification where required, to distinguish colonies from foreign matter. Arrange schedules of laboratory analysts to prevent eye fatigue and the inaccuracies that result from eyestrain.

1. **Normal plates** *(15 to 150 or less than 15 colonies):* Count all colonies, including those of pinpoint size, on selected plate(s). Record the dilution(s) used and the total number of colonies counted.
2. **Crowded plates** *(more than 150 colonies):* Do not record counts on crowded plates from the highest dilution as too numerous to count (TNTC). If the number of colonies per plate exceeds 250, count colonies in those portions of the plate that are representative of colony distribution, and calculate an estimated pectin gel plate count (EPGPC), from these counts. If there are fewer than 10 colonies per square centimeter, count colonies in 12 squares; select, if representative, 6 consecutive squares horizontally across the plate and 6 squares at right angles, being careful not to count a square more than once. When there are more than 10 colonies per square centimeter, count colonies in 4 such representative portions. In both instances, multiply the average number of colonies found per square centimeter by the area of the plate used to determine the estimated number of colonies per plate. Each laboratory must determine the area in square centimeters of the plates in use.

E. **Laboratory accidents or bacterial growth inhibitors:** When a plate from a sample is known to be contaminated or is otherwise unsatisfactory, record the plate as a laboratory accident (LA).

10. **Expression of Results:** Computing and recording counts is same as 7.020.9 Expression of Results.

11. **Precision:** See chapter 1: Precision Parameters.

12. **Test Report:** The test report identifies the method used and results obtained. The report will also identify any variation in the test not specified in this method as well as problems which may have impacted the test result. Each sample will be described in such a manner as to ensure traceability as to its origin.

7.090 *Enterobacteriaceae*

Dry rehydratable film method (3M Petrifilm™ *Enterobacteriaceae* count (PEB) plate method)

1. **Scope:** This method is applicable to dairy products including raw milk, pasteurized fluid milks, and dried milk products.

2. **References:** Chapter 2: Laboratory Quality Assurance and Safety.
   Chapter 3: Sampling Dairy and Related Products.
   Chapter 4: Preparation of Media, Dilution Water, and Sterilization.
   Chapter 6: Microbiological Count Methods.
   Chapter 9: Microbiological Methods for Dairy Products.

3. **Definition:** The Petrifilm™ *Enterobacteriaceae* count plate (PEB) method is a sample-ready culture medium system that consists of 2 plastic films coated with modified violet red bile glucose nutrients, a dehydrated cold water-soluble gelling agent, and a tetrazolium indicator that facilitates colony enumeration. The countable range of the plate is 15 to 100 colonies. Estimates can be made on plates containing less than 15 or greater than 100 colonies.

4. **Principle:** This method allows for the enumeration of *Enterobacteriaceae* as colony-forming units per milliliter or gram under conditions of the method as stated.The PEB plate is inoculated with 1 mL of sample. The sample is spread over approximately a 20-cm^2 growth area. The gelling agent is allowed to solidify, the plates are incubated and then enumerated.

   Enterobacteriaceae are oxidase-negative, gram-negative rods that ferment glucose. Colonies that produce acid and/or gas are considered to be *Enterobacteriaceae*. On PEB plates *Enterobacteriaceae* will appear as red colonies with yellow zones and/or red colonies with gas bubbles with or without yellow zones.

5. **Diluents, Culture Media, and Reagents:** See manufacturer's instructions for use (3M Microbiology Products, 3M Center, Bldg. 275-5W-05, St. Paul, MN 55144-1000).

   A. **Storage and disposal:** Store unopened Petrifilm plate pouches at temperatures ≤8°C (46°F). Just prior to use, allow pouches to come to room temperature before opening. Return unused plates to pouch. To prevent exposure to moisture, do not refrigerate or freeze opened pouches. Seal opened pouches by folding the end of the pouch over and taping shut. Store resealed pouches in a cool, dry place for no longer than one month. Exposure of Petrifilm™ plates to temperatures >25°C (77°F) and/or relative humidity >50% can affect the performance of the plates.

As with other microbial detection systems, PEB plates may contain viable bacteria that may be a biohazard. Follow current industry standards for disposal.

Expiration date and lot number are noted on each package of Petrifilm™ plates. The lot number is also noted on individual plates.

B. **Sterile diluent:** Butterfield's phosphate buffer (IDF phosphate buffer, 0.0425 g/L KH_2PO_4, adjusted to pH 7.2). Do not use buffers containing citrate, bisulfite, or thiosulfate with Petrifilm plates; they can inhibit growth.

C. **Reagents**
  1. NaOH solution (1.0*N*) for pH adjustment of diluted acidic products.
  2. HCl solution (1.0*N*) for pH adjustment of diluted alkaline products.
  3. Ethyl alcohol, 70%, for sample container decontamination.

6. Apparatus and Glassware

1. PEB spreader.
2. Refrigerator: Capable of ≤8°C (46°F).
3. Incubator: Capable of 32° ± 1°C.
4. Thermometer: ± 1°C accuracy.
5. Colony counter or other illuminated magnifier.
6. Hand tally.
7. Balance: Sensitive to 0.01 gram.
8. Dilution bottles: Capacity 150 mL with indelible mark at 99 ± 1 mL.
9. Pipets: 1 mL or pipeters that conform to APHA standards.
10. Stomacher blender with corresponding sterile stomacher bags or autoclaveable blender jars.
11. pH meter or pH paper.

7. Sampling: See chapter 3: Sampling Dairy and Related Products.

8. Preparation

A. **Pasteurized whole and reduced fat milks and raw milk:** [6.020.8.A, 6.020.9]. Depending on expected count, inoculate 1 mL direct or make appropriate serial dilutions by aseptically pipeting diluted sample into diluent to yield a dilution that gives 15 to 100 CFUs per mL of diluted sample plated. One mL of a direct yields a 1-coliform-per-gram sensitivity.

B. **Dry dairy products:** [6.020.8.C, 6.020.9]. Make a 1:10 minimum dilution (11 g/99 mL sterile diluent). Mix well and plate 1 mL on each of 2 plates. Multiply total of counts on 2 plates by 5 to obtain count/g.

For optimal bacterial growth or recovery adjust pH of the sample or diluted sample to 6.5 to 7.5. For acidic products, adjust pH with 1.0*N* NaOH. For alkaline products, adjust pH with 1.0*N* HCl.

C. **Other dairy or related food products:** See chapter 9: Microbiological Methods for Dairy Products for additional preparation instructions.

9. Procedure

A. **Method:** Make appropriate serial dilutions by aseptically pipeting mixed sample into phosphate buffer dilution blank to yield a dilution that gives 15-100 CFUs per mL of diluted sample.

Place the PEB plate on a flat, level surface.

Lift the top film and carefully inoculate 1 mL of undiluted or diluted sample by pipet or pipeter.

Roll the top film down onto the sample to prevent trapping air bubbles.

B. **Spread sample:** With the smooth side down, place the plastic spreader on the center of the plate. Press gently on the center of the spreader to distribute the sample evenly. Spread the inoculum over the entire Petrifilm™ growth area before gel is formed. Do not slide the spreader across the film.

Remove the spreader and leave the plate undisturbed for at least one minute to permit the gel to solidify.

C. **Incubation:** Incubate plates with the clear side up in stacks not exceeding 20 units at 35°C ± 1°C for 24 hours ± 2 hours. Alternative incubation temperatures may be used depending on the method.

D. **Counting colonies:** Count plates promptly after incubation period. Record the dilutions used and the number of colonies counted or estimated for each plate. When counting colonies on plates, proceed according to the directions given below. For each lot of samples, record the results of sterility tests on materials (dilution blanks, pipet/tips, air, etc.) used when pouring plates and the incubation temperature used.

E. **Manual counting of plates:** PEB plates can be counted on a standard colony counter or other illuminated magnifier. Coliform colonies are red and associated with entrapped gas. Colonies not associated with gas (greater than one colony diameter from gas bubble) are not counted as coliforms. Do not count colonies on the foam dam since they are removed from the selective influence of the medium. Do not count artifact bubbles that may be present.

Enterobacteriaceae are red colonies with yellow zones and/or red colonies with gas bubbles with or without yellow zones. Colonies not associated with gas (a distance greater than one colony diameter between colony and gas bubble) and not associated with a yellow zones are not counted as *Enterobacteriaceae*.

The circular growth area is approximately 20 cm^2. Estimates can be made on plates containing greater than 100 colonies by counting the number of colonies in one or more representative squares and determining the average number per square. Multiply the average number per square by 20 to determine the estimated count per plate.

Some *Enterobacteriaceae*, when present in large numbers, cause excessive gas formation and form small, indistinct colonies. When this occurs, record results as too numerous to count (TNTC). Occasionally, on plates containing greater than 100 colonies, colonies and gas will be indistinct; however, the acid produced by the *Enterobacteriaceae* colonies will change the color of the PEB plates to yellow. When any of these characteristics occurs, dilute the sample further to obtain a more accurate count.

F. **Laboratory accidents or bacterial growth inhibitors:** When a plate from a sample is known to be contaminated or is otherwise unsatisfactory, record the plate as a laboratory accident (LA).

10. **Expression of Results:** Computing and recording counts same as 7.020.9.

11. **Precision:** See chapter 1: Precision Parameters.

12. **Test Report:** The test report identifies the method used and results obtained. The report will also identify any variation in the test not specified in this method as well as problems that may have impacted the test result. Each sample will be described in such a manner as to ensure traceability as to its origin.

7.100 Cited References

1. BARTRAM, M.T.; BLACK, L.A. Detection and significance of the coliform group in milk: I. a comparison of media for use in isolation. Food Res. **1**:551-563; 1936.
2. BARTRAM, M.T.; BLACK, L.A. The detection and significance of *Escherichia-Aerobacter* in milk: III. correlation of total bacterial count and presence of the coli-aerogenes group. J. Dairy Sci. **20**:105-112; 1937.
3. COWELL, N.D.; MORISETTI, M.D. Microbiological techniques: some statistical aspects. J. Sci. Food Agric. **20**:573-579; 1969.
4. CUNNIFF, P., ed. *Official Methods of Analysis of AOAC International.* 16th ed. Gaithersburg, MD: AOAC International; 1998.
5. CURIALE, M.S.; FAHEY, P.; FOX; T.L.; McALLISTER, J.S. Dry rehydratable films for enumeration of coliforms and aerobic bacteria in dairy products: collaborative study. JAOAC **72**:312-318; 1989.
6. CURIALE, M.S.; GANGER, V.; D'ONORIAO, A.L.; GAMBREL-LENARZ, S.; McALLISTER, J.S. High-sensitivity dry rehydratable film method for enumeration of coliforms in dairy products; Collaborative study. JAOAC **80**:505-516; 1997.
7. CURIALE, M.S.; SONS, T.; McIVER, D.; McALLISTER, J.S.; HALSEY, B.; ROBLEE, D. Dry rehydratable film for enumeration of total coliforms and *Escherichia coli* in foods: collaborative study. JAOAC **74**:635-648; 1991.
8. DELAY, P.D. The significance of the coliform test in pasteurized milk. J. Milk Food Technol. **10**:297-299; 1947.
9. DE MAN, J.C. The probability of most probable numbers. European J. Appl. Microbiol. **1**:67-78; 1975.
10. DE MAN, J.C. MPN tables for more than one test. European J. Appl. Microbiol. **4**:307; 1977.
11. DRAUGHON, F.A.; NELSON, P.J. Comparison of modified direct plating procedures for recovery of injured *Escherichia coli.* J. Food Sci. **46**:1188-1191; 1981.
12. ENTIS, P. Enumeration of total coliforms, fecal coliforms, and *Escherichia coli* in foods by hydrophobic grid membrane filter: collaborative study. JAOAC **67**:812-823; 1984.
13. FENG, P.C.S.; HARTMAN, P.A. Fluorogenic assays for immediate confirmation of *Escherichia coli.* Appl. Environ. Microbiol. **43**:1320-1329; 1982.
14. FOURNELLE, H.J.; MACY. H. A comparative study of presumptive media for the coliform group. Am. J. Public Health. **40**:934-942; 1950.
15. GINN, R.E.; PACKARD, V.S.; FOX, T.L. Enumeration of total bacteria and coliforms in milk by dry rehydratable film methods; a collaborative study. JAOAC **69**:527-531; 1986.
16. GOEL, M.C.; KULSHRESTHA, D.C.; MARTH, E.H.; FRANCIS. D.W.; BRADSHAW, J.G.; READ, R.B., Jr. Fate of coliforms in yogurt, buttermilk, sour cream, and cottage cheese during refrigerated storage. J. Milk Food Technol. **34**:54-58; 1971.

17. HALL, H.E.; BROWN, D.F.; LEWIS, K.H. Examination of market foods for coliform organisms. Appl. Microbiol. **15:**1062-1069; 1967.
18. HARTMAN, P.A. Modification of conventional methods for recovery of injured coliforms and salmonellae. J. Food Prot. **42**:356-361; 1979.
19. HARTMAN, P.A.; HARTMAN, P.S.; LANZ, W.W. Violet red bile-2 agar for stressed coliforms. Appl. Microbiol. **29**:537-539, 865; 1975.
20. HITCHINS, A.D.; FENG, P.; WATKINS, W.D.; RIPPEY, S.R.; CHANDLER, L.A. Escherichia coli *and the coliform bacteria*. In: Food and Drug Administration. *Bacteriological Analytical Manual*, 8th ed. Washington, DC: U.S. Govt. Print. Off.; 1998.
21. MARSHALL, R.T., ed. *Standard Methods for the Examination of Dairy Products*, 16th ed. Washington, DC: APHA; 1992
22. MATNER, R.R.; FOX, R.L.; McIVER, D.E.; CURIALE, M.S. Efficacy of Petrifilm *E. coli* count plates for *E. coli* and coliform enumeration. J. Food Prot. **53**:145-150; 1990.
23. MAXCY, R.B. Non-lethal injury and limitations of recovery of coliform organisms on selective media. J. Milk Food Technol. **33**:445-48; 1970.
24. McCARTHY, J.A.; THOMAS, H.A., Jr.; DELANEY, J.E. Evaluation of the reliability of coliform density tests. Am. J. Public Health. **48**:1628-1635; 1958.
25. McCRADY, M.H. The numerical interpretation of fermentation tube results. J. Infect. Dis. **17**:183-212; 1915.
26. McCRADY, M.H.; ARCHAMBAULT, J. Examining dairy products for members of the *Escherichia-Aerobacter* group. Am. J. Public Health **24**:122-128; 1934.
27. McCRADY, M.H.; LANGEVIN, E.M. The coli-aerogenes determination in pasteurization control. J. Dairy Sci. **15**:321-329; 1932.
28. MORRIS, R.L.; CERNY, J. Significant abnormalities in the violet red bile technique for coliforms in milk. J. Milk Food Technol. **17**:185-187; 1954.
29. NELSON, F.E.; BAYER, M.P. The influence of time and temperature of plate incubation upon bacterial counts of market milk and related products, particularly after holding under refrigeration. J. Milk Food Technol. **17**:95-100; 1953.
30. NELSON, C.L.; FOX, T.L.; BUSTA, F.F. Evaluation of dry medium film (Petrifilm VRB) for coliform enumeration. J. Food Prot. **47**:520-525; 1984.
31. RAY, B. Methods to detect stressed microorganisms. J. Food Prot. **42**:346-355; 1979.
32. RAY, B.; SPECK, M.L. Plating procedure for the enumeration of coliforms from dairy products. Appl. Environ. Microbiol. **35**:820-822; 1978.
33. REBER, C.L.; MARSHALL, R.T. Comparison of VRB and VRB-2 agars for recovery of stressed coliforms from stored acidified half-and-half. J. Food Prot. **45**:584-585; 1982.
34. REINBOLD, G.W. Bacteriological testing of milk for regulatory purposes—usefulness of current procedures and recommendations for change: III. raw milk quality—where do we go from here? J. Milk Food Technol. **34**:260-263; 1971.
35. ROTH, L.A.; BENGSH, H.; DAVIDSON, C.; DICKSON, J.S. Extended incubation of LST and BGB tubes and the MPN estimates of coliforms. J. Food Prot. **57**:740-742; 1994.
36. ROTH, L.A.; STILES, M.E.; CLEGG, L.F.L. Communal growth response of a heat-injured strain of *Escherichia coli*. Can. J. Microbiol. **18**:1776-1777; 1972.
37. ROTH, L.A.; STILES, M.E.; CLEGG, L.F.L. Reliability of selective media for the enumeration and estimation of *Escherichia coli*. Can. Inst. Food Sci. Technol. J. **6**:230-234; 1973.
38. U.S. DEPARTMENT OF HEALTH AND HUMAN SERVICES. *Grade A pasteurized milk ordinance: Recommendations of the Public Health Service*, Publication No. 229 Washington, DC: U.S. Govt. Print. Off.; 1989 Rev.
39. WOODWARD, R.L. How probable is the most probable number? J. Am. Water Works Assoc. **49**:1060-1068; 1957.
40. YALE, M.W. Comparisons of solid with liquid media as a means of determining the presence of lactose fermenting bacteria in pasteurized milk. Am. J. Public Health. **27**:564-569; 1937.
41. ROTH, J.N.; BONTRAGER, G.L. (AOAC accepted precollaborative study report, unpublished). The enumeration of total coliforms and *Escherichia coli* in food and dairy products: a comparative study of the ColiChrome 2 Redigel method to MPN, Petrifilm EC and VRB Redigel methods. AOAC; 1995.

7.110 Other References

ASSOCIATION FRANCAISE DE NORMALISATION (AFNOR): Certificate N° 3M 01/5-03/97A, 3M™ Petrifilm™ P2000 rapid coliform count plates—reading after 14 hours. Tour Europe, 92049 Paris La Defense Cedex.

ASSOCIATION FRANCAISE DE NORMALISATION (AFNOR): Certificate N° 3M 01/5-03/97B, 3M™ Petrifilm™ P2000 rapid coliform count plates—reading after 24 hours of gas and non gas producing colonies. Tour Europe, 92049 Paris La Defense Cedex.

ASSOCIATION FRANCAISE DE NORMALISATION (AFNOR): Certificate N° 3M 01/5-03/97C, 3M™ Petrifilm™ P2000 rapid coliform count plates—reading of gas producing colonies after 24 hours. Tour Europe, 92049 Paris La Defense Cedex.

ASSOCIATION FRANCAISE DE NORMALISATION (AFNOR): Certificate N° 3M 01/6-09/97, 3M™ Petrifilm™ *Enterobacteriaceae* count plates. Tour Europe, 92049 Paris La Defense Cedex.

ASSOCIATION FRANCAISE DE NORMALISATION (AFNOR): Certificate N° 3M 01/7-03/99, 3M™ Petrifilm™ high-sensitivity coliform count plates—enumeration of gas producing coliform colonies. Tour Europe , 92049 Paris La Defense Cedex.

BETTS, G.D.; BETTS, R.P.; TAYLOR, R. Evaluation of 3M Petrifilm for aerobic plate count, yeast and mould count and *Escherichia coli* count. Campden Food and Drink Research Association. Technical Memorandum No. 703; 1994.

KINNEBERG, K.M.; LINDBERG, K.G. Dry rehydratable film method for the rapid enumeration of coliforms in foods (3M™ Petrifilm™ rapid coliform count plate): collaborative study. JAOAC Int.; at press.

MATUSHEK, M.G.; CURIALE, M.S.; McALLISTER, J.S.; FOX, T.L. Comparison of various plating procedures for the detection and enumeration of coliforms in ice cream and ice milk. J. Food Prot. **55**:113-115; 1992.

MACPHEE, S.; BENNETT, A.R.; BETTS, R.P. Evaluation of 3M Petrifilm count plates for enumeration of *Enterobacteriaceae* and coliforms from food samples.

McALLISTER, J.S. Part 1: Petrifilm—proprietary laboratory techniques—dry rehydratable film method. Bulletin 285/1993—Reference materials and interlaboratory collaborative studies. Brussels: Int. Dairy Fed.; 1993.

PITON, C.; GRAPPIN, R. A model for statistical evaluation of precision parameters of microbiological methods: application to dry rehydratable film methods and IDF reference methods for enumeration of total aerobic mesophilic flora and coliforms in raw milk. JAOAC **74**:92-103; 1991.

ROTH, J.N.; BONTRAGER, G.L. Temperature-independent pectin gel method for coliform determination in dairy products: collaborative study. JAOAC **72**:298-302; 1989.

SENYK, G.F.; KOZLOWSKI, P.S.; NOAR, P.S.; SHIPE, W.F.; BANDLER, D.K. Comparison of dry culture medium and conventional plating techniques for enumeration of bacteria in pasteurized fluid milk. J. Dairy Sci. **70**:1152-1158; 1987.

TORKAR, K.G.; TEGER, S.G. Vrednovanje primjene metode Petrifilm *Escherichia coli* za brojanje bakterije *Escherichia coli* u sirovom mlijeku. (Evaluation of Petrifilm *Escherichia coli* method for bacterial count of *Escherichia coli* in raw milk). Mlijekarstvo **47**:79-92; 1997.

U.S. DEPARTMENT OF HEALTH AND HUMAN SERVICES. *Grade "A" pasteurized milk ordinance: Recommendations of the Public Health Service,* Publication No. 229. Washington, DC: U.S. Govt. Print. Off.; 1999 Rev.

U.S. FOOD AND DRUG ADMINISTRATION. *Form 2400a—standard plate count, coliform, and simplified count methods.* Washington, DC: U.S. Govt. Print. Off.; 1999.

VAN HEDDEGHEM, A.; REYBROECK, W. Determination of the total bacteria and the coliform bacteria in raw milk with the Petrifilm method. Landbouwtijdschrift. **43**:839-848; 1990.

Chapter 8

Tests for Groups of Microorganisms

J. F. Frank and A. E. Yousef
(J. F. Frank, Tech. Comm.)

This chapter includes tests for groups of microorganisms that are particularly significant to ensure the quality and safety of dairy products. Microorganisms representing any given group may vary in significance, and dairy processors may become interested in testing for an individual microorganism rather than a group of microorganisms. Nevertheless, it is easier and often faster to test for these microorganisms as groups and use the results to make general inferences about the microbiological quality of the product.

8.010 Psychrotrophic Bacteria (Class O)

Psychrotrophic bacteria are those bacteria that grow at refrigeration temperatures (≤7°C) within 7-10 days regardless of their optimal growth temperature. Psychrotrophic bacteria that are commonly isolated from dairy products belong to a variety of genera that include but are not limited to *Pseudomonas, Flavobacterium, Alcaligenes, Acinetobacter, Klebsiella, Bacillus,* and *Lactobacillus*. The psychrotrophic bacteria most detrimental to dairy product quality are the oxidative, gram-negative rods belonging to the genus *Pseudomonas*. These are also the psychrotrophs most commonly isolated from milk. Some pathogenic bacteria isolated from milk (e.g., *Listeria monocytogenes* and *Yersinia enterocolitica*) are also psychrotrophic. With the exception of *Bacillus* spp.,[18] psychrotrophs are inactivated by pasteurization, so their presence in processed milk indicates either improper pasteurization or postpasteurization contamination. Growth of psychrotrophs in raw milk (to $\geq 10^6$ CFU/mL) can reduce the quality of the pasteurized product even though the cells are inactivated.

1. **Scope:** The psychrotrophic count procedure is used to estimate the level of microorganisms capable of growing during refrigerated storage and to predict product shelf life. This method is applicable to raw and pasteurized milk, cream, and cottage cheese.

2. **References:** Chapter 2: Laboratory Quality Assurance and Safety.
Chapter 3: Sampling Dairy and Related Products.
Chapter 4: Preparation of Media, Dilution Water, and Sterilization.
Chapter 6: Microbiological Count Methods.
Chapter 9: Microbiological Methods for Dairy Products.

3. **Definition:** Psychrotrophic bacteria are those bacteria capable of producing colonies on the specified medium during incubation at 7°C for 10 days.

4. **Principle:** Samples are plated using a rich, nonselective agar medium. Selection for psychrotrophic bacteria is accomplished by incubating the plates at refrigeration temperature.

5. **Diluents, Culture Media, and Reagents:** See chapter 6, Standard Plate Count Method (6.020).

6. **Apparatus and Glassware:** An incubator capable of being maintained at 7° ± 1°C. See chapter 6 for additional apparatus and glassware.

7. **Sampling:** See chapter 3, Sampling Dairy and Related Products.

8. **Preparation of Test Sample:** See chapter 6, Microbiological Count Methods.

9. **Procedure:** Prepare the test sample and primary dilution and pour-plate as described in chapter 6. Melted medium should be cooled to 45° ± 1°C before pouring plates to prevent destruction of some psychrotrophic bacteria.[25] Incubate plates at 7° ± 1°C for 10 days. At temperatures above 7°C, other nonpsychrotrophic organisms may grow, possibly yielding misleading results.

10. **Expression of Results:** Calculate results as described in chapter 6.

11. **Precision:** Precision parameters for this test are undefined.

12. **Test Report and Interpretation:** Specify the method used, results obtained, and any circumstance or deviations that may have affected the result. Report results as psychrotrophic bacteria count per milliliter or per gram.

8.020 Gram-Negative Bacteria (Class B)

1. **Scope:** This method is applicable to raw and pasteurized milk, cream, and cottage cheese.

2. **References:** Chapter 2: Laboratory Quality Assurance and Safety.
Chapter 3: Sampling Dairy and Related Products.
Chapter 4: Preparation of Media, Dilution Water, and Sterilization.
Chapter 6: Microbiological Count Methods.
Chapter 9: Microbiological Methods for Dairy Products.

3. **Definition:** For the purpose of this test, gram-negative bacteria are those bacteria capable of producing colonies in the presence crystal violet.[6]

4. **Principle:** Samples are plated using a selective agar medium. Selection for gram-negative bacteria is accomplished by including crystal violet in the medium and incubating at 21° ± 1°C.

5. **Diluents, Culture Media, and Reagents:** See chapter 6, Standard Plate Count and Associated Methods for diluents.

Crystal violet tetrazolium agar: Add 1 mL of 0.1% crystal violet (0.1 g/100 mL ethanol) to 1 L of molten standard method agar (SMA). Sterilize the mixture at 120° ± 1°C for 15 minutes. Cool to 45° ± 1°C. Add 5 mL of filter-sterilized 1% aqueous solution of 2,3,5-triphenyl tetrazolium chloride.

6. **Apparatus and Glassware:** An incubator capable of being maintained at 21°C ± 1°C.

   See chapter 6 for additional apparatus and glassware.

7. **Sampling:** See chapter 3, Sampling Dairy and Related Products.
8. **Preparation of Test Sample:** See chapter 6, Microbiological Count Methods.
9. **Procedure:** Prepare dilutions of the product and pour-plate [chapter 6]. Use crystal violet tetrazolium agar. Incubate plates at 21° ± 1°C for 48 ± 3 hours. Count red colonies.
10. **Expression of Results:** Calculate results as described in chapter 6.
11. **Precision:** Precision parameters for this test are undefined.
12. **Test Report and Interpretation:** Report as gram-negative CFU per milliliter or gram.

8.030 Thermoduric Bacteria (Class O)

The test for thermoduric bacteria is also known as a laboratory pasteurization count. High thermoduric counts are consistently associated with unhygienic production practices. The thermoduric count indicates thoroughness of equipment sanitation and assists in detecting sources of organisms responsible for high counts in pasteurized milk products. Thermoduric bacteria contribute appreciably to high standard plate counts in pasteurized milk and milk products since spores of psychrotrophic *Bacillus* spp. survive pasteurization. Vegetative cells resulting from these spores may grow during refrigerated storage of milk and adversely affect the shelf life of the pasteurized product.

1. **Scope:** This test is applicable to raw and pasteurized fluid milk products.
2. **References:** Chapter 2: Laboratory Quality Assurance and Safety.
   Chapter 3: Sampling Dairy and Related Products.
   Chapter 4: Preparation of Media, Dilution Water, and Sterilization.
   Chapter 6: Microbiological Count Methods.
   Chapter 9: Microbiological Methods for Dairy Products.
3. **Definition:** Thermodurics are microorganisms (vegetative cells or spores) that survive pasteurization treatment. Thermoduric bacteria can survive exposure to temperatures considerably higher than their maximum growth temperatures. Thermoduric bacteria isolated from milk usually include species of *Micrococcus, Microbacterium, Streptococcus, Lactobacillus*, coryneform group, *Bacillus*, and *Clostridium*.[24]
4. **Principle:** Milk in test-tubes is heated at 62.8° ± 0.5°C for 30 minutes to simulate the holding pasteurization method. Survivors are counted using the standard plate count method.

5. **Culture Media and Reagents:** See chapter 6.
6. **Apparatus and Glassware**
   1. Test tubes: Sterile, 20 × 125 mm, with rubber- or plastic-lined screw caps.
   2. Pipets: Sterile, graduated, for 5-mL or 11-mL delivery.
   3. Thermometers: 0.1°C graduations. Thermometers used in the water bath and in the pilot tube with milk should cover the critical range of temperature during pasteurization. These should be checked at least annually against a thermometer certified by NIST [chapter 2].
   4. Water bath: Electrically heated, thermostatically controlled at 62.8° ± 0.5°C, equipped with stirrer and thermometer. The volume of water should be sufficient to absorb the cooling effect of tubes placed in the bath without a drop in temperature below 62.8°C.
   5. Test tube rack: Metal, plastic, or wire.
7. **Sampling:** Normally, samples of milk from individual producers, trucks, and tankers are obtained. Samples of finished products may also be analyzed.
8. **Preparation of Test Sample:** See chapter 6, Microbiological Count Methods.
9. **Procedure:** Aseptically transfer 5 mL of a thoroughly mixed milk sample to a sterile test tube. Be careful to avoid contaminating the lip and upper portions of the tube with milk. During this step, all samples and filled tubes should be kept in ice water at 0° to 4.4°C. A temperature control tube containing a thermometer and 5 mL of milk should be placed in the test tube rack with the other samples so the temperature can be easily monitored. Place the rack of tubes in the pasteurizing bath at 62.8° ± 0.5°C. Immerse the closed, watertight tubes either completely or to approximately 4 cm above the level of milk in the bath. The temperature of the milk should reach 62.8°C *within 5 minutes*. If bubbles come from the immersed tubes during heating, the heat treatment is suspect because contaminants may be drawn into the tubes when they are cooled.

   Start timing the 30-minute holding period when the temperature in the pilot tube reaches 62.8°C. At the end of the holding period, immediately place the rack of tubes in an ice water bath and cool to 10°C or lower. Determine the laboratory pasteurization count by using the SPC procedure or an alternative method [chapter 6].
10. **Expression of Results:** Calculate results as CFU/mL as described in chapter 6.
11. **Precision:** Precision parameters for this test are unknown.
12. **Test Report and Interpretation:** Report results as laboratory pasteurization count per milliliter (LPC/mL). Where an alternative aerobic count method is used, add the appropriate designation to the reported count to identify the method.

8.040 Thermophilic Bacteria (Class O)

Thermophiles are usually spore-forming bacteria that enter milk from various sources on the farm, or from poorly cleaned equipment in the processing plant. These bacteria rapidly increase in numbers when present in milk or dairy products that are held at high temperatures. Thermophilic bacteria may accumulate in high-temperature short-time (HTST) pasteurizers or vacuum-concentration systems in continuous operation for lengthy periods.

1. **Scope:** In the dairy industry, the term thermophilic bacteria applies to microorganisms that grow in milk or milk products held at elevated temperatures (≥55°C) including low-temperature long-time (LTLT) pasteurization conditions.[6]
2. **References:** Chapter 2: Laboratory Quality Assurance and Safety.
   Chapter 3: Sampling Dairy and Related Products.
   Chapter 4: Preparation of Media, Dilution Water, and Sterilization.
   Chapter 6: Microbiological Count Methods.
   Chapter 9: Microbiological Methods for Dairy Products.
3. **Definition:** Thermophilic bacteria are those bacteria capable of producing colonies on the specified agar medium during incubation at 55°C.
4. **Principle:** Samples of dairy products are plated on SMA and incubated at 55° ± 1°C. Incubation at this temperature allows only for growth of thermophiles.
5. **Diluents, Culture Media, and Reagents:** See chapter 6 for diluents.
   Use 15 to 18 mL agar medium/plate.
6. **Apparatus and Glassware:** An incubator capable of being maintained at 55° ± 1°C.
   See chapter 6 for additional apparatus and glassware.
7. **Sampling:** See chapter 3, Sampling Dairy and Related Products.
8. **Preparation of Test Sample:** See chapter 6, Microbiological Count Methods.
9. **Procedure:** Prepare dilutions of the sample and pour-plate as described in chapter 6. Incubate plates at 55° ± 1°C for 48 hours. Maintain humidity during incubation to prevent drying of agar medium.
10. **Expression of Results:** Calculate results as described in chapter 6.
11. **Precision:** There are no precision parameters for this test.
12. **Test Report and Interpretation:** Report results as thermophilic bacterial count per milliliter or per gram (TBC/mL or /g).

8.050 Proteolytic Microorganisms

8.051 *Skim Milk Agar Method (Class O)*

Many bacteria responsible for spoilage of refrigerated dairy products are highly proteolytic and can cause flavor defects. Proteolytic enzymes produced by psychrotrophic bacteria during growth in milk often remain active after HTST and ultrahigh temperature (UHT) heat treatments, and thus reduce the quality of stored, heat-treated products. Tests for proteolytic bacteria may be useful in identifying practices during handling and storage of raw or processed milk that can cause contamination of products.

1. **Scope:** This test can be applied to raw and pasteurized fluid milk and other unfermented dairy products.

2. **References:** Chapter 2: Laboratory Quality Assurance and Safety.
   Chapter 3: Sampling Dairy and Related Products.
   Chapter 4: Preparation of Media, Dilution Water, and Sterilization.
   Chapter 6: Microbiological Count Methods.
   Chapter 9: Microbiological Methods for Dairy Products.
3. **Definition:** This method detects microorganisms that produce extracellular proteases capable of hydrolyzing casein and producing colonies at the incubation time and temperature used.
4. **Principle:** Skim milk is added to SMA to form skim milk agar. Proteolytic microorganisms in the plated sample hydrolyze the casein surrounding the colony. When colonies are flooded with acid, intact casein produces a white precipitate, whereas hydrolyzed casein does not precipitate and the agar remains translucent. Acid-producing organisms can cause false-positive reactions on skim milk agar.
5. **Diluents, Culture Media, and Reagents**
   A. **Skim milk agar:** Mix 100 mL of sterile skim milk (10% wt/wt solids) with 1 L of melted standard methods agar (SMA) adjusted to 49° ± 1°C.
   B. **Acid solution:** Prepare 1% HCL or 10% acetic acid.
   C. Diluents as described in Chapter 6.
6. **Apparatus and Glassware:** See chapter 6.
7. **Sampling:** See chapter 3, Sampling Dairy and Related Products.
8. **Preparation of Test Sample:** See chapter 6, Microbiological Count Methods.
9. **Procedure:** Proceed as for the SPC method [chapter 6] using skim milk agar. Incubate the poured plates for 48 to 72 hours at 32° ± 1°C or, to increase the recovery of psychrotrophic bacteria, for 72 hours at 21° ± 1°C. Flood the incubated plates for 1 minute with hydrochloric acid or acetic acid. Pour off the excess acid solution and count the colonies surrounded by clear zones.
10. **Expression of Results:** Calculate results as indicated in chapter 6.
11. **Precision:** Precision parameters for this test have not been defined.
12. **Test Report and Interpretation:** Report as proteolytic colony count per milliliter or per gram. Indicate the method used including medium, incubation time, and temperature.

8.052 *Standard Methods Caseinate Agar Method (Class B)*

1. **Scope:** See 8.051.1.
2. **References:** See 8.051.2.
3. **Definition:** See 8.051.3.
4. **Principle:** Proteolytic microorganisms hydrolyze caseinate surrounding the colony, causing the agar to clear. Caseinate agar is preferred over skim milk agar for enumerating this group of bacteria because caseinate agar is more sensitive when detecting weakly proteolytic organisms and rarely produces false-positive reactions.[16]

5. **Diluents, Culture Media, and Reagents**
   A. **Diluents:** See chapter 6.
   B. **Standard methods caseinate agar**
      1. Prepare standard methods caseinate agar using dehydrated SMA as a base.
      2. Prepare 0.015 M of trisodium citrate by dissolving 4.41 g of hydrated trisodium citrate in enough microbiologically suitable (MS) water to make 1 L.
      3. Dissolve 23.5 g of dehydrated SMA in 500 mL of the citrate solution. Dissolve 10 g of sodium caseinate in the other 500 mL of citrate solution, using a blender to aid in dispersion. Mix the 2 solutions and autoclave at 120° ± 1°C for 15 minutes.
      4. Prepare a 1-M calcium chloride solution by adding 218.99 g of calcium chloride hexahydrate to 1 L of MS water, and autoclave at 120° ± 1°C for 15 minutes.
      5. Before pouring plates, add 20 mL of the sterile 1-M calcium chloride solution to the molten agar and mix.
6. **Apparatus and Glassware:** See chapter 6.
7. **Sampling:** See chapter 3.
8. **Preparation of Test Sample:** See chapter 6, Microbiological Count Methods.
9. **Procedure:** Pour caseinate agar into plates so that the medium is 2 mm thick (e.g., 12 mL for an 8.5-cm plate).

   After the medium has hardened, plate 0.1-mL quantities of the sample or diluted sample on the agar surface and spread evenly with a sterile, bent-glass rod. To ensure absorption of the sample, allow inoculated plates to dry for 15 minutes

   Incubate plates (in inverted position) for 48 to 72 hours at 32° ± 1°C or for 72 hours at 21° ± 1°C. Colonies surrounded by a white or off-white zone of paracasein precipitate are proteolytic. Highly proteolytic bacteria will also produce a clear inner zone.

   Aerobic plate counts can be estimated using caseinate agar. However, to measure the proportion of proteolytic organisms in the total microflora, only uncrowded plates (fewer than 80 colonies per plate) can be read accurately. For best results, plates may have to be read twice—once at 48 ± 3 hours to estimate the total count and again after 72 ± 3 hours to ensure that slower-to-develop proteolytic colonies are included.
10. **Expression of Results:** Calculate results as indicated in chapter 6.
11. **Precision:** Precision parameters for this test have not been defined.
12. **Test Report and Interpretation:** Report as proteolytic colony count per milliliter or per gram. Indicate the method used including medium, incubation time, and temperature.

8.060 Lipolytic Microorganisms (Class B)[11,23]

1. **Scope:** This test can be applied to milk and high fat dairy products. It can be used to investigate the cause of flavor defects associated with fat hydrolysis.

2. **References:** Chapter 2: Laboratory Quality Assurance and Safety.
   Chapter 3: Sampling Dairy and Related Products.
   Chapter 4: Preparation of Media, Dilution Water, and Sterilization.
   Chapter 6: Microbiological Count Methods.
   Chapter 9: Microbiological Methods for Dairy Products.

3. **Definition:** This method detects microorganisms that produce extracellular lipase capable of hydrolyzing trybutyrin and able to produce colonies at the incubation time and temperature used. Many psychrotrophic bacteria as well as molds and some yeasts are lipolytic.

4. **Principle:** Sample dilutions are spread on spirit blue agar and plates are incubated under conditions that allow for colony formation. Colonies of lipolytic microorganisms hydrolyze the tributyrin, resulting in a clear zone and/or color change. The lipase reagent contains tributyrin as a substrate. It is the simplest triglyceride occurring in natural fats and oils. Some microorganisms that hydrolyze tributyrin will not hydrolyze other, more complex triglycerides or fats containing longer chain fatty acids. The result can be a misleading count.

5. **Diluents, Culture Media, and Reagents:** See chapter 6 for diluents.
   A. **Spirit blue agar:** Prepare spirit blue agar by hydrating the powdered medium and sterilizing the mixture at 120° ± 1°C for 15 minutes as instructed by the manufacturer. Cool the melted agar to 50° to 55°C and add 3% lipase reagent with thorough mixing. If desired, use 1% to 2% of the lipase reagent and sonicate the mixture to emulsify the reagent uniformly in the agar. Pour 10 to 12 mL of the medium into a sterile petri plate and allow the medium to solidify.
   B. Lipase reagent.

6. **Apparatus and Glassware:** See chapter 6.

7. **Sampling:** See chapter 3, Sampling Dairy and Related Products.

8. **Preparation of Test Sample:** See chapter 6, Microbiological Count Methods.

9. **Procedure:** Prepare 1:10 or other suitable dilutions of the product to be tested. Spread 0.1 mL of the desired dilution over the surface of solidified spirit blue agar.

   Invert the plate and incubate at 32° ± 1°C for 48 ± 3 hours. To increase the recovery of psychrotrophic bacteria, incubate for 72 ± 3 hours at 21° ± 1°C. The complete medium is light blue and translucent if it is not emulsified, or lighter blue and opaque if it is emulsified. Colonies of lipolytic microorganisms develop a clear zone and/or a deep blue color around and under each colony.

10. **Expression of Results:** Calculate results as indicated in chapter 6.

11. **Precision:** Precision parameters for this test have not been defined.

12. **Test Report and Interpretation:** Report as lypolytic colony count per milliliter or per gram. Indicate the method used including medium, incubation time, and temperature.

8.070 Lactic Acid Bacteria (Class B)

8.071 *Total Lactic Acid Bacteria*

Enumerating lactic acid bacteria in dairy products is useful when evaluating product quality including the cause of acid defects and in evaluating lactic starter cultures. There are numerous methods for enumerating lactic acid bacteria in dairy products. This group of microorganisms is diverse with different growth requirements and sensitivities to selective agents. Therefore, there is no growth medium that can be applied to all samples. In cases where significant populations of nonlactic microflora are present, media having greater selectivity may be required at the risk of inhibiting some of the lactic microflora. *Lactobacillus* selection agar[19] and MRS[4] broth with added agar are suitable when selectivity for lactobacilli is desired. Other useful media are described by Gilliland et al.[7] When selectivity is not required or when injured cells may be present, SMA [chapter 6] may be used. However, lactic acid bacteria grow slowly on SMA and pin-point colonies are observed after incubation. Dye indicators and sodium azide should be used with caution because some strains of lactic acid bacteria are inhibited by their presence.

Lactobacilli that survive pasteurization may be sublethally injured. Consequently, lactobacilli in young cheese should be enumerated by using a relatively nonselective medium followed by colony characterization.

1. **Scope:** The test for total lactic acid bacteria is applicable to products such as fluid milk, cottage cheese, cheese, cultured milks, uncultured products containing added cultures and lactic starter cultures.

2. **References:** Chapter 2: Laboratory Quality Assurance and Safety.
   Chapter 3: Sampling Dairy and Related Products.
   Chapter 4: Preparation of Media, Dilution Water, and Sterilization.
   Chapter 6: Microbiological Count Methods.
   Chapter 9: Microbiological Methods for Dairy Products.

3. **Definition:** Lactic acid bacteria found in dairy products are a diverse group consisting primarily of *Streptococcus, Lactococcus, Leuconostoc,* and homofermentative and heterofermentative *Lactobacillus* species.

4. **Principle:** Sample dilutions are plated on lactic (Elliker) agar[5] and incubated at 32° or 37°C for 48 hours. Since this medium is not highly selective, nonlactic microorganisms may produce colonies. Composition of this medium may be modified to aid in detecting acid-producing microorganisms. This is accomplished by adding 1 mL of a 1.6% alcoholic solution of bromcresol purple directly to 1 L of the medium before sterilization. Colonies producing a yellow halo are acid producers. To make SMA or lactic agar more selective, add 0.02% sodium azide before sterilization. Lactic acid bacteria are resistant to sodium azide, which inhibits *Enterobacteriaceae* and aerobic organisms.

5. **Diluents, Culture Media, and Reagents**
   1. **Diluent:** Use 0.1% peptone water sterilized at 120° ± 1°C for 15 minutes. Use of phosphate diluent [chapter 6] may reduce cell recovery.
   2. **Culture media:** Lactic (Elliker) agar and MRS are commercially available.

6. **Apparatus and Glassware:** See chapter 6, Microbiological Count Methods.

7. **Sampling:** See chapter 3, Sampling Dairy and Related Products.

8. **Preparation of Test Sample:** See chapter 6, Microbiological Count Methods.

9. **Procedure:** Samples must be handled with care because lactic acid bacteria are easily injured by adverse environments. Prepare dilutions of products using peptone water.

   Pour-plating of sample dilutions is done as described for the SPC method [chapter 6], but using lactic or MRS agar. Colony development is facilitated by either using an agar overlay or incubating plates in a reduced-oxygen atmosphere.

   Plates may be incubated for 48 ± 3 hours at either 32° or 37° ± 1°C, depending on whether mesophilic or thermoduric organisms are being enumerated.

   Because lactic and MRS agar are not highly selective, individual colonies should be tested for catalase reaction, gram reaction, and cell morphology. Gram-positive, catalase-negative cocci, or rods that produce acid are tentatively considered to be lactic acid bacteria.

10. **Expression of Results:** Report colony count as acid producers count per milliliter or per gram if acid production was visualized, or as CFU/mL or g if an acid indicator was not used.

11. **Precision:** Precision parameters for this test have not been defined.

12. **Test Report and Interpretation:** Report colony counts as in 8.071.10. Specify the medium used, the incubation conditions, and the results of colony testing.

    Injured cells may not be recovered on media specifically designed for growth of lactic acid bacteria. Acidified lactobacillus selection (LBS) agar is more selective than MRS and lactic agar and should be used with greater caution. However, MRS and lactic agar media are sufficiently inhibitory to prevent the recovery of some heat-injured lactobacilli that may be present in young cheese. SMA recovers injured lactobacilli, but this medium is not selective.

8.072 Rods and Cocci in Yogurt

1. **Scope:** This method is used for differentiating *Streptococcus thermophilus* and *Lactobacillus delbrueckii* in yogurt. It has not been evaluated for use on other products.

2. **References:** See 8.071.2.

3. **Definition:** Rods and cocci are *Lactobacillus* and *Streptococcus* spp. used in yogurt fermentation.

4. **Principle:** *L. delbrueckii* subsp. *bulgaricus* produces larger colonies and more acid on this medium than does *S. thermophilus*. The greater acid production results in a large white halo around colonies of *L. delbrueckii* subsp. *bulgaricus*.

5. **Diluents, Culture Media, and Reagents:** See chapter 6 for diluents.

   Culture media[17]**:** Prepare yogurt lactic agar as follows. Reconstitute nonfat dry milk to 11% (wt/wt) solids and autoclave at 120° ± 1°C for 12 minutes. Add the warm sterile reconstituted milk, 7% (vol/vol), to tempered lactic (Elliker) agar.

6. **Apparatus and Glassware**
   1. Apparatus for producing a low oxygen and enhanced carbon dioxide atmosphere.
   2. Incubator capable of maintaining 37°C.
7. **Sampling:** See chapter 3, Sampling Dairy and Related Products.
8. **Preparation of Test Sample:** See chapter 6, Microbiological Count Methods.
9. **Procedure:** Pour plates and allow the surfaces to dry.

   Prepare sample dilutions by aseptically blending 1 g of yogurt in 99 g of chilled, sterile 0.1% (wt/vol) peptone water at high speed for 2 minutes. This procedure breaks up chains of cells for a more accurate analysis.

   Prepare serial dilutions in sterile peptone water and surface plate 0.1-mL amounts onto poured, predried plates of yogurt lactic agar.

   Incubate the plates in a low-oxygen, carbon dioxide-enhanced atmosphere at 37° ± 1°C for 48 ± 3 hours. *Streptococcus thermophilus* colonies are small and white with no cloudy zone whereas *L. bulgaricus* colonies are large and white with a white cloudy zone.
10. **Expression of Results:** Report results as colony-forming units of rods or cocci per gram. Specify the medium used and whether results are confirmed by using gram stains.
11. **Precision:** Precision parameters for this test have not been defined.
12. **Test Report and Interpretation:** See 8.072.10.

8.080 Enterococci (Class B)

There are over 20 species in the genus *Enterococcus*. *Enterococcus faecalis* and *E. faecium* are found in dairy products; these species are recognized as being primarily of fecal origin and are the target microorganisms of this test. The *Enterococcus* count is more reliable than the coliform count as an index of the sanitary quality of churned butter since enterococci survive better than coliforms in the unfavorable microenvironment of salted butter.[22] In addition, the *Enterococcus* count may be a more reliable indicator of the sanitary quality of yogurt than the coliform count because coliforms are more readily inactivated in the low pH environment than are enterococci.

While KF streptococcal agar has been accepted by most industry and regulatory agencies for the quantitative estimation of enterococci in nondairy foods, more selective conditions are necessary in dairy products to reduce background growth of other streptococci and lactobacilli.[21] For example, m-enterococcus agar is suggested for membrane filtration procedures, and it has been used to select for enterococci in dried foods, including nonfat dry milk. However, this medium may not inhibit the growth of *Lactobacillus acidophilus* and *Streptococcus bovis*.

1. **Scope:** This method may be applied to all dairy products and environmental samples.

2. **References:** Chapter 2: Laboratory Quality Assurance and Safety.
Chapter 3: Sampling Dairy and Related Products.
Chapter 4: Preparation of Media, Dilution Water, and Sterilization.
Chapter 6: Microbiological Count Methods.
Chapter 9: Microbiological Methods for Dairy Products.

3. **Definition:** Enterococci enumerated by this method are primarily of the *E. faecium* and *E. faecalis* species.

4. **Principle:** This method employs citrate azide agar pour plates which are overlayed and incubated at 37°C for 48 to 72 hours. Enterococci colonies are stained blue by the tetrazolium blue in the medium.

5. **Diluents, Culture Media, and Reagents**

A. **Citrate azide agar:**

Base:

Yeast extract	10 g
Pancreatic digest of casein	10 g
Sodium citrate	20 g
Agar	15 g
MS water to make	1 L

Heat to boiling to dissolve ingredients. Disperse in 100-mL amounts and autoclave at 121° ± 1°C for 20 minutes.

Temper base medium 48°C and add 1 mL of 0.1% sterile (121° ± 1° for 20 minutes) aqueous tetrazolium blue and 1 mL of 4% sterile (121° ± 1° for 20 minutes) aqueous sodium azide to each batch of 100 mL. Final pH should be 7.0 ± 0.2 at 25°C.

B. Diluents as described in chapter 6.

6. **Apparatus and Glassware:** See chapter 6, Microbiological Count Methods.

An incubator capable of maintaining 37° ± 1°C.

7. **Sampling:** See chapter 3, Sampling Dairy and Related Products. See also chapter 13 for environmental samples.

8. **Preparation of Test Sample:** See chapter 6, Microbiological Count Methods.

9. **Procedure:** Inoculate petri dishes with 0.1 or 1 mL of appropriate sample dilutions.

Add 12 to 15 mL of sterile, citrate azide agar (tempered at 45°C) per plate. The medium must be allowed to solidify while the plates are on a level surface.

Add 3 to 4 mL of citrate azide agar as an overlay to cover the surface of the solidified agar completely.

After the overlay has solidified, incubate the plates at 37° ± 1°C for 48 to 72 hours.

To facilitate the counting of colonies, a thin sheet of white tissue paper may be placed under the petri dish on the illuminated colony counter. This enhances the contrast between the colonies and the background. Count only blue colonies.

10. **Expression of Results:** Calculate results as described in chapter 6.

11. **Precision:** Precision parameters for this test are undefined.

12. **Test Report and Interpretation:** Report as enterococci count per milliliter or per gram and specify the method used.

8.090 Aerobic Bacterial Spores (Class B)

1. **Scope:** This is a method for enumeration of psychrotrophic or mesophilic aerobic bacterial spores. It can be applied to raw or heated fluid milk, evaporated or other canned milk products, and milk and milk-derived powders.
2. **References:** Chapter 2: Laboratory Quality Assurance and Safety.
   Chapter 3: Sampling Dairy and Related Products.
   Chapter 4: Preparation of Media, Dilution Water, and Sterilization.
   Chapter 6: Microbiological Count Methods.
   Chapter 9: Microbiological Methods for Dairy Products.
3. **Definition:** Aerobic bacterial spores enumerated by this method are generally in the genus *Bacillus*. These spores can survive in products given mild to severe heat treatments and can cause defects such as sweet-curdling in pasteurized milk and coagulation of canned evaporated milk.
4. **Principle:** The sample is heated to 80° ± 1°C for 12 minutes to inactivate vegetative cells and activate bacterial spores. After cooling, serial dilutions of the sample are plated on SMA. These plates are incubated at either 32° ± 1°C to enumerate mesophilic spores or at 7° ± 1°C to enumerate psychrotrophic spores.[18]
5. **Diluents, Culture Media, and Reagents:** SMA (chapter 6) with 0.1% soluble starch added before sterilization.
   Diluents as described in chapter 6.
6. **Apparatus and Glassware**
   1. Erlenmeyer flasks: Sterile, 500-mL size, with rubber- or plastic-lined screw caps.
   2. Water or ethylene glycol bath: With thermostatic control for 80° and 82°C, equipped with shaker for constant agitation of flasks.
   3. Thermometers: For use in water or ethylene glycol bath and pilot flask.
   4. Plating equipment and supplies [chapter 6].
   5. Incubator capable of maintaining either 32° or 7°C.
7. **Sampling:** See chapter 3, Sampling Dairy and Related Products.
8. **Preparation of Test Sample:** See chapter 6, Microbiological Count Methods.
9. **Procedure:** Place 200 mL of each thoroughly mixed milk sample into a sterile Erlenmeyer flask and screw on the cap. Seal the outside of the cap with masking tape to prevent airborne contamination.
   Dispense 200 mL of milk in the pilot flask and seal it with a rubber stopper equipped with a thermometer.
   Place the pilot and test flasks in a water bath at 82° ± 1°C and agitate them throughout the heat treatment. When the contents of the control flask reach 79°C, lower the temperature of the bath to 80°C, or move the flasks to a second bath in which the water is set at 80° ± 1°C. After the

contents of the pilot flask reach 80°C, keep the samples in the bath for an additional 12 minutes.

Cool the samples immediately in an ice bath.

Dispense samples in petri plates, pour on SMA with starch, and incubate the plates, either at 32° ± 1°C for 48 hours for mesophilic spore counts, or at 7° ± 1°C for 10 days for psychrotrophic spore counts.

To detect low levels of psychrotrophic contamination, the heated milk can be incubated at 7° ± 1°C for 5 to 7 days before plating. If samples are to be taken during preincubation, a separate flask may be used for each sampling.

10. **Expression of Results:** Calculate results as described in chapter 6.
11. **Precision:** Precision parameters have not been determined for this test.
12. **Test Report and Interpretation:** Results should be reported as mesophilic or psychrotrophic aerobic spore count per milliliter. The preincubation time should be noted if applicable.

    High numbers of spore-forming bacteria in milk may indicate unsanitary production practices and may cause product defects, as previously noted. However, the initial mesophilic spore count of raw milk is not a good indicator of the keeping quality of the heated product.

8.100 Anaerobic Sporeformers (Class B)

Anaerobic sporeforming bacteria found in dairy products are in the genus *Clostridium*. No single method can provide an accurate estimate of anaerobic sporeformers, since some spores (*C. sporogenes*, *C. botulinum*, and related types) require heat activation for germination whereas others (*C. perfringens*, butyric anaerobes, and injured spores) are insufficiently heat resistant to survive the activation process. When using this method, the analyst must choose a spore activation heat treatment suitable for the population being analyzed. The method presented here will enumerate mesophilic anaerobic sporeformers and is not specific for *C. botulinum* or *C. perfringens*. Analysts should be aware that cultures produced from the described method may contain botulinum toxin, which is extremely toxic to humans. Botulinum toxin is inactivated by autoclaving.

1. **Scope:** The method has been applied to milk and cheese. The method is easily modified for determination of *Clostridium tyrobutyricum*, a common cause of late gas defect in cheese.[3,9]
2. **References:** Chapter 2: Laboratory Quality Assurance and Safety.
   Chapter 3: Sampling Dairy and Related Products.
   Chapter 4: Preparation of Media, Dilution Water, and Sterilization.
   Chapter 6: Microbiological Count Methods.
   Chapter 7: Coliform and Other Indicator Bacteria.
   Chapter 9: Microbiological Methods for Dairy Products.
3. **Definition:** Anaerobic bacterial sporeformers are defined for the purposes of this method as mesophilic *Clostridium* spp.
4. **Principle:** The most probable number (MPN) method gives more reproducible results than colony count methods and is therefore recommended.[20] Sample or sample slurry is heated to activate spores. Samples or

sample dilution is added to tubes of reinforced clostridial medium (RCM) (for total anaerobic spores) or RCM modified by substituting sodium lactate for glucose for estimating numbers of *C. tyrobutyricum*. Tubes are sealed and incubated at 37° ± 1°C for 7 days. Positive tubes show gas production. RCM and RCM-lactate are not highly selective media.

5. **Diluents, Culture Media, and Reagents:** See chapter 6 for diluents.
   A. Reinforced clostridial medium.
   B. Reinforced clostridial medium with lactate

Beef extract	10 g
Yeast extract	3 g
Tryptone	10 g
Sodium lactate (72% solution)	28 g
Sodium acetate	5 g
Cysteine hydrochloride	0.5 g
Soluble starch	1 g
Agar	1 g
MS water sufficient to make	1 L

   Adjust pH of the medium to 5.5 to 5.7 using 20% lactic acid. Sterilize by autoclaving at 120° ± 1°C for 15 minutes.
   C. **Agar plug:** Mix 20 g agar with 1 g sodium thioglycolate and dissolved in sufficient MS water to make 1 L. Sterilize by autoclaving at 120° ± 1°C for 15 minutes.

6. **Apparatus and Glassware**
   1. Narrow neck flasks or test tubes sufficient for 3-tube MPN [chapter 7]; no Durham tubes are needed.
   2. Other glassware as listed in chapter 6.
   3. Incubator capable of maintaining 37° ± 1°C.

7. **Sampling:** See chapter 3, Sampling Dairy and Related Products.

8. **Preparation of Test Sample:** See chapter 6, Microbiological Count Methods.

9. **Procedure:** Heat milk samples as described in 8.090.9 at 80°C for 10 minutes.

   If presence of injured spores is suspected (such as in fresh cheese) the heat treatment may be reduced to 62.5°C for 30 minutes.

   If analyzing 10-g samples, use flasks or tubes containing 10 mL of double strength medium. Otherwise add 1-g samples or sample dilutions to 9 mL of medium.

   Use RCM medium for total anaerobic sporeformers and RCM-lactate for *C. tyrobutyricum*. Just before use, media should be boiled or steamed for 10 to 20 minutes and quickly cooled to exclude oxygen.

   Distribute sample and sample dilutions into flasks or tubes of media as described for a 3-tube MPN [chapter 7]. Seal each tube or flask with an agar plug by pouring a small volume of melted agar containing sodium thioglycolate.

   Incubate at 37° ± 1°C for 7 days. Positive tubes are those that show gas production by raising the agar plug. Tubes may contain botulinum toxin, so there must be no human contact with tube contents until after autoclaving.

10. **Expression of Results:** Calculate results as MPN/g using the 3-tube MPN table [chapter 7].
11. **Precision:** Determine confidence limits from the MPN table [chapter 7].
12. **Test Report and Interpretation:** Report as MPN anaerobic sporeformers/gram or per milliliter. Give confidence limits associated with the result. Specify the medium used and the spore activation treatment.

8.110 Yeast and Mold Counts

8.111 Antibiotic Plate Count Method (Class A2)

1. **Scope:** This method is suitable for use with all dairy products. The method, however, may not recover osomotolerant fungi that are sometimes found in low water activity products.
2. **References:** Chapter 2: Laboratory Quality Assurance and Safety.
   Chapter 3: Sampling Dairy and Related Products.
   Chapter 4: Preparation of Media, Dilution Water, and Sterilization.
   Chapter 6: Microbiological Count Methods.
   Chapter 9: Microbiological Methods for Dairy Products.
3. **Definition:** For this method, yeasts and molds are defined as fungal cells capable of forming colonies under the specified conditions. Slow-growing yeasts and molds may not be enumerated by this method.
4. **Principle:** Sample or sample dilutions are spread plated on culture medium that employs antibiotics to inhibit growth of bacteria. Plates are incubated at 25°C for 5 days under aerobic conditions and under sufficient humidity to prevent the medium from dehydrating. The neutral pH of the culture medium provided for greater recovery of yeasts and molds than in the case of acidified media.[14,15]
5. **Diluents, Culture Media, and Reagents:** See chapter 6 for basic materials and diluents.
   A. **Culture medium:** See chapter 6, SMA.
   B. **Antibiotic solution:** Suspend 500 mg each of chlortetracycline hydrochloride and chloramphenicol (U.S. Biochemical Corp., Cleveland, OH; Sigma, St. Louis, MO) in 100 mL of sterile, phosphate-buffered diluent (chapter 4). (Chloramphenicol is highly toxic; skin contact should be avoided.) Filter-sterilization is generally not required. The suspension can be stored for 2 months at 5°C without loss of inhibitory activity.
6. **Apparatus and Glassware:** See chapter 6, Microbiological Count Methods.
7. **Sampling:** See chapter 3, Sampling Dairy and Related Products.
8. **Preparation of Test Sample:** See chapter 6, Microbiological Count Methods.
9. **Procedure**
   A. **Preparation of medium:** Prepare SMA according to the manufacturer's directions. Sterilize and cool to 45° ± 1°C. Add 2 mL of antibiotic solution per 100 mL of medium, and mix.

B. **Plating, incubation, and counting:** Prepare samples as for the SPC [chapter 6]. Use the surface (spread) plating technique by spreading 0.1 or 0.2 mL of the sample or the sample dilution over predried plates using a sterile, bent-glass rod. If agar surfaces are sufficiently dry, 1 mL of sample can be spread over 3 plates to increase the sensitivity of the method. Do not invert the plates during incubation. Incubate at 25°C for 5 days.

10. **Expression of Results:** Calculate results as described in chapter 6, but use plates that have between 15 and 150 colonies. If plates are outside this range, estimated counts can be reported.
11. **Precision:** Precision parameters are outlined in chapter 1.
12. **Test Report and Interpretation:** Report as yeast and mold per gram or per milliliter and specify the method used. If results must be obtained from plates containing colony numbers not within the recommended counting range, report the results as estimated yeast and mold per gram or per milliliter.

8.112 *Acidified Potato Dextrose (Glucose) Agar (Class O)*

1. **Scope:** This method is recommended only for dairy products that contain insignificant numbers of debilitated or injured fungal cells. These are products in which the microbial population has not been subject to processing stresses such as heat, acidification, or other antimicrobial treatments.[8]
2. **References:** See 8.111.2.
3. **Definition:** See 8.111.3.
4. **Principle:** See 8.111.4.

   The medium is acidified to pH 3.5 to inhibit the growth of bacteria.
5. **Diluents, Culture Media, and Reagents:** See chapter 6 for basic materials and diluents.

   A. **Culture medium:** Potato dextrose (glucose) agar (commercially available).

   B. **Acidifying agent:** Sterile 10% tartaric acid. Sterilize the tartaric acid solution at 120° ± 1°C for 10 minutes.
6. **Apparatus and Glassware:** See chapter 6, Microbiological Count Methods.
7. **Sampling:** See chapter 3, Sampling Dairy and Related Products.
8. **Preparation of Test Sample:** See chapter 6, Microbiological Count Methods.
9. **Procedure**

   A. **Preparation of medium:** Prepare potato dextrose (glucose) agar according to the manufacturer's directions. Sterilize and cool to 46°C. Add enough sterile 10% tartaric acid to adjust the pH of the medium to 3.5 ± 0.1.

   B. **Plating, incubation, and counting:** Prepare and plate samples as described in section 8.111.9. Incubate at 25° ± 1°C for 5 ± 0.5 days and count plates [chapter 6] that have between 15 and 150 colonies.

10. **Expression of Results:** See 8.111.10.
11. **Precision:** See 8.111.11.
12. **Test Report and Interpretation:** See 8.111.12.

8.113 *Yeast Extract-Glucose-Chloramphenicol Agar (Class B, IDF Recommended Medium[10]):*

1. **Scope:** See 8.111.1.

   This medium is especially useful for samples that are expected to contain predominantly yeasts or yeasts that have been injured.
2. **References:** See 8.111.2.
3. **Definition:** See 8.111.3.
4. **Principle:** See 8.111.4.
5. **Diluents, Culture Media, and Reagents:** See chapter 6 for basic materials and diluents.

   Culture medium:

   Yeast extract-glucose-chloramphenicol agar.

Yeast extract	5 g
Glucose	20 g
Chloramphenicol solution	1 mL
Agar	15 g
MS water to make	1 L

   Disperse ingredients in the water in the order listed, and boil or steam for about 30 minutes to dissolve agar. Sterilize for 15 minutes at 120° ± 1°C. Adjust the pH after sterilization to 6.6 ± 0.1.
6. **Apparatus and Glassware:** See chapter 6.
7. **Sampling:** See chapter 3, Sampling Dairy and Related Products.
8. **Preparation of Test Sample:** See chapter 6, Microbiological Count Methods.
9. **Procedure:** Prepare, inoculate, and count plates as described in 8.111.9 using yeast extract glucose chloramphenicol agar.
10. **Expression of Results:** See 8.111.10.
11. **Precision:** See 8.111.11.
12. **Test Report:** See 8.111.12.

8.114 *Dichloran-Rose Bengal-Chloramphenicol (DRBC) Agar (Class B)*

1. **Scope:** This method is suitable for all dairy products and environmental samples. The method is especially useful for enumerating molds when samples are expected to contain species of *Rhizopus* and *Mucor,* which tend to rapidly spread over plates made from other media.[12] Such plates are often not countable because slower-growing molds are overgrown. This medium may give lower yeast counts compared to yeast extract-glucose-chloramphenicol medium.
2. **References:** See 8.111.2.
3. **Definition:** See 8.111.3.
4. **Principle:** See 8.111.4.

The addition or rose bengal and dichloran (2,6-dichloro-4-nitroaniline) restricts the growth of spreading fungi without reducing fungal counts.

5. **Diluents, Culture Media, and Reagents**
See chapter 6 for basic materials and diluents.
Culture medium:
Dichloran-rose bengal-chloramphenicol (DRBC) agar

Glucose	10 g
Peptone, bacteriological	5 g
Potassium dihydrogen phosphate	1 g
Magnesium sulfate—$7H_2O$	0.5 g
Agar	15 g
MS water to make	1 L
Rose bengal	(0.5 mL of 5% wt/vol; 25 mg in water)
Dichloran	(1 mL of 2% wt/vol; 2 mg in ethanol)
Chloramphenicol	100 mg

Disperse ingredients in the water in the order listed and boil or steam about 30 minutes to dissolve agar. Sterilize for 15 minutes at 120° ± 1°C. Store prepared media in the dark to prevent decomposition of rose bengal. Stock solutions of rose bengal and dichloran need no sterilization and are stable for long periods.

6. **Apparatus and Glassware:** See chapter 6, Microbiological Count Methods.
7. **Sampling:** See chapter 3, Sampling Dairy and Related Products.
8. **Preparation of Test Sample:** See chapter 6, Microbiological Count Methods.
9. **Procedure:** Prepare, inoculate, and count plates as described in 8.111.9.
10. **Expression of Results:** See 8.111.10.
11. **Precision:** See 8.111.11.
12. **Test Report:** See 8.111.12.

8.115 *Dry Rehydratable Film Method*[1,2,13,26] *(3M™ Petrifilm™ Yeast and Mold Count) (Class A2)*

1. **Scope:** See 8.111.1.
2. **References:** See 8.111.2.
3. **Definition:** See 8.111.3.
4. **Principle:** The 3M™ Petrifilm™ yeast and mold count plate is a ready-made culture medium system that consists of 2 plastic films coated with nutrients, antibiotics, a cold-water-soluble gelling agent, and a phosphatase indicator that facilitates colony enumeration. The plate is inoculated with 1 mL of undiluted or diluted sample. The sample is spread over approximately a 30 cm^2 growth area. The gelling agent is allowed to solidify and the plates are incubated and then enumerated.
5. **Diluents and Reagents:** See chapter 6.
6. **Materials, Apparatus, and Glassware:** Refer to product literature (3M Microbiology Products, 3M Center, Building 275-5W-05, St. Paul, MN 55144-1000 USA) for use information.

A. **Equipment and supplies**

1. Petrifilm™ YM plates including plastic spreader (3M Microbiology Products, 3M Center, Building 275-5W-05, St. Paul, MN 55144-1000 USA).
2. Pipets: 1.0 mL or pipeter [chapter 6].
3. Diluent blanks: [chapter 6].
4. Incubator set at 25° ± 1°C.
5. Colony counters or tallies [chapter 6].

7. Sampling: See chapter 3, Sampling Dairy and Related Products.

8. Preparation of Test Sample: See chapter 6, Microbiological Count Methods.

9. Procedure: See product package insert for additional details.

Place the Petrifilm™ YM plate on a level surface and label.

Lift the top film and inoculate 1 mL of sample to the center of the bottom film with either a pipet or pipeter.

Drop the top film onto the innoculum.

Place the plastic spreader on the center of the plate.

Distribute the sample evenly by pushing downward on the center of the plastic spreader. Do not slide the spreader across the film.

Remove spreader and leave the plate undisturbed for at least one minute to permit the gel to solidify. Incubate plates in a horizontal position at 20° to 25°C for 5 days with the clear side up in stacks of no more than 20 plates.

10. Expression of Results: Report as yeast and mold per gram or per milliliter and specify the method used. If results must be obtained from plates containing colony numbers not within the recommended counting range, report the results as estimated yeast and mold per gram or per milliliter.

Yeasts appear as blue-green or off-white and form small, defined colonies. Mold colonies are often blue but may also assume their natural pigmentation (for example black, yellow, green). Molds tend to be larger and more diffuse than yeast colonies. Count and record the number of yeasts and molds on each plate counted. Use films containing between 15 and 150 colonies for calculating results.

The circular growth area is approximately 30 cm^2. Estimates can be made on plates containing greater than 150 colonies by counting the number of colonies in 1 or more representative squares and determining the average number per square. Multiply the average number per square by 30 to determine the estimated count per plate.

Estimates may be noted after 3 days of incubation of samples that are suspected to produce crowded plates or where sporulating molds may interfere with accurate colony enumeration.

11. Precision: See chapter 1.

12. Test Report and Interpretation: See 8.115.10.

8.120 Cited References

1. BEUCHAT, L.R.; NAIL, B.V.; BRACKETT, R.E.; FOX, T.L. Evaluation of a culture film (Petrifilm™ YM) method for enumerating yeasts and molds in selected dairy and high-acid foods. J. Food Prot. **53**:864-874; 1990.

2. BEUCHAT, L.R.; NAIL, B.V.; BRACKETT, R.E.; FOX, T.L. Comparison of the Petrifilm yeast and mold culture film method to conventional methods for enumerating yeasts and molds in foods. J. Food Prot. **54**:443-447; 1991.
3. DASGUPTA, A.P.; HULL, R.R. Late blowing of Swiss cheese: incidence of *Clostridium tyrobutyricum* in manufacturing milk. Austral. J. Dairy Technol. **44**:84-87; 1989.
4. DEMAN, J.C.; ROGOSA, M.; SHARPE, M.E. A medium for the cultivation of lactobacilli. J. Appl. Bacteriol. **23**:130-135; 1960
5. ELLIKER, P.R.; ANDERSON, A.W.; HANNESSON, G.W. An agar culture medium for lactic acid streptococci and lactobacilli. J. Dairy Sci. **39**:1611-1612; 1956.
6. FRANK, J.F.; CHRISTEN, G.L.; BULLERMAN, L.B. Tests for groups of microorganisms. In: MARSHALL, R.T., ed. *Standard methods for the examination of dairy products*, 16th ed. Washington, DC: APHA; 1992: 271-286.
7. GILLILAND, S.E.; SANDINE, W.E.; VEDAMUTHU, E.R. Acid-producing microorganisms. In: SPECK, M.L., ed. *Compendium of methods for the microbiological examination of foods*, 2nd ed. Washington, DC: APHA; 1984:184-196.
8. HENSON, O.E.; HALL, P.A.; ARENDS, R.E.; ARNOLD, E.A.,Jr.; KNECHT, R.M.; JOHNSON, C.A.; PUSCH, D.J.; JOHNSON, M.G. Comparison of four media for the enumeration of fungi in dairy products: a collaborative study. J. Food Sci. **47**:930-932; 1982.
9. HERLIN, A.H.; CHRISTIANSSON, A. Cheese-blowing anaerobic spores in bulk milk from loose-housed and tied dairy cows. Milchwissenschaft **48**:686-690; 1993.
10. INTERNATIONAL DAIRY FEDERATION. Method 94B. IDF-IDF; 1990.
11. INTERNATIONAL DAIRY FEDERATION. Standard method for the count of lipolytic organisms. FIL-IDF 41; 1966.
12. KING, A.D.; HOCKING, A.D.; PITT, J.L. Dichloran-rose bengal medium for enumeration and isolation of molds from foods. Appl. Environ. Microbiol. **37**:959-964; 1979.
13. KNIGHT, M.T.; NEWMAN, M.C.; BENZINGER, M.J.; NEUFANG, K.L.; AGIN, J.R. Dry rehydratable film and conventional culture methods for enumeration of yeasts and molds in foods. J AOAC International **80**:806-823; 1997.
14. KOBURGER, J.A. Fungi in foods: 1. Effect of inhibitor and incubation temperature on enumeration. J. Milk Food Technol. **33**:433-434; 1970.
15. KOBURGER, J.A. Fungi in foods: 5. Response of natural populations to incubation temperatures between 12° and 32°C. J. Milk Food Technol. **36**:434-435; 1973.
16. MARTLEY, F.G.; JAYASHANKAR, S.R.; LAWRENCE, R.C. An improved agar medium for the detection of proteolytic organisms in total bacterial counts. J. Appl. Bacteriol. **33**:363-370; 1970.
17. MATALON, M.E.; SANDINE, W.E. Improved media for differentiation of rods and cocci in yogurt. J. Dairy Sci. **69**:2569-2576; 1986.
18. MIKOLAJCIK, E.M.; SIMON, N.T. Heat resistant psychrotrophic bacteria in raw milk and their growth at 7°C. J. Food Prot. **41**:93-95; 1978.
19. ROGOSA, M.; MITCHELL, J.A.; WISEMAN, R.F. A selective medium for the isolation and enumeration of oral and fecal lactobacilli. J. Bacteriol. **62**:132-133; 1951.
20. ROSEN, B.; MERIN, U.; ROSENTHAL, I. Evaluation of clostridia in milk. Milchwissenschaft **44**:355-357; 1989.
21. SARASWAT, D.S.; CLARK, W.S., Jr.; REINBOLD, G.W. Selection of a medium for the isolation and enumeration of enterococci in dairy products. J. Milk Food Technol. **26**:114-118; 1963.
22. SARASWAT, D.S.; REINBOLD, G.W.; CLARK, W.S., Jr. The relationship between *Enterococcus*, coliform and yeast and mold counts in butter. J. Milk Food Technol. **28**:245-249; 1965.
23. SHELLEY, A.W.; DEETH, H.C.; MACRAE, I. C. Comparison of a simple butterfat agar medium with other media use for isolation and enumeration of lipolytic bacteria from dairy products. J. Dairy Res. **54**:413-420; 1987.
24. THOMAS, S.B.; DRUCE, R.G.; PETERS, G.J.; GRIFFITHS, D.G. Incidence and significance of thermoduric bacteria in farm milk supplies: a reappraisal and review. J. Appl. Bacteriol. **30**:265-298; 1967.
25. VANDERZANT, C.; MATTHYS, A.W. Effect of temperature of the plating medium on the viable count of psychrophilic bacteria. J. Milk Food Technol. **18**:383-388; 1965.
26. VLAEMYNCK, G.M. Comparison of Petrifilm and plate count methods for enumerating molds and yeasts in cheese and yogurt. J Food Prot. **57**: 913-914; 1994.

Chapter 9

Microbiological Methods for Dairy Products

S. E. Duncan, B. R. Yaun, and S. S. Sumner
(J. Bruhn, Tech. Comm.)

Determining the microbiological quality of milk and milk products typically involves performing various plate counts. These include, but are not limited to, the standard plate count (SPC) [6.020], the coliform count [7.080.1], the yeast and mold count [8.110], and the psychrotrophic bacteria count [8.010]. Plating techniques are the same for each test, but methods of sampling and the preparation of samples may differ. Additional testing for some products is necessary. For example, the SPC has limited value for cultured products and cheeses (except for directly acidified and hot-packed products) because numbers of viable microorganisms are large and are generally unrelated to quality. Because the procedures for performing the various plate counts are similar, this chapter details only those characteristics of products that make for unique analyses. Analysis for pathogens in these products also must be considered; refer back to chapter 5 for analysis procedures for particular pathogens. Methods for sampling and sample treatment also are discussed. Suggested dilutions for 6 of the most used tests are listed in Table 9.1.

9.010 Fluid Milk Products: Shelf Life

The main factors that affect the shelf life of pasteurized milk are raw milk quality, severity of heat treatment, postpasteurization contamination, and storage temperature. For most dairy products, controlling postpasteurization contamination and storage temperature are critical factors to improving shelf life. Microbiological methods for testing fluid milk products are the same regardless of fat content. Methods are described elsewhere for quantifying total aerobic numbers of microorganisms [chapter 6], coliforms [chapter 7], and specific groups of microorganisms [chapter 8]. The following tests are used to determine shelf life or keeping-quality for pasteurized products.

9.011 Moseley Keeping-Quality Test (Class B)

1. **Scope:** The Moseley keeping-quality test is often used as an indicator of keeping-quality of pasteurized products. It is not applicable to raw milk.

Table 9.1. Suggested Dilutions for Plating Dairy Products

	Type of Count					
Product	**Standard Plate**	**Coliform**	**Yeast and Mold**	**Proteolytic**	**Psychrotrophic**	**Thermoduric**
Evaporated milk	1:2	—	—	—	—	—
Concentrated milk	1:10 – 1:100	—	1:1 – 1:10	—	1:100	1:10
Sweetened condensed milk	1:10 – 1:100	—	1:1 – 1:10	—	—	1:10
Dry milk products	1:10 – 1:100	1:10	1:1 – 1:10	—	1:10	1:10
Butter and margarine	1:100	1:2 – 1:10	1:2 – 1:10	1:2 – 1:10	1:2 – 1 :10	—
Cheese	—	1:10	—	—	—	—
Cottage cheese						
Cultured	—	1:1	1:10	1:10 – 1:100	1:10 – 1:100	—
Acidified	1:10 – 1:100	1:1	1:10	1:10 – 1:100	1:10 – 1:100	—
Soft or semi-fluid products						
Cultured	—	1:1	1:10	1:10 – 1:100	1:10 – 1:100	—
Acidified	1:10 – 1:100	1:1	1:10	1:10 – 1:100	1:10 – 1:100	—
Frozen desserts	1:10 – 1:100	1:1	1:10	—	—	—
Unfrozen dessert mixes	1:10 – 1:100	1:1 – 1:100	1:10	—	1:10 – 1:100	—
Coloring						
Dry form	1:100	1:100	1:100	—	—	1:100
Solubilized	1:10 – 1:100	1:1	1:1	—	—	1:1
Extracts, flavors	1:1 – 1:10	1:1	1:1	—	—	—
Fruits, nuts	1:10 – 1:100	1:10	1:10	—	—	—
Pastry, cake, and confections	1:10 – 1:100	1:10	1:10	—	—	—
Stabilizers and emulsifiers	1:100	1:100	1:100	—	—	—

2. **Definition:** This test provides an estimation of the bacteria that are potential causes of short shelf life.
3. **References:** Chapter 3: Sampling Dairy and Related Products.
   Chapter 4: Preparation of Media, Dilution Water, and Sterilization.
   Chapter 6: Microbiological Count Methods.
4. **Principle:** A standard plate count is obtained for fresh samples and samples stored at 7°C ± 1°C for 5 or 7 days. The increase in colony counts is an indicator of shelf life.
5. **Diluents, Culture Media, and Reagents:** See 6.020.5.
6. **Apparatus and Glassware:** See 6.020.6.
   Incubator: Capable of 7°C ± 1°C.
7. **Sampling:** See chapter 3.
8. **Procedure:** After SPC procedure [6.020.8], store containers of freshly processed fluid produce in a refrigerator at 7°C ± 1°C for 5 or 7 days. Repeat SPC procedure on stored samples. Many processing plants have eliminated the initial SPC and plate samples only after 5 or more days of storage at 7°C.
9. **Expression of Results:** Large increases in the bacterial count between the first and second plating indicate limited shelf life of refrigerated products. For examples of results under various conditions of plant sanitation, see Elliker et al.[5]
10. **Precision:** The precision with which this test estimates shelf life is undetermined.
11. **Test Report:** The test report should identify the method used and results obtained. The report should also identify any variation in the test not specified in this method as well as problems that may have impacted the test result. Each sample will be described in such a manner as to ensure traceability as to its origin.

9.020 Preliminary Incubation Method for Processed Milk Products (Class B)

1. **Scope:** See 9.011.1.
2. **Definition:** See 9.011.2.
3. **References:** See 9.011.3.
4. **Principle:** Samples are preincubated at 21°C for 18 hours before analysis for total aerobic count. Potential spoilage microorganisms may be present at very low levels in fresh samples and will increase in number before plating.
5. **Diluents, Culture Media, and Reagents:** See SPC [6.020.5] or Petrifilm™ aerobic count method [6.040.5].
6. **Apparatus and Glassware:** See 6.020.6.
   1. Incubator, capable of 21°C ± 1°C.
   2. Petrifilm™ supplies if using this method for enumeration.
7. **Sampling:** See chapter 3.
8. **Procedure:** Incubate 10 mL of a fresh, well-mixed pasteurized sample in a sterile test tube at 21°C for 18 hours ± 10 minutes.

Plate the sample using the SPC [6.020] or the Petrifilm™ aerobic count method [6.040]. Incubate SPC plates for 25 hours and Petrifilm™ plates for 48 hours at 21°C.

Count all colonies including pinpoint types. Colonies on Petrifilm™ are red.

9. **Expression of Results:** For an estimate of shelf life, the Virginia Tech shelf life study demonstrated the following relationship between the PI count and shelf life as determined by sensory tests:

PI Count / mL	Estimated Shelf Life (Days)
< 1000	> 14
1000–200,000	10–14
200,000	< 10

10. **Precision:** See 9.012.9.

11. **Test Report:** The test report should identify the method used and results obtained. The report should also identify any variation in the test not specified in this method as well as problems that may have impacted the test result. Each sample will be described in such a manner as to ensure traceability as to its origin.

9.030 Concentrated Milk Products

9.031 Introduction

Evaporated milk is obtained by removing a portion of the water from milk. Following homogenization, evaporated milk is further processed by heat (either before or after sealing in a can) to prevent spoilage. The resulting product is commercially sterile or microbiologically stable. Heat-resistant spores are usually found in canned, evaporated milk spoiled by pure cultures. Mixed cultures indicate gross under processing, contamination after heat processing, or contamination during microbiological examination.

Concentrated (condensed) milk is also obtained by removing a portion of the water from milk. To prevent spoilage, the milk may have sugar added and may be pasteurized. Proper heat processing destroys all coliform bacteria in concentrated products. Because bulk concentrated milk is usually exposed to contamination more often than canned milk and because canned milk, once opened, is subject to recontamination, the coliform test may be used to indicate possible recontamination after processing or opening the can. Yeasts and molds are the most common cause of spoilage of sweetened condensed milk. The presence of yeast or mold indicates a lack of proper sanitation.

9.032 Collection and Preparation of Test Sample

The preferred work area when examining samples in hermetically sealed containers (e.g., evaporated milk) is a class 100 laminar-flow work station. This equipment can provide an environment free of particles 0.3 mm in diameter or smaller at an efficiency of 99.99%.

Before use, disinfect the interior of the unit with iodophor or quaternary ammonium compound at the concentration recommended by the manufacturer. After chemical disinfection, operate the blower for at least 1 hour before doing analyses within the unit. Monitor the air quality within the unit by exposing sterile media in control plates during the transfer period. Place 1 plate each at the left, center, and right of the work area.

Alternatively, the transfer of material from hermetically sealed containers may be made on a counter surface that has been thoroughly scrubbed with detergent solution and disinfected with iodophor or quaternary ammonium compound.

Open hermetically sealed cans using a sanitized Bacti-Disc cutter can opener (Wilkins-Anderson Co., 4525 W. Division St., Chicago, IL 60651) [Figure 9.1].

Personnel performing tests for commercial sterility should scrub their hands thoroughly with germicidal hand soap before doing the analyses, wear clean laboratory clothing, and restrain long hair and beards.

Collect samples using the apparatus and procedures given in 9.033, except as follows: When necessary to ensure the uniformity of contents immediately before plating—as with viscous, sweetened condensed milk—heat contents in a water bath to a temperature not above 45°C, mix thoroughly, and transfer promptly to plates or dilution blanks.

Weigh 11 g of the sample into a wide-mouthed bottle and add 99 mL dilution water [6.020.8]. Optionally, with evaporated milk and products no more viscous than evaporated milk, transfer the sample to a dilution blank volumetrically.

For direct plating, transfer 0.5-mL portions of the sample or 5 mL of a 1:10 dilution to each of 2 petri dishes. If the sample is coagulated, use MS water containing 2% sodium citrate as the first dilution blank to dissolve the sample. Use MS water to prepare additional dilutions of any product. Suggested dilutions are given in Table 9.1.

9.033 Microbiological Analysis

A. **Plate counts:** Use the SPC or an alternative method [6.020], except as follows:

For samples in hermetically sealed containers, prepare 4 sets of plates in duplicate for each dilution. Incubate 2 sets at 32°C for 48 ± 3 hours: 1 aerobically and 1 anaerobically. Similarly incubate 2 sets at 55°C for 48 ± 3 hours. Use 15 to 18 mL of agar in plates incubated at 55°C and provide high humidity in the incubator by placing a shallow container of water inside if high humidity is not otherwise provided.[1] For samples in unsealed containers, make only the counts of aerobic microorganisms at 32°C and 55°C. Count plates [6.020.K] and record the number of colonies on the control plates.

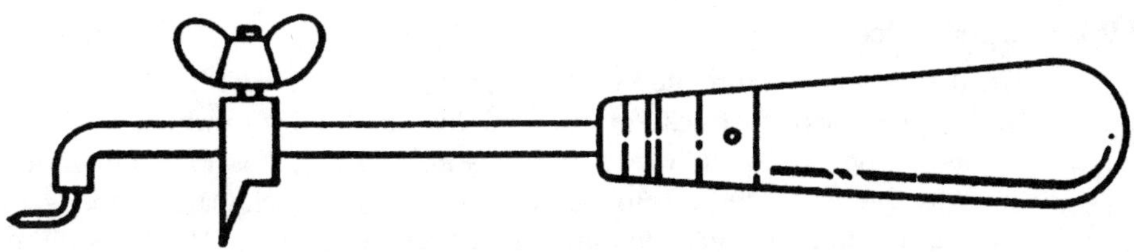

Figure 9.1. Bacti-Disc cutter for opening hermetically sealed cans prior to microbiological examination.

1. Report counts according to the incubation method as follows:
   a. **SPC:** 32°C, aerobic.
   b. **Anaerobic plate count:** 32°C, anaerobic
   c. **Thermophilic plate count:** 55°C, aerobic.
   d. **Thermophilic anaerobic plate count:** 55°C, anaerobic. Plates having few colonies should be considered possibly contaminated and additional tests should be performed on the same lot of the product.

B. **Coliform count:** Divide 10 mL of a 1:10 dilution approximately equally among 3 petri dishes and proceed as per 7.020. Apply the test to heat-treated but not to sterilized, concentrated products.

C. **Yeast and mold count:** Make 1:1, 1:10, or other suitable dilutions. For 1:1 dilutions, divide 10 mL of a 1:10 dilution approximately equally among 3 petri dishes. Prepare plates as per 8.110 with 15 to 18 mL of antibiotic-supplemented agar. Invert and incubate the plates at 23° ± 2°C for 5 days. Count colonies [8.110] after 3 days if colonies are numerous.

D. **Thermoduric count:** Dilute as per Table 9.1 and proceed as per section 8.030.

E. **Determination of sterility of sterilized product:** Commercial sterility of the product can be determined by incubating unopened cans at 32° ± 2°C and 55° ± 2°C for 1 week and then analyzing for microorganisms by using SPC [6.020]. If the contents have an abnormal appearance after incubation, large numbers of organisms are probably present. The presence of nonsporeforming organisms usually indicates poststerilization contamination, which is often caused by imperfect cans. Cans containing milk that appears normal after incubation and yields no colonies on plates may be assumed to be commercially sterile. Negative controls are required for agar, plates, and pipets used in plating.

   Alternatively, test for the presence of viable anaerobes by aseptically transferring 1 mL of sample to each of 4 tubes containing 9 mL of cooked meat medium. Incubate anerobically at 32°C and 55°C for 2 days. Prepare smears, stain, and examine under a light microscope for bacilli. The presence of spore-formers is presumptive evidence of survivors of the heating process.

   Where it is desirable to establish the significance of microorganisms from hermetically sealed cans, consult the chapters on canned foods in the *Compendium of Methods for the Microbiological Examination of Foods.*[4]

9.040 Ultra-High-Temperature Processed, Aseptically Packaged, Low-Acid Products (Class B)

9.041 Introduction

The primary concern related to the microbiology of ultra-high-temperature (UHT) processed, aseptically packaged, low acid dairy products is sterility of the finished product. These products are regulated as low acid canned foods by the FDA. Methods for testing sterility of low acid canned foods and for examination of packages are described in Chapter 21 of the FDA's *Bacteriological Analytical Manual.*[6] A description of these methods is beyond the scope of this chapter.

A rapid method for detecting lack of sterility of UHT processed dessert mixes has been developed by Celsis-Lumac (Celsis LTD, Cambridge, UK). This method utilizes ATP bioluminescent technology, which allows the microbial contamination within 48 hours.

1. **Scope:** Spoilage of any low acid UHT treated, aseptically packaged products should be investigated using these procedures.
2. **Definition:** Lack of sterility is defined as the presence of any microorganisms capable of growing in the product under normal storage conditions.
3. **References:** Chapter 3: Sampling Dairy and Related Products.
   Chapter 4: Preparation of Media, Dilution Water, and Sterilization.
   Chapter 6: Microbiological Count Method.
4. **Principle:** Containers are physically examined for defects. Containers are then opened without introducing microbial contaminants. The contents are examined microscopically for the presence of microorganisms, cultured in various liquid media, and examined for pH, odor, and appearance. The interior surface of the container is examined for discoloration.
5. **Diluents, Culture Media, and Reagents:** See chapter 21 in the FDA publication, *Bacteriological Analytical Manual.*[6]
6. **Apparatus and Glassware:** See chapter 21 in the FDA publication, *Bacteriological Analytical Manual.*[6]
7. **Sampling:** Select packaged products representative of the lot and transfer them to the laboratory in unopened, clean containers. Keep the product temperature at 0° to 40°C. See chapter 3 and chapter 21 in the FDA publication, *Bacteriological Analytical Manual.*[6]
8. **Preparation of Test Sample:** Swab a flat surface of the container thoroughly with 70% alcohol. Insert the needle of a sterile, single-service hypodermic syringe through the package wall, staying within the disinfected area and away from any seam. Operate the plunger to obtain the required amount of sample.

   Because the usual purpose of sampling is to determine whether contents are sterile, it is normally unnecessary to make precise measurements of each sample. When accuracy of the volume dispensed is important, it may be necessary to expel entrained air from the syringe. This must be done carefully to avoid contaminating the sample.

   Examine the contents of packages using applicable methods published in the chapter "Examination of Canned Foods" in *Bacteriological Analytical Manual.*[6]

9.050 Dairy Products

9.051 Introduction

Dry dairy products are often incorporated into ice cream mix to provide the required milk solids. They also are used in cottage cheese and cheese-food preparations and for reinforcing lowfat milk and yogurt. These products may also be reconstituted in the home for beverage or culinary use. They may be made from grade A or manufacturing-grade raw milk.

The coliform group, when present in dry dairy products, has the same significance as it has when present in pasteurized milk [8.010]. Food poisoning outbreaks caused by coagulase-positive staphylococci have been associated with dry milk and special foods prepared from it. Although not all coagulase-positive cocci in foods are toxigenic, their presence in large numbers in milk suggests a need for additional tests to determine if enterotoxin is present. Occurrence of salmonellae in dry milk and related products has been the object of intensive study. Salmonellae entering dry milk during the final stages of processing are quite heat resistant. The mold content of dry dairy products is influenced by exposure and handling during and after drying.

Standard tests for dry milk include the SPC, the coliform count, and the direct microscopic count. These methods are generally applicable to all types of dry milk products, including those sold for infant feeding and for special diets. Product users may set limits on numbers of coagulase-positive staphylococci, salmonellae, and *Enterobacteriaceae* in products they purchase

Instant-type dry milk is processed to encourage particle agglomeration, resulting in a product that is easily rehydrated. Nonfat dry milk may be classified by heat treatment based on the use of the whey-protein nitrogen test. This is of practical importance in indicating the suitability of spray-process, nonfat dry milk for specific purposes.

1. **References:** Chapter 3: Sampling Dairy and Related Products.
   Chapter 4: Preparation of Media, Dilution Water, and Sterilization.
   Chapter 5: Pathogens in Milk and Milk Products.
   Chapter 6: Microbiological Count Methods.
   Chapter 7: Coliform and Other Indicator Bacteria.
   Chapter 8: Tests for Groups of Microorganisms.

2. **Collection and Preparation of Test Sample:** Collect samples using the apparatus and procedures given in 3.072.

3. **Microbiological Analyses:** Using appropriate dilutions [Table 9.1], determine counts by one or more of the following methods, reporting results as the count per gram of the specific dry dairy product
   A. **Standard plate count:** See 6.020.
   Incubate SPC plates for 72 hours at 32° ± 2°C for dry milk. Optionally pour 3 to 5 mL of agar overlay on surfaces of solidified plates before incubation. This reduces the spread of colonies. If colonies cannot be discerned from undissolved particles of dry product, verify the identity of objects in doubt under low-power microscopic or magnifying lens. Because determinations by the agar plate method do not reveal all the sanitary conditions of production, processing, and storage, the direct microscopic method and one or more of the following microbiological tests may be of value.
   B. **Coliform count:** See 7.020, 7.030, 7.040, 7.050, 7.060, and 7.080.
   C. **Yeast and mold count:** See 8.110.
   D. **Psychrotrophic, thermoduric, and thermophilic bacteria counts:** See 8.010, 8.030, and 8.040.

9.060 Butter, Margarine, and Related Products

1. **Introduction:** Methods to measure the microbiological quality of butter or similar foods must be designed to account for their composition and physical structure. The water content is relatively low (16% to 17%) and, in well-worked butter or margarine, is distributed in numerous microscopic droplets throughout the product. If salt is added and distributed evenly in the water phase, the relatively high sodium chloride concentration in the dispersed aqueous phase effectively inhibits microbial growth. The fine dispersion of water limits the availability of nutrients providing significant protection against microbial spoilage of butter or margarine. However, in lowfat and unsalted spreads, the inhibitory effect of salt is less.

   Low fat spreads are usually water-in-oil plastic solids. As a result, microorganisms that survive the heat treatment are confined in the small water droplet. Droplet size less than 20 μm do not harbor bacteria. Some growth is expected to occur when droplet size reaches 20 to 30 μm in diameter, and poorly worked spreads may have droplets with diameters from 50 to 100 μm. Microbial spoilage in butter will depend on the microorganisms present in the water phase, the amount of salt present, and the storage temperature.

   Butter may be contaminated in the manufacturing process from contaminated water sources, air, or unsanitary equipment. Conditions such as poor water or salt dispersion and high temperature favor microbial growth. Uneven distribution of water droplets can result in a nonhomogeneous distribution of microorganisms, and appropriate sampling is important. Spoilage, primarily putridity or hydrolytic rancidity, may occur from proteases and lipases produced by microbial organisms. Psychrotrophic bacteria are prominent in this type of deterioration. Mold growth also may cause color changes. Butter recalls occurred in 1991 and 1992 because of *L. monocytogenes* contamination. Contamination with *Salmonella* and *S. aureus* may occur under poor sanitary conditions.

   Yeasts, molds, and coliforms do not survive pasteurization and are rarely found in butter made under sanitary conditions. Estimates of the numbers of coliforms, yeasts, and molds or enterococci in samples of cream or butter taken at various stages of processing are useful in detecting the source of contamination. Enterococci are more salt-tolerant and survive cold storage better than do coliform bacteria. The SPC method can be used as a measure of processing sanitation because viable cultures of lactic acid bacteria are seldom used during the processing of commercial butter or margarine. Plating methods to detect lipolytic, proteolytic, and psychrotrophic bacteria are useful in evaluating the keeping-quality of butter.

   Microbiological methods described here are also applicable to butter—margarine combinations and lowfat spreads.

2. **References:** Chapter 3: Sampling Dairy and Related Products.

3. **Principle:** Samples are melted and mixed with diluent to break the emulsion and release microrganisms entrapped in water droplets. These microorganisms can then be enumerated.

4. **Diluents, Culture Media, and Reagents:** Warm dilution blanks [6.020.5].
5. **Apparatus**
   1. Water bath set at 40°C.
   2. Pipet.
6. **Sampling:** Follow instructions for sampling given in 3.073.
7. **Procedure:** Before plating, warm dilution blanks [6.020.5.B] and pipets to 40° to 45°C. Rotate the containers, which are filled to not more than 50% of capacity with butter or a similar product, in a water bath at not more than 40°C (for usually less than 15 minutes) until the product is fluid enough to pipet. Avoid separating fat and serum fractions.

   Wet the pipet by drawing into it 11 mL of sterile, warm water from the dilution blank and discharging the contents back into the blank. With a minimum of product adhering to the exterior of the pipet, immediately transfer 11 g of thoroughly mixed, melted sample into 99 g of warm (40°C) dilution water. Shake the dilution bottle [6.020.8]. Pipet immediately to avoid the uneven sampling of serum and fat.

   To prepare a 1:2 dilution, divide 5 mL of 1:10 dilution equally into 2 petri dishes. For 1:10, 1:100, and higher dilutions follow the procedure for milk described in Figure 6.1. Plating of undiluted butter or a similar product is unsatisfactory because it prevents the breakup of clumps of cells and the uniform dispersal of fat in the plates.

   Using appropriate dilutions [Table 9.1], determine counts by one or more of the following methods, reporting results as the count per gram of butter, margarine, or similar product.

   A. Standard plate count: See 6.020.
   B. Coliform count: See 7.020.
   C. Proteolytic count: See 8.050.
   D. Psychrotrophic count: See 8.010.
   E. Lipolytic count: See 8.060.
   F. Enterococcus count: See 8.080.
   G. Yeast and mold count: See 8.110.
   H. Enterobacteriaceae: See 7.090.

9.070 Cheese

1. **Introduction:** Cheese making generally depends on the natural presence in milk, or the addition to milk or curd, of specific types of microorganisms. The sequence of changes that usually occurs during manufacturing can be predicted within biological limitations; however, growth and activity of microorganisms are influenced by time, temperature, salt, pH, nutrient requirements, and oxygen-reduction potential during the ripening process. Different groups of bacteria may develop sequentially. Growth of one group often enhances the growth of others, but the metabolic by-products of many microbial species eventually inhibit their own growth. Some of these changes are essential for the development of the characteristic flavor in certain types of cheese. The microbial flora vary among different types of cheese and even among different cheeses of the same type. Numbers of bacteria in natural or processed cheeses are not generally related to public health or safety. For example, the absence of

coliforms should not be used as an indicator of good sanitation because growth and death rates of coliforms are not easily predicted during ripening. Although comparatively few cheese-borne disease outbreaks have been reported, some have occurred in recent years. From 1990 through 1997, a total of 62 FDA recalls of cheese have been reported. The majority (46) have been from *L. monocytogenes* contamination. *C. botulinum* (7), *Salmonella* (3), mold (2), *E. coli* (2) and *Cryptosporidium* (1) have also been found in cheese.

2. **References:** Chapter 3: Sampling Dairy and Related Products.
   Chapter 4: Preparation of Media, Dilution Water, and Sterilization.
   Chapter 7: Coliform and Other Indicator Bacteria.
3. **Principle:** Cheese samples are blended with warm sodium citrate to melt fat and dissolve the curd matrix. This releases microorganisms entrapped within the curd matrix so that they can be enumerated using plate count procedures.
4. **Diluents, Culture Medium, and Reagents:** 2% sodium citrate.
5. **Apparatus**
   A. Spatula: Sterile.
   B. Blender: Electromechanical.
   C. Container for blender: Sterile, stainless steel, or other nontoxic metal or glass, with leakproof blending-blade assembly. The unit may be autoclaved (preferred) or sanitized with a 200-ppm chlorine solution for 5 minutes. Rinse the chlorine solution from the container with an ample, single rinse of sterile 0.1% aqueous sodium thiosulfate. Select a blender to produce the rapid and complete emulsification of cheese.
   D. Balance: With the capacity and pan size to accommodate the sample, container, and container cover with a precision of ± 0.1 g.
6. **Sampling:** Use the apparatus and procedures in 3.074 and 3.075.
7. **Sample Preparation**
   A. **Preparation for cheese other than cottage:** Using aseptic technique, thoroughly comminute or mix each sample until representative portions can be removed. Heat 99 mL of sterile, freshly prepared, aqueous 2% sodium citrate to 40° to 45°C. Aseptically transfer 11 g of cheese to a sterile blender container previously warmed at 40° to 45°C and add the contents of a warmed citrate dilution blank. Mix for 2 minutes at a speed sufficient to emulsify the sample thoroughly. Invert the container to rinse particles from the interior walls and remix for approximately 10 seconds. Determine the extent of the temperature rise during the 2 minutes of blending, and when temperatures exceed 40°C, take corrective action such as chilling the blender containers. If heating is unavoidable with the equipment available, mixing for periods of less than 2 minutes may be used provided complete emulsification is obtained. Plate or further dilute the 1:10 dilution immediately, taking care to exclude foam from the pipet.

      A second alternative method of preparing cheeses for plating is to place 11 g of the sample and 99 mL of diluent in an 18- × 30-cm polyethylene bag. Lock the bag into the jaws of a Stomacher 400 (Dynatech Laboratories Inc., 900 Slaters Lane, Alexandria, VA 22314) and blend for 2 minutes.

B. **Preparation for cottage cheese:** Place the sterile blender-container on the balance and tare. With a sterile spatula, mix the contents of the cottage cheese container or, if contents are in a tightly closed, plastic sample pouch, gently knead and mix the enclosed curd. Aseptically remove the cover of the blender and place it upside down on the balance beside the container.

Weigh 11 g of cottage cheese into the sterile container, add 99 mL of warmed (40° to 45°C), sterile 2% sodium citrate solution, and proceed as described in 9.070.7.A. The alternative bag or Stomacher method described above may also be used.

C. **Preparation for cultured and acidified milk and cream products:** After thoroughly mixing sample, weigh 11 g of the product into a sterile, wide-mouthed container. Add 99 mL of sterile MS water (40° to 45°C).

Shake until a homogenous dispersion is obtained and withdraw appropriate amounts of this 1:10 dilution for plating or further dilution. Alternatively, the same may be dispersed in 2% sodium citrate with a mechanical blender or Stomacher [9.070.7]

8. **Procedure:** Using appropriate dilutions [Table 9.1], determine counts by one or more of the following methods, reporting results as the count per gram of cheese.

9. **Microbiological Analysis**

A. **SPC** *(applicable only to cultured products that are heat treated after culturing and to acidified products):* Make suitable dilutions [Table 9.1] and proceed as per sections 6.020.9 to 6.020.10.

B. **Coliform count:** Make suitable dilutions [Table 9.1] and proceed as described in 7.020 or 7.010. Samples of cultured or acidified cottage cheese, sour cream, yogurt, and milk products must be plated within 24 hours after manufacture to obtain meaningful results. Coliform-like colonies in violet red bile agar should be confirmed for yogurt and other products containing fruit or added sweetener.

Alternatively, inoculate a series of tubes of brilliant green bile (2%) broth with appropriate volumes of the diluted sample and proceed as described in 7.030. Report as coliform most probable number per gram or other appropriate quantity.

C. **Psychrotrophic count:** Make suitable dilutions [Table 9.1] and proceed as described in 8.010.

D. **Yeast and mold count:** Make appropriate dilutions [Table 9.1] and proceed as described in 8.115. Where counts are expected to be low, distribute 10 mL of the 1:10 dilution about equally among 3 plates. Include in the count the total number of colonies appearing on the 3 plates.

E. **Lactobacillus count** *(Class B):* Because the usual purpose of determining counts of lactobacilli is to ensure that numbers are high in products to which they are added, it is common to plate at 10^{-4}

through 10^{-6} dilutions. Prepare sterile dilution blanks containing 0.1% nonfat dry milk (0.1 g/100 mL of buffered MS water). Plate samples according to 6.020, except pour plates with lactobacillus selective agar and then overlay with 3 to 5 mL of this agar.

9.080 Yogurt and Other Fermented Milk Products

1. **Introduction:** The pattern of microbial growth in other cultured products is less complex than it is in ripened cheese. In cottage cheese, cultured milks, yogurt, sour cream, and similar products, the specific organisms producing lactic acid are present in large numbers and may provide, to some degree, an index of culture development. Organisms such as coliform bacteria and yeasts and molds are present as contaminants and may be used as indices of sanitary conditions.

   The pH of yogurt should not allow for bacterial spoilage and will instead select for growth of yeast and mold. Gas production by yeast can swell packages and limit shelf life when levels reach 10^5 to 10^6 yeast/gram. Common sources for yeast spoilage are contaminated ingredients such as fruits, nuts, and sweeteners.

   Isolated outbreaks have been attributed to pathogens. In 1991 16 cases of *E. coli* O157:H7 were linked to farm-produced yogurt. A study by Boor[2] reports that *E. coli* O157:H7 can survive for 60 days when retail samples of yogurt, buttermilk, sour cream, and cottage cheese were inoculated with 10 CFU/g and stored at 4°C.

   Certain dairy foods are produced by adding food-grade acids directly to pasteurized milk or milk products. Lactic acid-producing cultures are normally not added to these foods and the expected microflora of the freshly prepared food is that of the pasteurized milk product from which the food was made. Viability of acid-sensitive bacteria, however, decreases with time after acidification.

2. **References:** Chapter 4: Preparation of Media, Dilution Water, and Sterilization.
   Chapter 6: Microbiological Count Methods.
   Chapter 7: Coliform and Other Indicator Bacteria.

3. **Collection and Preparation of Samples:** Use the apparatus and procedures in 3.074 and 3.075.

4. **Microbiological Analysis**
   A. **Coliform count:** See 9.070.9.A.
   Samples of cultured or acidified sour cream, yogurt, and milk products must be plated within 24 hours after manufacture to obtain meaningful results. Coliform-like colonies in violet red bile agar should be confirmed for yogurt and other products containing fruit or added sweetener.

   Alternatively, inoculate a series of tubes of brilliant green bile (2%) broth with appropriate volumes of the diluted sample and proceed as described in 7.020. Report as coliform most probable number per gram or other appropriate quantity.

   B. **Yeast and mold counts:** See 9.070.9.D.

C. **Enumeration of Characteristic Microorganisms [chapter 8]:** According to IDF Method 117:2003.

The test is performed to determine viable microorganisms in yogurt by means of a colony count technique at 37°C. Enumeration is carried out in selective media for *Lactobacillus delbrueckii* ssp. *bulgaricus* and for *Streptococcus thermophilus.*

5. **Reagents, Diluents, and Culture Media**
   1. M-17 for enumeration of *Streptococcus thermophilus.*
   2. Acidified MRS for enumeration of *Lactobacillus delbrueckii* spp. *bulgaricus.*
   3. Acetic acid for addition to MRS agar (to reduce pH to 5.4 ± 0.1) after sterilization.
   4. 10% lactose solution for addition to molten M-17 (add 5 mL of a sterile 10% lactose solution to 95 mL M-17).
   5. 0.1% non-fat dry milk dilution blanks (add 0.1 g/100 mL MS water).

6. **Apparatus and Glassware**
   1. Anaerobic incubator jar.
   2. Blender (Stomacher or rotary).
   3. Test tube agitator (Vortex mixer).
   4. Colony counting equipment.
   5. Water bath set at 45° ± 1°C.
   6. pH meter accurate to ± 0.1 pH unit at 25°C.
   7. Flasks or bottles for media.
   8. Dilution blanks.
   9. Graduated pipets.
   10. Petri dishes.
   11. Sterile spatula.

7. **Sampling:** See chapter 3.
   Use the apparatus and procedures in 3.074 and 3.075.

8. **Procedure:** Prior to opening sample, aseptically clean the external surface with a 70% (v/v) solution of ethanol.

For non-fruit yogurts: Carefully mix the contents with a sterile spatula; weigh 10.0 ± 0.1 g of sample into appropriate container. For fruit yogurts, blend the contents of the container for 1 minute prior to sampling. Weigh 10.0 ± 0.1 g of sample into an appropriate container.

Prepare sterile dilution blanks containing 0.1% nonfat dry milk (0.1 g/100 mL of buffered MS water). Prepare decimal dilutions in duplicate (for *S. thermophilus* and *L. delbrueckii*) and transfer 1 mL using a sterile pipet into appropriately labeled petri dishes. Because the usual purpose of determining counts of lactobacilli is to ensure that numbers are high in products to which they are added, it is common to plate at 10^{-4} through 10^{-6} dilutions. Plate samples according to section 6.020, except pour plates with a selective agar (M-17 or MRS).

Pour the 15 mL of the appropriate media (acidified MRS for *L. delbrueckii*, M-17 with 10% lactose for *S. thermophilus*) into the appropriate petri dish. Mix carefully by swirling the petri dish and allow to solidify.

Incubate acidified MRS inverted at 37°C anaerobically for 72 hours. Incubate M-17 inverted at 37°C for 48 hours.

After the appropriate incubation times, count typical colonies on plates containing between 30 and 300 colonies. Confirm colonies on MRS as gram-positive, catalase-negative rods and on M-17 as gram-positive, catalase-negative chains of cocci or diplococci.

Enumeration of bile-resistant lactobacilli (primarily *Lactobacillus acidophilus*). Add 0.15% oxgal to lactobacillus selective agar and proceed as described in section 9.050. Record results as bile-resistant lactobacillus count per gram or per milliliter.

9.090 Ice Cream and Related Food Products

1. **Introduction:** Methods to determine the sanitary quality of frozen dairy foods are similar in application and limitations to those used for fluid milk and cream. Directions for determining the bacteriological quality of certain dairy product ingredients are given elsewhere as follows: fluid milk and cream [chapters 6, 7, and 8]; evaporated, concentrated, and sweetened condensed milk [9.030]; dry milk products [9.050]; and butter [9.060].

   Microbiological methods described here are also applicable to frozen dairy foods in which vegetable fats (e.g., Mellorine and Parevine) have been substituted for milkfat and to water ices, popsicles, and nondairy creamers.

   SPCs of bacteria in frozen dairy foods and ingredients, as in other dairy products, are indices of plant sanitation and of processing and handling conditions. The method may be applied to samples taken at successive stages of manufacture to detect bacterial contamination, growth, or both. Growth is inhibited in ice cream and frozen desserts when storage is below –10°C; however, contamination of these products is often an indicator of sanitation and raw ingredient quality. Pathogens that have been found in significant numbers in frozen dairy products include *Staphylococcus aureus* and *Bacillus cereus*. The recent popularity of homemade ice creams containing eggs has led to an increase in outbreaks associated with *Salmonella*. In 1994 an estimated 240,000 cases of *Salmonella enteritidis* were linked to commercially produced ice cream. The pasteurized ice cream mix was transported to a plant in a tanker that had previously been used to haul liquid raw eggs and was not repasteurized once reaching the plant. The tankers were the likely source of *S. enteritidis.*

   Ingredients added to frozen dessert mixes before pasteurization normally contribute little to the microbial flora of the pasteurized mix except as these ingredients contain bacterial spores. However, microbiological analysis may be important in establishing the quality of ingredients such as chocolate, cocoa, eggs, milk, cream, other dairy ingredients and stabilizers, emulsifiers, and other food additives. The SPC, coliform count, yeast and mold count, and thermoduric count are useful tests to determine the quality of such ingredients. With coliforms, the problem of false counts in fruit ice cream should be recognized. There can be microorganisms other than coliforms present in fruit ice cream that give positive results with the coliform test. Therefore, confirmed tests and caution are required when interpreting positive presumptive coliform tests.

Coloring materials, extracts and flavors, fruits, nuts, cakes, pastries, and confections (ingredients often added to pasteurized ice cream mix or to the partially frozen product) may be important sources of bacterial contamination of frozen dairy foods.

2. **References:** Chapter 3: Sampling Dairy and Related Products.
   Chapter 4: Preparation of Media, Dilution Water, and Sterilization.
   Chapter 6: Microbiological Count Methods.
   Chapter 7: Coliform and Other Indicator Bacteria.
   Chapter 8: Tests for Groups of Microorganisms.
3. **Sampling:** Use the apparatus and procedures in 3.076.
   Preparation of samples: Use the equipment and supplies described in section 6.020.6, except as specified in the following: Whereas the following calls for adding diluent to the sample weighed into a sample container, optionally weigh the sample on sterile foil or hard-surface paper and transfer it quantitatively and aseptically to a dilution blank.
4. **Sample Preparation**
   A. **Mixes and frozen desserts:** Aseptically weigh 11-g portions of the frozen or unfrozen product into a sterile, wide-mouthed container and add 99 mL of MS dilution water. Thaw frozen samples at a temperature of up to 40°C for no more than 15 minutes; stir to make homogeneous before weighing.
   B. **Coloring, flavoring, or other added material:** When necessary to ensure homogeneity, warm samples in a water bath at 40°C for up to 15 minutes. To improve solubility of some samples, use dilution blanks tempered to 40° to 45°C for the initial dilution. Weigh 1 g of well-mixed dry colors into a sterile, wide-mouthed container; then add 99 mL of dilution water. Mix liquid samples [6.020.8] before pipeting to plates or dilution blanks. Owing to the inhibitory properties of some components of extracts and flavors, more colonies may appear on plates of higher rather than lower dilutions. Weigh representative 11-g portions of nuts, cake, pastry, confection, or fruits directly into a wide-mouthed container before adding 99 mL of dilution water. Allow the mixture to soak for 5 minutes and shake vigorously; then plate.
   C. **Stabilizers and emulsifiers:** Mix the contents of the sample container thoroughly by stirring and shaking. Where materials are coarse (e.g., 10-mesh), aseptically grind or pulverize the sample sufficiently so that it will pass through a sterile sieve of 40-mesh or smaller. Weigh 1 g into a wide-mouthed container and add 99 mL of MS dilution water. Shake the diluted sample vigorously for 15 seconds; then allow hydration at 20° to 40°C for up to 20 minutes, shaking intermittently. Optionally, hold the diluted sample(s) at 0° to 4.4°C for up to 4 hours to allow hydration.
5. **Procedure:** Using appropriate dilutions [Table 9.1], determine counts by one or more of the following methods, reporting results as the count per gram or per milliliter.
   A. **Standard plate count:** Proceed with the general instructions for diluting and plating samples, and for incubating and counting plates [6.020].

Because of the relatively long time required to prepare initial dilutions of frozen dairy foods, the number of samples in a single series of plating ordinarily should be limited to 6 to 8. This is so that exposure of mixtures to temperatures that might permit bacterial growth will not exceed 20 minutes.

B. **Coliform count:** Proceed with the general instructions in chapter 7 for diluting and plating samples and for incubating and counting plates. Confirm representative colonies for solid media [7.050] or for liquid media [7.040], because false-positive results may arise when certain microorganisms ferment the sucrose or glucose in frozen desserts and grow rapidly at 32°C.

C. **Psychrotrophic count:** Using procedures in 8.010, evaluate ice cream mixes, milk shake mixes, and other mixes intended for freezing or semi-freezing and sold as refrigerated products.

D. **Yeast and mold count:** Using appropriate dilutions [Table 9.1], proceed as per 8.110

Where molds are suspected to be present in products such as frozen, crushed, and pureed fruit, prepare a homogeneous mixture of pulp from a representative portion of sample and examine it microscopically. Test for mold filaments according to the methods outlined in the AOAC's *Official Methods of Analysis.*[3]

9.100 Cited References

1. ALEXANDER, R.N.; MARSHALL, R.T. Moisture loss from agar plates during incubation. *J. Food Prot.* **45**:162-163; 1982
2. BOOR, K.J. Survival of *Escherichia coli* O157:H7 in fermented dairy products. Seattle, WA: Abstracts Annual Meeting of the International Association of Milk, Food, and Environmental Sanitarians, July 2, 1996. In: MARTH, E.H., STEELE, J.L. eds. *Applied dairy microbiology.* New York, NY: Marcel Dekker, Inc.; 1998:323.
3. CUNNIFF, P., ed. *Official methods of analysis,* 16th ed., 4th Revision. Gaithersburg, MD: AOAC International; 1998.
4. DOWNES, F.P.; ITO, K., eds. *Compendium of methods for the microbiological examination of foods,* 4th ed. Washington, DC: APHA; 2001.
5. ELLIKER, P.R.; SING, E.L.; CHRISTENSEN, L.J.; SANDINE, W.E. Psychrophilic bacteria and keeping quality of pasteurized dairy products. J. Milk Food Technol. **27**:69-75; 1964.
6. U.S. FOOD AND DRUG ADMINISTRATION. *Bacteriological analytical manual,* 8th ed. Gaithersburg, MD: AOAC International; 1998.

9.110 Other References

ALEXANDER, R.N.; MARSHALL, R.T. Moisture loss from agar plates during incubation. J. Food Prot. **45**:162-163; 1982

ALLEN, V.D.; STOVALL, W.D. Laboratory aspects of staphylococcal food poisoning from Colby cheese. J. Milk Food Technol. **23**:271-274; 1960.

AMERICAN DAIRY PRODUCTS INSTITUTE. *Standards for grades of dry milks, including methods of analysis.* ADPI Bull. 916. (Revised) Chicago, IL: Amer. Dairy Products Inst.; 1990.

ANDERSON, P.H.R.; STONE, D.M. Staphylococcal food poisoning associated with spray-dried milk. J. Hyg. **53**:387-397; 1955.

ANONYMOUS. Federal Standard 209a. No. 252-522/290. Washington, DC: U.S. Govt. Print. Off.; 1967.

ARMIJO, R.; HENDERSON, D.A.,TIMOTHEE, R.; ROBINSON, H.B. Food poisoning outbreaks associated with spray-dried milk—an epidemiologic study. Am. J. Public Health and the Nation's Health **47**:1093-1100: 1957.

BARBER, F.W.; FRAM, H. The problem of false coliform counts on fruit ice cream. J. Milk Food Technol. **18**:88-90; 1955.

BISHOP, J.R. A simple shelf-life estimation method as an integral part of a total dairy quality assurance program. Dairy, Food and Environ. Sanit. **9**:698-701; 1989.

BISHOP, J.R.; WHITE, C.H. Estimation of potential shelf-life of cottage cheese utilizing bacterial numbers and metabolites. J. Food Prot. **48**:1054-1057; 1985.

BISHOP, J.R.; WHITE, C.H. Estimation of potential shelf-life of pasteurized fluid milk utilizing bacterial numbers and metabolites. J. Food Prot. **48**:663-667; 1985.

BISHOP, J.R.; WHITE, C.H.; FIRSTENBERG-EDEN, R. Rapid impedimetric method for determining the potential shelf-life of pasteurized whole milk. J. Food Prot. **47**:471-475; 1984.

BLACKBURN, B.O.; ELLIS, E.M. Lactose-fermenting *salmonella* from dried milk and milk-drying plants. Appl. Microbiol. **26**:672-674; 1973.

BUCHBINDER, L.; ALFF, E.C. Studies of coliform organisms in dairy products. Mycopathol. Mycol. Appl. **35**:281-289; 1947.

BYRNE, R.D.; BISHOP, J.R. Estimation of potential shelf-life of pasteurized fluid milk utilizing a selective preliminary incubation. J. Food Prot. **52**:805-807; 1989.

CUSTER, E.W.; KNIGHT, H. An evaluation of the reliability of the C.V.T., early detection, and Moseley tests as predictors of shelf-life of pasteurized fluid milk. J. Dairy Sci. **63** (Suppl. 1):169; 1980. Abstract.

FELINGHAM, D.; JUFFS, H.S. Comparison and evaluation of keeping quality tests for pasteurized milk and cream products. Austral. J. Dairy Technol. **32**:158-162; 1977.

FLEET, G.H. Yeast in dairy products. J. Appl. Bacteriol. **68**:199-211; 1990.

FOOD AND DRUG ADMINISTRATION. Enforcement Report. Recalls and field corrections. August 7, Foods—Class I, 1991. p. 1. In: KORNACKI, J.L.; FLOWERS, R.S. Microbiology of butter and related products. Ch. 5. In: MARTH, E.H.; STEELE, J.L., eds. *Applied dairy microbiology*. New York: Marcel Dekker, Inc.; 1998:109-130.

FOSTER, E.M.; NELSON, F.E.; SPECK, M.L.; DOETSCH, R.N.; OLSON, J.C., Jr. Microbiology of cream and butter. Dairy Microbiology. Englewood Cliffs, NJ: Prentice-Hall. 1957. In: KORNACKI, J.L.; FLOWERS, R.S. Microbiology of butter and related products. Ch. 5. In: MARTH, E.H.; STEELE, J.L., eds. *Applied Dairy Microbiology*. New York, NY: Marcel Dekker, Inc.; 1998:109-130.

GALESLOOT, T.H.E.; STADHOUDERS, J. The microbiology of spray-dried milk products with special references to *Staphylococcus aureus* and salmonellae. Neth. Milk Dairy J. **22**:158-172; 1968.

GILLILAND, S.E.; SPECK, M.L. Enumeration and identity of lactobacilli in dietary products. J. Food Prot. **40**:760-762; 1977.

GOEL, M.C.; KULSHRESTHA, D.C.; MARTH, E.H.; FRANCIS, D.W.; BRADSHAW, J.G.; READ, R.B., Jr. Fate of coliforms in yogurt, buttermilk, sour cream and cottage cheese during refrigerated storage. J. Milk Food Technol. **34**:54-58; 1971.

HALL, H.E. The significance of *Escherichia coli* associated with nut meats. Food Technol. **25**:230-232; 1971.

HEINEMANN, B. Factors affecting the direct microscopic clump count of nonfat dry milk. J. Dairy Sci. **43**:317-328; 1960.

HENDRICKS, S.L.; BELKNAP, R.A.; HAUSLER, W.J., Jr. Staphylococcal food intoxication due to Cheddar cheese: I. Epidemiology. J. Milk Food Technol. **22**:313-317; 1959.

INTERNATIONAL DAIRY FEDERATION STANDARDS. Yoghurt: enumeration of characteristic microorganisms colony count technique at 37°C. IDF Standard 117B:1997. Brussels, Belgium: IDF, 1993: 6-8.

JAY, J.M. *Modern food microbiology.* 6th ed. New York: Chapman and Hall. 2000.

KEOGH, M.K. Chemistry and technology of milk fat spreads. Ch. 6. In: FOX, P.F., ed. *Advanced dairy chemistry*, vol. 2., 2nd ed. New York, NY: Chapman and Hall; 1995: 215-217.

KORNACKI, J.L.; FLOWERS, R.S. Microbiology of butter and related products. In: MARTH, E.H., STEELE, J.L. eds. *Applied Dairy Microbiology*. New York, NY: Marcel Dekker, Inc.; 1998:109-130.

MACY, H.; COULTER, S.T.; COMBS, W.B. Observations on the quantitative changes in the microflora during the manufacture and storage of butter. Minn. Agric. Exper. Sta.

Tech. Bull. 82. St. Paul, MN: University of Minnesota; 1932.

MARTH, E.H. Salmonellae and salmonellosis associated with milk and milk products: a review. J. Dairy Sci. **52**:283-315; 1969.

MARTLEY, F.G. The effect of cell numbers in streptococcal chains on plate-counting. New Zealand J. Dairy Sci. Technol. **7**:7-11; 1972.

MATALON, M.E.; SANDINE, W.E. Improved media for differentiation of rods and cocci in yogurt. J. Dairy Sci. **69**:2569-2576; 1986.

McALLISTER, J.S. Proprietary laboratory techniques—dry rehydratable film method, Part 1: Petrifilm®. IDF Bulletin No. 285, 1993. Brussels, Belgium: IDF, 1993: 6-8.

McDONOUGH, F.E.; HARGROVE, R.E. Heat resistance of salmonella in dried milk. J. Dairy Sci. **51**:1587-1591; 1968.

MINOR, T.E.; MARTH, E.H. *Staphylococcus aureus* and staphylococcal food intoxications: a review: III. Staphylococci in dairy foods. J. Milk Food Technol. **35**:77-82; 1972.

MONTVILLE, T.J. Rapid automated methods. In: MONTVILLE, T.J., ed. *Food microbiology,* vol. 2: *New and emerging technologies*. Boca Raton, FL: CRC Press, Inc.; 1987.

MORGAN, D.; NEWMAN, C.P.; HUTCHINSON, D.N.; WALKER, A.M.; ROWE, B.; MAHID, F. Verotoxin producing *Escherichia coli* O157 infections associated with consumption, yoghurt. Epidemiol Infect. **111**:181; 1993.

NORRIS, J.R.; RIBBONS, D.W., eds. *Methods in microbiology.* New York, NY: Academic Press; 1969: 79-115.

OLIVERIA, J.S.; PARMALEE, C.E. Rapid enumeration of psychrotrophic bacteria in raw milk and pasteurized milk. J. Milk Food Technol. **39**:269-272; 1976.

PARK, H.S.; MARTH, E.H.; OLSON, N.F. Fate of enteropathogenic strains of *Escherichia coli* during the manufacture and ripening of Camembert cheese. J. Milk Food Technol. **36**:543-546; 1973.

PEDRAJA, R.; CHOI, R.; MENGELLIS, A.; SMALL, E. Joint collaborative study of the direct microscopic clump count method in dry milks and its statistical considerations. J. Dairy Sci. **46**:810-818; 1963.

PETTIPHER, G.L. *The direct epifluorescent filter technique for the rapid enumeration of microorganisms*. New York, NY: John Wiley and Sons, Inc.; 1983

PETTIPHER, G.L.; MANSELL, R.; MCKINNON, C.H.; COUSINS, C.M. Rapid membrane filtration-epifluorescent microscopy technique for direct enumeration of bacteria in raw milk. Appl. Environ. Microbiol. **39**:423-429; 1980.

RODRIGUES, U.M.; PETTIPHER, G.L. Use of the direct epifluorescent filter technique for predicting the keeping quality of pasteurized milk within 24 hours. J. Appl. Bacteriol. **57**:125-130; 1984.

RYSER, E.T. Public health concerns. Ch. 11. In: MARTH, E.H., STEELE, J.L., eds. *Applied Dairy Microbiology*. New York, NY: Marcel Dekker, Inc.; 1998:263-404.

SARASWAT, D.S.; REINBOLD, G.W.; CLARK, W.S., Jr. The relationship between enterococcus, coliform and yeast and mold counts in butter. J. Milk Food Technol. **28**:245-249; 1965.

SCHAERTEL, B.J.; TSANG, N.; FIRSTENBERG-EDEN, R. Impedimetric detection of yeast and mold. Food Microbiol. **4**:155-163; 1987.

SMITH, K.L.; JEZESKI, J.J.; WILKINS, D.W. The Moseley test as predictor of the shelf-life of pasteurized milk. J. Dairy Sci. **65:**221; 1982. Abstract.

SMITTLE, R.B. Foods, quality control. In: *Encyclopedia of Microbiology.* Vol. 2. New York: Academic Press; 1992:219-229. In: KORNACKI, J.L.; FLOWERS, R.S. Microbiology of butter and related products. Ch. 5. In: MARTH, E.H.; STEELE, J.L. eds. *Applied dairy microbiology*. New York: Marcel Dekker, Inc.; 1998:109-130.

THRASHER, S.; RICHARDSON, G.H. Comparative study of the Stomacher and the Waring blender for homogenization of highfat dairy foods. J. Food Prot. **43**:763-764; 1980.

TODD, E.; SZABO, R.; ROBERN, H.; GLEESON, T.; PARK, C.; CLARK, D.S. Variation in counts, enterotoxin levels and TNase in Swiss-type cheese contaminated with *Staphylococcus aureus.* J. Food Prot. **44**:839-848; 1981.

U.S. DEPARTMENT OF HEALTH AND HUMAN SERVICES. Grade A condensed and dry milk products and condensed and dried whey. Suppl. 1 to the grade A pasteurized milk ordinance. Washington, DC: U.S. Govt. Print. Off.; 1978.

U.S. FOOD AND DRUG ADMINISTRATION. *Code of federal regulations.* 21 CFR 116.110. Washington, DC; 2002.

U.S. FOOD AND DRUG ADMINISTRATION. Enforcement Report. Recalls and field corrections. July 22, Foods—Class I, 1992, pp. 1-2. In: KORNACKI, J.L.; FLOWERS, R.S. Microbiology of butter and related products. Ch. 5. In: MARTH, E.H.; STEELE, J.L., eds. *Applied dairy microbiology*. New York: Marcel Dekker, Inc.; 1998:109-130.

U.S. FOOD PROCESSORS INSTITUTE. *Canned foods: principles of thermal process control, acidification, and container closure evaluation,* 6th ed. Washington, DC: The Food Processors Inst.; 1995:134.

VANDERZANT, C.; SPLITTSTOESSER, D., eds. *Compendium of methods for the microbiological examination of foods,* 3rd ed. Washington, DC: APHA; 1992.

VASAVADA, P.C.; COUSIN, M.A. Dairy microbiology and safety. Ch. 5. In: Hui, Y.H., ed. *Dairy Science and Technology Handbook,* vol. 2: Product Manufacturing. New York: VCH Publishers, Inc.; 1993: 385-386.

WILKINSON, R.F.; RICHARDSON, G.H. Comparative and collaborative studies on the preparation of hard cheese samples for microbiological assay using a plastic pouch technique. J. Milk Food Technol. **38**:583-585; 1975.

Chapter 10

Direct Microscopic Methods for Bacteria or Somatic Cells

J. E. Fitts and D. Laird
(R. T. Marshall, Tech. Comm.)

10.010 Introduction

The direct microscopic method makes it possible for milk or certain milk products to be examined for numbers of bacterial clumps or somatic cells. In the former application, the direct microscopic clump (DMC) count, bacterial clumps may be counted and, at the same time, an evaluation made of the distinctive morphology and arrangement of bacteria.[2] To a limited extent, cell morphology and configuration of clumps allow the analyst to assess the cause(s) of quality problems. In the latter instance, large numbers of somatic cells indicate mastitis or other abnormal conditions of the udder. (Over the years, the term *somatic cells* has come to replace the word *leucocytes* as a more meaningful expression of those body cells that are usually associated with inflammation of the udder.) Accordingly, the microscopic method as regards somatic cells is referred to as the direct microscopic somatic cell count (DMSCC). As such, it reflects the research findings of several investigators[8,15-18] and is applied as one of the officially recognized procedures for confirming somatic cell counts, which were previously estimated by one of several screening tests. Test results are reported in actual counts of bacterial clumps or individual somatic cells.

The microscopic method has limited, but possibly beneficial, application in determining the extent of bacterial contamination in pasteurized fluid milk and cream. Because dead cells lose some of their ability to take up stain and because numbers of bacteria are generally low in pasteurized milk products, this method is not used to determine compliance with finished product standards. But because large numbers of bacteria in uncultured products give evidence of unsanitary conditions, no matter what type of organisms are present or whether they are viable (living) cells, this method does have value as a quality control procedure.

10.020 Direct Microscopic Count

The microscopic method offers a rapid technique for determining the extent of the bacterial contamination of raw milk or cream samples taken directly from the dairy farm bulk tank or from pooled supplies in tankers or storage tanks. Individual samples may be examined in 10 to 15 minutes. The causes of high counts may be suggested by evaluating the morphology of cells, the configuration of clumps, or the presence of somatic cells. Such interpretations of cause, however, need to be made cautiously—even by well-trained analysts.

Most dry milk contains relatively few viable bacteria. Nonetheless, microscopic examination of films prepared from reconstituted samples can provide meaningful information on the previous sanitary history of the product. Such evaluation can serve a quality control program.[5] The DMC has been incorporated into both government[1] and industry standards.[2] Arguments have been made against such application, however,[3] as evidence[14] suggests a potential for wide interlaboratory differences ($RSD_R = 3.7$) in counts made on the same sample of milk. In addition, research indicates that bacterial counts made on skim milk do not necessarily correlate well with counts made on corresponding dry products.[6] Cells in heat-treated products do not stain well with the Levowitz-Weber stains,[11] whereas periodic acid-bisulfite toluidine blue stain has yielded substantially higher counts.[12]

The number of somatic cells in raw milk provides a measure of the presence and the extent of mastitis or certain other abnormal milk secretions. Stained cells are discernible under the microscope and can be enumerated as a way of assessing one aspect of raw milk quality. In this method, only intact somatic cells are counted and then only those cells that meet specific morphological characteristics. The method has been found to have a relative standard deviation within laboratories (RSD_r) of 1.7, and among and within laboratories (RSD_R) of 3.2 [1.110].

1. **Scope:** This method is applicable to raw milk and to dry milk products, with limited application to processed fluid milk products.

2. **Definition:** Direct microscopic counts and direct microscopic somatic cell counts are, with certain limitations as noted above, the number of bacteria and somatic cells, respectively, per milliliter or per gram of dairy product.

3. **Principle:** Bacteria or somatic cells contained in a representative and specific quantity of sample of dairy product are transferred to a microscopic slide, stained, and counted using quantitative microscopic techniques to yield the number of bacterial or somatic cells per milliliter or gram of dairy product.

4. **Reagents:** Chemical reagents must be reagent grade unless otherwise specified. Keep containers of stock reagents tightly closed.
   A. **Methylene blue chloride, certified:** Use commercially available liquid stains.
   B. **Immersion oil:** Immersion oil should have a refractive index of 1.51 to 1.52 at 20°C and be of a nondrying type. Type B (medium viscosity) is preferred.

5. **Apparatus and Glassware**

A. **Microscope slides:** Use only *clean* microscope slides. Optional sizes include 2.5 × 7.50 cm, 5.0 × 7.50 cm, or 5.0 × 11.25 cm. Each slide should have 1 or more clear, circular, 1-cm^2 (diameter 11.28 mm) areas delineated by etched surfaces or painted rings. Clear glass slides with a guide are unacceptable.

Slides that have horizontal and vertical centering markings at the perimeters of the 1-cm^2 areas are available from various sources. These slides should be used where a high degree of accuracy is desired, as they allow for confirmation of the correct reading area when performing the field-wide single strip method.

Slides may be cleaned for repeated use. Several procedures are reported to be satisfactory for cleaning slides. Slides may be submerged in a hot detergent solution until free of residue, rinsed thoroughly in flowing tap water, and dried. Alternatively, new (or used) slides may be cleaned using appropriate commercial alkaline and/or acid cleaners followed by rinsing in distilled water. To avoid fingerprints on clean surfaces, use steel or glass holders for transferring slides.

Always store slides with minimal exposure to dust, insects, or other contaminants. Slides may be stored dry or in alcohol. If stored in 95% alcohol, slides can be dried by flaming just prior to use. Otherwise, they must be drained and air-dried. Still another method of slide storage involves applying a surface coating of BonAmi (Faultless Starch/BonAmi Co., Kansas City, MO 64104)[10] or other comparable detergent. Just prior to using the slide, wipe off the detergent with a clean, dry cloth.

B. **Instruments for transferring 0.01-mL quantities**

1. **Metal syringe:** These instruments are still in use; however, they are not the preferred method due to the problems discussed below.

   Allowing for the rapid and convenient transfer of milk or cream, this instrument comes equipped with a semiautomatic, spring-actuated plunger and a stainless steel piston fitted closely to a stainless steel measuring tube.

   Note: The mechanical principle of the syringe makes possible a positive measurement of 0.01-mL portions without manually adjusting the sample column. It also provides for an accurate measurement of cold, viscous cream. Problems may occasionally be encountered in metal syringes, however, because particles of metal oxide can create artifacts in the milk film. Do not allow residues to dry on the instrument. Immediately after use, disassemble and clean the measuring tube and piston. To disassemble, unscrew the tip assembly from the barrel. If it is necessary to remove the spring, reassemble it with the larger end toward the tip. Except when it is unavoidable, do not unscrew the barrel at the finger-grip joint. Handle parts carefully when they are disassembled. Clean all residues from the piston and the lower part of the plunger by wiping the exposed portions with a dry paper tissue or cloth. Use soapless detergents and fat solvents *sparingly but as needed.* Metal is not as resistant to corrosion as glass; unless the syringe is properly maintained, metal can contribute both bacterial cells and artifacts (metallic oxide particles) to a sample.

Do not submerge the barrel and finger grip in detergents or solvents. With forced suction or pressure from a close-fitting rubber bulb applied at the *delivery* end of the measuring tube, clean the interior by submerging the opposite end in soapless detergent. Then, in a similar manner, rinse the interior in clean water before air-drying. Do not use acids, alkalis, or ordinary soap solutions for cleaning (as may be the custom with glassware). Use chemical cleaners only in low concentrations at or near pH 7.0. Clean new instruments before first use.

Before reassembling the syringe, make certain that both the detergent and the milk residues have been removed from the instrument. To reassemble, slide the spring (if removed) over the piston and plunger; *carefully* insert the piston into the measuring tube at the countersunk opening and tighten the threaded joint. Be sure that threaded joints are always tightened to identical positions (scribe syringes at each joint). *Do not interchange parts from one syringe with parts from another.* When assembled, the instrument is reasonably sturdy; however, it should not be dropped or handled carelessly.

Syringes need to be tested for accuracy annually. If certification is required, the appropriate regulatory agency must verify the accuracy. After repeated use, all syringes that are tested and found not to conform to milk deliveries as specified above should be replaced.

Calibration of the volumetric load of the syringe is indirectly determined by weight measurements. Withdraw a representative test charge of milk and wipe the exterior of the tip. Weigh the

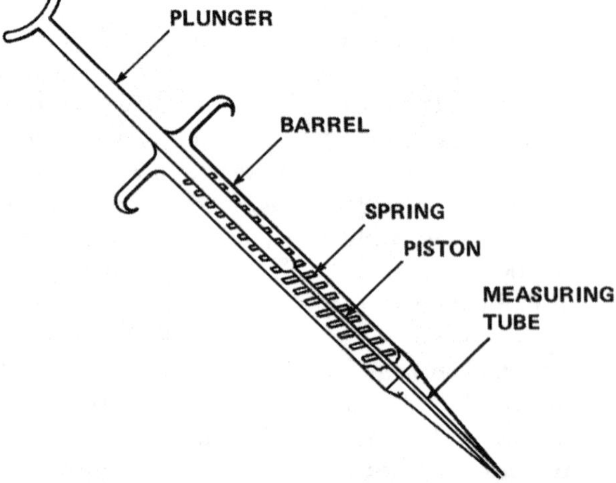

Figure 10.1. Metal syringe for transfer of 0.01-mL amount.

charged instrument on an analytical balance. Expel the charge near the center of the 1-cm^2 area of a slide and touch off on a dry spot. Weigh the discharged instrument. Over 10 such trial weighings, the difference of the charged and uncharged instrument should average 0.0103 ± 0.0005 g. (See Figure 10.1.)

2. **Micro pipeters:** There are several manufacturers of these devices and are the preferred instruments for measuring the 0.01-mL milk test portion.
3. **Micro syringes:** Many makes of these devices are available and may be used if they meet calibration standards to deliver 0.01 mL of milk.

C. **Bent-point needle:** A bent-point biological dissecting needle is used for spreading milk or cream delivered from a 0.01-mL pipet or syringe over the square centimeter area.

D. **Drying surface:** A clean, dust-free, level surface should be provided with a suitable regulated heat source for drying films at 40° to 45°C. Metal heating blocks that provide uniform heat distribution should be considered. Use of a cross-test or round level is suggested to ensure that the surface on which the films are made and dried is perfectly level.

E. **Forceps and partitioned slide holders:** Forceps and partitioned slide holders are required for dipping and holding slides.

F. **Trays or jars:** Trays or jars should be equipped with tight-fitting covers and should be large enough to hold solvents and stains and/or slides held in partitioned racks for submergence.

G. **Slide-storage boxes, cases, or files:** Slide-storage boxes, cases, or files must be clean, dust-free, and insect proof.

H. **Compound microscope:** A binocular microscope with a 1.8-mm oil-immersion objective and a substage actuated by a rack-and-pinion gear is preferred. It should carry an Abbe condenser; have a numerical aperture of 1.25 or higher; and be equipped with an iris diaphragm, a mechanical stage, and oculars (single for monocular or paired for binocular, 10 × magnification is recommended, 12.5 × to 15 × is permitted). If a mirror is used, it should be flat. For both enumerative and grading-purposes, the ocular(s) should be selected to provide a microscopic factor (MF) of less than 600,000. Wide-field oculars with high eyepoint are advantageous, especially for those who wear eyeglasses.

When determining the numbers of bacterial clumps or somatic cells in milk on a per milliliter basis, the microscopic field area is fundamentally important because it determines the amount of milk that can be examined in any one field. MFs are values by which the average number of bacterial clumps or somatic cells per field is multiplied to calculate the respective count. The area of a single field determines the amount of milk film that can be seen at any one time.

Tube length and paired oculars are normally adjusted by the manufacturers of binocular microscopes for use at the most common interpupillary distance (65 mm), or they may be specifically adjusted for a given individual. When estimates are to be made by an individual whose interpupillary distance varies substantially from that for which the microscope was set up, the individual needs to use paired oculars with diaphragms especially adjusted for him or her; otherwise, counts must be corrected accordingly to the diameter of the field actually observed.

Currently available binocular and trinocular microscope bodies are of a constant tube length. With this feature, the resultant calibrated field and magnification also remain constant, regardless of changes in interpupillary settings.

Although the recognized counting procedure uses the field-wide single strip, an analyst may wish to estimate a count by observing a small number of fields. This is especially true when cell numbers are as high as 10 per field. In such cases, it is convenient to know the MF.

To determine the MF, first adjust the microscope lamp to maximize optical resolution. Place a stage micrometer slide, ruled in 0.01-mm divisions, on the microscope stage. Measure the field diameter under the oil-immersion objective, estimate to the third decimal (e.g., 0.160 mm). Use the following formula to calculate the MF:

$$MF = \frac{40{,}000}{3.1416 \times d^2}$$

$$MF = \frac{40{,}000}{3.1416 \times 0.160^2} = 497{,}358$$

d = diameter.

Express the MF to 2 significant figures (e.g., 500,000).

Because the distance from the eye to the ocular affects the MF and possible physical changes to the microscope, each analyst should determine his or her MF for each microscope annually. The reciprocal of the MF represents the fraction of 1 mL of milk observed in 1 microscopic field.

I. **Ocular disc subdivided into quarters:** To use the disc, place it in the ocular so that it rests on the edge of the reducing diaphragm. Face the etched surface of the disc according to directions provided by the microscope manufacturer. Only 1 disc is required for a binocular microscope.

J. **Mechanical stage:** A regular mechanical stage (as supplied with the microscope) or a special stage for slides 5.0 × 11.25 cm may be used.

K. **Stage micrometer slide:** A stage micrometer slide ruled in 0.1- and 0.01-mm divisions is needed.

L. **Hand tally:** A single or double hand tally must be used.

6. **Sampling:** See applicable sections in chapter 3.

7. **Preparation of Test Sample:** Warm samples to be tested for a DMSCC to 40°C immediately before transferring them to slides. *Do not* warm samples to be used for a DMC of bacteria, or for any other purpose.

   Mix sample by shaking 25 times in 7 seconds with a 1-foot (30-cm) movement. Allow it to stand until the foam disperses (but no more than 3 minutes) to obtain a virtually foamless test portion. Legibly and indelibly identify each film as it is prepared; that is, place a number or other symbol on the etched margin of the slide.

8. Procedure

A. **Using transfer instruments and preparing films:** Always keep instruments and glassware scrupulously clean and free of foreign materials. Cleanliness of milk or cream contact surfaces is especially important; however, sterility is not necessary.

Work carefully but as rapidly as possible to avoid bacterial growth while preparing the films. Dry the films at 40° to 45°C within 5 minutes on a level surface protected from dust. Heat them slowly to prevent them from cracking or peeling. Protect them from exposure to dirt, dust, insects, or other damage at all times through the actual counting.

After thoroughly mixing the sample, measure 0.01-mL portions by the following procedures:

1. **0.01-mL syringe:** Before each use and between successive samples, rinse the measuring tube in fresh tap water (at 25° to 35°C) by dipping the tip slightly beneath the surface and repeatedly drawing in and expelling water. Before transferring test portions to the slide, dip the tip of the tube not more than 1 cm below the surface (excluding foam) of well-mixed milk or cream and repeatedly rinse the tube by drawing in and expelling portions. Holding the tip beneath the surface, fully release the plunger and withdraw a test portion. While holding the syringe with the tip upward, wipe downward with a clean paper tissue or cloth to remove excess milk or cream from the exterior of the tip. Do not wipe over the tip. Holding the instrument in a nearly vertical position, place the tip near the center of the area designated for the film and, while touching the glass, expel the 0.01-mL test portion and touch off on a dry spot. Spread the milk film with the tip of a bent-point needle (hold the needle as vertically as possible, do not lay down, as a hockey stick), then dry on a level surface at 40° to 45°C within 5 minutes, but do not heat rapidly. Protect from contamination by dust, etc., during drying.
2. **Micro pipeters:** Use a separate (new) tip for each sample. Insert tip not more than 1 cm below surface of the sample, avoiding foam, and then depress the plunger to the first stop. Slowly release the plunger completely. With the tip still below dilution surface, depress plunger to the first stop again and slowly and completely release the plunger and then remove the tip from the sample. Hold the pipeter horizontally and carefully remove the excess milk from exterior of tip by wiping away from the tip. Do not wipe over the tip. Hold the pipeter vertically and discharge the test portion near the center of the test area and touch off on a dry spot. Discharge used tips into disinfectant, or biohazard bags, or containers to be sterilized. Spread the milk film with the tip of a bent-point needle (hold the needle as vertically as possible, do not lay down, as a hockey stick), then dry on a level surface at 40° to 45°C within 5 minutes, but do not heat rapidly. Protect from contamination by dust, etc., during drying.

3. **Micro syringes:** Follow the manufacturer's recommendations. With a clean bent-point dissecting needle, promptly spread the sample over the square centimeter area. Between samples, wipe the needle on a clean, dry tissue or towel. Spread the milk film with the tip of a bent-point needle (hold the needle as vertically as possible, do not lay down, as a hockey stick), then dry on a level surface at 40° to 45°C within 5 minutes, but do not heat rapidly. Protect from contamination by dust, etc., during drying.

B. **Handling of slides during staining:** For handling multiple slides containing dried films, use holders of glass, stainless steel, or other suitable material partitioned to permit the multiple transfer of slides. Such holders must be maintained free from residues that might subsequently contaminate the staining solution in which the slides are dipped.

C. **Preparation and use of stains:** Always avoid using liquid reagents that contain suspended foreign matter. After a stain has been formulated, handle it in a manner that minimizes evaporation of solvents and the consequent formation of a precipitate that might introduce artifacts into the stained films. Solvent loss must be minimized at all times to allow for proper staining.

Three different stains may be used for cow's milk. One is the Levowitz Weber modification of the Newman-Lampert stain using tetrachlorethane (LW/NL-T).[9] Another is similar to the modified Newman-Lampert stain but substitutes xylene, a less toxic compound, for tetrachlorethane (LW/NLX). The third, a Canadian modification, uses basic fuchsin dye (LW/NL-F).

The LW/NL-T stain has produced highly variable results with, and is unreliable for, staining goat's milk for a somatic cell count.[4] Pyronin Y methyl green stain, however, when used with Carnoy's fixative (PG/CF), has been found to be a suitable replacement for staining somatic cells in goat's milk.[4]

Use one or the other of the three stain formulations given below.

CAUTION: Prepare the stain under a fume hood to avoid toxic fumes.

1. **LW/NL-T stain:** Add 0.6 g of certified methylene blue chloride to 52 mL of 95% ethyl alcohol and 44 mL of tetrachlorethane (technical) in a 200-mL flask. Swirl to dissolve. Let the solution stand for 12 to 24 hours at 4.4° to 7.2°C, add 4 mL of glacial acetic acid, and filter through fine filter paper (Whatman No. 42 or equivalent). Store in a clean, tightly closed bottle with a closure that is not affected by stain reagents.
2. **LW/NL-X stain:** Prepare in the same manner as LW/NL-T, but with 0.5 g of methylene blue chloride, 56 mL of 95% ethyl alcohol, 40 mL of xylene, and 4 mL of glacial acetic acid.
3. **Canadian modification of the modified Newman-Lampert stain:** This stain has been subjected to a comparative study for the somatic cell counting of cow's milk.[7] The stain is formulated the same as the LW/NL-T stain, except that, in addition to the reagents specified for the latter, 0.14 g of basic fuchsin (basic violet 14) is added.

4. **PG/CF fixative and stain for goat's milk:** For Carnoy's fixative, combine 60 mL of chloroform, 20 mL of glacial acetic acid, and 120 mL of 100% ethyl alcohol. For pyronin Y stain, combine 1 g of pyronin Y, 0.56 g of methyl green, and 196 mL of water.[13] Filter the stain through Whatman No. 1 paper before use. NOTE: This stain is sensitive to light and is best stored in brown bottles. This stain is available commercially.
5. **Use any one of the three Levowitz-Weber stains for cow's milk:** Place the stain in a container that can be covered to prevent evaporation while the slides are in the stain solution. Repeated use of stain in an uncovered vessel may result in the formation of precipitate. Flood or submerge slides of the fixed, dried films, singly or in multiples, into the stain for 2 minutes. Remove and drain off the excess stain by resting the edge of the slide in a near vertical position on absorbent paper. Dry the slides thoroughly. Rinse the dried, stained slides in 3 changes of tap water at 35° to 45°C, and then drain and air dry before examining the films under the microscope. Proceed as above in preparing and staining cream films. When small numbers of raw milk films are to be stained, flooding the slides may be more practical than submerging them. Care must be taken to limit flooding exposure so that evaporation does not progress to the point where precipitation of dye occurs. Use adequate ventilation. (A fume hood is recommended.)
6. **New York (Fitts/Davis) modification of the pyronin Y-methyl green stain procedure:** Use of a fume hood is required for this procedure. Fix a prepared film in Carnoy's fixative for 5 minutes. Hydrate the films for 1 minute each in 50% ethyl alcohol, 30% ethyl alcohol, and MS water, respectively. Stain for 6 minutes in pyronin Y-methyl green. Keep the stain covered with aluminum foil. Briefly flush with n-butyl alcohol, then with xylol.

D. **Storage of staining solution:** Discard used stain whenever the solution becomes contaminated or otherwise unsuitable. When solution is not in use, keep containers tightly closed to prevent evaporation. This applies to surplus supplies as well as to working batches of stain. Avoid using containers or closures that may dissolve or disintegrate and thus contaminate staining solutions. Store solutions in a relatively dark, cool place but do not refrigerate.

E. **Storage of slides:** After the slides have been examined, remove the immersion oil on the films by dipping each slide in xylene or Hemo-De (Scientific Safety Solvents, 2000 H Whitley Road, Keller, TX 76248) for 15 to 20 seconds. Allow the films to air dry. Store the slides in dust-free, slide-storage boxes for future observations. Avoid accumulation of pencil marks on slides because their presence will interfere with the staining procedure or with future re-examination of milk films.

F. **Examining films for bacteria or somatic cells:** To obtain estimates of the bacteria or somatic cell count per milliliter, examine each film with an oil-immersion objective after placing 1 drop of immersion oil on the film. When counting bacteria, count as separate clumps any 2 single cells or clumps of cells (apparently of the same type) that are separated by a distance equal to or greater than twice the smallest diameter of the 2 cells nearest each other. Regardless of the proximity to each other of the cells of different types, count each type as a separate unit.

When making DMSCCs, count only those somatic cells with an identifiable stained nucleus. The nucleus is stained dark blue (bovine) or blue or blue-green (caprine). For polymorphonucleated cells, count as a single cell any that has two or more discernible nuclear lobes; for other somatic cells, count any that has a nucleus that appears to be essentially intact. Do not count if the nucleus is less than 8 microns in diameter. If in doubt about a cell, which may in fact be only a fragment, do not count it.

G. **Field-wide single strip method (Class O)**

1. **Determining the counting factor:** This counting method uses as boundaries a single strip that runs the width of the microscopic field and across the diameter of the milk film. A single strip factor (SSF) must first be calculated:

   $$\text{Area of a single strip (mm}^2\text{)} = 11.28 \text{ mm} \times D \text{ (in mm)},$$

   where D is the diameter of the field. The field diameter is measured using a stage micrometer calibrated in 0.01-mm divisions. Determine the number of single strips in the 0.01-mL milk film by dividing 100 mm^2 (area of the 0.01-mL milk film) by the strip area:

   $$\text{Number of single strips} = 100 \text{ mm}^2/\text{area of single strip.}$$

   Convert the number of single strips in 0.01 mL of milk to a 1-mL basis by multiplying the number of single strips in 0.01 mL by 100:

   $$\text{SSF} = \text{Number of strips in 0.01 mL} \times 100.$$

   Example:

   Diameter of microscopic field = 0.160 mm.
   Length of strip (diameter of a 1-cm^2 circle) = 11.28 mm.
   Area of single strip: 11.28×0.160 = 1.80 mm^2.

   Number of single strips in area of milk film (0.01 mL of milk):
   $100 \div 1.80 = 55.6$.
   SSF = $55.6 \times 100 = 5{,}560$.

2. **Counting procedure:** To make a single-strip count, focus on the film edge in the oil-immersion field that appears to be at the maximum horizontal or vertical excursion. Traverse the entire diameter of the milk film, counting those cells within the strip and also those cells touching one edge of the strip (top or bottom if reading horizontally, or left or right if reading vertically). Do not count bacteria or somatic cells that touch the other edge. During scanning of the strip, continually make fine focusing adjustments.

9. **Expression of Results:** Count per milliliter = Number of somatic cells and/or bacterial clumps in a single strip × SSF.

Example:

Assuming an SSF of 5,560, if an analyst counts 84 cells or clumps in a field-wide strip, the count is computed as follows:

$$\text{Count per milliliter} = 84 \times 5{,}560 = 467{,}040.$$

Round off the result to 2 significant figures. The reported count becomes 470,000 per milliliter.

10. **Precision and Performance Parameters:** As in other methods of enumerating bacteria or somatic cells, results of the direct microscopic method are to be considered as estimates only. In general, the most important factors in determining accuracy, precision, and reproducibility are the training and skill of the analysts.[5] Even with exacting techniques, however, replicate estimates may vary appreciably. The extent of variations in counts made by different analysts as well as by the same analyst has been reported for certain screening and confirmatory methods.[16]

    Among factors responsible for such variation are inaccuracy in measuring 0.01-mL quantities of sample, faulty preparation and staining of slides, failure of some bacteria to stain, the minute amount of milk actually examined in counting, irregularity in the distribution of bacteria or somatic cells in the films, failure to count a sufficient number of cells, poor microscopy due to inadequate or excessive illumination of the microscope, poor focusing or improper use of colored filters, failure to dry the films on a level surface, eye fatigue, analyst inexperience, and errors in observation and calculation.

11. **Test Report and Interpretation:** Report counts only to the first 2 left-hand digits of the estimate, followed by the appropriate number of zeroes. If the third digit is 5, round according to the following rules:
    A. If the second digit is odd, round up, and raise the second digit by 1. For example, 235 becomes 240.
    B. If the second digit is even, round down, and delete the 5 and report the second digit as is. For example, 225 becomes 220.

    A way to summarize these rules is to round the second number to the nearest even digit when the third digit is 5.

    Save slides for future reference, especially those with violative counts.

10.030 Cited References

1. AGRICULTURAL MARKETING SERVICE, DAIRY DIVISION. Milk for manufacturing purposes and its production and processing: recommended requirements. Effective June 17, 2002. United States Department of Agriculture, Washington, DC. Available at http://www.ams.usda.gov/dairy/manufmilk.pdf.
2. BREED, R.S. The determination of the number of bacteria in milk by direct microscopic examination. Centralb. f. Bakt. Part II **30**:337-340; 1911.
3. COULTER, S.T. Quality considerations. J. Dairy Sci. **40**:1012-1015; 1957.
4. DULIN, A.M.; PAAPE, M.I.; WERGIN, W.P. Differentiation and enumeration of somatic cells in goat milk. J. Food Prot. **45**:435-439; 1982.
5. FOREST, H.L.; SMALL, E. The direct microscopic clump count as a measure of quality of non-fat dry milk. 15th Proc. Intem. Dairy Cong. **3**:1883-1889; 1959.
6. HEINEMANN, B. Factors affecting the direct microscopic clump count of nonfat dry milk. J. Dairy Sci. **43**:317-31-8. 1960.

7. HINZ, C. Comparison of two stains for use in making direct microscopic somatic cell counts. Dairy Food Sanit. **8**:57; 1988.
8. LEVOWITZ, D. Reproducible data by microscopic method. Bull. Intem. Assoc. Milk Dealers: 198; 1944.
9. LEVOWITZ, D.; WEBER, M. An effective "single solution" stain. J. Milk Food Technol. **19**:121, 127; 1956.
10. MARSHALL, R.T., ED. *Standard Methods for the Examination of Dairy Products*, 16th ed. Washington, DC: APHA; 1992.
11. MOATS, W.A. Chemical changes in bacteria heated in milk as related to loss of stainability. J. Dairy Sci. **44**:1431-1439; 1961.
12. MOATS, W.A.; MARSHALL, R.T. Relationship between direct microscopic counts of nonfat dry milk by two staining methods. J. Dairy Sci. **62** (Suppl 1): 45; 1979. Abstract.
13. PAAPE, M.J.; HAFS, H.D.; SNYDER, W.W. Variation of estimated numbers of milk somatic cells stained with Wright's stain or pyronin Y-methyl green stain. J. Dairy Sci. **46**:1211-1216; 1963.
14. PEDRAJA, R.; CHOI, R.; MENGELIS, A.; SMALL, E. Joint collaborative study of the direct microscopic clump count method in dry milks and its statistical considerations. J. Dairy Sci. **46**:810-818; 1963.
15. PRESCOTT, S.C.; BREED, R.S. The determination of the number of body cells in milk by a direct method. J. Infect. Dis. **7**:362; 1910.
16. READ, R.B., JR.; BRADSHAW, J.G.; PEELER, J.T. Collaborative study of confirmatory testing procedures for somatic cells in milk. J. Milk Food Technol. **34**:285-288; 1971.
17. SMITH, J.W. Development and evaluation of the direct microscopic somatic cell count (DMSCC) in milk. J. Milk Food Technol. **32:**434–441; 1969.
18. SUBCOMMITTEE ON SCREENING TESTS. Direct microscopic somatic cell count in milk. J. Milk Food Technol. **31**:350-354; 1968.

10.040 Other References

AMERICAN DAIRY PRODUCTS INSTITUTE. Standards for grades of dry milks, including methods of analysis, 1st ed. Bull. 916. Chicago, IL: Amer. Dairy Products Inst.; 1990.

MILONE, N.A. Retention of milk and milk-product films on glass slides during staining, defatting and rinsing for microscopic examination. J. Milk Food Technol. **15**:195; 1952.

SCHULTZE, W.D.; SMITH, J.W.; JASPER, D.E.; KLASTRUP, O.; NEWBOULD, F.H.S.; POSTLE, D.S.; ULLMAN, W.W. The direct microscopic somatic cell count as a screening test for control of abnormal milk. J. Milk Food Technol. **34**:76-77; 1971.

FDA Form 2400e-Direct Microscopic Somatic Cell Count. Washington, DC: U.S. Govt. Print Off.; 1987.

Chapter 11

Methods to Detect Abnormal Milk

P. Nierman
(J. Fitts, Tech. Comm.)

11.010 Introduction

Regulations in all areas of the U.S. require that raw milk for commercial sale be derived from one or more healthy cows or goats, that it be practically free of colostrum, and that abnormal milk not be offered for sale. Abnormal milk includes milk from cows or goats with mastitis; milk from cows or goats treated with medicinal agents that may be secreted in the milk; and milk containing pesticides, herbicides, or other agents judged hazardous to the consumer.

Cows in very early or very late lactation, or cows with a low-grade or latent udder infection, are likely to produce milk having an excessive number of somatic cells. Concentrations of somatic cells in excess of 300,000 per milliliter are generally considered indicative of mastitis or other abnormality.

Screening and confirmatory tests described in this chapter estimate the number of somatic cells (including leucocytes) in milk. Although polymorphonuclear leucocytes are the cells principally associated with inflammation of mammary glands, enumeration of all nucleated somatic cells has generally been found to be more feasible when determining the normality or abnormality of milk. The tests are not intended for the diagnosis of mastitis.

11.020 Cowside Tests

11.021 California Mastitis Test (Class O)

1. **Scope:** The California mastitis test (CMT) is applicable to test raw milk from individual quarters of the cow.[26,27] The test may also be applied to bulk-tank milk and other blended supplies.
2. **References:** See chapter 3, Sampling Dairy and Related Products.

3. **Definition:** *Gel formation:* A measure of the extent of reaction (gel formation) between the detergent and DNA of cell nuclei. The greater the extent of gel formation, the greater the number of somatic cells in the milk.

4. **Principle:** The CMT reagent consists of a detergent plus a pH indicator (bromcresol purple). When combined with milk, the detergent and DNA of cell nuclei react to form a gel that is first evidenced as a precipitate at a concentration of 150,000 to 200,000 somatic cells per milliliter. Thicker gels occur in samples with larger number of cells. The grading system is based on the amount of gel formation, but assignment of test scores is subjective. This test has the advantages of simplicity, rapidity, low cost, and convenience.

5. **Reagents and Diluents:** CMT Reagent (from Dairy Research Products, Inc., 5345CR68, Spencerville, IN 46788; and Nasco, Inc., 901 Janesville Ave., Fort Atkinson, WI 58538, and other suppliers).

   Cold rinse water.

6. **Apparatus and Glassware**
   1. Cornwall continuous pipeting device.
   2. Cornwall 2-mL syringe.
   3. Cornwall metal pipet holder.
   4. Special CMT plastic paddle.

7. **Sampling:** Test samples within 36 hours of collection.[12] Samples may be tested immediately after collection. If samples are to be tested later, they should be placed on ice and/or refrigerated until testing begins.

8. **Preparation of Test Sample:** No additional requirements other than those outlined in chapter 3.

9. **Procedure:** *Mix sample:* Somatic cells tend to migrate with milkfat; therefore, a thorough mixing of milk just before testing is essential to ensure a representative sample.

   Place 2 mL of milk in a cup of the paddle. Add 2 mL of CMT reagent. Gently rotate the paddle (or cup) in a circular pattern for 10 seconds so that the milk and reagent mix thoroughly. Immediately score the reaction per manufacturer's instruction. Rinse the paddle and shake off any excess moisture. The paddle need not be dried.

10. **Expression of Results:** Record results in reaction categories[22,23,29,31] as:
    1. Negative: 0-200,000 cells per mL.
    2. Trace (T): 150,000-500,000 cells per mL.
    3. Weak Positive: 400,000-1,500,000 cells per mL.
    4. Distinct Positive: 800,000-5,000,000 cells per mL.
    5. Strong Positive: generally >5,000,000 cells per mL.

    Do not report numbers of somatic cells in place of test reaction categories.

    If milk is kept refrigerated, reliable readings can be obtained for up to 36 hours. Thereafter, DNAse activity causes milk to lose its reactivity. Unrefrigerated milk cannot be tested accurately after about 12 hours.

11. **Precision and Performance Parameters:** None reported.

12. **Test Result and Interpretation:** See (10) above.

11.022 *Conductivity Measurement (Class B)*

Microelectronics has allowed the production of small, accurate conductivity meters for cowside measurement of milk conductivity.[16] Readings from these instruments correlate with the lactose content, somatic cell count, and protein content of milk.[16,30] Because high conductivity readings do not always correlate with the presence of primary pathogens, the technique is for screening only. Instrumentation has provided expanded readout scales to allow for the evaluation of milks from breeds that produce milk of either high or low fat content.[16]

1. **Scope:** This method is applicable to milk from individual quarters of infected or potentially infected cows. Combined milk from individual cows may also be tested. The method is for screening purposes only and confirmatory methods are necessary to establish the significance of the readings.
2. **References:** See chapter 3 for sampling and transporting conditions.
3. **Definition:** *Milk conductivity:* The extent to which milk conducts an electrical current. Milk conductivity can be correlated to somatic cell count levels.
4. **Principle:** Inflamed mammary glands produce milk with a reduced amount of lactose.[24] The osmolality of milk must remain comparable to that of blood; thus, the mammary membranes allow the transfer of salts from the blood to maintain osmotic equilibrium.[2,24] Because lactose is nonconductive and serum salts conduct electrical current, the conductivity of milk increases as the milk becomes abnormal.[5]
5. **Reagents:** Standardized salt solution: 123 μm sodium chloride for checking the instrument operation.
6. **Apparatus**
    1. Handheld, portable conductivity meter: Approximate readout range of 5,000 to 12,000 microsiemens, with the scale divided into 10 subranges.[16]
    2. Appropriate 9-V battery power source.
7. **Sampling:** No additional requirements other than those outlined in chapter 3.
8. **Preparation of Test Sample:** No additional requirements.
9. **Procedure:** Manually inject a stream of foremilk from 1 teat of a cleaned and dried cow's udder into the funnel of the conductivity meter.

    Push the button and observe the reading (0 to 9) on the LED scale.

    Immediately follow this with sequential foremilk streams from each of the other 3 teats.

    Instrument should be rinsed with a mild detergent solution and then water.

    Check the instrument at least weekly by pouring the standardizing sodium chloride solution at 25°C into the funnel. The light-emitting diode (LED) reading should be 5. If this reading is not obtained, the unit should be recleaned or checked for leaks. Replace the battery when the low-battery indicator shows. If the unit fails to read out the proper values, return it to the manufacturer for repair.

10. **Expression of Results:** Conductivity readings are generally on a scale of 0 to 9. Record the number.
11. **Precision and Performance Parameters:** None reported.
12. **Test Report and Interpretation:** Absolute readings of 5 or above in either low- or high-fat breeds indicate abnormal conductivity. Care in interpretation is needed because some individual animals may produce consistently high readings in all quarters although appearing normal in other respects.[17] Herd conductivity must also be considered during interpretation.

11.023 *Charm Somalite Analyzer (Class B)*

1. **Scope:** The "Somalite" test is a quantitative somatic cell test kit for field applications applicable to raw milk products.[25] The luminator gives results in less than 2 minutes with good correlation compared to the direct microscopic somatic cell count (DMSCC). The test should be used for screening purposes only. Samples with bacterial levels in excess of 1,000,000/mL may give high test results. This test is not for milk treated with preservatives.
2. **References:** See chapter 3, Sampling Dairy and Related Products.
3. **Definition:** *Luminescence:* The extent of light signal created by ATP released from lysed somatic cells when reacted with firefly enzyme. The light signal (luminescence) that is converted to a somatic cell count per mL (SCC/mL).
4. **Principle:** Somatic cells are trapped on a filter while passing other milk constituents and bacteria. The somatic cells on the filter are rinsed and then broken. ATP released from the disrupted cells is analyzed with firefly enzyme to create a light signal (luminescence) that is converted to a somatic cell count per mL (SCC/mL) value.
5. **Reagents and Diluents**
    1. **Negative control milk:** Fresh pasteurized homogenized milk should test less than 200,000 SCC/mL.
    2. **Buffer S:** Use Buffer S at room temperature. Buffer S is stable for up to 1 week at room temperature. For longer storage, refrigerate at 0° to 4.4°C between use.
    3. **ATP positive control tablets:** Store at –15°C or below.
6. **Apparatus and Glassware**
    1. **Somalite:** Store Somalites at 0° to 4.4°C for long-term storage. Sealed Somalites can be stored for up to 8 hours at room temperatures (15° to 25°C).
    2. **Charm Luminator:** (Charm Sciences, Inc. 36 Franklin St., Malden, MA 02148-4120) The cell assay channel of the luminator is calibrated to measure luminescence in units of somatic cells per mL.
7. **Sampling:** No additional requirements other than those outlined in chapter 3.
8. **Sample Preparation:** No additional requirements.

9. **Procedure:** Buffer S and Somalite units should be at room temperature. Observing manufacturer's instructions, remove the plunger from a 3-mL syringe and assemble filter and bivalve on the syringe. (NOTE: Use a new filter for each sample, rinse syringe and bivalve with warm water after each use, and use a new syringe every 25 tests). Add 2 mL of buffer S to the syringe. Shake milk sample and, using a 1.0-mL pipet, add 1.0 mL milk sample directly to the buffer S in the syringe. (Keep the syringe assembly upright during the following filtration steps). Insert plunger and slowly filter dropwise into waste container. Somatic cells are captured on the filter surface.

   Remove plunger and add 2 mL Buffer S. Reinsert plunger and slowly filter dropwise into waste container. Remove plunger. Add another 2 mL Buffer S, reinsert plunger, and slowly filter dropwise into waste container. Pass air through the filter by fully raising and depressing the plunger 3 times. Remove the plunger and shake excess moisture off the filter outlet.

   Following manufacturer's handling instructions, check that barrier is intact. Unscrew cap from the tube containing the barrier and tablet. Save this cap and avoid contact with the inside of the cap. Position the syringe/filter over the microtube containing the barrier and tablet. Unscrew the cap from the tube containing the liquid, pour the liquid from this microtube into the syringe, and discard the empty microtube and cap.

   Holding the syringe and tube upright, reinsert the plunger and slowly filter dropwise into the microtube containing the barrier and tablet. Depress the plunger fully, being careful not to spill liquid. Cap the microtube, shake and tap vigorously until barrier dissolves and tablet disperses in the liquid. Then shake tube vigorously for 10 seconds. Within 10 seconds, count on the cell assay channel. For Lum-T, remove cap, replace with Lum-T holder, and insert microtube into the chamber; for other luminators, insert microtube into the chamber, and close chamber. Press Start or Enter. Discard used filter.

10. **Expression of Results:** The relative light unit (RLU) reading is obtained from the instrument. The reading (RLU) from the instrument is equivalent to somatic cell count/mL (SCC/mL).

11. **Precision and Performance Parameters:** None reported.

12. **Test Report and Interpretation:** See 11.023.10.

11.030 Laboratory Tests

11.031 *Direct Microscopic Somatic Cell Count (DMSCC)*

Refer to procedures in chapter 10 for performing the DMSCC on cow and/or goat milk.

11.032 *Electronic Somatic Cell Counting (Fluorescent Dye)*

Somatic cells in milk have been counted electronically by using chemical methods to disperse the fat globules and provide somatic cell counting by flow cytometry or by placing the cells on a rotating disc, which serves as the object plane for the microscope. Cell-size distribution from electronic counting devices offers additional important information. A high degree of correlation has been confirmed between results of the chemical procedure and the microscopic counts.[1,3,7,15,18-21] Samples of unpreserved or preserved milk can be tested successfully by the electronic somatic cell count method. Unpreserved samples can be held up to 72 hours at 0°C to 4.4°C before examination.

1. **Scope:** This method is applicable to commingled raw milk, bulk tank milk, individual cow milk, individual quarter milk samples, and as a screening tool for goat milk.
2. **References:** See chapter 3: Sampling Dairy and Related Products.
3. **Definition:** *Fluorescence:* The extent of light emitted from somatic cells stained with a fluorescent dye. The emitted light is converted to a somatic cell value in an instrument calibrated to the standard DMSCC method.
4. **Principle:** A preheated milk sample is mixed with preheated buffer and dye. Part of the mixture is transferred to a rotating disc or transferred into a flow cytometry channel. The mixture on the disc or in the flow cytometry cell is illuminated by a lamp or laser light that excites the somatic cell-nuclear dye complex, causing it to fluoresce. Each cell produces an electrical pulse that is counted, and the total cell content is printed out or transmitted to a computer.
5. **Reagents and Diluents**
   A. **Foss semiautomatic model 90 (Class A1), and automated model Foss 215 (Class A1)**
      1. **Stock solutions**
         a. **Dye solution:** Ethidium bromide, 0.1%. Dissolve 1 g of ethidium bromide in 1 L of LG water by heating to 40° to 50°C. Store in a lightproof, airtight bottle for no longer than 60 days. CAUTION: TOXIC.
         b. **Triton X-100:** 1%. Dissolve 10 mL of Triton X-100 in 1 L of LG water by heating to about 60°C. Store in an airtight container for no longer than 25 days.
         c. **Buffer:** 0.025 M of potassium hydrogen phthalate. Dissolve 51 g of potassium hydrogen phthalate and 13.75 g of potassium hydroxide in 10 L of LG water by heating to 50°C. Add 10 mL of 1% Triton X-100. Store for less than 7 days in an airtight container.
      2. **Working solutions:** Foss semiautomatic model 90 (Class A1).[6,10,13] Use working solution within 7 days. Mold may develop and can cause inaccurate results.
         a. **Dye solution:** Add 26 mL of 0.1% ethidium bromide solution to 2.5 L of buffer.
         b. **Rinsing liquid:** Add 10 mL of 1% Triton X-100 and 25 mL of 25% ammonia solution to 10 L of LG water. NOTE: Working solutions should not be used if they are more than 7 days old.
         c. **Alternative:** Prepare from manufacturer's kits.

3. **Working solutions:** Foss 215 (Class A1).[6,10,13,14] Use working solution within 7 days. Mold may develop and can cause inaccurate results.
    a. **Dye solution:** Dilute 20 mL of 0.1% stock dye solution to 1 L with stock buffer solution.
    b. **Rinsing solution:** Add 10 mL of 1% Triton X-100 solution and 25 mL of a 25% ammonia solution to 10 L of LG water.
    c. **Alternative:** Prepare from manufacturer's kits.

B. **Foss automated models 250, 300, 360, 400, 5000 (Class A1)**[6,10,13,14]

1. **Stock solution**
    a. **Dye-buffer solution:** Dissolve 2.5 g of ethidium bromide (10 dye tablets) in 1 L of LG water in a 5-L container. Stir gently and heat to 40° to 60°C until the ethidium bromide is completely dissolved. Pour 1 plastic bag (415 g) of Fossomatic buffer into the container and add 4 L of LG water, stirring gently until the solids are completely dissolved. Add 50 mL of Triton X-100 concentrate while stirring. Keep dye-buffer solution in a lightproof, airtight container, and keep cool. Use for not longer than 90 days. This quantity, prepared as above, is adequate for about 14,500 samples.
    b. **Triton X-100, 1%:** Dissolve 10 mL of Triton X-100 in 1 L of LG water at about 60°C and cool. This solution can be stored for 30 days when kept in an airtight container.
2. **Working solutions:** Use working solution within 7 days. Mold may develop and can cause inaccurate results.
    a. **Dye-buffer working solution:** Mix 1 part dye-buffer solution [11.032.5.B.1] with nine parts LG water. Mix the dye-buffer working solution in a 10-L steel container. The 10-L mixture of working solution will be sufficient for 2,700 samples. Use the working solution for up to 21 days.
    b. **Cleaning solution:** Add 10 mL of 1% Triton X-100 and 25 mL of a 25 % ammonia solution to 10 L of LG water. Place the cleaning solution in a 50-L steel container.

C. **Bentley Instruments models 150, 300, 500 (Class A1)**

1. **Stock solution:** Using forceps, put 10 Glocount tablets (ethidium bromide, also labeled Homidium bromide) in a 1.0-L container. Add 500 mL deionized/distilled water. Heat the solution to 50°C. Stir gently to dissolve the tablets. Add deionized/distilled water to make a 1.0-L solution. Store refrigerated in a lightproof, airtight container.
2. **Buffer concentrate**
    a. Heat 1.0 L of deionized/distilled water to 50°C. Add one 10-L packet of buffer chemical; gently stir to mix thoroughly. Add 10 mL of Triton X-100 concentrate. Mix thoroughly.
    b. **To prepare 20 L of buffer concentrate:** Add one 20-L packet of buffer chemical to prepare 20 L. Add 20 mL of Triton X-100 concentrate to prepare 20 L.
    c. **To prepare 50 L of buffer concentrate:** Heat 2.0 L of deionized/distilled water to 50°C. Add one 50-L packet of buffer

chemical to prepare 50 L. Stir to mix. Add 50 mL of Triton X-100 concentrate to prepare 50 L. Mix thoroughly.

3. **Working solutions:** Use working solution within 7 days. Mold may develop and can cause inaccurate results.
   a. **10-L volume:** Put 1.0 L of dissolved buffer concentrate in a container large enough to hold 10 L of solution. Add 100 mL of the dye concentrate. Mix well. Add 9.0 L of deionized water.
   b. **20-L volume:** Put 1.0 L of dissolved buffer concentrate in a container large enough to hold 20 L of solution. Add 200 mL of the dye concentrate. Mix well. Add 19 L of deionized water.
   c. **50-L volume:** Put 2.0 L of dissolved buffer concentrate in a container large enough to hold 50 L of solution. Add 500 mL of the dye concentrate. Mix well. Add 48 L of deionized/distilled water.
4. **Carrier fluid:** Add 20 mL of RBS 35 detergent concentrate to each liter of deionized/distilled water. For larger quantities, increase RBS 35 detergent concentrate and water proportionately. Use carrier fluid solution within 7 days.

D. Delta also manufactures the Somascope™ instrument, which measures the total somatic cell count in raw milk. The Somascope has been approved for use in the NCIMS.

6. **Apparatus**
   1. Fossomatic 90, 215, 250, 300, 360, 400 , 5000 (Class A1). Foss Electric Company, Hillerod, Denmark.
   2. Bentley Instruments 150, 300, 500 (Class A1) (REF 5.27). Bentley Instruments, P.O. Box 150, Chaska, MN 55318.
7. **Sampling:** Samples may be tested preserved or unpreserved. If not preserved, samples should be analyzed within 72 hours of collection. Properly preserved samples may be analyzed up to 7 days after preservation with proper transportation and handling.
8. **Sample preparation:** No additional requirements.
9. **Procedure**

A. **Foss 90 (Class A1):** Heat the samples to 40°C ± 2° and hold for not more than 15 minutes. Mix the heated sample carefully by gently turning it over a few times. Carefully fill a 500-µL pipet with the sample. Press down the intake chamber and dispense the sample into the chamber. Releasing the intake chamber initiates a measuring cycle. Results are obtained after approximately 40 seconds and should be multiplied by 1000 to give the results per mL of sample. Calibrate using 3 to 5 samples (Notes 14.1, 14.2) from each of 4 ranges of concentration (100,000 to 200,000; 300,000 to 500,000; 600,000 to 800,000; and 900,000 to 1.2 million). Maintain the routine calibration as specified in the operating manual.

B. **Foss 215, 250, 300, 360, 400, 5000 (Class A1):** Heat samples from 37°C to 42°C and hold for not more than 15 minutes. Complete the systems operational check as directed in the Foss operating manual for zero check, pilot check, repeatability check, and carryover check. Calibrate using 3 to 5 samples (Notes 14.1, 14.2) from each of 4 ranges of concentration (100,000 to 200,000; 300,000 to 500,000; 600,000 to 800,000; and 900,000 to 1.2 million). Maintain calibration as specified in the operating manual. Check the instrument against the reference sample hourly, or use the automatic pilot programs to monitor instrument performance for comparison with encoded pilot values and limits. Coefficient of variation (CV) may not vary more than 5% from the established DMSCC value. Invert heated samples and place them on the automatic instrument rack and conveyer system.

C. **Bentley Instruments models 150, 300, 500 (Class A1):** Heat samples from 37° to 42°C and hold for not more than 15 minutes. Sample should be inverted or agitated by gently turning it over a few times. Sample can then be placed under the pipet manually or placed on an automatic rack and conveyer system. Calibrate using 3 to 5 samples (Notes 14.1, 14.2) from each of the 4 ranges of concentration (100,000 to 200,000; 300,000 to 500,000; 600,000 to 800,000; and 900,000 to 1.2 million). Follow manufacturer's guidelines. Coefficient of variation (CV) may not vary more than 5% from the established DMSCC value. Check the instrument against the reference sample hourly. Maintain the instrument as specified in the operating manual.

10. **Expression of Results:** Report as somatic cell count per mL.

11. **Precision and Performance Parameters:** See chapter 1.

12. **Test Result and Interpretation:** See 11.032.10.

Technicians using the Foss 90 and Foss 215 electronic somatic cell instruments may see counts of unpreserved samples typically increase for 24 to 48 hours and then stay constant.[11] Therefore, holding samples for this time period prior to testing will improve the day-to-day repeatability of specific milk samples. This increase in counts is most noticeable on milk samples in the range of 400,000 to 800,000 cells per mL.

Technicians using any of the other electronic somatic cell counters using the fluorescent dye methods can test unpreserved or preserved samples immediately upon receipt of the samples. The improved dye buffer solutions readily react with the DNA portion of the somatic cell, resulting in excellent repeatability and consistent results from one day to the next.

13. **Notes**

1. DQCI Services, Inc., 5205 Quincy St., Mounds View, MN 55112-1400.
2. Dairy One Laboratory, 730 Warren Road, Ithaca, NY 14850.

11.040 Laboratory Tests to Detect Abnormal Goat's Milk

Tests for the detection of somatic cells in goat's milk differ from routine procedures used for cow's milk because the apocrine secretory system of the goat differs from the merocrine secretory system of the cow. The normal secretion pattern of the goat results in the shedding of cytoplasmic particles into the milk. Methods acceptable for testing goat's milk must be specific for DNA, which differentiates nucleated cells from cytoplasmic particles.[4,8,9,27]

1. **Scope:** Applicable to raw goat's milk.
2. **References:** See chapter 3.

3. **Definition:** See definitions above under CMT [11.021], ESCC [11.032], and for DMSCC [chapter 10].
4. **Principle:** See principles above under CMT [11.021], ESCC [11.032], and for DMSCC [chapter 10].
5. **Reagents:** See reagents above under CMT [11.021], ESCC [11.032], and for DMSCC [chapter 10].
6. **Apparatus and Glassware:** See apparatus and glassware above under CMT [11.021], ESCC [11.032], and for DMSCC [chapter 10].
7. **Sampling:** No additional requirements other than those outlined in chapter 3.
8. **Preparation of Test Sample:** No additional requirements.
9. **Procedure:** CMT: see 11.021.

   Electronic somatic cell count (Official on counts of 1 million or less on goat milk). See 11.032.

   DMSCC (Official): see chapter 10.
10. **Expression of Results:** See expression of results above under CMT [11.021], ESCC [11.032], and for DMSCC [chapter 10].
11. **Precision and Performance Parameters:** None reported.
12. **Test Report and Interpretation:** See test report above under CMT [11.021], ESCC [11.032], and DMSCC [chapter 10].

    When the CMT is used for goat's milk, the cell count ranges for the various reactions are different from the ranges reported for cow's milk. CMT score of trace (T) is interpreted to have a somatic cell range of 0 to 630,000 cells per mL. CMT score of (1) has a range of 240,000 to 1,440,000 cells per mL. CMT score of (2) has a range of 180,000 to 5,850,000 cells per mL. CMT score of (3) denotes more than 10,000,000 cells per mL.

    Electronic somatic cell counters used in testing cow's milk can be used to determine the somatic cell count in goat's milk. The counts received from equipment used for this procedure [11.032] will possibly include counts of nucleated cells along with counts of the cytoplasmic particles. Therefore, in most instances, goat milk counts by current electronic equipment may have higher values for somatic cells detected in the milk. Somatic cell counts greater than 1 million require direct microscopic somatic cell count confirmation for reporting under NCIMS.

    DMSCC [chapter 10]: The Pyronin Y-methyl green stain differentiates between nucleated cells and cytoplasmic particles. The DMSCC with the pyronin Y stain is the confirmatory test for somatic cells in goat's milk.

11.050 Cited References

1. CULLEN, G.A. The use of electronic counters for determining the number of cells in milk. Vet. Rec. **77:**858; 1965.
2. DAVIS, J.G. The detection of sub-clinical mastitis by electrical conductivity measurements. Dairy Indus. Intern. **40:**286; 1975.
3. DUKMAN, A.J.; SCHIPPER, C.J.; BOOY, C.J.; POSTHUMUS, G. The estimation of the number of cells in farm milk. Neth. Milk Dairy J. **23:**168-181; 1969.
4. DULIN, A.M.; PAAPE, M.J.; WERGIN, W.P. Differentiation and enumeration of somatic cells in goat milk. J. Food Prot. **45:**435-439; 1982.
5. FERNANDO, R.S.; RINDSIG, R.B.; SPAHR, S.L. Electrical conductivity of milk for detection of mastitis. J. Dairy Sci. **65:**659-664; 1982.

6. GRAPPIN, R.; JEUNET, R. Premiers essais de L'appreil "Fossomatic" pour la determination automatique du nombre de cellules du lait. Le Lair (Nov.-Dec.): 627-644; 1974.
7. HAUSLER, W.J., JR., ED. *Standard methods for the examination of dairy products*, 13th ed. Washington, DC: APHA; 1972: 127-132.
8. HINCKLEY, L.S. The somatic cell count issue. Dairy Goat J. **62(8):**672; 1984.
9. HINCKLEY, L.S. Somatic cell count in relation to caprine mastitis. Vet Med. **78:**1267-1271; 1983.
10. MADSEN, P.S. Fluoro-opto-electronic cell-counting on milk. J. Dairy Res. **42:**227-239; 1975.
11. MADSEN, P.S. Influence of storage and preservation of milk samples on microscopic and fossomatic somatic cell counts. Nord. Vet. Med. **31:**449-454; 1979.
12. MARSHALL, R.T.; BRECHBUHLER, J.D. Change in WMT score with time of milk storage. J. Food Prot. **40:**195; 1977.
13. MOCHRIE, R.D.; DICKEY, D.A. Comparison of semi automated method with official optical somatic cell counting method III for determining somatic cells in milk. JAOAC **67:**615-617;1984.
14. MOCHRIE, R.D.; MONROE, R.J. Collaborative study of somatic cell counting: Fossomatic method. Proc. 91st Annual Meeting of the AOAC. Washington, DC; 1977.
15. NEWBOULD, F.H.S. *A technique for differential somatic cell counts in milk. Document 85. Proc. seminar on mastitis control.* Brussels, Belgium: Intern. Dairy Fed.; 1975: 136-141.
16. OKIGBO, L.M.; SHELAISH, M.A.; RICHARDSON, G.H.; ERNSTROM, C.A; BROWN, R.J.; TIPPETTS, E.L. Portable conductivity meter for detecting abnormal milk. J. Dairy Sci. **76:**1510-1516; 1984.
17. PEAKER, M. The electrical conductivity of milk for the detection of subclinical mastitis in cows: comparison of various methods of handling conductivity data with the use of cell counts and bacteriological examination. Br. Vet. J. **134:**467-480; 1970.
18. PEARSON, J.K.L.; WRIGHT, C.L.; GREER, D.O. A study of methods for estimating the cell content of bulk milk. J. Dairy Res. **37:**467-480; 1970.
19. PEARSON, J.K.L.; WRIGHT, C.L.; GREER, D.O.; PHIPPS, L.W.; BOOTH, J.M. Electronic counting of somatic cells in milk: a recommended procedure. Belfast, Northern Ireland, Northern Ireland Minis. Agric.; 1970.
20. PHILLPOT, W.N.; PANKEY, J.W., Jr. Comparison of four methods for enumerating somatic cells in milk with an electronic counter. J. Milk Food Technol. **36:**94-100; 1973.
21. PHIPPS, L.W.; NEWBOULD, F.H.S. Isolation and electronic counting of leucocytes in cow's milk. Vet. Res. **77:**1377-1379; 1965.
22. POSTLE, D.S.; BLOBEL, H. Studies of bulk milk screening procedures for mastitis. Amer. J. Vet. Res. **26:** 90-96; 1965.
23. READ, R.B., Jr.; REYES, A.L.; BRADSHAW, J.G.; PEELER, J.T. Evaluation of seven procedures for detection of abnormal milk due to mastitis. J. Dairy Sci. **52:** 1359-1367; 1969.
24. RENNER, E. Possibility of determination of udder diseases with the infra-red milk analyzer (IRMA). Deutche Milkeri-Zeitung (Kempten-Allgau) f. **3**:71; 1972.
25. SALTER, R.S.; ANGSTADT, T. Field applied somatic cell determination (Somalite) in comparison to foss (ESCC). National Mastitis Council 36th Annual Mtg. Feb. 1997.
26. SCHALM, O.W.; NOOLANDER, D.O. The California mastitis test. California Vet. (October): unpaginated; 1956.
27. SCHALM, O.W.; NOORLANDER, D.O. Experiments and observations leading to development of the California mastitis test. J. Amer. Vet. Med. Assoc. **130:** 199-207; 1957.
28. SCHALM, O.W.; CARROLL, E.J.; JAIN, N.C. *Bovine mastitis*. Philadelphia, PA: Lea and Febiger; **94:**150-151; 1971.
29. SCHULTZE, W.D.; SMITH, J.W. The cellular content of cows milk: II. Comparison of the CMT and microscopic count for estimating cell concentrations in quarter samples. J. Milk Food Technol. **29:** 126-129; 1966.
30. SHELDRAKE, R.F.; MCGREGOR, G.D.; HOARE, R.J.T. Somatic cell count, electrical conductivity, and serum albumin concentration for detecting bovine mastitis. J. Dairy Sci. **66:**548-555; 1983.

31. SMITH, J.W.; SCHULTZE, W.D. The cellular content of cows milk: I. an evaluation of the California mastitis test as a method for estimating the number of cells in milk. J. Milk Food Technol. **29:** 84-87; 1966.

11.060 Other References

READ, R.B., JR.; REYES, A.L.; BRADSHAW, J.G.; PEELER, J.R. Electronic counting of somatic cells in milk. J. Dairy Sci. **50:**669-674; 1967.

Chapter 12

Detection of Antibiotic/ Drug Residues in Milk and Dairy Products

M. Bulthaus [Tech. Comm.]

12.010 Introduction

Common management practice for dairy animals worldwide includes antibiotic therapy. Residues of these antibiotics—whether infused, injected, or added to the diet—may enter the milk supply from the treated animals. Regulations for use of antibiotics require that milk from treated animals be withdrawn from sale for a prescribed time. When proper procedures for use of a drug and withdrawal of the milk are not followed, milk containing drug residues may be sent to the marketplace. Testing programs intend to keep such milk from the human food supply—the smaller the identified lot size of milk tested and kept from further pooling, the smaller the volume of milk to be discarded. Contamination incidents are, at the very least, undesirable, and in most instances, illegal. Public health professionals strictly enforce the regulations prohibiting the sale of milk with drug residues. Such residues may trigger hypersensitivity reactions in susceptible individuals, cause quality problems for cultured products manufacturers, and promote resistance in bacteria populations.

Early test methods were cumbersome and time consuming and, because results were not available for several hours, not suited to screening of milk prior to receipt. A number of manufacturers now market test kits that are in widespread routine use throughout the world. These test kits enable handlers to screen milk for drug residues prior to pickup and/or receipt at the milk plant. Regulatory standards and customer specifications can be met by use of these tests on individual producer supplies and finished products. Tests are available for specific drug families and/or drugs within families. These kits are generally rapid assays of a qualitative nature. Some tests are required, while others are performed on a voluntary basis by all facets of the industry. Since the public health emphasis has favored beta lactam testing, these methods are the most widely used. A number of test types exist, however, and there is not one best test for all products and all situations. There are assays no longer accepted in the U.S. still routinely used in other countries and some newer tests routinely used elsewhere that have no approved U.S. status. For regulatory use in the U.S., procedures for screening or confirmation must be approved for this use and used under specific conditions. Unofficially, tests are often used under conditions for which no approval exists, and unapproved tests are routinely used where conditions warrant use. Any test result for a product for which the test is not recommended may or may not be valid, and the same may be true if the conditions of usage are different from those recommended by the test kit manufacturer. Other countries approve test methods differently than the U.S., so there is a lack of uniformity of testing between countries.

12.020 Growth Inhibition Tests

Growth inhibition tests were the first routinely and widely used antibiotic tests. The earlier common, official test (*Sarcina lutea*) was time consuming and not easily performed by some laboratories. Later, growth inhibition tests were developed that were easy to do, relatively inexpensive, and, therefore, adopted for routine use on raw milk as well as selected finished and intermediate dairy products. For large-volume testing, these tests are still the most cost effective choice. The time to obtain results is longer than for rapid screening tests, and some rapid screening tests are sensitive to lower residue levels than the growth inhibition tests. Growth inhibition tests have an added benefit of *some* sensitivity to multiple drug families and are required for some regulatory testing in the U.S. for finished products.

12.021 Bacillus Stearothermophilus *Disc Assay (BSDA): Generic*[1,2,6-8] *(Class A1 for penicillin only; Class B for other beta lactams and other inhibitors)*

This method no longer has status in the U.S. Interstate Milk Shippers (IMS) program and is not used for regulatory testing. It is sometimes used for testing individual cows and products other than raw milk. This method is still routinely used in Canada and other countries both for regulatory and informational testing. Details not found in 12.021 may be found in AOAC Official Methods of Analysis.

1. **Scope:** This method is applicable to bulk raw milk. Samples that have developed acidity, contain high levels of solids, are extremely viscous, or contain flavorings or other ingredients that may be growth inhibitory to the spores should not be tested with this method.
2. **References:** Chapter 3: Sampling Dairy and Related Products.
   CUNNIFF, P. ed. *Official Methods of Analysis*, 16th ed. Washington, DC: AOAC; 1995.
3. **Definition:** This test detects beta lactam antibiotics and other antibiotics that inhibit germination of *B. stearothermophilus* spores or growth of vegetative cells.
4. **Principle:** The presence of antibiotics is detected by the inhibition of growth of specific bacteria. A zone of no growth of specific bacterial

spores in an agar medium around a milk sample indicates the presence of inhibitors. A paper disc saturated with milk is placed on the surface of a specific agar medium in a petri dish. The medium contains a lawn of spores of *B. stearothermophilus* that will grow out with incubation at 64°C. If no inhibitors are present, the spores grow, produce acid, and turn the indicator in the media from purple to yellow. Inhibitory substances, if present, diffuse into the agar and prevent the growth of the spores around the disc. The agar remains purple and a zone of inhibition exists around the paper disc. The larger the zone, the more inhibitor is present. For this assay, only zones equal to or greater than 16 mm after the confirmation step are considered positive.

5. **Reagents**
   1. PM indicator agar.
   2. *Bacillus stearothermophilus* spores.
   3. Positive control: Penicillin G, 5 ± 0.5 ppb.
   4. Negative control milk.
   5. Beta lactamase: Optional.
6. **Apparatus**
   1. Dry incubator: Capable of maintaining 64° ± 2°C without significant moisture loss.
   2. Tweezers/forceps.
   3. Paper discs: 0.5 inch.
   4. Calipers: Vernier.
   5. Pipet: 90 µL, fixed-volume with disposable tips.
   6. Water bath: 82° ± 1°C.
   7. Test tubes and racks.
   8. Petri dishes: 100 mm, flat-bottom, at least 85 mm ID.
   9. Refrigerator for storing samples and freezer for storing controls.
   10. Timer.
7. **Sampling:** See chapter 3.
8. **Preparation of Test Sample:** Test portion is to be removed within 3 minutes of sample agitation.
9. **Procedure**

   A. **Method**
   1. Prepare PM indicator agar as indicated on label and sterilize at 120° ± 1°C for 15 minutes. If not to be used immediately, let solidify and store at room temperature protected from heat and light. For immediate use, cool the media to 64° ± 2°C. Add *B. stearothermophilus* spores to the media to achieve a level of 1,000,000/mL. Each lot of spores must be tested prior to use to determine the correct amount of spores to add to the agar.
   2. Distribute 6 mL of agar per standard petri dish (100 × 15 mm) and allow to solidify on a level surface with the cover of the dish slightly open. Use plates immediately or store inverted and sealed in containers at 0.5° to 4.4°C for no more than 5 days. Allow plates to come to room temperature before use.
   3. Mix sample well. Insert a new tip onto the fixed-volume 90-µL pipet. Remove a paper disc from the container with the tweezers.

While holding the disc with the tweezers, measure 90 µL of a well-mixed sample with the fixed-volume pipet. Place the disc gently on the agar surface and immediately add the 90 µL of sample to the disc, holding the pipet vertical to the agar surface. Touch off.

4. Repeat the steps in 12.021.9.A.3, placing no more than 5 samples around the perimeter of the petri dish. Be careful not to place the discs too close to one another or to the edge of the dish. Repeat the above steps for the positive and negative controls and place them on the dish with the samples. No more than 7 discs should then be on each dish.
5. Incubate the dish at 64°C for 2.5 to 3 hours or until well-developed zones of inhibition are noted around the positive control and the agar has turned from purple to yellow. Remove plates from the incubator and allow to equilibrate to room temperature on a flat surface. Measure zones of inhibition around positive control and any samples showing a zone.
6. Positive control should have a zone size of 16 to 20 mm for test to be valid. Confirm any positive result by heating an aliquot of the sample to 82° ± 1°C for 2 minutes, cooling in ice water and repeating above steps on the heated sample.

B. **Optional:** The optional addition of beta lactamase to a portion of the heated sample or to a second heated aliquot and testing that portion as outlined will determine if the residue present is a beta lactam.

Positive and negative control samples must be run with each plate and must give appropriate results for the test results to be valid.

10. Expression of Results: Samples with no zones should be recorded as *no zone*. Actual zone sizes of positive control and any samples showing a zone should be recorded in millimeters and only if the positive control has a zone 16 to 20 mm. Samples with a positive response are recorded as presumptive positive.

11. Precision and Performance Parameters: Information on sensitivity and collaborative studies is available in the references.[10,18]

12. Test Report: Samples with no zone of inhibition should be reported as *negative* or *not found*.

Samples with zones of inhibition greater than or equal to 16 mm on a heated sample or sample aliquot should be reported as *positive for inhibitors*. If beta lactamase was used, the result may be further defined as *positive for beta lactams*.

Samples with zone sizes greater than 16 mm that are partially reduced using beta lactamase (≥to 4 mm reduction) are positive for both beta lactams and non-beta lactam inhibitors.

Samples that demonstrate zone sizes less than 16 mm on a heated sample are reported as nonactionable positives or below actionable level. Microbial counts on such samples are invalid.

Reports list the testing site, analyst, date sampled, date tested, temperature control information, and results obtained.

12.022 *Charm Sciences* Bacillus stearothermophis *Disc Assay (BSDA) (Class A4)*

1. **Scope:** This method is applicable to raw milk, pasteurized white milk, raw goat milk, other fluid dairy products, dry milk, and individual cow milk.

   This method is approved for use in the IMS program for screening and confirmation of beta lactam residues in raw supplies. The method has also been evaluated by the FDA and found acceptable for use on pasteurized white milks and goat milk for beta lactam residues.

2. **References:** Chapter 3: Sampling Dairy and Related Products.

   AOAC INTERNATIONAL RESEARCH INSTITUTE. AOAC referee, vol. 19-1. Gaithersburg, MD: AOAC; 1995.

   AOAC INTERNATIONAL RESEARCH INSTITUTE. AOAC referee, vol. 20-1. Gaithersburg, MD: AOAC; 1996.

   CUNNIFF, P., ed. *Official Methods of Analysis*, 16th ed. Washington, DC: AOAC; 1995.

   FOOD AND DRUG ADMINISTRATION. 2400 forms for appendix N drug testing procedures in accordance with PMO. Washington, DC: U.S. Govt. Print. Off.; 1995: revisions, 1995 and 1998.

   U.S. DEPT. OF HEALTH AND HUMAN SERVICES. FDA milk safety, M-I-85, revision 5. Washington, DC: Public Health Services, Food and Drug Administration; 1996.

   U.S. DEPT. OF HEALTH AND HUMAN SERVICES. FDA milk safety, M-I-92-11. Washington, DC: Public Health Service, Food and Drug Administration; 1992.

   U.S. DEPT. OF HEALTH AND HUMAN SERVICES. FDA milk safety, M-I-98-8. Washington, DC: Public Health Service, Food and Drug Administration; 1998.

3. **Definition:** See 12.021.

4. **Principle:** See 12.021.

5. **Reagents**
   1. PM indicator agar: Charm Sciences.
   2. Spores: *Bacillus stearothermophilus*, tablet form.
   3. Negative control milk.
   4. Positive control milk containing penicillin G at 0.008 IU/mL.
   5. Beta lactamase R tablets or liquid, optional.
   6. Distilled or deionized water (or equivalent).

6. **Apparatus and Glassware:** See 12.021.6.

7. **Sampling:** Samples with developed acidity, those containing flavorings or additives that may be growth inhibitory, and viscous samples such as creams are not suitable for testing with this method (without modifications recommended by Charm Sciences).

8. **Preparation of Test Sample:** Test portion must be removed from sample within 3 minutes of sample mixing. Dry samples are to be reconstituted prior to testing as recommended by Charm Sciences. High solids and/or high fat samples (such as creams) are to be diluted as recommended prior to testing. Consult test manufacturer for testing other sample types.

9. **Procedure**

A. **Method**

1. Prepare PM indicator agar as instructed on label. DO NOT AUTOCLAVE. Cool to 64° ± 2°C after boiling. Add spores as recommended by manufacturer to a level of 1,000,000/mL. Charm Sciences provides spore counts on each lot of spore tablets that may be used to determine the level of addition. Distribute 6 mL of agar per standard flat bottom petri dish (100 × 15 mm), and allow to solidify on level surface with the cover of the dish slightly open. Air dry for 15 minutes until condensate on upper lid dissipates. Use plates immediately or store inverted and sealed in containers at 0.5° to 4.4°C for no more than 5 days. Allow plates to come to room temperature before use.
2. Mix sample or prepare as necessary. Insert a new disposable tip onto the fixed-volume 90-µL pipet. Remove a paper disc from the container with the tweezers. While holding the disc with the tweezers, measure 90 µL of a well-mixed sample with the fixed volume pipet. Place the disc gently on the agar surface and immediately add the 90 µL of sample to the disc, holding the pipet vertical to the agar surface. Touch off.
3. Repeat the steps in 12.022.9.A.2 for each sample, placing no more than 5 samples around the perimeter of the petri dish. Be careful not to place the discs too close to one another or to the edge of the dish. Repeat steps again for the positive and negative control and place them on the dish with the samples. No more than 7 discs should then be on each dish.
4. Incubate the dish inverted at 64°C until well-developed zones of inhibition are evident around the positive control and the agar has turned from purple to yellow (about 2.5 hours). Remove plates from the incubator and allow them to come to room temperature on flat surface. Measure zones of inhibition around the positive control and any samples showing a zone. Positive control should have a zone size of 16 to 20 mm for test to be valid. Confirm any positive results by heating an aliquot of the sample to 82° ± 1°C for 2 minutes, cooling in ice water, and repeating steps in 12.022.9.A.2 on the heated sample. Presence of zone after heating confirms antibiotic presence.

B. **Optional:** Addition of beta lactamase to a portion of the heated sample or to a second heated aliquot and testing that portion as outlined will determine if the residue present is a beta lactam. Elimination of zone with beta lactamase confirms the antibiotic is beta lactam.

Control samples should be run with each plate and must give appropriate results for the test to be valid.

10. **Expression of Results:** Samples with no zones should be recorded as *no zone*. Zone sizes of the positive control and any sample showing a zone should be recorded in millimeters and only if the zone on the positive control is 16 to 20 mm. Samples with a positive response should be recorded as *presumptive positive* on the initial assay and confirmed with a repeat analysis on a heated sample.

11. **Precision and Performance Parameters:** Performance parameters are available from the AOAC International Research Institute, Gaithersburg, MD. Dose response data from the approval process is available on the package insert from Charm Sciences.
12. **Test Reports:** Samples with no zone of inhibition are reported as *not found.*

    Samples with zones of inhibition ≥16 mm on a heated sample or sample aliquot are reported as positive for inhibitors. If beta lactamase was used, the results may be further defined as being positive for beta lactam.

    Samples with zone sizes >16 mm that are partially reduced using beta lactamase (≥4 mm reduction) are positive for both beta lactam and non-beta lactam inhibitors.

    Samples that demonstrate zone sizes <16 mm on a heated sample are reported as nonactionable positives or below actionable level. Microbial counts on such samples are invalid.

    Test reports to show the testing site, analyst, date sampled, date tested, temperature control information, and results obtained.

12.023 *Delvotest® P, Gist-Brocades*

1. **Scope:** Class A4 beta lactams for raw milk and raw goat milk. Class B for individual cow milk, other dairy products, pasteurized white milk, and milk from other species. This method is also applicable to dry milk and dry whey, concentrated whey, and other dairy products.
2. **References:** Chapter 3: Sampling Dairy and Related Products.

    AOAC International Research Institute. AOAC referee, vol. 19-1. Gaithersburg, MD: AOAC; 1995.

    AOAC International Research Institute. AOAC referee, vol. 20-1. Gaithersburg, MD: AOAC; 1996.

    AOAC International Research Institute. AOAC referee, vol. 19-8. Gaithersburg, MD: AOAC; 1995.

    Cunniff, P., ed. *Official Methods of Analysis*, 16th ed. Washington, DC: AOAC; 1995.

    Food and Drug Administration. 2400 forms for appendix N drug testing procedures in accordance with PMO; 1995.

    U.S. Dept. of Health and Human Services. FDA milk safety, M-I-85, revision 5. Washington, DC: Food and Drug Administration; 1996.

    U.S. Dept. of Health and Human Services. FDA milk safety, M-I-92-11. Washington, DC: Food and Drug Administration; 1992.

    U.S. Dept. of Health and Human Services. FDA milk safety, M-I-98-8. Washington, DC: Food and Drug Administration; 1998.
3. **Definition:** See 12.021.
4. **Principle:** Delvotest® P agar medium contains a standardized number of spores of the bacterial strain *B. stearothermophilus* var. *calidolactis* C 953. This selected strain is very sensitive to many antibiotics, especially beta lactams. Addition of selected nutrients and incubation of the agar (with spores) at 64°C results in growth of the spores with the production of acid. After sufficient acid is produced, the indicator in the medium

changes from purple to yellow. If the sample contains an inhibitory substance, the substance will diffuse into the media, growth of the spores will be inhibited, and no acid production will occur. No color change will be observed indicating a level of inhibitor above the detection limit.

5. **Reagents**
   1. Delvotest® P ampules containing agar with a standardized number of spores and a pH indicator available from Gist-Brocades.
   2. Bottles with a nutrient tablet and a silicagel capsule (to absorb moisture).
   3. Positive control of penicillin G at 5 ± 0.5 ppb.
   4. Negative control milk.
   5. Beta lactamase: Optional.
   6. Deionized/distilled water.
6. **Apparatus and Glassware**
   1. Pair of plastic tweezers.
   2. 0.1-mL syringe with disposable pipet tips.
   3. Dry incubator: Heater block or water bath, 64° ± 1°C.
   4. Calibrated thermometer appropriate for designated use.
   5. Rack or floater to accommodate ampules if water bath is used.
   6. Cool space (<15°C) for storage of test kits.
   7. Refrigerator and freezer for storage of milk samples and controls.
   8. Timer.
   9. Analytical balance (if preparing positive controls in house).
7. **Sampling:** Samples should accurately reflect the product to be tested. Samples with developed acidity, those with very high solids, and samples that may contain ingredients known to be inhibitory are not suitable for this test.
8. **Preparation of Test Sample:** Remove sample aliquot within 3 minutes of mixing. Dry milk or dry whey to be reconstituted to the solids level of the original fluid, milk, or whey. Samples with high solids or high viscosity should be diluted or assayed by another method
9. **Procedure**

   A. **Method**
      1. Remove test kit from storage and let it come to room temperature. NOTE: This is especially important for the bottle containing the nutrient tablets. Allow sufficient time for the dry incubator, heater block, or water bath to stabilize at the temperature of 64° ± 1°C.
      2. Remove the required number of ampules from the kit and mark each with sample identity. Open ampules carefully, taking care not to damage the foil of adjacent ampules. Any ampule with a torn foil seal should be used immediately or discarded. Place 1 nutrient tablet in each ampule using the plastic tweezers. Place a disposable pipet tip on the syringe, taking care not to touch the ends. Draw 0.1 ± 005 mL of each milk sample to be tested. Dip the pipet tip about 1 cm into the milk and draw slowly. Transfer the milk to the correct ampule by emptying the syringe slowly and completely. Use new tip for each sample.

3. When all tests are prepared, place ampules in the prewarmed water bath, dry incubator, or heater block. Record time and set timer for 2 hours and 30 minutes. At end of incubation, remove the ampules and determine the color of the positive and negative controls. If these are appropriate, the test is complete.
4. Presumptive positive results are confirmed by heating the sample or a portion of the sample to 82° ± 1°C for 2 minutes. Cool immediately to 4.4°C and repeat steps in 12.023.9.A.2 and 12.023.9.A.3.

B. **Option:** The optional addition of beta lactamase to the heated sample allows for the confirmation of beta lactam inhibitors. Positive and negative controls must give expected results in each assay or sample set for valid results.

10. **Expression of Results:** Use color chart test results provided by the manufacturer to determine results. Examine the ampules and record the color as yellow, purple, or yellow-purple.

11. **Precision and Performance Parameters:** Contact AOAC International Research Institute, Gaithersburg, MD, for performance parameters.

12. **Test Report and Interpretation:** Samples with normal spore growth and yellow color development are negative for residues at or above the detection limits provided on the package insert from the manufacturer. These results should be reported as *not found*.

Samples that remain purple denoting failure of spore growth should be reported as *positive for inhibitor*. Reversal of the inhibition with beta lactamase treatment defines the inhibitor as a beta lactam, and the result is reported as positive for beta lactam.

Samples that are yellow-purple after heating are negative and reported as *not found*.

Test reports to show the testing site, analyst, date sampled, date tested, temperature control information, and results obtained.

12.024 *Delvotest® P 5 Pack (Class A4 for raw bovine and goat milk, pasteurized white milk; Class B for other dairy products)*

1. **Scope:** See 12.023.

This method is accepted by the FDA for use in the IMS program for screening and confirmation of beta lactam residues in raw supplies. This method has also been evaluated by FDA and found acceptable for use on pasteurized white milks for beta lactam residues.

2. **References:** See 12.023.
3. **Definition:** See 12.021.
4. **Principle:** See 12.023.
5. **Reagents:** Delvotest® P: 5-pack square blocks containing media and indicator, 96 tests per block. These blocks may be broken down into smaller test batches, but no fewer than 16.

All other items in 12.023.

6. **Apparatus:** See 12.023 and include a nutrient tablet dispenser.
7. **Sampling:** See 12.023.

8. **Preparation of Test Sample:** See 12.023.
9. **Procedure:** Trays have letters and numbers across the outside edges of the trays to identify samples; otherwise, the procedure is the same as indicated in 12.023.
10. **Expression of Results:** See 12.023.
11. **Precision and Performance Parameters:** See 12.023.
12. **Test Reports:** See 12.023.

12.025 *Delvotest® SP (Class A4 for raw milk, pasteurized white milk; Class B for other dairy products)*

This method is identical to 12.023 with these minor variations:

1. The *B. stearothermophilus* organism has been modified to have a higher sensitivity to compounds in the sulfonamide family. The level of detection is above the current U.S. safe tolerance level (10 ppb) for drugs in this family.
2. The incubation time has been modified to 3 hours at 64° ± 1°C.
3. Minimum sensitivities to individual beta lactams are slightly different than those noted on the package insert for the Delvotest® P.

12.030 Enzyme Substrate Tests—Beta Lactam Specific

12.031 *Penzyme® Milk Test* [5,9] *(Class A4 for raw milk and raw goat milk; Class B for other dairy products and individual cow milk)*

1. **Scope:** This method is applicable to raw commingled cow and goat milk, pasteurized white milk, and individual cow milk.

   This method has been approved for use in the NCIMS Appendix N program for screening and confirmation of beta lactams in raw commingled bovine milk and by the FDA for beta lactams in pasteurized white milk and for beta lactams in raw goat milk.

2. **References:** Chapter 3, Sampling Dairy and Related Products.

   AOAC International Research Institute. AOAC referee, vol. 19-1. Gaithersburg, MD: AOAC; 1995.

   AOAC International Research Institute. AOAC referee, vol. 20-1. Gaithersburg, MD: AOAC; 1996.

   AOAC International Research Institute. AOAC referee, vol. 19-8. Gaithersburg, MD: AOAC; 1985.

   Food and Drug Administration. 2400 forms for Appendix N drug testing procedures in accordance with PMO; 1985, revisions 1995 and 1998.

   U.S. Dept. of Health and Human Services. FDA milk safety, M-I-85, revision 5. Washington, DC: Public Health Service, Food and Drug Administration; 1996.

   U.S. Dept. of Health and Human Services. FDA milk safety, M-I-92-11. Washington, DC: Public Health Service, Food and Drug Administration; 1992.

   U.S. Dept. of Health and Human Services. FDA milk safety, M-I-98-8. Washington, DC: Public Health Service, Food and Drug Administration; 1998.

3. **Definition:** Antibiotics, primarily beta lactams, that are able to inhibit caroxypeptidase activity are detected by this test.
4. **Principle:** Beta lactam antibiotics inhibit, on an equimolar basis, the release of D-alanine from a substrate by DD-carboxypeptidase. The D-alanine is further oxidized to pyruvic acid by d-amino acid oxidase simultaneously forming hydrogen peroxide. Hydrogen peroxide oxidizes an organic redox indicator, the amount of which is related to the concentration of beta lactam in the milk.
5. **Reagents**
   1. Vials: Each containing a DD-carboxy-peptidase isolated from the *Actinomadura* strain R-39.
   2. Vial of 25 reagent tablets containing the active ingredients of the substrate and the D-amino acid oxidase.
   3. Negative control milk.
   4. Positive control of penicillin G at 5 ± 0.5 ppb.
6. **Apparatus and Glassware**
   1. Tweezers.
   2. Spring syringe with disposable tips.
   3. Standard color chart.
   4. Incubator capable of maintaining 46° to 48°C.
   5. Timer.
   6. Analytical balance (optional, for making the positive control of penicillin G at 5 ± 0.5 Gin-house).
7. **Sampling:** No additional requirements from those outlined in chapter 3.
8. **Preparation of Test Sample:** Remove test portion within 3 minutes of sample agitation.
9. **Procedure:** Preheat incubator to 46° to 48°C. Allow tablets to come to the ambient temperature (4° to 37°C) before opening bottle. Keep tablet bottle covered at all times except to remove a tablet for testing purposes. Take an enzyme vial and tap gently on base to dislodge any enzyme from cap. Remove tear-off seal and rubber cap from vial carefully. Place new tip on syringe and draw up sample portion by placing end of tip about ½ inch in to milk sample. Level of milk should almost fill the tip. (Volume is 0.18 to 0.22 mL.)

   Completely transfer sample volume to vial. Replace cap. Roll and shake vial so that all enzyme goes into solution. Place capped vial into preheated incubator and incubate 5 minutes at 47° ± 1°C. (This initial time must be at least 5 minutes, but no longer than 15 minutes.) After 5 minutes, remove vial from incubator. Remove cap and, using tweezers, add 1 tablet to vial. Replace cap and shake 5 seconds until yellow begins to appear in milk. Do not invert. NOTE: Ensure that tablet is covered by milk and at bottom of vial.

   Incubate 15 minutes at 47° ± 1°C. After 5 minutes have elapsed, remove vial and shake contents approximately 5 seconds to aid tablet disintegration. Return vial to incubator. Remove vial from incubator and read color immediately. For consistent color determination, incubate a minimum of 15 minutes to a maximum of 16 minutes. Swirl vial contents gently to aid in color determination.

A positive and negative control should be run at least daily with appropriate results obtained on each for results of testing to be valid

10. **Expression of Results:** Record observed color of vial. Compare color to those on color chart. Color should be either pink (same or darker than chart), yellow, or intermediate color.
11. **Precision and Performance Parameters:** Contact AOAC International Research Institute for information on performance parameters. Package inserts detail the sensitivity of the assay for the detectable beta lactams. A collaborative study has been reported.[9]
12. **Test Report and Interpretation:** A pink color indicates a negative result and should be reported as *negative* or *not found.*

    Any color other than a color corresponding to the negative is a presumptive positive and should be retested. Under NCIMS regulations, retests are in duplicate and are performed with positive and negative controls. If either or both results on the retest are positive, the sample is positive and results are reported as positive for beta lactams.

    Test reports should show testing site, date sampled, date tested, analyst, temperature control information, and results obtained.

12.032 *Penzyme® III*

1. **Scope:** This method is Class A4 for raw commingled bovine milk; Class A4 for pasteurized white milk; and Class B for raw goat milk, dry milk, and other fluid dairy products.

   This method has been accepted for use in the NCIMS Appendix N testing program for raw bovine and goat milk. It has also been found suitable for pasteurized white milk.
2. **References:** See 12.031.
3. **Definition:** See 12.031.
4. **Principle:** See 12.031.
5. **Reagents**
   1. Test kit for 100 tests containing: Vial 1 with DD-carboxypeptidase isolated from the Actinomadura R-39 strain, and vial 2 containing tablets, each of which contain the active ingredients of the substrate and the amino acid oxidase.
   2. Negative control milk.
   3. Positive control of penicillin G at 5 ± 0.5 ppb.
   4. Distilled or deionized water.
6. **Apparatus and Glassware**
   1. Fixed-volume pipets: 10 µL and 50 µL, and disposable tips.
   2. Pipet to deliver 1.5 mL.
   3. 1.5 mL clear microcentrifuge tubes.
   4. Dry bath incubator to maintain 46° to 48°C with a heat block with holes specially designed for microcentrifuge tubes.
   5. Mechanical vortex.
   6. Timer.
7. **Sampling:** No additional requirements from those outlined in chapter 3.

8. **Preparation of Test Sample:** Remove test portion within 3 minutes of sample agitation.

9. **Procedure:** Preheat incubator to 46° to 48°C. Allow tablets to come to ambient temperature (4° to 37°C) before opening bottle. Keep tablet bottle covered at all times except to remove a tablet for testing purposes. Reconstitute contents of vial 1 with 1.5 mL of cold distilled water. Shake gently and allow 10 minutes for contents to dissolve properly. Refrigerate if not used immediately.

   Add 10 µL of vial 1 to the bottom of a clean, empty microcentrifuge tube. Add 50 µL of sample. Thoroughly mix enzyme and milk sample with vortex or by tapping at the base of the tube for 3 seconds. Volumes must be ± 10%. Incubate tube with cap closed for 5 minutes at 47° ± 1°C. (This initial incubation must be at least 5 minutes, but no more than 15 minutes.)

   Remove sample from incubator and add 1 tablet from vial 2. Mix sample vial by using a vortex or by tapping at the base of the tube for 3 seconds. This will start tablet disintegration. Incubate vial for 10 minutes at 47° ± 1°C. After the elapse of 5 minutes, remove vial and mix contents to aid tablet disintegration. Return vial to incubator.

   Remove vial from incubator. For consistent color determination, incubate for a minimum of 10 minutes to a maximum of 11 minutes. Mix vial thoroughly before reading to aid color development and read results immediately.

   Positive and negative controls must give appropriate results on each new lot of reagents and at any time they are tested for results to be valid. Initial positive results on a sample are presumptive and confirmation with positive and negative controls will determine if the sample is positive or not.

10. **Expression of Results:** Read and record color of vial. Compare color obtained to those on color chart and record as negative or positive. Colors should be dark peach to a brilliant yellow.

11. **Precision and Performance Parameters:** Contact AOAC International Research Institute for information on performance parameters.[9]

12. **Test Report and Interpretation:** Results that are of a color corresponding to the negative should be reported as *negative* or *not found*.

    Results that are found to be positive after retesting should be reported as *positive for beta lactams.*

    Reports should list the testing site, the analyst, date sampled, date tested, temperature control information, and the results obtained.

12.040 Receptor Assay Tests—Beta Lactam Specific

12.041 *Charm II® (Sequential, Competitive, Quantitative), Charm I®, Cowside II® (Modification using tablet reagents)*

1. **Scope:** Class A4 for raw bovine milk, raw goat milk (sequential), and pasteurized white milk (competitive); Class B for other dairy products. These methods are applicable for routine use for high fat products (>5%) and individual cow milk.

These methods are accepted for use in the beta lactam NCIMS Appendix N testing program.

2. **References:** Chapter 3: Sampling Dairy and Related Products.

AOAC INTERNATIONAL RESEARCH INSTITUTE. AOAC referee, vol. 19-1. Gaithersburg, MD: AOAC; 1995.

AOAC INTERNATIONAL RESEARCH INSTITUTE. AOAC referee, vol. 20-1. Gaithersburg, MD: AOAC; 1998.

AOAC INTERNATIONAL RESEARCH INSTITUTE. AOAC referee, vol. 19-8. Gaithersburg, MD: AOAC; 1995.

CUNNIFF, P., ED. *Official Methods of Analysis*, 16th ed. Washington, DC: AOAC; 1995.

FOOD AND DRUG ADMINISTRATION. 2400 forms for Appendix N Drug Testing Procedures in accordance with PMO; 1995, revisions 1995 and 1998.

U.S. DEPT. OF HEALTH AND HUMAN SERVICES. FDA milk safety, M-I-85, Revision 5. Washington, DC: Public Health Service, Food and Drug Administration; 1996.

U.S. DEPT. OF HEALTH AND HUMAN SERVICES. FDA milk safety, M-I-92-11. Washington, DC: Public Health Service, Food and Drug Administration; 1992.

U.S. DEPT. OF HEALTH AND HUMAN SERVICES. FDA milk safety, M-I-98-8. Washington, DC: Public Health Service, Food and Drug Administration; 1998.

3. **Definition:** These assays test for beta lactam antibiotics or other compounds that will bind to specific bacterial receptor sites.

4. **Principle:** Charm beta lactam tests use bacteria with specific receptor sites that bind all beta lactam drugs. The bacteria are added to a milk sample along with a small (exempt from regulation) quantity of ^{14}C labeled penicillin (tracer). Any beta lactam drug already in the milk competes for the binding sites with this tracer. The amount of tracer that binds to the receptor sites is measured and compared to a previously determined control point or to a standard curve. The greater the amount of tracer measured, the lower the beta lactam drug concentration in the sample.

5. **Reagents**

   1. Beta lactam reagents: Yellow tracer reagent and green binding reagent.
   2. Penicillin G standard at 4.5 ppb (0.008 IU/mL). This is reconstituted with negative raw milk or zero control milk.
   3. Zero control standard: Powdered milk based buffer representative of commingled bovine milk from untreated herd. This is reconstituted with 100 mL of 37°C water.
   4. Optifluor scintillation fluid for Charm II®.

6. **Apparatus and Glassware**

   1. Charm II® (6000 or 6600 models) or Charm I® (9150, 160, 210, Cowside® 2000 models) analyzer.
   2. Planchets and hot plate for Charm I®.
   3. 13- × 100-mm test tubes, disposable, of borosilicate glass, with 13-mm caps.

4. Cotton swabs.
5. Fixed-volume dispenser/pipeter at 5.0 mL.
6. Positive volume dispenser to dispense 300 µL.
7. Positive dispenser for 3.0 mL (Optifluor).
8. Incubator block for 13 × 100 test tubes maintained at a temperature of 65° ± 2°C (Charm I® and Charm II® sequential) or 85° ± 2°C (competitive) or 55° ± 2°C (quantitative).
9. Centrifuge for 13- × 100-mm test tubes capable of 1200 g.
10. Test tube mixer (vortex).

7. **Sampling:** For individual cow samples or samples with high fat (>5%), centrifuge the sample at 1200 × g for 3 minutes prior to testing the skim portion. For pasteurized and other dairy products, refer to the general sample preparation and test validation procedure for Charm II® test analysis from the manufacturer. Observe precautions and regulations for handling and disposing of low levels of ^{3}H and ^{14}C radioactivity.

8. **Preparation of Test Sample:** Remove test portion within 3 minutes of sample agitation. Remove skim portion of centrifuged samples by inserting pipet tip into the skim portion and withdrawing sample volume. Avoid transferring cream to sample tube.

9. **Procedure:** Establish a control point by testing positive control sample 6 times and taking the average. Multiply the average by 1.25 (sequential) or 1.15 (competitive) or 1.35 (Charm I®). This is the control point. All 6 tests should be less than the control point. If not, the control point should be redetermined.

   Determine a negative average by testing zero control 3 times and taking an average (for quantitative assay, test 6 times). Multiply the average by 0.85. Establish control point and negative average for each new lot of reagents. In addition, a daily performance check should include an assay of the known negative milk with results ± 20% of the average (15% quantitative), and of the positive control with results less than the control point. If these conditions are not met, redo the control point and zero average.

   Label empty test tube, 1 for each sample, and add 1 green tablet to empty tube. Add 300 µL of water to each tube. Break up tablets in tubes by mixing tubes 10 times for 10 seconds each on mixer using a rise and fall motion. Mix samples and draw 5.0 mL milk using new pipet tip for each sample. Add drawn sample to appropriately labeled test tube.

   See 12.044 for the expression of results, precision and performance parameters, and references.

12.042 *Charm II® Competitive Procedure*

See 12.041 for scope, references, definition, principle, reagents, apparatus, sampling, and preparation of test sample.

Add yellow tablet to tube and mix 15 times for 15 seconds each on mixer in rise and fall motion. Incubate tubes for 3 minutes at 85° ± 2°C. Remove tubes and centrifuge for 3 minutes. Pour off milk. While still draining tubes, remove fat ring with 2 or more cotton swabs, continue until dry. Do not touch pellet.

Using water pipet, add 300 µL of water to tubes and break up pellets using mixer. Pellets must be completely suspended. Add 3.0 mL scintillation fluid (optifluor) to each tube and vortex to mix. Count tubes in scintillation counter for 1 minute using ^{14}C channel. Record counts as counts per minute (CPM).

See 12.044 for the expression of results, precision and performance parameters, and bibliography.

12.043 *Charm II® Sequential, Charm I®, Cowside II® Procedure*

See 12.041 for scope, references, definition, principle, reagents, apparatus, sampling, and preparation of test sample.

Incubate tubes for 2 minutes at 65° ± 2°C. Remove tubes and add yellow tablet to each tube and mix on vortex 10 times for 10 seconds in a rise and fall motion on vortex mixer. Incubate tubes for 2 minutes at 65° ± 2°C. Remove tubes and centrifuge for 3 minutes. Pour off milk. While still draining tubes, remove fat ring with 2 or more cotton swabs, continue until dry. Do not touch pellet.

Using water pipet, add 300 µL of water to tubes and break up pellet using mixer. Pellets must be completely suspended. For Charm II®, add 3.0 mL scintillation fluid to each tube, cap, and vortex to mix. For Charm I® and Cowside II®, pour into planchett, rinse 2 or more times with 200 µL of water, and bake dry on hot plate. For Charm II®, count tubes on scintillation counter for 1 minute using ^{14}C channel. For Charm I® and Cowside II, count planchettes in analyzer for 2 minutes and record count.

See 12.044 for the expression of results, precision and performance parameters, and bibliography.

12.044 *Quantitative Procedure*

See 12.041 for scope, references, definition, principle, reagents, apparatus, sampling, and preparation of test sample.

Incubate tubes for 7 minutes at 55° ± 2°C. Add yellow tablet to tube and mix 10 times for 10 seconds each on mixer in rise and fall motion. Incubate tubes for 2 minutes at 55° ± 2°C. Remove tubes and centrifuge for 3 minutes. Pour off milk. While still draining tubes, remove fat ring using 2 or more cotton swabs, continue until dry. Do not touch pellet.

Using water pipet, add 300 µL of water to each tube and break up pellet using mixer. Pellets must be completely suspended. Add 3.0 mL of scintillation fluid to each tube, cap, and vortex to mix. Count tubes on scintillation counter for 1 minute using ^{14}C channel. Record counts.

1. **Expression of Results:** Record test results as CPM.
2. **Precision and Performance Parameters:** These tests have been verified to have at least a 90 to 95% selectivity of negative samples in blind studies and minimum 90 to 95% sensitivity to the specific beta lactam antibiotics listed on package inserts.[3,4]
3. **Test Report and Interpretation:** If the CPM in the analyzer is more than the control point (50 points greater with Charm II®), the sample is negative (contains less than the ppb level used to calculate the control point). These results should be reported as *not found*.

If the CPM is less than or equal to the control point the sample is presumptive positive.

If the CPM of a Charm II® test is within 50 points of the control point, the sample should be recounted. If the recount is less than or equal to the control point, the sample is a presumptive positive. If the recount is greater than the control point, the sample is negative. Positive results obtained on a retest in duplicate are reported as *positive*.

Test reports include sample date, test date, temperature, analyst, testing site, and method.

12.045 *Charm Cloxacillin® Determination in Milk-Immuno-Assay Method*

1. **Scope:** Class A4 for raw bovine milk and pasteurized white milk; Class B for other dairy products. The method may also be applied to individual cow milk.
2. **References:** See 12.041.
3. **Definition:** The assay tests for cloxacillin and antibiotics with similar specific binding ability.
4. **Principle:** Antibodies with specificity to cloxacillin drugs are added to a milk sample along with an exempt amount of ^{14}C labeled cloxacillin (tracer). Any cloxacillin drug already in the milk competes for the binding sites with this tracer. The amount of tracer that binds to the antibody is measured and compared to a previously determined control point or to a standard curve. The greater the amount of tracer measured, the lower the cloxacillin drug concentration in the sample. The lower the amount of tracer measured, the greater the concentration in the sample.
5. **Reagents**
    1. Cloxacillin tablet reagents: Blue tracer reagent and white binding reagent.
    2. Cloxacillin standard: 10 ppb positive control standard reconstituted with 100 mL negative milk or zero control to make concentration of 10 ppb.
    3. Zero control standard-powdered milk based buffer representative of commingled bovine milk from untreated herd. Reconstituted with 100 mL of 37°C water.
    4. Optifluor (Charm II®).
6. **Apparatus and Glassware:** Identical to those required for Charm I®/Cowside II® and Charm II® beta lactam testing. See 12.041.
7. **Sampling:** Observe precautions and regulations for handling and disposing of low levels of ^{3}H and ^{14}C radioactivity.
8. **Preparation of Test Sample:** For all samples, the sample must be centrifuged at 1200 g for 3 minutes. For pasteurized milk and other dairy products, refer to the general sample preparation and test validation procedure for Charm II® test analysis provided by the manufacturer.
9. **Procedure:** Establish a control point by testing as outlined in 12.041.9. For Charm II®, multiply the average by 1.15; for Charm I®, multiply the average by 1.35. This is the control point. All 6 tests should be less than the

control point or the control point needs to be redetermined. Follow steps in Charm II®/Charm I® in 12.041.

Fill labeled test tubes ¾ full with milk sample and centrifuge at 1200 g for 5 minutes. Remove from centrifuge and cool to 0.5° to 4.4°C in ice bath. Label empty test tubes, 1 for each sample, and add 1 white tablet to each. Add 300 µL of water to each tube and mix 15 times for 15 seconds each on mixer using a rise and fall motion. Draw 5.0 mL of milk from below fat layer using new pipet tip for each sample and add to appropriate labeled tube. Add blue tablet to each tube and mix 15 times for 15 seconds each using a rise and fall motion on the mixer.

Incubate tubes for 3 minutes at 35° ± 2°C. Remove tubes and centrifuge for 5 minutes.

Pour off milk. While still draining tubes, remove fat ring with 2 or more cotton swabs; continue until dry. Do not touch pipet. Using water pipet, add 300 µL of water to tubes and break up pellets using mixer. Pellets must be completely suspended. Add 3.0 mL of scintillation fluid to each tube, cap, and vortex to mix (Charm II®). For Charm I®, pour contents to planchette. Dry on hot plate. Count tubes on scintillation counter for 1 minute using ^{14}C channel or planchette on Geiger-Mueller counter for 1 minute.

10. **Expression of Results:** Results are expressed as a CPM for either test.

11. **Precision and Performance Parameters:** The Charm II® cloxacillin test and the Charm I® cloxacillin test have been validated to have at least a 90 to 95% selectivity of negative samples in a blind study and a minimum 90 to 95% sensitivity of cloxacillin at 8.5 ppb (Charm II®) and 9.5 ppb (Charm I).

12. **Test Report and Interpretation:** If the CPM of the analyzer is more than the control point, the sample is negative. This result should be reported as *not found for cloxacillin*. If the CPM is less than or equal to the control point, the sample is a presumptive positive.

    If the CPM of a Charm II® test is within 50 points of the control point, the sample should be recounted. If the recount is less than or equal to the control point, the sample is a presumptive positive. If the recount is greater than the control point, the sample is negative and should be reported as *not found for cloxacillin*.

    Samples that are presumptive should be retested in duplicate using positive and negative controls. If controls perform appropriately, results are valid. If not, the test is invalid and the control point and instrument function must be verified. If either duplicate retest results in a positive, sample is positive and should be reported as *positive for cloxacillin*. If both retests are negative, sample is negative and should be reported as *not found for cloxacillin*.

    Test reports should show test site, test name, date sampled, date tested, analyst, temperature control information, and result.

12.046 *Charm SL® Test and Charm SL-6, Beta Lactams*

1. **Scope:** These methods are Class A4 for raw commingled bovine milk and raw producer bulk tank milk. It has been approved under the NCIMS

program for use on raw commingled bovine milk and raw producer bulk tank milk. Charm SL is also validated in commingled raw goat's milk.

2. **References:** See 12.041.
3. **Definition:** See 12.041.
4. **Principle:** This test uses receptors that bind to beta lactam drugs. As milk flows through the device, a line forms in the T (test) portion when the sample contains beta lactam. A weaker intensity T-line forms when beta lactam is present in the sample. The T-line is compared to the C (control) line, which is designed to discriminate beta lactam close to the current U.S. safe levels. If the T-line is darker than or equal to the C-line, the sample is negative. If the T-line is lighter than the C-line, or if the T-line does not form, the sample is positive. If the C-line does not form, the test is flawed and must be repeated. A ROSA reader or LUM-T imager converts the line comparison to a reading and provides the result. The SL-6 also has an X-line that is treated the same as the T-line and detects cloxacillin at lower levels than the T-line.
5. **Reagents:** Unless otherwise specified, reagents should be of analytical grade.
   1. SL and SL-6 test strips: Packaged in plastic canisters.
   2. Positive control: Standard 5.0 ppb, penicillin G for SL and 10 ppb cloxacillin/5 ppb penicillin G for SL6.
   3. Negative milk.
   4. Deionized or distilled water or water of equivalent purity.
6. **Apparatus and Glassware**
   1. For SL strip incubator at 56° ± 1°C with built-in timer light. For SL-6 strip incubator at 45°C ± 2°C.
   2. Fixed-volume pipet: 300 µL.
   3. SL strip reader or LUM T reader adapter.
   4. Pipet and/or glassware to reconstitute the standard and negative milk as directed on label.
   5. Analytical balance (optional, for making positive control from scratch).
   6. Centrifuge (for samples >5% fat and individual cow samples).
7. **Sampling:** No additional information other than that outlined in chapter 3.
8. **Sample Preparation:** Carefully mix the sample as directed in chapter 8. For frozen samples, heavy fat samples (>5%), and individual cows, centrifuge the sample at 1200 g for 3 minutes prior to testing the skim.
9. **Test Procedure:** Reconstitute the positive control as directed on the label. Freeze aliquots at –15°C, or use within 48 hours (stored at 0.5° to 4.4°C). Negative milk may be subsampled and stored at –15°C, or held at 0.5° to 4.4°C for up to 72 hours. Turn incubator on and allow to come to temperature. Temperature indicator should be green at 55°C, indicating that the temperature is 56° ± 1°C. Place a labeled test strip in incubator with flat side up. Use tab to peel tape back to edge of white label exposing sample pad. Slowly, to avoid spilling, pipet 300 µL of milk into either side well of the sample pad compartment. Reseal tape over sample pad compartment by pressing.

Close cover on incubator and tighten latch. Solid red timer light will automatically start when lid is closed. If desired, set a different timer for 8 minutes. Incubate for 8 minutes (10 minutes maximum). The green light (test complete) will start blinking at 8 minutes. Read test strips by placing strip in reader per manufacturer's instructions, being careful to hold strip so that the sample pad is in the down position.

10. **Expression of Results:** The reader compares the C-line and the T-line (and X-line with SL-6) and displays either a positive or a negative numerical result. Record or store this information. The results are stored in memory and may be subsequently recalled by the operator, or they may be downloaded to a printer or computer.

    Initial positive results should be retested in duplicate for NCIMS use along with positive and negative control samples. If control conditions are not correct, the test results are invalid. If controls are appropriate, the results on the retest are used.

11. **Precision and Performance Parameters:** This test has been validated to have at least a 90 to 95% selectivity of negative samples in blind studies, and a minimum of 90 to 95% sensitivity to the beta lactams listed on the package insert. Information on the sensitivity for other beta lactams is available from the manufacturer.

12. **Test Report and Interpretation:** Samples with negative values on the reader should be reported as *negative* or *not found (for beta lactams).* Samples with positive values after retesting in duplicate with appropriate positive and negative controls should be reported as *positive for beta lactams.*

12.050 ELISA Tests—Beta Lactam Specific

12.051 *Delvo X-Press®, Beta Lactam Specific (Class A4)*

1. **Scope:** This method is applicable to raw milk and pasteurized white milk. It has been accepted for use in the NCIMS Appendix N program for screening raw milk for beta lactam residues. It has also been evaluated by the FDA and found acceptable for pasteurized white milk. It is not recommended for testing milk from species other than cows as interference may be noted.

2. **References:** See 12.041.

3. **Definition:** This assay detects beta lactam antibiotics.

4. **Principle:** Delvo X-Press® is an enzyme-linked competitive qualitative assay for detecting residues of beta lactams at or below the U.S. current safe tolerance levels in raw, commingled bovine milk. Samples are incubated with a tracer in tubes coated with beta lactams. The tracer will bind either the beta lactams on the tubes or beta lactams in the milk sample. After incubation, a color developer is added. Residual tracer in the tubes is more intense the greater the concentration of beta lactam in the milk sample. A standard is run with each bank of samples as the first sample, and each sample is compared to the standard in the reader to provide a pass or fail response.

5. **Reagents**
   1. Tracer: Bottle containing enzyme-linked receptor protein in buffered saline solution of goat serum with 4-aminoantipyrine preserved with thimersol (bottle 1).
   2. Standard bottle containing beta lactam in buffered saline solution of milk, lyophilized (bottle S).
   3. Bottles of diluent for the lyophilized standard containing an aqueous solution preserved with thimersol (bottle D).
   4. Bottle of color developer containing an enzyme substrate, an aqueous solution of color developer (bottle 2).
   5. Bottle of stop solution reagent for the color reaction containing a diluted salt solution (bottle 3).
   6. Bottle of 50x wash solution to be diluted with deionized or distilled water containing a buffered solution of glycerol preserved with benzalkonium chloride (bottle W).
   7. Deionized or distilled water.
   8. Positive control containing penicillin at 5 ppb ± 10%
   9. Negative control milk (milk with no detectable beta lactam).
6. **Apparatus and Glassware**
   1. Ampules for first reaction in bags labeled A.
   2. Coated tubes with beta lactam in bags labeled T.
   3. Pipeters: 200 µL and 500 µL.
   4. Disposable pipet tips.
   5. 5-mL measuring beaker.
   6. Tube rack.
   7. Wash bottle (squeeze bottle).
   8. ISRP work station (containing incubator).
   9. Jet washer (optional).
7. **Sampling:** No additional requirements other than those outlined in chapter 3.
8. **Preparation of Test Sample:** Avoid foam when mixing sample. Milk sample and reagents should be at the same temperature. Be sure not to take in air bubbles when pipeting sample volume.
9. **Procedure:** At least 30 minutes prior to beginning of testing, remove test kit from refrigerator. Remove all necessary ampules, tubes, and reagents and allow them to warm to room temperature (15° to 25°C). Standard and milk ampules must be at same temperature range (e.g., standard 0.5° to 4.4°C, sample 0.5° to 4.4°C).

   Turn on ISRP work station for at least 15 minutes to warm to set temperature, 64° ± 2°C. Prepare sufficient wash solution for entire day by diluting 1 part of wash solution (50x) with 49 parts deionized or distilled water (about 250 mL is needed for 10 tubes). Fill a squeeze bottle or jet washer with this diluted wash solution.

   A. **Prepare standard:** Remove seal from standard diluent and standard (lyophilized) bottle. Carefully lift stoppers, releasing vacuum; remove stoppers and carefully avoid contaminating the plug end of the stoppers by contact with fingers, bench, etc. Pour entire contents of diluent bottle into the lyophilized bottle and replace stopper. Gently mix by inverting 20 times, holding the stopper in place. Standard should be allowed to equilibrate for 20 minutes at room temperature and gently remixed 10 times. Date and store at 0.5° to 8.0°C for no more than 2 weeks, or for no more than 1 day at room temperature.

Prepare required number of ampules, 1 for standard, and 1 for each sample. No more than 6 samples should be processed together. Label an equal number of coated tubes for each. (ISRP display prompts analyst at each step.) Pipet 0.2 ± 0.01 mL standard into ampule labeled *standard*. Pipet 0.2 ± 0.01 mL of sample into corresponding ampules using new pipet tip for each. Pipet 0.2 ± 0.01 mL tracer into all ampules. Incubate ampules for 2 minutes (+12 seconds max.) in the incubator row A at 64° ± 2°C.

Transfer ampules from the incubator to tube rack and place the coated tubes on top of the corresponding ampules. Transfer the contents from the ampules to the tubes by inverting the combined coated tube plus ampule. Tap ampule to transfer all contents.

Incubate coated tubes with the ampules still on top for 2 minutes (± 12 seconds) in the incubator row A at 64° ± 2°C. Remove coated tubes from the incubator and discard ampules. Pipet 0.5 ± 0.025 mL of color developer into each tube. Incubate tubes for 4 minutes ± 24 seconds in incubator row B (15° to 25°C, room temperature). Pipet 0.05 ± 0.025 mL of stop solution into each tube. Shake tubes to mix contents by using ISRP work station.

Read results in ISRP work station. Check positive and negative controls on a daily basis. Each new lot should show correct results on positive and negative controls before use. When used in the NCIMS program, NCIMS regulations require that all initial positives be retested in duplicate with positive and negative controls before the result is reported.

10. **Expression of Results:** ISRP work station gives numerical result and automatically interprets reading.

    Reader numbers +00 or greater are positive and shown as +, ++, or +++.

    Reader numbers –01 and less are negative and shown as OK.

11. **Precision and Performance Parameters:** Contact the AOAC International Research Institute for information on performance parameters.

12. **Test Report and Interpretation:** Samples testing negative should be reported as *not found*. Samples testing positive in duplicate should be reported as *positive (for beta lactam)*.

    Test reports should show sample date, test date, test type, test site, analyst initials, and temperature control information.

12.052 *IDEXX SNAP® B/L (Beta Lactam) (Class A4 for raw bovine milk, raw goat milk, and pasteurized white milk)*

1. **Scope:** This method is applicable to raw commingled bovine milk, pasteurized white milks, and raw goat milk. Application has been made to milk from individual cows.

2. **Reference:** See 12.041.

3. **Definition:** This assay tests for beta lactam antibiotics.

4. **Principle:** Milk is preincubated with conjugate A. Beta lactams, if present, will bind to conjugate A. The sample is then added to the SNAP device, allowing unbound enzyme-labeled conjugate A to bind to the sample spot and enzyme-labeled conjugate B to bind to the control spot. The sample flows and begins to turn the blue activation circle white. The activator is depressed, puncturing the foil in the base of the device, allowing substrate to be absorbed and drawn across the sample and control spot in the results window. Substrate is cleaved by the enzyme portion of the conjugate to form a blue precipitate, causing color development. The more drug in the sample, the less color in the sample spot.

5. **Reagents**
   1. Positive control milk at 5 penicillin G ± 0.5 ppb.
   2. Negative control milk (containing no detectable beta lactam residues).
   3. Penicillin G (optional for making positive control in-house).

6. **Apparatus and Glassware**
   1. SNAP beta lactam test kit containing individual foil packets, each containing a SNAP device, sample tube with reagent pellet, and a pipet.
   2. Heater block capable of maintaining operating temperature of 45° ± 5°C with insert for SNAP device and tubes.
   3. Single-use 450-µL pipet with incubator line as supplied or fixed-volume pipet to dispense 450 µL.
   4. Timer.
   5. IDEXX SNAP® image reader (optional).
   6. Analytical balance (optional for making positive control).

7. **Sampling:** No additional requirements other than those outlined in chapter 3.

8. **Preparation of Test Sample:** Remove test portion within 3 minutes of sample agitation.

9. **Procedure:** Store test kit at 0° to 7°C (32° to 45°F) until day of use. Kits may be left at room temperature (64° to 84°F) during day of use. Allow test kit to reach room temperature before use. Remove SNAP device, pipet, and sample tube from foil packet. Ensure that the heat block has been preheated and that the temperature has maintained 45° (113°F) ± 5°C for at least 5 minutes.

   Verify that the reagent pellet is at the bottom of the sample tube (if not, tap tube to return pellet to the bottom). Place SNAP device in test block. Remove and discard sample tube cap. Draw up milk sample (450 ± 50 µL) to the indicator line.

   Carefully add the entire milk sample from pipet to tube. Shake sample tube to dissolve reagent pellet. Incubate sample tube in preheated heat block (45°C) for 5 minutes. (Incubation must occur for a minimum of 5 minutes and for no longer than 6 minutes.) Pour entire contents of sample tube into sample well of SNAP device and discard tube. The sample will flow across the results window toward the blue activation circle.

When the blue activation circle begins to disappear, push the activator firmly until it snaps flush with the body of the SNAP device. NOTE: When the edge of the circle nearest the sample well begins to turn from dark blue to white, activation should occur. Do not let the circle completely disappear.

The device should be left on the heater block for 4 minutes for color development. Read results immediately, visually or optionally, with the SNAP Image Reader®. Each new lot should be tested with positive and negative controls and appropriate results obtained prior to use. Daily performance checks of a positive and negative control are also recommended.

10. **Expression of Results:** Position the SNAP device with the sample well to the left. If using reader, insert sample well first as shown on decal over the sample port of reader. If the sample spot is darker than or equal to that of the control spot, the sample is negative. If the sample spot is lighter than the control spot, the sample is positive. The SNAP Image Reader® automatically prints the ratio reading and interpretation.

11. **Precision and Performance Parameters:** Contact the AOAC International Research Institute for performance parameter information. Dose response and sensitivity data is published in table format by the FDA. Product inserts also show this information.

12. **Test Report and Interpretation:** Results on negative samples should be reported as *not found*. Results on positive samples should be reported as *positive for beta lactam*. Initial positive results should be confirmed in duplicate with positive and negative controls. Results are valid only if controls give appropriate results. Test reports should show sample date, test date, test type, test type, results obtained, analyst initials, and temperature control information.

12.060 Sulfonamide Assays

12.061 *Charm II® Sulfonamide*[19,20,23]

1. **Scope:** This method is applicable to raw, whole, and commingled bovine milk (Class A4). Application has also been made to milk from individual cows. The method is accepted for use in the U.S. for use under the Pasteurized Milk Ordinance Appendix N drug monitoring program for the detection of sulfonamide residues.

2. **References:** See 12.041.

3. **Definition:** This assay determines the presence of sulfonamide antibiotics.

4. **Principle:** Bacteria with specific receptor sites that bind all sulfonamide antibiotics are added to a milk sample along with an exempt quantity of ^{3}H labeled sulfamethazine (tracer). Any sulfonamide antibiotic already in the milk sample competes for the binding sites with this tracer. The amount of tracer that binds to the receptor sites is measured and compared to a previously determined control point or to a standard curve. The greater the amount of tracer measured, the lower the antibiotic concentration in the sample. (Results are inversely proportional to concentration.)

5. **Reagents**
   1. Sulfa reagents, pink tracer, and beige binding reagent tablets packed in blister packs.
   2. Sulfamethazine standard 10 ppb or multiantimicrobial standard containing sulfa drug. Positive control standard reconstituted with 100 mL negative milk or zero control to make a concentration of 10 ppb.
   3. Zero control standard: Powdered milk-based buffer representative of commingled bovine milk from untreated herd. Reconstituted with 100 mL of 37°C water.
6. **Apparatus and Glassware**
   1. Charm analyzer (Charm II® 6000 or 6600).
   2. Optifluor scintillation fluid.
   3. 13- × 100-mm test tubes: Disposable, of borosilicate glass with 13-mm caps.
   4. Fixed-volume dispenser or pipet: 5.0 mL ± 0.25 mL.
   5. Fixed-volume dispenser or pipet: 300 µL.
   6. Incubator block, dry-well bath, maintained at 85° ± 0.5°C (sized for 13- × 100-mm tubes).
   7. Centrifuge for 13 × 100-mm test tubes capable of 1200 g.
   8. Test tube mixer (vortex).
7. **Sampling:** Observe precautions for handling and disposing of exempt levels of radioactive chemicals.
8. **Sample Preparation:** For individual cow samples or for heavy fat samples (>5%), centrifuge the sample at 1200 for 3 minutes prior to testing skim portion. For pasteurized and other dairy products, refer to general sample preparation and test validation procedure for Charm II® test analysis.
9. **Procedure**
   A. **Establish control point:** Test positive control 6 times. Average results and multiply average by 1.24. This is the control point. All 6 tests should be less than control point. If not, redo control point. This procedure must be done for each new reagent lot and if daily checks are unacceptable.

   B. **Determine a negative average:** Test zero control 3 times and average. Check control point and equipment operation daily. Test positive and negative control. Negative control should be ± 30% of negative average and positive should be less than the control point. Label empty test tubes and add 1 beige tablet to each. Add 300 µL water to each tube. Break up tablets in tubes by mixing tubes 10 times for 10 seconds each on mixer in a rise and fall motion. Mix sample and draw 5.0 mL using new pipet tip for each sample. Add drawn sample to labeled tube. Add pink tablet to each tune and mix 15 times for 15 seconds each on mixer in a rise and fall motion. Incubate tubes for 3 minutes at 85° ± 2°C. Remove tubes and centrifuge for 3 minutes. Pour off milk. While still draining tubes, remove fat ring with 2 or more cotton swabs. Continue until dry. Do not touch pellet.

   Using water pipet, add 300 µL of water to tubes and break up pellets using mixer. Pellets must be completely suspended. Add 3 mL of scintillation fluid to each tube, cap, and vortex to mix. Do not add fluid until just before counting. Count tubes on scintillation counter for 1 minute using ^3H channel. Daily performance analyses of positive and negative controls are recommended. Each new lot must be tested to establish the performance and positive control for that lost of test kits.

10. **Expression of Results:** Numerical value is a CPM. Record numerical readout of CPM.
11. **Precision and Performance Parameters:** Contact the AOAC International Research Institute and consult manufacturer's operator's manual for performance parameter information.
12. **Test Report and Interpretation:** If the CPM of the sample is greater than the control point, the sample is negative (contains less than the level used to calculate the control point) and should be reported as *not found for sulfonamides*.

    If the CPM is less than or equal to the control point, the result is positive. Initial positive results should be confirmed by retesting in duplicate using positive and negative controls. Control conditions must be met on a repeat assay for the results to be valid. If one or both of the repeat assays are positive, the sample is positive and should be reported as *positive for sulfonamides*.

    Test report should show the test site, test type, date sampled, date tested, initials of analyst, results obtained, and appropriate temperature control information.

12.070 Tetracycline Assays

12.071 *Charm II® Tetracycline*

1. **Scope:** This method is applicable to raw, whole commingled bovine milk (Class A4). The method is also often applied to milk from individual cows and other dairy products. This method is acceptable for use under the NCIMS program.
2. **References:** See 12.041.
3. **Definition:** This method tests for tetracycline and related antibiotics.
4. **Principle:** This test uses antibodies that bind all tetracycline drugs. The antibodies are added to a milk sample along with a small (regulatory exempt) quantity of ^3H labeled tetracycline. Any tetracycline in the milk competes for the antibodies with this labeled tetracycline. The amount of ^3H tetracycline that binds to the antibodies is measured and compared to a previously determined control point. The greater the amount of labeled tetracycline measured, the lower the concentration of drug in the sample.
5. **Reagents**
    1. Tetracycline reagents: Tableted orange tracer reagent and white binding reagent.
    2. Positive control: Multiantimicrobial standard containing 30 ppb oxytetracycline. Positive control standard reconstituted with 100 mL zero control to make 30 ppb oxytetracycline. Store at 0° to 4.4°C for 48 hours or –15°C for 2 months or less.

3. Zero control standard: Powdered milk based buffer representative of commingled bovine milk from untreated herd. Reconstitute with 100 mL of 37°C water

6. **Apparatus and Glassware**
   1. Charm analyzer: Charm II® 6000 or 6600.
   2. Optifluor scintillation fluid.
   3. 13- × 100-mL test tubes: Disposable, borosilicate glass with 13-mm caps.
   4. Fixed-volume pipet/dispenser: 5.0 mL.
   5. Pipet: 300 μL.
   6. Incubator block, dry well bath for holding 13- × 100-mm test tubes. Must be able to maintain 85° ± 0.5°C.
   7. Centrifuge for 13- × 100-mm test tubes capable of 1200 g.
   8. Test tube mixer (vortex).

7. **Sampling:** Observe precautions for handling exempt quantities of radioactive chemicals.

8. **Preparation of Test Sample:** For individual cow samples or for heavy fat samples (>5%), centrifuging the samples at 1200 g for 5 minutes is recommended prior to testing the skim portion. For pasteurized and other dairy products, refer to general sample preparation and test validation procedure for Charm II® test analysis.

9. **Procedure:** Establish a control point by testing positive control 6 times. Average results. Multiply the average by 1.25. All 6 tests should be less than the control point. If not, repeat determination. Determine a negative average by testing zero control 3 times. Average results. Test positive and negative control daily. Negative control should be ± 30% of average, and positive should be less than the control point. If these conditions are met, establishing the control point and averaging the results need only be done with each new lot. If conditions are not met, recalibrate equipment and redo control point and average.

   Label test tube for each sample. Add 1 white tablet to each. Add 300 μL of water to each tube. Break up tablets in tubes by mixing 10 times for 10 seconds each in rise and fall motion on vortex. Dilute milk sample 1 part sample plus 9 parts zero control standard (ZCS). Mix well. Draw 5.0 mL of diluted sample (using new pipet tip for each sample) and add to labeled tube. Add orange tablet to each tube. Mix 20 times for 20 seconds each in rise and fall motion on vortex mixer. Incubate tubes for 3 minutes at 35° ± 2°C. Remove tubes and centrifuge for 5 minutes.

   Pour off milk. While still draining tubes, remove fat ring with 2 or more cotton swabs. Continue until dry. Do not touch pellet. Using water pipet, add 300 μL of water to tubes and break up pellets using mixer. Pellets must be completely suspended. Add 3 mL of scintillation fluid to each tube, cap, and vortex to mix. Count tubes on scintillation counter for 1 minute using (^3H) channel.

10. **Expression of Results:** Record the CPM for each sample. Record the positive and negative control CPM.

11. **Precision and Performance Parameters:** Contact the AOAC International Research Institute and manufacturer's operator's manual for information on performance parameters. FDA has accepted the modification to the sample preparation to test more closely to the increased tolerance levels for drugs in this family.[3]

12. **Test Report and Interpretation:** If the CPM of the sample is greater than the control point, the sample is negative and should be reported as *not found for tetracycline*. If the CPM is less than or equal to the control point, the sample is positive.

    Test reports should show the test date, test site, date sampled, analyst initials, and temperature control information.

12.080 Chloramphenicol Assays

12.081 *Charm II® Chloramphenicol Assay (Class A4)*

1. **Scope:** This method is applicable to raw whole bovine milk. This test has been accepted by the FDA for use in monitoring milk for residues of chloramphenicol at or below 1 ppb.

2. **References:** See 12.041.

   FDA 2400 forms for laboratory evaluation and approval for detecting chloramphenicol: 1995 and later.

3. **Definition:** This assay tests for chloramphenicol and similar antibiotics.

4. **Principle:** A binding reagent containing antibodies to the chloramphenicol family of drugs is added to a milk sample. If the sample contains amphenicols, the drug binds to the antibodies. When labeled ^{3}H chloramphenicol is then added to the sample, it is prevented from binding to these sites. Unbound ^{3}H chloramphenicol is then absorbed onto charcoal. The more ^{3}H chloramphenicol is then bound and left in solution, the less amphenicols there are in the sample. The amount of ^{3}H left in solution is measured with a Charm II® analyzer.

5. **Reagents**
   1. Tableted reagents for chloramphenicol and other amphenicols.
   2. Zero control standard.
   3. Multiantimicrobial standard containing 1 ppb chloramphenciol (positive control).
   4. Optifluor scintillation fluid.

6. **Apparatus and Glassware**
   1. Charm Analyzer (6000 or 6600).
   2. Pipet: 1.0 mL, fixed-volume.
   3. Dispenser: 3.0 mL.
   4. 13- × 100-mL test tubes, borosilicate glass, disposable, with 13-mm caps.
   5. Vortex mixer.
   6. Pipet: 300 µL.
   7. Centrifuge capable of 1200 g.
   8. Timer.
   9. Test tube rack

7. **Sampling:** Observe precautions for handling of exempt quantities of radioactive chemicals. Exercise extreme caution when handling chloramphenicol (tablets or solutions).
8. **Preparation of Test Sample:** Remove test portion within 3 minutes of sample agitation.
9. **Procedure:** Establish control point by testing 6 replicates of the positive control standard. Average results and add 25%. All 6 assays should be within 25% of this average. Test 3 replicates of the zero milk (negative control) and average. This must be above the highest value contributing to the positive control average. Label each test tube and add 1 white tablet to each tube. Add 300 µL of water to each tube and mix 10 seconds on vortex to break up tablet. Add 1.0 ± 0.05 mL of sample to each tube using a new tip for each sample. Milk temperature is to be at 4.0° ± 2°C. Mix tubes up and down on vortex mixer 10 times.

   Add black tablet and immediately mix up and down 10 times on vortex. Place tubes in ice bath (50% ice, 50% water) for 3 minutes. Centrifuge at 1200 g for 5 minutes. After centrifugation, remove tubes carefully and place in test tube rack. Carefully transfer 300 µL of skim portion (from below fat layer) to clean test tube without disturbing pellet. Discard test tubes containing remaining milk and pellet.

   Add 3.0 ± 0.5 mL scintillation fluid to the skim portion in the tube. Cap and invert (or shake) until mixture has uniform cloudy appearance. Count in analyzer for 60 seconds on (^3H) channel. Analyze positive and negative control samples daily. Values for negatives must agree with those established in the original test kit check. Values for positive control must be within 25% of control point.
10. **Expression of Results:** Results are in CPM values. Record the PM for each sample and for the positive and negative controls.
11. **Precision and Performance Parameters:** Validated to detect less than 1.0 ppb chloramphenicol; consult operator's manual for other performance information.
12. **Test Report and Interpretation:** If the sample CPM is greater than the control point, the sample is negative and reported as *not found for chloramphenicol.* If the sample CPM is less than or equal to the control point, the sample is positive. If the CPM is less than 50 points above the control point, the tube should be recounted. If the recount is above the control point, the sample is negative. If the recount is less than or equal to the control point, the sample is positive.

    Test reports should show test type, test site, sample date, test date, analyst initials, results, and appropriate temperature control information.

12.090 High-Performance Liquid Chromatography (HPLC)

Most of the tests available for testing milk for the presence of drug residues are screening tests that provide only a presence/absence determination. In some instances, more information may be required. HPLC methods to confirm the presence and identify the specific beta lactams in milk are available.[11-17,21-23] At least 2 methods have been used successfully. One method, typically referred to as the Moats method, is currently the method of choice for the FDA. A newer method, the Boison method, is receiving extensive evaluation by FDA and is viewed favorably by the agency at this time. At least one other method (Charm Sciences HPLC Recptogram) has been used successfully by laboratories doing identification work. Estimates of concentration of the residue(s) are possible with either method, but a number of other factors need to be considered when these data are examined. At present, it is not acceptable to identify the residue, determine a concentration, and use the level to accept or reject a positive sample based on the limit for the residue. A method to identify both the specific residue (out of the 6 legal beta lactam drugs for lactating cows in the U.S.) and also a concentration of the residue with one analysis is not currently available. Generally, HPLC analysis is used to provide identification of the positive residue in the belief that this additional information will be helpful in avoiding future similar incidents.

12.100 Assays for Other Inhibitors

There are a number of quick tests available for screening milk for other drug families or specific drugs within a family. These test are generally modifications of the tests described above and do not require additional equipment. Results from these tests are qualitative in nature and do not have official status in the U.S. Information obtained from these assays may be useful for testing individual cows or tanks, but results should be viewed as information only.

Some residues for which tests may be performed are Macrolides, Gentamicin, (Aminoglycosides), Streptomycin, and Novobiocin. Generally, these tests are positive or negative in nature and have sensitivities at or below the tolerance for a specific drug or family.

12.110 Cited References

1. ARRET, B.; KIRSHBAUM, A. A Rapid disc assay method for detecting penicillin in milk. J. Milk Food Technol. **22:** 329-331;1959.
2. CERNY, J.; MORRIS, R.I. A modified disc assay method for detecting antibiotics in milk. J. Milk Food Technol. **18:** 281-283;1953.
3. CHARM, S.E.; CHI, R.K. Microbial receptor assay for rapid detection and identification of seven families of antimicrobial drugs in milk: collaborative study. JAOAC **71:** 304-316; 1988.
4. CHARM, S.E.; CHI, R.K., Rapid screening assays for beta lactam antibiotics in milk: collaborative study. JAOAC **65:**1186-1192; 1982.
5. FRERE, J.M.; KLEIN, D.; GHUYSON, J.M. Enzymatic method for rapid and sensitive determination of beta lactam antibiotics. Antimicrobial. Agents Chemother. **18:** 506-510; 1980.
6. GINN, R.E.; CASE, R.A.; PACKARD, V.S.; TATINI, S.R. Quantitative assay of beta lactam residues in raw milk using a disc assay method. J. Food Prot. **45:** 571-573; 1982.
7. GINN, R.E.; CASE, R.A.; PACKARD, V.S.; TATINI, S.R. Quantitative estimates of beta lactam residues in raw milk around a reference standard: collaborative study. JAOAC **65:** 1407-1412; 1982.
8. IGARASHI, R.T., BAUGHMAN, R.W., NELSON, F.E., HARTMAN, P.A. Rapid antibiotic assay methods using *Bacillus stearothermophillus*. J. Milk Food Technol. **34:** 143-146; 1961.
9. KNIGHT, A.H.; SHAPTON, N.; PRENTICE, G.A. Collaborative trail of the Penzyme assay: a rapid method for the detection of beta lactam antibiotic compounds in the fluid milk supply of New York state. J. Dairy Technol. **40:** 30-33; 1987.

10. MESSER, J.W.; LESLIE, J.E.; HOUGHTBY, G.A.; PELLER, J.T.; BARNETT, J.E. *Bacillus stearothermophillus* disc assay for detection of inhibitors in milk: collaborative study. JAOAC **65:** 1208-1214; 1982.
11. MOATS, W.A.; HARIK-KHAN, R. Rapid HPLC determination of tetracycline antibiotics in milk. Agri. and Food Chem. **43:** 931-934; 1995.
12. MOATS, W.A. Determination of Cephapirin and Desacetylcephapirin in milk using automated liquid chromatographic cleanup and ion-pairing liquid chromatography. JAOAC **76:** 535-540; 1993.
13. MOATS, W.A. Determination of lincomycin and lincomycin in milk and tissues by reversed-phase liquid chromatography. J. Agri. and Food Chem. **39:** 1812-1816; 1991.
14. MOATS, W.A. Determination of penicillin G in milk by high-perfromance liquid chromatography with automated liquid chomatographic clean-up. J. Chromatography. **507:** 177-185; 1990.
15. MOATS, W.A.; HARIK-KHAN, R. Rapid HPLC determination of tetracycline antibiotics in milk. J.Agri. and Food Chem. **43:** 931-934; 1995.
16. MOATS, W.A. Determination of ampicillin and amoxicillin in milk with an automated liquid chromatographic clean-up. JAOAC **77:** 41-45; 1994.
17. MOATS, W.A.; HARIK-KHAN, R. Liquid chromatographic determination of beta lactam antibiotics in milk: a multi-residue approach. JAOAC **78:** 49-54; 1995.
18. PARKS, O.W., DOAN, F.J. Sensitivities of the disc assay and triphenyltetrazolium methods for antibiotics in milk. J. Milk Food Technol. **22:** 74-76; 1959.
19. WEBER, J.D.; SMEDLY, M.D. Liquid chromatographic determiniation of sulfamethazine in milk. JAOAC **72:** 445; 1989.
20. ZOMER, et al. HPLC receptogram: a method for confirmation and identification of antimicrobial drugs by using liquid chromatography with microbial receptor assay, 1. sulfonamides in milk. JAOAC 987-993; 1992.
21. ZOMER, et al. LC receptogram: A method for confirmation and identification of antimicrobial drugs by using liquid chromatography with microbial receptor assay 1. Sulfonamides in milk. JAOAC **75:**8; 1992.
22. ZOMER, et al. HPLC receptogram: A method for identification and quantitation of beta lactams in milk by liquid chromatography with microbial receptor assay. JAOAC **78:** 5; 1995.
23. ZOMER, E.; QUINTANA, J.; SCHEEMAKER, J.; SAUL, S.; CHARM, S.E. High-performance liquid chromatography-receptogram: A comprehensive method for identification of veterinary drugs and their active metabolites. In: *Veterinary drug residues*. Washington, DC: American Chemical Society; 1996.

Chapter 13

Microbiological Tests for Equipment, Containers, Water, and Air

R. L. Dyer, J. F. Frank, B. Johnson, and P. Hickey
(J. Fitts, Tech. Comm.)

13.010 Introduction

Plant hygiene and product safety are of critical importance to dairy manufacturers. Sources of the microorganisms that may deposit onto equipment surfaces and containers include air, water, manufacturing activities, waste, and personnel. The relative importance of these sources will vary with each situation. The significance of any deposition that occurs will be influenced by both the numbers and the variety of organisms. The inside of closed cooling systems and the outside of milk containers and crates have been shown to support the growth and survival of pathogenic microorganisms, as have drains, floors, and food contact surfaces.[5,13,16,17,32,39,48,54]

Microbiological monitoring programs for the environment may be designed and carried out to minimize the risk of product contamination. For example, a priority rating system may be established with critical and noncritical zones or sampling sites. Critical priority rating refers to equipment near the product or critical environmental points situated near the production line where there is a high potential risk for heat-treated products to be contaminated. Noncritical priority rating refers to sites close to the production line where the risk of direct contamination of heat-treated products is low. These sites include warehouse and storage areas.

13.020 Tests for the Microbiological Quality of Air

Microorganisms are carried in air on dust particles, on water droplets, and as dehydrated clumps or single cells. Microbial aerosols originate from floor drains, worker activity, water spraying, air conditioning systems, and air movement over dusty surfaces. Microbial contamination from air may limit the shelf life of pasteurized and cultured products[10] and may add to the total microflora of products in which air is used as a processing aid (ice cream and dairy powders), or that have postprocess exposure to air before packaging.[24] Aseptic packaging systems require a source of high-quality air.

The microbiological quality of air is controlled by limiting the aerosol forming practices of personnel, maintaining a clean processing environment, and installing and maintaining an appropriate air handling system. Testing the microbiological quality of air can be used to determine if acceptable control over these factors has been achieved. There are no standards for acceptable microbiological content of air in dairy processing facilities, so interpretation of results should be based on historical data. Limited survey data of microbial aerosols in dairy processing facilities have been published.[41-43]

13.021 *Selection of Method*

There are no standardized methods for determining viable particles in the air of dairy processing facilities. Methods that have been successfully used are based on sedimentation, impaction on solid surfaces, or impingement in liquid.[27] Sedimentation relies on particles settling onto the surface of an agar plate. Results are greatly influenced by particle size and weight, as only large viable particles (>10 µm diameter) will settle onto the agar surface, with smaller particles detected on a random basis depending on air flow. Viable particle counts obtained by sedimentation have, at best, only weak correlation with counts determined by other more quantitative methods.[40]

Impaction methods collect particles by directing air over an agar surface so that particles collide and stick to the surface. The air can be forced through a sieve or series of sieves placed over agar plates or through a slit under which an agar plate is rotated. These devices employ a vacuum pump. Centrifugal air samplers use a spinning rotor to propel particles onto an agar strip or plate.[44] In either case, the amount of air flowing over the agar is controlled so that viable particles per volume of air can be calculated. Impaction methods provide high recovery because the microorganisms are collected with minimal stress. However, some centrifugal samplers do not generate sufficient force to efficiently collect small particles. For all impaction samplers, if large volumes of air must be sampled, the agar surface will dehydrate, reducing collection efficiency and inhibiting colony development. To overcome this problem, cover the poured media with a monolayer of oxyethylene docosanol.[34] Allow the surface of agar to dry, then pour onto it a sterile emulsion of 0.2% oxyethylene docosanol. The emulsion may be poured from plate to plate. Excess emulsion should be allowed to drain from the plate for a few seconds. Although this treatment reduces drying during impactions sampling, it does not significantly reduce the rate of evaporation during storage in static air.[23]

Impinger methods use a liquid to collect the particles. An air jet is directed at the liquid surface where the air and liquid mix, resulting in entrapment of the particles in the liquid. Liquids used may be buffers, salt, or nutrient solutions. Antifoam or antifreeze agents may need to be added if long sampling times are employed. Microorganisms collected by the impinger are quantified by plating the fluid on appropriate solid media. High-velocity air impingers provide efficient recovery of small particles, but the forces involved in collection may injure vegetative cells, resulting in low counts, or break up clumps of cells, producing a high count. Glass impingers break easily and should be used with caution in food processing plants.

The viability and number of microorganisms in air is influenced by temperature, relative humidity, and light. Consequently, results may reflect factors not related to plant sanitation practices. Use of selective media for bacteria is not recommended as many vegetative cells are sublethally injured upon collection and will lack the ability to form colonies on these media.[28] Therefore, the use of selective media will underestimate the true microbiological content of the air.

13.022 *Agar Plate Preparation*

Using procedures described for SPC [chapter 6], for psychrotroph counts [chapter 8], or for yeast and mold count [chapter 8], aseptically pour 10- to 12-mL portions of sterilized, tempered (45° ± 1°C) agar into sterile petri plates. Replace covers and allow the agar to solidify on a level surface. Hold plates at 2° to 7°C under conditions that minimize dehydration of the agar. These plates can be used for sedimentation or impaction methods.

13.023 *Sedimentation Method*[37] *(Class O)*

Set the agar plate on a new paper towel or parchment paper on a flat surface at the location where air is to be sampled. SMA [6.020] or antibiotic supplemented agar [8.110] is generally used. Expose the agar by removing the plate cover and, without inversion, placing it on the paper beside the bottom of the petri plate. After exposing the agar medium for 15 minutes, replace the cover and incubate the plate according to the appropriate procedure. Count colonies and express results as colonies per square meter or square foot per minute. Because a standard plastic petri plate bottom is approximately 60 cm^2, the number of colonies divided by 60 gives the estimated count per square centimeter.

13.024 *Impaction onto Agar*[1,2,6,14,29] *(Class B)*

Various commercial samplers are available (Andersen Instruments, Inc., Atlanta, GA; Biotest Diagnostics Corp., Denville, NJ; Pool Bioanalysis Italiana, Milano, Italy). For information on selection of a specific design see Griffiths and DeCosemo.[20] Use each instrument according to manufacturers' directions, with particular attention to airflow rate and placement of the device. Sample volumes should be adjusted to account for expected contamination level.

13.025 *Liquid Impingement*[12] *(Class B)*

The AGI-30 (Ace Glass, Inc., Vineland, NJ) was designated the standard for aerosol collection by the First International Symposium on Aerobiology in 1963.[20] Connect the impinger to a vacuum pump using adequate tubing. Adjust the airflow rate as specified for the unit. Remove unit; add sterile, buffered MS water that contains silicon antifoam; and sterilize. There should be a 30-mm gap between the impinger orifice and the collection liquid. Connect the impinger to the suction tube and sample for 0.5 hours. Collection time may be adjusted in accordance with the number of microorganisms expected in the air. Prepare dilutions and plate, and incubate as previously described [chapters 6, 7, and 8]. Count colonies and record as viable particles per volume of air.

13.030 Tests for Water Supplies

To be suitable for use in dairy operations, water must be of a safe, sanitary quality and practically free of microorganisms that could initiate product spoilage. Spoilage of refrigerated milk and milk products has been caused by contamination with waterborne organisms (primarily psychrotrophs).[53] This contamination occurs either directly, through product contact with the water itself (e.g., by milk traversing a surface that was freshly rinsed with water, or by cheese curd or butter having been washed in water), or indirectly, by microbes growing on nutrient residues on incompletely cleaned equipment surfaces. Because most of the microorganisms in water are destroyed by chlorination or heat, many plants treat water to keep spoilage at a minimum.

Procedures to sample and test water supplies for the presence of coliform organisms by the multiple tube fermentation, membrane filter, and presence absence methods are presented in the 20th edition of *Standard Methods for the Examination of Water and Wastewater.*[11] This volume also contains useful information regarding the heterotrophic plate count (HPC) using pour plate, spread plate, and membrane filter methods and tests for pathogenic organisms. Information regarding the numbers of organisms developing at various incubation temperatures is helpful in classifying untreated waters and in assaying the efficiency of treatment procedures. The HPC also provides a means for measuring potential bacterial interference with coliform recovery.

Refer also to the latest FDA Milk Laboratory Evaluation 2400 Series Form.[51]

13.040 Tests for Equipment and Containers

13.041 *Rinse Solution Methods*

1. **Scope:** This method is applicable to firm-walled uncapped items, flexible-walled items, individual items of equipment, and CIP assemblies.
2. **References:** Chapter 2: Laboratory Quality Assurance.
   Chapter 3: Sampling Dairy and Related Products.
   Chapter 4: Media and Reagent Preparation.
   Chapter 7: Coliform and Other Indicator Bacteria.
   Chapter 8: Tests for Groups of Microorganisms.
3. **Definition:** This method allows for the enumeration of microorganisms on the surface of containers and various types of equipment.
4. **Principle:** The effectiveness of cleaning and sanitizing containers and equipment is assessed by repeatedly flushing a measured volume of sterile, buffered sanitizer-neutralizing solution or nutrient broth over the product contact surface and then determining the bacterial population of

the rinse solution by plating or membrane filter techniques.[11] Large equipment assemblies can be checked by circulating water that has been either chlorinated and neutralized, or sterilized by membrane filtration.[33] The increase in the bacterial population is determined by membrane filter techniques.[11] Sanitation of assemblies may also be checked by sampling milk at successive points of access along the processing lines.[47]

5. **Reagents**
   A. **Media:** Standard methods agar (SMA) [chapter 4], violet red bile agar [chapter 4], m-Endo broth MF or m-Coliform broth or equivalent [chapter 7].
   B. **Stock phosphate solution:** [chapter 4].
   C. **Rinse solution:** *Sterile:* Add 1.25 mL of stock phosphate solution, 5 mL of 10% aqueous sodium thiosulfate, 4 g of Azolectin (Associated Concentrates, 32-60 61st St., Woodside, NY 11377), and 10 g of Tween 20 (monolaurate; Sigma Chemical Co., P.O. Box 14508, St. Louis, MO 63178-9916) to MS water and make to 1 L. Adjust to pH 7.2 and dispense sufficient quantities into screw-capped vials made up to contain 20 mL, 50 mL, 100 mL, or other suitable volumes following sterilization. Azolectin is hygroscopic and should be stored in a desiccator. Weigh the Azolectin and rapidly dissolve it by heating it over boiling water.

      Nutrient broth (available commercially) may be used for the testing of containers.[55]
   D. **Rinse water for large-volume rinsing of cleaned-in-place (CIP) equipment:** Large volumes of water may be treated or sanitized by chlorinating to a residual concentration of 25 mg/L and holding for 10 minutes, and then neutralized by adding an excess of 10% sodium thiosulfate solution.

      Tap water may also be sterilized by membrane filtration followed by the addition of sodium thiosulfate (1 mL of 10% solution per liter of water) to inactivate the residual disinfectant.[33]
   E. **Sodium thiosulfate solution, 10%:** Dissolve 100 g of sodium thiosulfate in MS water and make up to 1 L. Filter and store in the refrigerator in a dark place or in an amber bottle.
   F. **Ethyl alcohol, 70%.**

6. **Apparatus and Glassware**
   A. Petri dishes: Sterile [chapter 2].
   B. Transfer pipets: Sterile [chapter 2].
   C. Hypodermic syringe and needles: Sterile.

7. **Sampling:** Sample containers shall be obtained as directed in chapter 3. For 1-L or smaller containers, aseptically introduce 20 mL of rinse solution [13.041.5.D] into each container; for 1.89-L containers, use 50 mL; and for 3.78-L or larger containers, use 100 mL.

8. **Preparation of Test Sample:** See 13.041.9.

9. **Procedure**
   A. **Firm-walled uncapped items:** Swab a portion of the side surface of the containers with 70% ethanol; aseptically fill a sterile hypodermic

syringe with sterile, buffered rinse solution; and inject the solution into the container. Aseptically apply a piece of cellophane tape to cover the area punctured by the needle. Proceed as in section 13.041.9.B.

B. **Shaking firm-walled containers:** Grasp the container firmly with its long axis in a horizontal position. Shake vigorously 10 times, each shake being a to-and-return thrust of about 20 cm. Turn the container 90° and repeat the horizontal shaking treatment; turn the container 90° twice more, repeating the horizontal shaking treatment each time. Grasp the container by the neck and swirl it vigorously 20 times in a small circle with its long axis in a vertical position, then invert and repeat. Stand the container upright for 1 minute before removing the sample.

C. **Flexible-walled items:** Swab all caps on fill tubes of collapsed liners with a soft paper towel moistened with 70% ethanol, then remove and aseptically introduce the required amount of buffered rinse solution [13.041.5.C] with a sterile pipet. Where tubes are sealed, swab an area of the tube adjacent to the liner with 70% ethanol and introduce the rinse solution with a sterile hypodermic syringe. Apply cellophane tape to the puncture area.

   Arrange the collapsed liner on a smooth, clean, firm horizontal surface as flat as its construction permits. With hands or a roller, work the rinse solution back and forth 10 times so that it contacts all interior surfaces completely. Lift the liner and hang it with the fill tube down. Place the fill tube over a sterile container. Transfer the rinse solution to the sterile container by cutting the fill tube with sterile scissors.

D. **Equipment assemblies:** The rinse solution method may be used on individual items of equipment or on hookups designed for cleaning in place [chapter 3]. Obtain a control (approximately 1 L) of treated rinse water [13.041.5.D] before rinsing. Add a sufficient volume of this water to a storage vat or tank at the upstream end of the assembly and then pump it or allow it to flow by gravity through the assembly. Collect samples at the equipment's point of discharge from the first, middle, and final portions of rinse water. Samples may also be collected at various points throughout the assembly.

E. **Plating rinse solutions and counting plates**

   1. **Container sample measurements:** For 236-mL containers, distribute 5 mL of the rinse solution equally between 2 sterile petri dishes. For all larger containers, place 2 mL of the rinse solution in a single plate. Pour 15 to 20 mL of SMA into each plate. Incubate the plates at 32°C for 48 ± 3 hours and count all colonies. To calculate the residual bacterial count (RBC) per specified container capacity, multiply the total number of colonies by the volume of the rinse solution divided by the volume of the sample plated. For example, if the volume of rinse is 20 mL, the volume of sample plated is 5 mL, and the number of colonies is 10, the RBC is $10 \times (20 \div 5) = 40$.

      Determine the numbers of coliforms in rinse solutions by dividing 10 mL of rinse solution among 3 plates and culturing [chapter 7]. To calculate the coliform count per specified size of container, multiply the number of coliform colonies by the volume of rinse solution divided by the volume of the sample plated. Membrane filter procedures[11] may also be used with the rinse solutions to enumerate coliforms, fecal coliforms, and fecal streptococci. Yeasts, molds, proteolytic bacteria, or other specific microorganisms may be determined similarly by using appropriate differential media and incubation temperatures and times [chapter 8].

2. **Equipment samples (Class B):** All rinse solutions that are obtained from CIP systems or processing assemblies and control samples require the use of the membrane filter procedure[11] for analysis. Average the yields of rinse samples taken at the beginning, middle, and end of drainage, and subtract the yield (if any) of the control samples. The result is the corrected yield. Calculate the ratio of the sample volume to the rinse volume and multiply by the corrected yield to obtain an indication of the numbers of organisms present in the entire system. The presence of specific types of organisms can be determined by using appropriate differential media and incubation conditions (e.g., m-Endo medium would be used for coliform counts).[11]

F. **Screening method (nutrient broth modification) for retail milk containers (Class O):** Plates poured from 3 containers, using either rinse solution or nutrient broth, sometimes yield no colonies. To determine the frequency with which such containers are encountered, a large number of samples must be examined. Inoculate 20-mL portions of nutrient broth into 50 containers and shake them to rinse their surfaces thoroughly. It is preferable to incubate the containers at 32°C; otherwise, room temperature is acceptable. After 48 hours, note the percentage of containers with turbid broth, an indication of bacterial growth. Calculate the percentage of containers exhibiting growth.

G. **In-line processing samples (Class O):** Milk samples obtained from points along processing lines may be plated directly to determine where significant changes in counts occur. The presence of psychrotrophic bacteria may be determined by incubating milk samples at 7°C for 5 days and then replating [8.010]. A substantial increase in count indicates the presence of psychrotrophs. Points of entry of other types of microorganisms can be determined by plating with appropriate selective media.

10. **Expression of Results:** Report computed bacterial count as residual bacterial count (RBC)/specified container capacity in mL.

    Report computed coliform count as residual coliform count (RCC)/container.

11. **Precision Parameters:** No precision parameters have been determined for this method.

13.042 *Disintegration Method (Class O)*

1. **Scope:** The disintegration method is applicable to paper, paperboard, or molded pulp items in intermediate or complete stages of conversion. Except as noted below, the method is not applicable to items fabricated

from plastic, dry or wet-waxed paper, metal, or combinations of these materials where the plastic or metal is the food-contacting surface. For these latter items, the rinse or swab method should be used. Microbiological tests with paperboard that is laminated or coated with foil or plastic may be performed if the paperboard is cut into pieces 6 mm^2 or smaller before blending [13.042.9].[38,55]

2. **References:** Chapter 2: Laboratory Quality Assurance.
   Chapter 3: Sampling Dairy and Related Products.
   Chapter 4: Media and Reagent Preparation.
   Chapter 6: Microbiological Count Methods.
3. **Definition:** This method allows for the enumeration of microorganisms in raw materials used to manufacture containers of certain types, such as paperboard milk cartons.
4. **Principle:** The purity of packaging materials is determined by dividing the material into small pieces, blending those pieces with sterile dilution water, and plating portions of the water.
5. **Reagents**
   1. Plating medium: SMA [chapter 4].
   2. Phosphate dilution water: Sterile [chapter 4].
6. **Apparatus and Glassware**
   1. Pipets: Sterile, capacity 10 mL, with tip opening cut to about 3 mm for the passage of pulp. A 20-mL large-bore pipet is preferable for plating paper pulp [chapter 2].
   2. Petri dishes: Sterile [chapter 2].
   3. Scalpels or scissors: Sterile.
   4. Forceps: Sterile.
   5. Balance [chapter 2].
   6. Kraft paper or envelopes: Sterile, for protecting samples in transit to laboratory.
   7. Disintegrator blender: Sterile interior, high speed, electrically operated, with corrosion-resistant metal (preferably stainless steel) or glass cup (preferably with a screw cover), capacity about 500 to 1000 mL.
7. **Sampling:** See chapter 3.
8. **Preparation of Test Sample:** With a sterile scalpel or other sterile cutting device, cut representative portions of at least 10 g from rolls of paper or paperboard, sheeted stock, nested containers, blanks, or closure discs. With sterile forceps, transfer the cut portions to sterile Kraft wrappers or envelopes. Also using sterile forceps, place bottle caps, hoods, and other similar closures directly into sterile envelopes. Protect the samples from moisture or other contamination during transit to the laboratory. Because some papers contain few bacteria, take great precautions to avoid dust or other contamination of samples.
9. **Procedure:** With sterile scissors, cut the middle portion of the sample sheet into pieces (maximal size 1.3 cm) and collect the pieces in a sterile petri dish. Using sterile forceps to handle the stock, weigh 3.0 g of the sample directly into a sterile petri dish. Put 300 mL of sterile, phosphat-

ed dilution water into a large sterile mixer cup, add 3.0 g of paper, and recover the mixer. In larger cups, use 500-mL portions of sterile, phosphated dilution water and 5.0 g of paper. Place the cup on the blender-driving mechanism and operate at high speed so that the total time of operation does not exceed 2 minutes. The time of operation will depend on the type of paper, however, and some grades of paper may require further blending. After 30 seconds of high-speed operation, stop the machine. By revolving the cup at a slight angle, rinse all pieces of paper or paperboard from the cup walls into the water. Resume disintegration at high speed, but re-examine the interior at intervals to be sure that no pieces of material that have not been disintegrated remain on the sides of the cup.

With a sterile 10- or 20-mL pipet having a large bore at the tip, divide 10 mL of the paper or paperboard suspension (representing 0.1 g of disintegrated stock) approximately equally among 3 sterile petri dishes. Pour with 15 to 20 mL SMA, incubate plates at 32° ± 1°C for 48 ± 3 hours, and count colonies [6.020]. When introducing the medium, rotate the plate so that the medium is thoroughly mixed with the disintegrated paper or paperboard. When board that contains secondary stock is being analyzed, higher dilutions are usually required. Optionally, use 5 instead of 3 plates per sample.

The procedure to test for coliforms is outlined in the *Manual of Recommended Laboratory Methods for Sampling and Microbiological Testing of Single-Service Food Packages and Their Components.*[38]

10. **Expression of Results:** Multiply the sum of the colonies developing on 3 or 5 plates from 0.1 g of paper or paperboard stock by 10 and report the result as the number of colonies per gram of stock. A specification of not more than 250 colonies per gram has also been established.[51] This is calculated as the logarithmic average of plate counts of the last 4 analyses.
11. **Performance Parameters:** No precision parameters have been determined for this method.

13.043 *Surface Contact Methods*

For the microbiological examination of surfaces, the replicate organism direct agar contact (RODAC) procedure, the Petrifilm™ aerobic count (PAC) plate procedure, the swab procedure, and the ATP bioluminescence procedure are the methods of choice. The swab technique, including the ATP bioluminescence procedure, should be used for surfaces with cracks, corners, or crevices—areas of such dimensions that the swab is more effective at recovering microorganisms. The RODAC and Petrifilm™ procedures are better used on flat surfaces such as walls, floors, ceilings, and some equipment surfaces. Selection of the proper technique is essential for meaningful results.[18]

13.044 *RODAC Plate (Agar Contact) Method*[4,7,21,46,52] *(Class O)*

The RODAC plate method provides a simple agar contact tool for sampling surfaces. It is of value in estimating the sanitary quality of surfaces encountered in food-processing plants. Comparative studies[4] have indicated that the mean percent recovery of aerosolized *Bacillus subtilis* spores from stainless steel surfaces is 47% for the swab contact method and 41% for the RODAC plate method. Results for the RODAC plate method, however, are more reproducible than those for the swab technique. Studies[46] with food contact surfaces that are naturally contaminated with a mixed flora and sanitized by food service personnel have shown higher recoveries with the RODAC procedure than with the swab contact procedure, possibly owing to bacterial retention in swab fibers. The RODAC plate method is particularly recommended when quantitative data are sought from flat, nonporous surfaces. It should not be used for porous, creviced, or irregular surfaces.

Product contact surfaces amenable to RODAC sampling necessarily will be flat and nonporous and thus relatively easy to clean and disinfect. Other environmental surfaces, such as floors, are more likely to be heavily contaminated. In either event, a sufficient number of spots should be sampled to obtain representative data.

1. **Scope:** This method is applicable to flat, nonporous food contact surfaces and clean environmental surfaces.
2. **References:** Not applicable.
3. **Definition:** This method allows for the enumeration of microorganisms on the tested surface.
4. **Principle:** Microorganisms on the test surface are transferred to an agar plate by bringing the agar plate into direct contact with the surface and then incubating the plate and enumerating the resulting colonies.
5. **Reagents:** Disposable plastic RODAC plates may be filled in the laboratory or purchased prefilled with test medium. They should be prepared with 15.5 to 16.5 mL of SMA, and the meniscus of the agar should rise above the rim of the plate. When surfaces to be sampled have been subjected to germicidal treatment, incorporate the appropriate neutralizers into the medium. Use 0.5% polysorbate (Tween 80) to neutralize substituted phenolic disinfectants and 0.07% soy lecithin to neutralize quaternary ammonium compounds. Dey-Engley medium may also be used as it contains a variety of ingredients able to neutralize germicides that are likely to be used on surfaces. [15]

   If qualitative data on different types of microorganisms are sought, selective media may be used, or, preferably, colonies should be transferred to selective media from the original broad-spectrum medium. Following preparation, plates should be incubated at 32° ± 1°C for 18 to 24 hours as a sterility check. They should then be used within the succeeding 12 hours unless appropriately wrapped and refrigerated to retard dehydration.
6. **Sampling:** See applicable sections in chapter 3 and in the bibliography.[8,49]
7. **Preparation of Test Sample:** See 13.044.9.
8. **Procedure:** Remove the plastic cover and carefully press the agar surface to the surface being sampled. Make certain the entire agar meniscus touches the surface, and use a rolling uniform pressure on the back of the

plate to effect contact. Replace the cover and incubate the plate in an inverted position for 24 to 48 hours at 32°C. When heavy contamination is present, incubate for 24 hours to prevent overgrowth. When contamination is light, 48 hours should be allowed for growth of colonies.

9. **Expression of Results:** Count colonies and record as either the number of colonies per RODAC plate or the number of colonies per square centimeter.

10. **Precision and Performance Parameters:** No precision parameters have been determined for this method.

13.045 *Swab Contact Method (Class O)*

1. **Scope:** This method is applicable to food contact surfaces, including those that are not smooth or readily accessible.
2. **References:** Chapter 2: Laboratory Quality Assurance and Safety.
   Chapter 7: Coliform and Other Indicator Bacteria.
3. **Definition:** This method allows for the enumeration of microorganisms on the surface of containers and various types of equipment.
4. **Principle:** The swab technique consists of taking a sterile swab moistened in an appropriate solution and brushing it over a measured surface area. The swab is then rinsed thoroughly in a measured amount of sterile solution, and the liquid is plated. Select areas for swabbing that appear to be unclean or difficult to clean. Equipment surfaces that are regular, smooth, ground, polished, large, or accessible are easier to clean than those that are irregular, rough-seamed, ridged, small, rounded on small radii, or less conveniently reached. If these latter areas are not properly cleaned, residues will accumulate and surfaces will not be sanitized when chemical solutions are applied.
5. **Reagents**
   A. **Screw-capped vials:** If insoluble swabs are used, dispense the rinse solution [13.045.5.C] in small, screw-capped vials (7 to 10 cm long) containing 5 mL of solution after autoclaving. If calcium alginate swabs are used, prepare vials with 4.5 mL of solution after autoclaving.
   B. **Insoluble swabs:** Sterile, nonabsorbent cotton or dacron,[26] firmly twisted to approximately 5 mm in diameter by 2 cm long over one end of a wooden applicator stick 12 to 15 cm long. Package as individuals or multiples in convenient, protective containers (glassine envelopes, test tubes, or vials) with swab heads away from the closure and autoclave. If toxicity of cotton swabs is suspected, autoclave a representative sample of swabs in MS water (5 mL per swab) at 121° for 15 minutes and perform a water quality test for MS water [chapter 2] to show the absence or presence of toxicity.
   C. **Calcium alginate swabs:** Swabs made of calcium alginate fibers[3,5,9,25,50] are soluble in aqueous solutions (rinse, culture media, etc.) containing 1% sodium hexametaphosphate, sodium glycerophosphate, or sodium citrate (not to be used with Petrifilm™). All organisms dislodged from swabbed surfaces are thus liberated.

D. **Solubilizing solution for calcium alginate swabs:** Prepare a 1% solution of sodium hexametaphosphate or other solubilizing compound and package it in appropriate vials and autoclave.

6. **Apparatus and Glassware:** Mechanical shaker: Optional.
7. **Sampling:** See applicable sections of chapter 3.
8. **Preparation of Test Sample:** See 13.044.4.
9. **Procedure:** At the laboratory, remove the vial from refrigerated storage. Shake it vigorously, making 50 complete cycles of 15 cm in 10 seconds, striking the palm of the other hand at the end of each cycle. Groups of vials may be put into appropriate racks and shaken manually, or they may be shaken mechanically for a time interval, as long as the cotton swab heads are treated similarly to the manual procedure. Plate 1 mL of rinse solution for the RBC. Plate additional decimal dilutions if deemed necessary. Pour plates with SMA, incubate, count colonies, and then calculate the number of colonies recovered from 50 cm^2 (equivalent to 1 mL of rinse).
10. **Expression of Results:** Divide the number of organisms in 1 mL of rinse by 50 and report the RBC as the number of organisms per square centimeter.

    For the residual coliform count (RCC), plate 3 mL of rinse solution and culture using one of the methods described in chapter 7. Report the RCC as the number of colonies counted (equivalent to the RCC per 150 cm^2; to determine the coliform count per square centimeter, divide by 150).

    Tests for other microorganisms may be determined similarly by using appropriate differential media and incubation temperatures and times.
11. **Precision and Performance Parameters:** No precision parameters have been determined for this method.

13.046 *Modified Swab for Flat Lids (Class O)*

Sample size is 35 lids. Use sterile forceps to remove lid from package. Aseptically remove sterile swab from container. Open vial containing 9 mL of sterile rinse solution [13.041.5.C], wet swab, and press out excess solution. Holding swab at a 30° angle to the surface, rub over entire food contact area. Repeat this process for remainder of lids using the same swab and vial of rinse solution. After swabbing all lids, position swab's head in vial and break the stick, leaving the head in the vial. Add 1 mL of sodium citrate [13.045.6.C] to vial, cap, and shake vigorously until swab dissolves. Transfer 2 mL of vial contents to each of 2 petri dishes. Pour 15 to 20 mL of SMA into one dish and 15 to 20 mL of VRB into the other dish. Overlay the VRB plate and incubate at 32° ± 1°C for 24 ± 2 hours. Count and confirm all colonies. Incubate the SMA plate at 32° ± 1°C for 48 ± 3 hours and count all colonies. To calculate counts determine food contact area of lid in square cm, multiply number of colonies on each plate by dilution factor 5 and divide by area of lid. Report plate count and coliform as number of colonies/sq.cm.

13.047 *Cellulose Sponge Method*[45] *(Class B)*

Food-processing equipment and other environmental surfaces may be sampled using the cellulose sponge swab technique. Retail sponges often contain bacterial inhibitors.[31]

Only sponges that are known to be free of inhibitors should be used. The sponge sample may be subjected to various analytical procedures such as the aerobic plate count or counts of coliforms, yeasts and molds, and pathogens (*Listeria, Salmonella, Staphylococcus* species, etc.). For quantitative analyses, add 50 to 100 mL of diluent to the bag containing the sponge. Then vigorously massage the sponge with the diluent for 1 minute or more. Remove portions of the diluent from the bag, plate on the desired medium, and incubate under appropriate conditions. Calculate the numbers of microorganisms per unit of surface area on the basis of the area swabbed, the amount of diluent used, and the size of the sample plated. For example, if 50 colonies are obtained from a 1-mL sample derived from a sponge in 100 mL of diluent that swabbed 1 m^2, the aerobic plate count per square meter will be 5,000.

Because of the large areas that can be sampled with the cellulose sponge, this technique is particularly useful in detecting salmonellae and *Listeria* on food plant equipment and in the environment. When testing for pathogens, introduce the sponge directly into the enrichment or preenrichment broth and proceed with the test procedure as described in chapter 5.

Cellulose sponges are cut into 5-cm^3 pieces, placed in individual Kraft paper bags and steam sterilized at 120° ± 1°C for 20 minutes. The sterile sponge is then removed from the bag using sterilized or sanitized crucible tongs and is moistened with 10 mL of phosphated rinse solution or 0.1% peptone water. A 1% solution of Tergitol Anionic-7 (Sigma Chemical Co.) should be used if test surfaces have visible residues of fat. Tergitol Anionic-7 should not be used in the absence of fat because of its possible deleterious effect on gram-positive bacteria.

Sterile or sanitized rubber or plastic gloves should be worn to handle the sponge. Use of disposable gloves with frequent changing during sample collection is recommended.

Sample the surface by vigorously rubbing the sponge over the designated area until the soil is removed. An area of several square meters may be efficiently swabbed. If the surface is flat, the rinse solution may be applied directly to the surface and then taken up into the sponge by the rubbing action. After sampling, introduce the sponge into a sterile plastic bag and transport it under refrigeration to the laboratory.

13.048 *ATP Bioluminescence-ATP Specific Luciferin/Luciferase Reaction*[35] *(Class B)*

Sampling and testing the environment or equipment on a preoperative basis for plate counts is not immediately useful due to the time required to obtain microbiological results. Generally, sites with unacceptable numbers or types of microorganisms are not identified prior to beginning production. The benefits of using the ATP bioluminescence method are that not only is the method rapid, sensitive, and simple, but swabbing is changed from being a retrospective exercise into a proactive measure. The use of ATP measurements as an index of microbial level and food residues is generally based on 3 premises: 1) All living organisms as well as some food residues contain ATP; 2) with highly purified reagents and a sensitive luminometer, ATP can be selectively measured in very low concentrations; and 3) intracellular concentrations of ATP are maintained in a constant range in all microorganisms.[30]

Various commercial systems are available. Instruments should be used according to the manufacturers' directions. Systems contain dilution buffer for washing of ATP from the applicator tip, a wetting agent to dislodge residue from the swabbed surface and release ATP from the sample, and luciferin/luciferase for the bioluminescent reaction that is then measured using a luminometer. Flowers et al.[19] provides comparative information on relative sensitivity and repeatability for the systems mentioned above.

13.050 Cited References

1. ANDERSEN, A.A. New sampler for the collection, sizing and enumeration of viable airborne particles. J. Bacteriol. **76:**471-484; 1958.
2. ANDERSEN, A.A.; ANDERSEN, M.R. A monitor for airborne bacteria. Appl. Microbiol. **10:**181-194; 1962.
3. ANGELOTTI, R.; FOTER, M.J.; BUSCH, K.A.; LEWIS, K.H. A comparative evaluation of methods for determining the bacterial contamination of surfaces. Food Res. **23:**175-185; 1958.
4. ANGELOTTI, R.; WILSON, J.L.; LITSKY, W.; WALTER, W.G. Comparative evaluation of the cotton swab and RODAC methods for the recovery of *Bacillus subtilis* spore contamination from stainless steel surfaces. Health Lab. Sci. **1:**289-296; 1964.
5. BARNES, J.M. The removal of bacteria from glass surfaces with calcium alginate, gauze and absorbent cotton-wool swabs. Proc. Soc. Appl. Bacteriol. **15:**34; 1952.
6. BENBOUGH, J.E.; BENNETT, A.M.; PARKES, S.R. Determination of the collection efficiency of a microbial air sampler. J. Appl. Bact. **74:**170-173; 1993.
7. BOND, R.G.; HALBERT, M.M.; KEENAN, K.M.; PUTNAM, H.D.; RUSCHMEYER, O.R.; VESLEY, D. Development of a method for microbial sampling of surfaces, with special reference to reliability. Final report under contract PH-86-62-182. Washington, DC: U.S. Dept. of Health, Education, and Welfare; 1963.
8. BUCHBINDER, L.; BUCK, T.C., JR.; PHELPS, P.M.; STONE, R.V.; TIEDEMAN, W.D. Investigations of the swab rinse technique for examining eating and drinking utensils. Amer. J. Public Health and the Nation's Health. **37:**373-378; 1947.
9. CAIN, R.M.; STEELE, H. The use of calcium alginate soluble wool for the examination of cleansed eating utensils. Can. J. Public Health 44:464-467; 1953.
10. CANNON, R.Y.; REDDY, K.K. Contamination of milk with airborne microorganisms through the vacuum defoamer. J. Milk Food Technol. **33:**197-201; 1970.
11. CLESCERI, L.S.; GREENBERG, A.E.; EATON, A.D.; eds. *Standard methods for the examination of water and wastewater,* 20th ed. Washington, DC: APHA; 1998.
12. COWN, W.B.; KETHLEY, T.W.; FINCHER, E.L. The critical-orifice liquid impinger as sampler for bacterial aerosols. Appl. Microbiol. **5:**119-124; 1957.
13. COX, L.J.; KLEISS, T.; CORDIER, J.L.; CORDELLANA, C.; KONKEL, P.; PEDRAZZINI, C.; BEUMER, R.; SIEBENGA, A. *Listeria* spp. in food processing, non-food and domestic environments. J. Food Microbiol. **6:**49-61; 1989.
14. DECKER, H.M.; KUEHNE, R.W.; BUCHANAN, L.M.; PORTER, R. Design and evaluation of a slit-incubator sampler. Appl. Microbiol. **6:**389-400; 1958.
15. DEY, B.P.; ENGLEY, F.B., JR. Methodology for recovery of chemically treated *Staphylococcus aureus* with neutralizing medium. Appl. Environ. Microbiol. **45:**1533-1537; 1983.
16. DONNELLY, C.W. Listeria and U.S. dairy products: The issues in perspective. J. Dairy and Food Sanitation. **8:**297-299; 1988.
17. DUMOULIN, G.C.; DOYLE, G.O.; MACKAY, J.; HEDLEY-WHYTE, J. Bacterial fouling of a hospital closed-loop cooling system by *Pseudomonas sp.* J. Clin. Microbiol. **13:**1060-1065; 1981.
18. FAVERO, M.S.; MCDADE, J.J.; ROBERTSEN, J. A.; HOFFMAN, R.K.; EDWARDS, R.W. Microbiological sampling of surfaces. J. Appl. Bacteriol. **31:**336-343; 1968.
19. FLOWERS, R.; MILO, L.; MYERS, E.; CURIALE, M.S. An evaluation of five ATP bio-

luminescence systems. Food Quality March: 23-33; 1997.
20. GRIFFITHS, W.D.; DECOSEMO, G.A.L. The assessment of bioaerosols: a critical review. J. Aerosol Sci. **25:**1425-1458; 1994.
21. HALL, L.B.; HARTNETT, M.J. Measurement of the bacterial contamination on surfaces in hospitals. Public Health Rep. **79:**1021-1024; 1964.
22. HARPER, W.J.; HALL, C.W. *Dairy technology and engineering.* Westport, CT: AVI Publishing Co., Inc.; 1976:545.
23. HARTMAN, P.A.; WEBER, J.A. Negligible evaporation retardation by oxyethylene docosanol under static conditions. Appl. Microbiol. **24:**508-509; 1972.
24. HEDRICK, T.I.; HELDMAN, D.R. Air quality in fluid milk and manufactured milk products plants. J. Milk Food Technol. **32:**265-269; 1969.
25. HIGGINS, M. A comparison of the recovery of organisms from cotton-wool and calcium alginate wool swabs. Great Britain: Monthly Bull. Minis. Health and Public Health Lab. Serv. **9:**50-51; 1950.
26. HOLLINGER, N.F.; LINDBERG, L.H. Delayed recovery of streptococci from throat swabs. Amer. J. Public Health and the Nation's Health **48:**1162-1169; 1958.
27. KANG, Y.J.; FRANK, J.F. Biological aerosols: A review of airborne contamination and its measurement in dairy processing plants. J. Food Prot. **52:**512-524; 1989.
28. KINGSTON, D. Selective media in air sampling: a review. J. Appl. Bacteriol. **34:**221-232; 1971.
29. LACH, V. Performance of the surface air system air samplers. J. Hospital Inf. **6:**102-107;1985.
30. LAROCCO, K.A.; LITTLE, K.J.; PIERSON, M.D. The bioluminescent ATP assay for determining the microbial quality of foods. In: PEARSON, M.D.; STERN, N.J., EDS. *Foodborne microorganisms and their toxins: developing methodology.* New York, NY: Marcel Dekker, Inc.; 1986.
31. LLABRES, C.M.; ROSE, B.E. Antibacterial properties of retail sponges. J. Food Prot. **52:**49-54; 1989.
32. LOFGREN, J.P.; KONIGSBERG, C.; RENDTORFF, R.; ZEE, V.; HUTCHESON, R.H.; RAUSA, A.; BROWER, D.; RIECKEN, W.E. Multi-state outbreak of yersiniosis. Morbid. Mortal. Weekly Rep. **31:**505-506; 1982.
33. MARSHALL, R.T.; APPEL, R. Sanitary conditions in twelve fluid milk processing plants as determined by use of the rinse filter method. J. Milk Food Technol. **36:**237-241; 1973.
34. MAY, K.R. Prolongation of microbiological air sampling by a monolayer on agar gel. Appl. Microbiol. **18:**513-514, 1969.
35. MCELROY, W.D.; SELIGER, H.H.; WHITE, E.H. Mechanism of bioluminescence, chemiluminescence, and enzyme function in the oxidation of firefly luciferin. J. Photochem. Photobiol. **10:**153-170; 1969.
36. MCGOLDRICK, K.F.; FOX, T.L.; MCALLISTER, J.S. Evaluation of a dry medium for detecting contamination on surfaces. Food Technol. **40:**77-80; 1986.
37. OLSON, H.C.; HAMMER, B.W. Numbers of microorganisms falling from the air in dairy plants. J. Dairy Sci. **17:**613-623; 1934.
38. PARROW, T. *Manual of recommended laboratory methods for sampling and microbiological testing of single-service food packages and their components.* Syracuse, NY: Syracuse University Res. Corp.; 1978:22
39. PETRAN, R.; ZOTTOLA, E.A. Survival of *Listeria* monocytogenes in simulated milk cooling systems. J. Food Protection. **51:**172-175; 1988.
40. RADMORE, K.; LUCK, H. Microbial contamination of dairy factory air. S. Afr. J. Dairy Technol. **16:**119-123; 1984.
41. REN, T.J.; FRANK, J.F. A survey of four fluid milk processing plants for airborne contamination using various sampling methods. J. Food Prot. **55:**38-42; 1992a.
42. REN, T.J.; FRANK, J.F. Measurement of airborne contamination in two commercial ice cream plants. J. Food Prot. **55:** 43-47; 1992b.
43. REN, T.J.; FRANK, J.F. Sampling of microbial aerosols at various locations in fluid milk and ice cream plants. J. Food Prot. **55:**279-283; 1992c.
44. SAWYER, K.F.; WALTON, W.H. The conifuge: a size separating sampling device for airborne particles. J. Sci. Instr. **27:**272; 1950.

45. SILLIKER, J.H.; GABIS, D.A. A cellulose sponge sampling technique for surfaces. J. Milk Food Technol. **38:**504; 1975.
46. SILVERMAN, G.J.; ROSS, E.W.; KAUTZ, W.P. Assessment of the sanitary quality food preparation surfaces. J. Foodservice Sys. **4:**285-301; 1981.
47. SING, E.L.; ELLIKER, P.R.; CHRISTENSEN, L.J.; SANDINE, W.E. Effective testing procedures for evaluating plant sanitation. J. Milk Food Technol. **30:**103-111; 1967.
48. STANFIELD, J.T.; JACKSON, G.J.; AULISIO, C.C.G. *Yersinia enterocolitica:* survival of a pathogenic strain on milk containers. J. Food Prot. **48:**947-948; 1985.
49. TIEDEMAN, W.D., Chairman. Technic for the bacteriological examination of food utensils, part 2. New York, NY: Amer. J. Public Health Yearbook; 1947-48:68-70.
50. TREDINNICK, J.E.; TUCKER, J. The use of calcium alginate wool for swabbing dairy equipment. Proc. Soc. Appl. Bacteriol. **14:**85; 1951.
51. U.S. DEPARTMENT OF HEALTH AND HUMAN SERVICES, PUBLIC HEALTH SERVICE, U.S. FOOD AND DRUG ADMINISTRATION. Milk Laboratory Evaluation Forms 2400 Series. Washington, DC: U.S. Govt. Print. Off.; 1995.
52. U.S. PUBLIC HEALTH SERVICE, FOOD AND DRUG ADMINISTRATION. Grade A pasteurized milk ordinance: recommendations of the Public Health Service. Publication No. 229. Washington, DC: U.S. Govt. Print. Off.; 1999.
53. WALTER, W.G.; POTTER, J. Bacteriological field studies on eating utensils and flat surfaces. J. Environ. Health **26:**187-197; 1963.
54. WITTER, L.D. Psychrophilic bacteria: a review. J. Dairy Sci. **44:**983-1015; 1961.
55. ZOTTOLA, E.A.; SMITH, L.B. Survival of salmonellae in refrigerated, agitated water and water/glycol mixtures. J. Food Prot. **49:**467-470; 1986.

Chapter 14

Alkaline Phosphatase Methods

R. M. Rocco
(J. Fitts, Tech. Comm.)

14.010 Introduction

Alkaline phosphatase (ALP, EC 3.1.3.1) is an enzyme that is widely distributed in nature. It has been found in blue-green algae, slime molds, bacteria, and in the tissues of all members of the animal kingdom.[23] Its exact function within cells is unknown; however, *in vitro* it cleaves, with a high degree of specificity, the monophosphoric ester bond from a wide variety of substrates releasing phosphate radicals. In 1933, Kay and Graham initially demonstrated that ALP activity in bovine milk was heat labile and that ALP measurements could be used to monitor the effectiveness of pasteurization.[15] They found that ALP is inactivated at a time and temperature that are slightly greater than normal pasteurization conditions. This first method described for ALP in milk used beta glycerophosphate as substrate followed by measurement of the liberated phosphorus. The detection limit of the assay was about 5.0% in raw milk.

In 1935, Kay and Graham went on to develop a more sensitive assay using phenyl phosphate as substrate.[16,17] In this assay, ALP cleaves off phosphorus from phenyl phosphate and leaves free phenol and phosphorus in solution. The liberated phenol was measured by means of Folin and Ciocalteu color reagent. The detection limit was 0.2% raw milk contamination following a 24-hour incubation. For the first time, it was possible to use a laboratory test to ensure that milk had been heated to the required temperature or that it had not been contaminated with raw milk during manufacture.[18]

In 1938, Scharer modified the Kay and Graham phenyl phosphate procedure and obtained a detection limit of 0.2% raw milk after only a 1-hour incubation.[35] In this assay the liberated phenol was measured using Gibb's reagent (BQC, 2,6-dibromoquinone-4-chloroimimide) after protein precipitation of the reaction mixture with lead acetate. Improved sensitivity was obtained when Scharer reported on the use of n-butanol extraction to remove the BQC-phenol complex from the reaction mixture.[36] Butanol extraction of the colored complex made it possible to read the assay visually.

Procedures for the measurement of ALP appeared for the first time in the 7th edition of *Standard Methods for the Examination of Dairy Products* published in 1939.[4] A total of 4 different methods was presented for consideration—all using phenyl phosphate as the substrate. In the 5th edition of the *Official and Tentative Methods of Analysis* of the AOAC published in 1940, the first ALP method in this series of reference manuals was presented.[3] In 1944 Scharer received U.S. Patent No. 2,359,052 for the use of the phenyl phosphate method employing either BQC or CQC (2,6-dichloroquinone-4-chloroimide) for measuring ALP activity.[38] Scharer's visual rapid method using CQC and a 1-hour incubation gained wide acceptance over the next few years.[39] In 1953, the Public Health Service Milk Ordinance and Code included this method in its code and required that health inspectors run the rapid field test at the plant.[37,41]

In 1949, Aschaffenburg and Mullen published the first ALP assay for milk using p-nitrophenyl phosphate (PNP) as a substrate.[5] PNP has the advantage over phenyl phosphate in that it is self-indicating. Self-indicating substrates do not require secondary color reactions in order to measure the product formed. PNP is colorless to pale yellow in alkaline solution, but when ALP cleaves off the phosphate radical, the product, p-nitrophenol, is deep yellow in color with an absorbance maximum of about 405 nm. With a 2-hour incubation, the detection limit of the Aschaffenburg and Mullen assay for whole milk was 0.1% raw milk. In the U.K., the Aschaffenburg and Mullen procedure is widely used and has been given official status by the IDF.[11]

Stiven was the first to publish a milk ALP method using the self-indicating substrate phenolphthalein diphosphate.[40] When phosphorus is cleaved from phenolphthalein phosphate compounds, phenolphthalein produces a distinct pink to red color in alkaline buffer. Babson and Greeley in 1967 described the synthesis and use of a stable phenolphthalein monophosphate (PMP) for measuring milk ALP.[2,6] Using visual indication of the formation of the pink color at the end of a 30-minute incubation, a detection limit of 0.1% raw milk was obtained. Over the next few years Kleyn and others from Rutgers University conducted various collaborative studies for the AOAC, and the PMP method became known as the Rutgers method.[19,20]

The first fluorometric procedure for the determination of ALP in dairy products was reported in 1990.[33] In this assay, the self-indicating substrate is a monophosphorylated benzothiazole derivative that is nonfluorescent in alkaline solution. When its single phosphate is cleaved by ALP it gives rise to a highly fluorescent product with an excitation of 430 nm and an emission of 560 nm. In this assay, the production of the fluorescent product is monitored continuously in a dedicated fluorometer, making this the first real-time kinetic assay for dairy products. The assay described was completed in 3 minutes and a detection limit for raw milk of 0.003% was reported. Reports of an AOAC collaborative study appeared,[34] and it received IDF recognition in 1992[13] and ISO approval in 1997.[14]

In 1993 a chemiluminescent method for the measurement of ALP in dairy products was approved by the NCIMS.[30] In this assay, a 1,2-dioxetane substrate is modified to contain a single ortho monophosphoric radical that undergoes rearrangement when the phosphorus is cleaved by ALP. This intermediate product has a very short half life during which it decomposes and emits light at about 477 nm. A fluorescein molecule in solution acts as an acceptor of the blue light and gives off a bright yellow luminescent signal at 525 nm that can be read by a scintillation counter as a burst of light. The amount of light is directly related to the enzyme activity of the sample being tested. Detection limits equivalent to the fluorometric procedure have been reported.[30]

The ALP assay in milk products has served the dairy industry well for over 60 years. It is a sensitive monitor of the completeness of pasteurization as well as an indicator of raw milk contamination in finished products. Under proper pasteurization conditions, ALP activity in raw milk is reduced by log orders of magnitude down to stable consistent levels when measured by current analytical methods. In addition, ALP levels in milk following pasteurization are quite sensitive to deviations in process temperatures and can be used to monitor as little as a 1°C drop in treatment temperature or as little as 0.01% or less of raw milk contamination.[1,9]

ALP levels in dairy products, despite their utility and widespread acceptance in the dairy industry, have limitations. False-positive and false-negative results must be prevented by use of good laboratory practice along with the running of proper controls with each batch of unknowns. False-positives, for example, can occur when a finished dairy product contains reactivated ALP. Milk and cream products processed at 87.8°C or higher by high-temperature, short-time (HTST) pasteurization will give acceptable low levels of ALP activity by current methods if the product has been cooled and stored at 4.4°C or below. During storage, however, ALP in these products can undergo reactivation, especially in products stored at higher temperatures for extended periods of time. The mechanism of reactivation is not well understood,[10] despite the fact that it was described in cream products as early as 1943[7] and was studied extensively in the 1950s by Wright.[42,43] Fortunately, controls are available for checking for reactivated ALP in the product.[32]

Reagent controls or interference controls run with the assay will also prevent false-positives due to contamination of the reagents with chemicals that are known to interfere with the measurement of ALP. Phenol, for example, is a common contaminant of laboratory glassware as well as being the end product measured in the Scharer ALP methods. Procedures for reagent controls are described in this manual.

False-positives may also occur because of the presence of heat stable microbial ALP in the product.[8,21,31] No current methods for ALP can distinguish between native bovine enzyme and the more heat stable enzyme produced by bacteria in milk. A positive ALP result in any dairy product must be confirmed with a microbial control to help distinguish between native bovine ALP and microbial ALP. Normally, bacterial ALP is inactivated during pasteurization, as is native bovine ALP. However, there are bacteria in raw milk that produce a heat stable form of ALP that survives the pasteurization process. Murthy and Kaylor[25] were able to differentiate bovine ALP from microbial enzyme in butter using agarose-gel electrophoresis.

Finally, the ALP assay has limited usefulness in high-acid dairy products such as buttermilk and yogurt due to the inactivation of the enzyme by the acid conditions. This results in reduced levels of ALP activity that may not reflect alterations in the processing temperature.

14.020 Scharer Rapid Visual ALP Method (Class O)

1. **Scope:** The Scharer rapid visual method is an end-point qualitative, visual, colorimetric assay for the determination of ALP activity in milk, skim milk, cream, flavored milk, cultured buttermilk, sour cream, yogurt, ice cream, cheese, butter, casein, and concentrated and dry milk products.[24,26-29,37]

2. **References:** Chapter 3: Sampling Dairy and Related Products.

3. **Definition:** ALP activity is the µg phenol liberated per mL of sample in 15 minutes. A value of 1 µg phenol liberated per mL of milk or milk product or per gram of butter or cheese extract per 15-minute incubation is indicative of improper pasteurization or of contamination with underpasteurized product. The 1 µg/mL standard used for visual comparison is approximately equivalent to 0.1% raw milk. Positive results with this method should be confirmed with a quantitative procedure.

4. **Principle:** Phenyl phosphate as substrate is enzymatically cleaved by ALP to yield phenol that reacts with Gibbs reagent to form a CQC-phenol complex. The complex is extracted by butanol and read visually against phenol standards developed with the CQC color reagent.[37]

5. **Reagents:** All reagents and supplies are available in kit form from Weber Scientific, Inc., Hamilton, NJ 08691 or Applied Research Institute, Newtown, CT 06482. Reagents and equipment from these suppliers must not be mixed. Individual chemicals may be purchased from suppliers such as Sigma Chemical Company (St. Louis) or Fisher Scientific Inc., (Pittsburgh). All chemicals must be reagent grade.
   1. **DI water or equivalent LG water.**
   2. **Stock carbonate buffer:** *pH 9.8.* Dissolve 46.89 g of sodium carbonate and 37.17 g of sodium bicarbonate in DI water and make up to 1 liter with additional DI water. Stable 6 months in the refrigerator.
   3. **Working carbonate buffer:** *Single strength, pH 9.8.* Dilute 5 mL stock carbonate buffer [14.020.5.2] to 100 mL with DI water. Stable 6 months in the refrigerator.
   4. **Working carbonate buffer:** *Double strength, pH 9.8.* Dilute 10 mL stock carbonate buffer [14.020.5.2] to 100 mL with DI water. Stable 6 months in the refrigerator.
   5. **Working CQC solution.** Dissolve 30 mg of reagent grade CQC (2,6-dichloroquinone-4-chloroimide) in 10 mL of methanol. Stable in

amber glass in the refrigerator for 3 months. Do not use if the solution turns brown.

6. **Copper sulfate catalyst.** Dissolve 200 mg cupric sulfate anhydrous in 100 mL of DI water. Store in glass in the refrigerator.
7. **Butanol neutralized (for indophenol extraction).** Add 10 mL of stock carbonate buffer pH 9.8 [14.020.5.2] to 3.785 L of n-butyl alcohol. Use reagent grade or better butanol with a boiling point of 116° to 118°C. Mix thoroughly and store in the refrigerator at 4°C. The addition of the stock carbonate buffer neutralizes any free acids that may be present in the butanol.

   To test, shake alcohol with an equal quantity of neutral MS water, allow them to separate, and add a few drops of indicator solution to the water layer.
8. **Butanol:** *7.5% (v/v) in DI water (for substrate preparation and casein extraction).* Mix 75 mL of butanol neutralized [14.020.5.7] with 925 mL of DI water. Store in amber glass in the refrigerator.
9. **Butanol:** *8.3% (v/v) in DI water (for cheese extraction).* Mix 83 mL of butanol neutralized [14.020.5.7] with 917 mL of DI water. Store in amber glass in the refrigerator.
10. **Working substrate in carbonate buffer:** *Single strength.* Dissolve 0.5 g disodium phenyl phosphate in 10 mL DI water contained in a 100 mL separatory funnel. Add 25 mL of stock carbonate buffer pH 9.8 [14.020.5.2]; 0.1 mL of CQC reagent [14.020.5.5] and 0.1 mL of the copper catalyst reagent [14.020.5.6]. Mix and allow to stand for 5 minutes. Add 3 mL of butanol neutralized [14.020.5.7] and mix. Allow the butanol layer to separate; draw off the aqueous bottom layer into a 500-mL volumetric flask and dilute to the mark with DI water. It may be necessary to repeat this extraction step. Stable 1 month in the refrigerator.
11. **Working substrate in carbonate buffer:** *Double strength.* Prepare exactly as above except use 50 mL of the stock carbonate buffer. [14.020.5.2].
12. **Hydrochloric acid:** *0.1 N.* Add 8.3 mL of concentrated hydrochloric acid to about 500 mL of DI water in a 1-L volumetric flask. Mix and bring to the 1-L mark with additional DI water.
13. **Stock phenol:** *Standard, 1 mg/mL.* Dissolve 1.00 g of molecular biology grade or better anhydrous phenol in 0.1 N hydrochloric acid in a 1-L glass volumetric flask. Dilute to the mark with additional 0.1 N hydrochloric acid. Store in amber glass in the refrigerator. Solution is stable for 3 months.
14. **Intermediate A phenol:** *Standard, 10 µg/mL.* Dilute 5.0 mL of the stock phenol standard [14.020.5.13] to 500 mL with DI water in a 500-mL volumetric flask. Prepare fresh daily.
15. **Intermediate B phenol:** *Standard, 1 µg/mL.* Dilute 10 mL of the intermediate 10 µg/mL phenol standard [14.020.5.14] to 100 mL with DI water in a volumetric flask. Prepare fresh daily.
16. **Working phenol:** *Standard, 0 to 10 µg phenol/5 mL.* Into labeled test tubes add the following:

Phenol Std. B (1 µg/mL)	DI Water	Concentrations: Phenol Std. µg/0.5 mL	1.0 mL Sample µg/mL Equivalent[a]
0.0 mL	5.0 mL	0.0	0.0
0.5	4.5	0.5	1.0
1.0	4.0	1.0	2.0
2.5	2.5	2.5	5.0
5.0	0.0	5.0	10.0

Prepare fresh daily.

[a] NOTE: In the Scharer rapid method presented a sample of 0.5 mL fluid milk or 0.5 g of solid sample is used in the assay. However, the final results for this ALP assay are reported as µg phenol produced/mL or per g of sample. The above standards by historical convention are made to contain HALF the amount of phenol so that the final results do not have to be converted to 1 mL of sample from the 0.5 mL that was used in the assay (see below).

17. **Magnesium acetate solution (for cheese):** *1 mg Mg/0.1 mL.* Dissolve 8.82 g of magnesium acetate $Mg(C_2H_3O_2)_2\ 4H_2O$ in about 50 mL of DI water in a 100-mL volumetric flask. Warm to completely dissolve the salt then bring to 100 mL with additional DI water.
18. **Magnesium acetate solution (for reactivation control):** *35.4 mg/1 mL.* Dissolve 35.4 grams of $Mg(C_2H_3O_2)_2\ 4H_2O$ in about 50 mL of DI water. Warm to dissolve completely then bring to 100 mL with additional DI water. Stable for 6 months at 4°C.

6. Apparatus

1. Test tubes: 12 × 144 mm, calibrated at 5 mL, 5.5 mL, and 8.5 mL to the top of the meniscus with screw caps with phenol-free lining.
2. Test tube stoppers phenol-free to fit the 12 × 44 mm test tubes.
3. Pipets: 1 mL, 5 mL and 10 mL graduated in 0.1-mL divisions.
4. Thermometer: Calibrated to 110°C and accurate to ± 0.5°C or better.
5. Beakers.
6. Erlenmeyer and volumetric flasks at 100, 500 and 1,000 mL; separatory funnel, 100 mL, all cleaned with phenol-free detergent.
7. Water baths accurate to within 0.5°C of the set points of 34°, 40°, 63°, and 66°C.
8. Mechanical blender.
9. A light source against which to take the visual readings such as a dental X-ray viewer.
10. Whatman filter paper: No. 4, 9-cm diameter.
11. Ice water bath.
12. Glass stir rods.
13. Centrifuge capable of at least 1,000 × g.
14. Vortex mixer.
15. Test tubes for cheese extraction 18 × 150 mm with phenol-free stoppers.

7. Sampling: All samples of milk and milk products must be held at 0° to 4.4°C or less from the time of collection until sampling and analysis. ALP must be measured within 36 hours of collection.

8. Sample Preparation

A. **Milk, skim milk, cream, and flavored milk:** Mix in an Erlenmeyer flask with a swirling motion until homogenous.

B. **Cultured buttermilk and sour milk products:** Homogenize in a blender at low speed for a few seconds, avoiding whipping. Use double-strength buffered substrate [14.020.5.11]. Adjust the pH of the mixture to 9.5 to 10.0 with solid buffer [14.020.5.2] as necessary.

C. **Ice cream:** Melt a portion of the sample and let it stand for 1 hour to release entrapped air. Remove fruits and nuts from the ice cream before sampling.

D. **Cheese:** Measure the pH of the cheese using any pH meter calibrated for surface pH measurements. Freeze portions of the cheese sample at –15° ± 1°C. Weigh 5-g portions of the frozen cheese directly into each of two 18 × 150 mm test tubes labeled *blank* and *test*.

For cheese samples with a pH above 7.0 add 2.0 mL of water to the *blank* and *test* samples. For samples with a pH below 7.0 add 1.0 mL of DI water and 1.0 mL of stock carbonate buffer [14.020.5.2] pH 9.8. Macerate the samples in the *blank* and *test* tubes with a glass rod. Heat the macerated sample mixture in the *blank* tube in a boiling water bath to 95°C for 1 minute followed by cooling in an ice bath.

To both the *blank* and *test* tubes add 18.0 mL of butanol 8.3% [14.020.5.9] and vortex mix for 30 seconds and let stand for 5 minutes. Filter the extracted samples through Whatman No. 4 filter paper into clean labeled test tubes that are immersed in an ice bath. For every mL of extract in both the *blank* and *test* add 0.2 mL of magnesium acetate solution: 1 mg Mg/0.1 mL [14.020.5.15]. These are the extracts that are run in the Scharer rapid visual assay presented below.

E. **Butter:** Freeze portions of the butter as for cheese in [14.020.8.4]. Weigh 0.5-g portions of the frozen butter directly into 2 test tubes labeled *blank* and *test*. Heat the blank tube to 95°C in a boiling water bath exactly as was done for the cheese sample in [14.020.8.D]. After heating, cool both the *blank* and *test* tubes in an ice bath for a few minutes.

Before running the assay, place both the *blank* and *test* tubes into a water bath at 40° ± 1°C for a few minutes to melt the butter.

F. **Casein:** Add 3.0 g of the casein sample into a 100-mL glass volumetric flask containing 25 mL of butanol 7.5% [14.020.5.8] and shake for 1 minute. Let stand for 1 minute then dilute to the 100-mL mark with additional butanol 7.5%. Invert and shake the flask until the casein dissolves or use an ultrasonic bath to hasten the dissolution of the casein. Store the solution in the refrigerator overnight.

Place 5.0-mL samples of the above casein extract into 2 tubes labeled *blank* and *test*. Heat the tube labeled *blank* to 95°C for 1 minute in a boiling water bath. Cool the tubes in an ice bath. For every mL of extract in both the *blank* and *test* add 0.2 mL of the magnesium acetate solution: 1 mg Mg/0.1 mL [14.020.5.15].

G. **Concentrated and dry milk products:** Dilute 1.0 mL of evaporated milk with 1.25 mL of DI water. Dilute 1.0 mL of condensed milk with 2.0 mL of DI water. Disperse 10 g of dry milk product into 90.0 mL of DI water in a blender and process.

9. Procedure

A. **Calibration:** Prepare a set of working phenol standards as given in 14.020.5.16. To each of the above working standard tubes add 0.5 mL of stock carbonate buffer [14.020.5.2]; 0.1 mL CQC reagent [14.020.5.5]; and 0.1 mL of the copper sulfate catalyst [14.020.5.6]. Mix the tubes and immediately incubate them in a water bath at 40° ± 1°C for 5 minutes after coming to temperature.

Optionally, standards are available commercially.

At the end of the incubation, cool the tubes in an ice bath for at least 10 minutes. Add 3.0 mL of butanol neutralized [14.020.5.7] to each tube and extract the indophenol by inverting the tubes through 6 full turns. Allow the butanol layer to separate. These extracted standards can now be used for visual comparison in the Scharer rapid visual method.

B. **Controls:** A positive and negative control must be run with every batch of unknown samples.

1. **Negative control:** Heat a sample of the liquid milk product or a 5-gram sample of the solid product to 95°C for 1 minute followed by rapid cooling to room temperature. Heat transfer within the solid product is promoted best when the solid is macerated in saline or alkaline buffer. In all cases use a thermometer to measure the temperature of the sample during heating. Record the 1-minute heating time only after the product reaches 95°C. This control must show no color in the assay. If desired, distribute 1.0-mL quantities in small tubes, seal, and freeze for later use.

2. **Positive control:** Add 0.1 mL of a fresh sample of mixed herd raw milk to a 100-mL volumetric flask containing about 50 mL of negative control. Mix the flask gently and then add more negative control to the 100-mL mark.

   This positive control contains 0.1% raw milk (equivalent to about 1 µg/phenol per mL/15 minutes) and may be stored in aliquots in the freezer for at least 1 month. This control must be equal in color intensity to the 1 µg/mL phenol standard.

   NOTE: 0.1 mL of raw milk may not always give the desired color intensity, in which case 0.2 mL or other appropriate amount of raw milk must be used.

3. **Interfering-substance and reagent control:** Test an interfering-substance control with chocolate milk, cheese, ice cream, or other flavored products. For this control use 5 mL of single strength buffer control [14.020.5.3] for chocolate milk, ice cream, and other flavored products, or 5 mL of double-strength buffer control [14.020.5.4] for cheese; *do not* use buffered substrate [14.020.5.10]. Any color in this control sample that is equal to or less than the color obtained with the negative control sample [14.020.9.B.1] is due to interfering substances and not to milk ALP. The interference is from contamination of the sample or reagents with free phenol. If the color of the test sample containing the buffered substrate is greater than the color obtained in the interfering-substance control, underpasteurization or contamination with raw product is indicated.

   NOTE: Vanillin, a flavoring agent used in many dairy products, may undergo oxidation to vanillic acid, which will react with CQC to yield a blue color. Also, free phenol that is present as a contaminant will react with CQC to yield a blue color. On the other hand, chocolate or cocoa added to milk, may contain enzyme-inhibiting substances. Therefore, analysis may result in a false-negative test.

4. **Microbial control:** A microbial control should be analyzed with all positive samples to help confirm the source of the ALP activity being measured. First, heat a sample of the product in a water bath to 63° ± 1°C (or 66° ± 1°C if the fat content is over 10%) for exactly 30 minutes. Use a thermometer immersed in the sample and start the 30-minute timing after the sample reaches the required temperature. This sample is the repasteurized sample. Heat a second sample of the product to 95°C exactly as was done to prepare the negative controls above [14.020.9.B.1]. Analyze both the repasteurized sample and the heated (95°C) sample. The heated sample will confirm that the initial positive result with the sample was due to ALP activity. The results from this sample must be negative and show little or no color development. The repasteurized sample will be negative if the source of the ALP is bovine raw milk or underpasteurization during manufacture. If the repasteurized sample is positive, this indicates the possibility of a heat stable bacterial ALP that was not inactivated during the manufacturing pasteurization process. Further investigation should be undertaken in order to find and eliminate the bacteria (usually psychrotrophs) responsible for producing the heat stable microbial ALP.[24]
5. **Reactivated control:** This control should be run with all positive samples especially high-temperature, short-time (HTST) processed products such as milk, cream, and buttermilk.
   a. Heat a 15-mL sample of the product to 95°C for exactly 30 minutes as was done to prepare the negative control [14.020.9.B.1]. Set aside for use as indicated.
   b. Into labeled test tubes add the following:

		Sample	Test
Positive sample to be tested	mL	5.0	5.0
DI water [14.020.5.1]	mL	0.1	—
Magnesium acetate [14.020.5.18]	mL	—	0.1

   c. Incubate all tubes for 1 hour at 34° ± 1°C with occasional mixing.
   d. At the end of the incubation remove 1.0 mL of the mixture from the above tube labeled Test and mix in a separate tube with 5.0 mL of the product which has been heated from the first step above. Label this tube *x 6 test dilution*.
   f. Run a sample of the product from the sample tube and a sample of the product from the tube labeled *x 6 test dilution*.
   g. If the results of the ALP assay for the x 6 test dilution are equal to or greater than the results of the sample tube then the original sample contains reactivated ALP and does not contain residual ALP from raw milk contamination.

      If the results of the ALP assay for the x 6 test dilution are less than the results of the sample tube then the original sample contains no reactivated ALP and the original positive result was due to raw milk contamination.[27]

C. **Assay procedure**

1. Into labeled 12 × 144 mm test tubes add 0.5 mL of the sample or sample extract and 5.0 mL of the working substrate as indicated below:

Sample	Substrate 5.10 Single	Substrate 5.11 Double
Milk, skim milk, cream, flavored milk [14.020.8.A]	5.0 mL	—
Cultured buttered milk, sour cream, yogurt [14.020.8.B]	—	5.0 mL
Ice cream [14.020.8.C]	5.0 mL	—
Cheese [14.020.8.D]		
Filtrate for *blank* and *test*	—	5.0 mL
Butter [14.020.8.D]		
Filtrate for *blank* and *test*	5.0 mL	—
Casein [14.020.8.E)		
Extract for *blank* and *test* 5.0 mL	—	
Concentrated and dry products [14.020.8.F]		
Evaporated milk dilution	5.0 mL	—
Condensed milk dilution	5.0 mL	—
Dry milk blended dilution	5.0 mL	—

2. Mix all tubes by inversion and immediately place into a water bath for 15 minutes at 40° ± 1°C. Make sure the liquid in the tubes is below the water line in the bath. Use a temperature control blank to ensure the correct temperature. Incubation time and temperature are critical and must not exceed or be less than what is indicated. If large batches of tubes are being run, add the substrate to the sample and place the tubes into the water bath in a timed sequence.
3. Remove the tubes from the water bath and add 0.1 mL of the CQC reagent [14.020.5.5] followed by 0.1 mL of the copper sulfate catalyst [14.020.5.6]. Mix the tubes by inversion and immediately place back into the water bath at 40° ± 1°C for 5 minutes.
4. Remove the tubes from the water bath and cool them in an ice bath to below 10°C. Add 3.0 mL of cold (–20°C) butanol neutralized reagent [14.020.5.7].
5. Restopper the test tubes and mix gently by inverting the tubes 4 times through a half circle. Take about 1 second to invert the tubes, pause about 1 second, take another 1 second to return the tubes upright, pause 1 second, and then proceed. The purpose of the slow turns for the extraction step is to prevent formation of emulsions. Lay the tubes on their sides on a flat surface for 2 minutes to permit the separation of the butanol layer then repeat the mixing and separating steps a second time before reading.
6. If the butanol layer has emulsified so that no clear alcohol layer remains, cool the tubes for 5 minutes in an ice bath and then centrifuge them for 5 minutes at 1000 × g.

   Observe the tubes by placing them in an observation rack and read against a light source such as an X-ray reader box.

a. Place a sample to be read in a center position in the rack with a 0 µg phenol standard behind it and the increasing concentration of standards next to it.
b. For samples that have a *blank* and *test* (cheese, butter, and casein) place these side by side with the zero phenol standard behind the *blank* and the increasing concentration standards next to the test sample.
c. Compare the unknown samples with the 1, 2, and 5 µg/mL standards by holding them up to the light source and viewing through each tube.

10. **Expression of Results:** Results from the Scharer rapid visual assay are reported as below or above the 1 µg/mL phenol standard. A value of 1 µg/mL or above for milk or milk product or 1 µg/g for butter or cheese extract is indicative of improper pasteurization or of contamination with unpasteurized products. A value of 1 µg/mL/15 minutes is approximately equal to 0.1% raw milk contamination.

11. **Test Report:** Test reports should identify the method used and the results obtained. Each report should also contain the sample identification number, sample type, and sufficient information for complete sample traceability. Report results with this method as above or below 1 µg/mL. Sample results confirmed as above 1 µg/mL are considered to be underpasteurized or contaminated with raw milk.

14.030 Scharer Spectrophotometric ALP Method

1. **Scope:** This is a quantitative modification of the Scharer rapid visual ALP method [14.020] and is applicable to the same products listed in 14.020. The method is: 1) Class A1 for casein; 2) Class A2 for cheese; and 3) Class O for other dairy products.
2. **References:** Chapter 3: Sampling Dairy and Related Products.
3. **Definition:** *ALP activity:* µg phenol formed per mL or per g of sample per 15 minutes at the specified temperature. A value of 1 µg phenol liberated per mL of liquid product or per gram of solid product per 15 minutes incubation is indicative of improper pasteurization or of contamination with underpasteurized product. The 1 µg/mL standard is approximately equivalent to 0.1% raw milk contamination.[28]
4. **Principle:** This procedure employs the same principle as the Scharer rapid visual method [14.020], but has been modified to allow the extracted phenol complex to be spectrophotometrically read against known phenol standards to provide for quantitation of the ALP units of activity in the product.
5. **Reagents:** See 14.020.5.
6. **Apparatus:** *Apparatus in 14.020.6 plus*
   1. Borosilcate glass test tubes: 16 × 125 mm with glass stoppers.
   2. Precision 1.0-mL pipette graduated in 0.1- or 0.01-mL divisions.
   3. Any colorimeter or spectrophotometer capable of absorbance readings at 650 nm.
   4. Matched cuvettes for the spectrophotometer.

7. **Sampling:** All samples of milk and milk products must be held at 0° to 4.4°C from the time of collection until analyzed. ALP must be measured within 48 hours of collection.

8. **Sample Preparation:** See 14.020.8.

9. **Procedure**

   A. **Calibration:** Prepare the 0 to 10 µg/5 mL phenol standards according to [14.020.5.16] except that after the butanol extraction step, centrifuge all the tubes for 5 minutes at 1000 × g to obtain a clear upper alcohol layer. Carefully remove the butanol layer after the centrifugation step using a Pasteur transfer pipet and place the alcohol layer into labeled matched spectrophotometer cuvettes. Zero the spectrophotometer with the 0-µg phenol standard to zero absorbance at 650 nm. Read and record the absorbance of each of the other standards. Construct a calibration curve with absorbance versus µg phenol using best fit or a regression equation.

   B. **Controls:** Results for a positive and negative control must be obtained for every batch of unknown samples or at least once per shift. Each positive result for a test sample should be repeated with additional controls as required.

      1. **Negative control:** See 14.020 for preparation. This control must show no color.
      2. **Positive control:** See 14.020 for preparation. This control must give a result that is equivalent to 0.1% or 1 µg/mL/15 minutes.
      3. **Interfering substance and reagent control:** See 14.020 for preparation and interpretation.
      4. **Microbial control:** See 14.020 for preparation and interpretation.
      5. **Reactivated control:** See 14.020 for preparation and interpretation.

   C. **Assay procedure:** The procedure for the unknown samples is given in 14.020.9.3, except that the butanol layer is read in a spectrophotometer after centrifugation of the final reaction mixture for 5 minutes at 1000 × g. Read each sample including the blank and test for that unknown sample if it has one in the spectrophotometer at 650 nm against the 0-µg phenol standard set to zero absorbance. Record all of the absorbance values.

      Read the final result for each sample in µg phenol/mL or per g of sample from the calibration curve constructed above. For samples that have a blank and test sample (cheese, butter, and casein), subtract the absorbance of the blank tube from the test tube and then read the final result off the calibration curve.

      NOTE: The final result for the following sample types must be multiplied by a correction factor to account for the dilutions in the sample preparation procedures [14.020.8] and to give µg phenol per mL or per µg of product.

Product	Dilution Factor
1. Milk, skim milk, cream, and flavored milk	none
2. Cultured buttermilk and sour cream	none
3. Ice cream	none
4. Cheese	x 8
5. Butter	none
6. Casein	x 33.3
7. Condensed and dry milk products	
Evaporated milk	x 2.05
Condensed milk	x 3
Dry milk products	x 10

10. **Expression of Results:** The results from the Scharer spectrophotometric ALP assay are reported as µg/mL or µg/g of product. A value of 1 µg/mL or 1 µg/g or above is indicative of improper pasteurization or of contamination with unpasteurized products.
11. **Precision:** A coefficient of variation from 4.4 to 13.4% has been reported over the analytical range of the assay.[28]
12. **Test Report:** Test reports should identify the method used and the results obtained. Each report should also contain the sample identification number, sample type, and sufficient information for complete sample traceability. Report the results by this method as a quantitative result in µg/mL for fluid dairy products or µg/g for solid products. Results of 1.0 µg/mL or greater are considered to be underpasteurized or contaminated with raw milk.

14.040 Rutger's Visual ALP Method

1. **Scope:** The Rutger's ALP visual assay is an end-point colorimetric assay for the measurement of ALP activity, applicable to milk, skim milk, heavy cream, light cream, cheese, plain ice cream mix, butter, concentrated milk, and dry milk. The method is: 1) Class A1 for milk, skim milk, light cream; 2) Class A2 for cheese; and 3) Class B for heavy cream, plain ice cream mix, butter, concentrated milk, and dry milk.
2. **References:** Chapter 3: Sampling Dairy and Related Products.
3. **Definitions:** ALP activity is measured in units of phenolphthalein released per mL under specified time and temperature conditions. In the Rutger's ALP assay, visual comparison is made between a sample run in the assay and an aliquot of the same sample to which an amount of phenolphthalein has been added to give an equivalent contamination of 0.1% raw milk.
4. **Principle:** A sample of the product being tested is incubated with an alkaline buffered phenolphthalein monophosphate substrate at pH 10.15 with and without the addition of phenolphthalein. After addition of sodium hydroxide to stop the reaction and develop the color the liberated phenolphthalein turns pink to red in direct relation to the ALP activity in the sample. All positive results should be confirmed using a quantitative method.

5. **Reagents:** Complete reagent test kits are available from Applied Research Institute, Newtown, CT 06482. Individual chemicals may be purchased from suppliers such as Sigma Chemical Company (St. Louis) or Fisher Scientific, Inc. (Pittsburgh).
   A. **Substrate.** Dissolve 3.9 g of the dicyclohexylamine salt of phenolphthalein monophosphate and 73.2 g of 2-amino-2-methyl-1-propanol in 21.9 mL of hydrochloric acid. The pH is 10.15 at 25°C. Stable for 1 year in the refrigerator.
   B. **Calibrator.** Dissolve 10.0 mg of phenolphthalein, 40.0 mg of tartrazine, and 73.2 g of 2-amino-2-methyl-1propanol in 21.9 mL of hydrochloric acid. The pH is 10.15 at 25°C. Additional standards may be prepared exactly as above but using 20 or 50 mg of phenolphthalein.

Phenolphthalein mg/total volume	Equivalent to % raw milk
10 mg	0.1
20 mg	0.2
50 mg	0.5

   Calibrators are stable for 1 year in the refrigerator.
   C. **Color developer.** Dissolve 10 g of sodium hydroxide in about 50 mL of DI water and mix. Bring up to 100 mL with additional DI water. Stable for 1 year in the refrigerator.
6. **Apparatus:** Clean dry 5-mL test tubes.
7. **Sampling:** All samples of milk and milk products must be held at 0° to 4.4°C or less from the time of collection until sampling and analysis. ALP must be measured within 48 hours of collection.
8. **Sample Preparation:** See 14.020.8.
9. **Procedure**
   A. **Calibration:** No separate calibrators are required. In the assay, an amount of phenolphthalein is added to an aliquot of each sample of dairy product being tested, making that sample equivalent to a 0.1% raw milk positive. The corresponding test (dairy) sample is analyzed and compared to this spiked sample.
   B. **Controls:** Results for a positive and negative control should be obtained with every batch of test samples, or at least once per shift. Each positive test sample result should be repeated with additional controls as required.
      1. **Negative control.** See 14.020 for preparation. Analyze this control exactly as a sample. The test sample should contain less color than the negative control sample to which phenolphthalein was added.
      2. **Positive control.** See 14.020 for preparation. Analyze this control exactly as a sample. The test sample should contain as much color as the positive control sample to which phenolphthalein was added.
      3. **Reagent (interfering-substance) control.** Prepare calibrator exactly according to [14.040.5.2]; however, do not add any phenolphthalein. Add 0.04 mL of this 0-µg calibrator to 1.0 mL of the milk sample. Incubate for 30 minutes at 37°C. Add 0.04 mL of color

developer at the end of the incubation. This sample should contain no visible color.

4. **Microbial control.** See 14.020 for preparation and interpretation.
5. **Reactivated control.** See 14.020 for preparation and interpretation.

C. **Assay procedure**

1. Pipet 1.0 mL of sample into each of 2 test tubes labeled test and control.
2. Place both tubes into a water bath at 37° ± 1°C for at least 2 minutes to bring the samples to temperature.
3. Into the tube labeled *test* add 1 drop (0.04 mL) of the substrate [14.040.5.1] and into the tube labeled *control* add 1 drop (0.04 mL) of the phenolphthalein calibrator [14.040.5.2].
4. Vortex mix the tubes and incubate in the water bath for 30 minutes at 37° ± 1°C.
5. At the end of the incubation add 1 drop (0.04 mL) of color developer [14.040.5.3] to each tube. Mix and compare the colors visually.

10. **Expression of Results:** The tube labeled control contains the milk sample and an equivalent amount of phenolphthalein to give a pink color equivalent to what this sample would give if it had 0.1% raw milk contamination. Compare the color in the tube labeled test to the color in the control tube and report results as below or above 0.1% raw milk contamination.

11. **Precision:** This method gives results comparable to the Scharer visual method.[18,19]

12. **Test Report:** Test reports should identify the method used and the results obtained. Each report should also contain the sample identification number, sample type, and sufficient information for complete traceability. Report the results with this method as above or below the 0.1% control point.

14.050 Fluorophos® Fluorometric ALP Method

1. **Scope:** This is a quantitative kinetic fluorometric assay for ALP applicable to whole milk, skim milk, flavored milk, cream, and milk-based drinks. It is Class A1 for milk, skim milk, flavored milk, and cream.

   The method has been accepted by the IDF (155A:1999 for whole milk, semi-skimmed milk, and flavored milks) and ISO (DIS 11816 for milk and milk-based drinks).

2. **References:** Chapter 3: Sampling Dairy and Related Products.

3. **Definition:** *ALP activity:* mU/L or mU/kg, which are derived from the international convention of reporting enzyme activity in terms of micromoles of substrate catalyzed per liter or per kilogram of sample per minute at the specified temperature.

4. **Principle:** The sample is incubated at 38°C with a nonfluorescent benzothiazole orthophosphoric monoester substrate (Fluorophos®). When the phosphate is cleaved, the product released (Fluoroyellow®) is highly fluorescent with an excitation of 440 nm and an emission of 560 nm. The formation of Fluoroyellow® is monitored kinetically during a 3-minute

incubation period and the ALP units of activity are calculated from the slope of the reaction.[33,34]

5. **Reagents:** All reagents are available in test kit form from Advanced Instruments, Inc., 2 Technology Way, Norwood, MA 02062.
   1. **Substrate diluent:** *pH 10.0.* Diethanolamine (DEA) buffer: 2.4 M, pH 10.0. Stable for 2 years in the refrigerator.
   2. **Fluorophos substrate.** Each vial contains 144 mg of substrate (2′-[2-benzothiazoyl]-6′-hydroxybenzothiazole phosphate). Stable for 2 years in the refrigerator. To prepare working substrate, add the contents of 1 substrate diluent vial to 1 vial of Fluorophos® substrate vial. Mix by gentle inversion to dissolve. Stable for 60 days at 4°C and for 8 hours at 38°C.
   3. **Fluoroyellow® calibrators.** Ready-to-use liquid calibrators of (2′-[2-benzothiazoyl]-6′-hydroxybenzothiazole) labeled A, B, and C (30 mL each) containing 0, 3.44×10^{-5}, and 6.89×10^{-5} µM Fluoroyellow®/2 mL respectively. Stable for 1 year in the refrigerator.
   4. **Cheese extraction buffer.** Diethanolamine buffer, pH 8.0 with magnesium and Triton X-100. Stable for 3 years in the refrigerator.

6. **Apparatus**
   1. Advanced filter fluorometer thermocuvetted at 38° ± 1°C. Excitation is at 440 nm and emission is at 560 nm.
   2. Cuvettes: Disposable, nonfluorescent, round glass, 12 × 75 mm.
   3. Positive displacement pipeters: Fixed-volume at 75 µL (0.075 mL) and reagent dispenser with a fixed volume of 2.0 mL.
   4. Incubator block dry bath set to 38° ± 1°C.
   5. Test tubes: 16 × 100 mm with screw cap.

7. **Sampling:** All samples of milk and milk products must be held at 0° to 4.4°C or less from the time of collection until sampling and analysis. ALP must be measured within 48 hours of collection.

8. **Sample Preparation**
   A. **Milk, skim milk, low-fat milk, chocolate milk, half and half cream, heavy cream:** Mix the sample thoroughly; remove a sample and test.
   B. **Buttermilk, sour cream, and creamed cottage cheese:** Homogenize in a mechanical blender; remove a sample and test.
   C. **Concentrated and dry milk products:** Reconstitute the product with DI water to the concentration that existed before the water was removed; remove a sample and test.
   D. **Cheese:** To labeled 16- × 100-mm screw-cap glass test tubes, add 0.5 g of the cheese sample followed by 5.0 mL of the cheese extraction buffer [14.050.5.5]. Macerate with a glass rod, vortex mix, and centrifuge for 10 minutes at 1000 × g. Remove a sample from the top clear layer and test.

9. **Procedure**
   A. **Calibration:** Each type of dairy product being tested requires its own calibration curve. Calibration for a particular dairy product needs to be performed only when the lots of the calibrators or reagents are changed.

1. Into labeled 12- × 75-mm glass cuvettes, dispense in duplicate 2.0 mL of the A, B, and C calibrators. Place each cuvette into the incubator block and prewarm to 38° ± 1°C for 5 minutes.
2. To all 6 tubes, add a 75-µL (0.075-mL) sample of the well-mixed dairy product being tested. For cheese calibration, prepare an extract of the cheese [14.050.8.D].
3. Mix all tubes by gentle inversion and return to the incubation block. Starting with the A calibrator, set the fluorometer to zero fluorescence and then read the amount of fluorescence obtained with the B and C calibrators. Follow the instructions on the display of the fluorometer and perform the calibration routine.

B. **Controls:** Both a positive and negative control should be run with every batch of unknown samples or at least once per shift. Each positive result should be repeated with additional controls as required.

1. **Negative control.** See 14.020 for preparation.
   Results should be less than 10 mU/L.
2. **Positive control.** See 14.020 for preparation.
   Results should be 350 to 500 mU/L.
3. **Interfering-substance and reagent control.** Test for the presence of an interfering substance in the products or reagents by adding 75 µL of the dairy product to 2.0 mL of the zero calibrator A instead of the working substrate. Place this tube in the Fluorometer and run the 3-minute read-out routine. Final results of less than 10 mU/L indicate no interfering substances are present.
4. **Microbial control.** See 14.020 for preparation and interpretation.
5. **Reactivated control.** See 14.020 for preparation and interpretation.

C. **Assay procedure**

1. Bring 2.0 mL of the working Fluorophos® substrate [14.020.5.1] to 38° ± 1°C in labeled 12- × 75-mm cuvettes by placing them in the dry-bath incubator block. Allow to prewarm for at least 20 minutes.
2. Add 75 µL (0.075 mL) of the well-mixed sample or cheese extract to the 2.0 mL of substrate. Immediately mix by gentle inversion, wipe the outside of the cuvette with tissue paper, and place the cuvette into the fluorometer.
3. After 1 minute of temperature equilibration time, measure the rate of increase of fluorescence (F/minute) over the next 1 or 2 minutes. The milliunits per liter (mU/L) of ALP activity is displayed on the fluorometer and is printed out.

10. **Calculation and Expression of Results:** ALP activity in finished dairy products: Results are reported in milliunits per liter (mU/L) or mU/kg of finished dairy product. Final results are automatically calculated and printed on the fluorometer and are calculated from the following:

$$\frac{\text{(Increase in Fluorescence)(Sample Volume) (459.7)}}{\text{Fluorescence of Calibrator}} = \text{mU/L}$$

OR

$$\frac{(\Delta F/\text{min})\ (0.075\ \text{mL})\ (459.7)}{\text{F of Calibrator}} = \text{mU/L}$$

The factor 459.7 converts the μMoles of product formed per minute by the sample tested into mU/L final result. For calculation of cheese results obtain the mU/L from the printout. Convert the mU/L value obtained using the × 10 dilution in the extraction procedure by multiplying the mU/L by 10.

mU/L in extract (10) = mU/kg

11. **Precision:** The between-run CV's for a pool sample of milk with 190 mU/L (~ 0.04% raw milk) of ALP activity was reported as 2.6%.[33,34] The absolute difference in test results for duplicate assays within the same run on the same samples was shown to not exceed 62 mU/L for whole milk, 55 mU/L for skimmed milk, and 79 mU/L for flavored (chocolate) milk.[12]
12. **Test Report:** Test reports should identify the method used and the results obtained. Each report should also contain the sample identification number, sample type, and sufficient information for complete traceability. The results for the Fluorophos® ALP method are reported in mU/L for fluid milk samples or mU/kg for solid samples. A value of 350 mU/L indicates improper pasteurization or contamination of the finished product with raw milk.

14.060 Charm Chemiluminescent ALP Method (Class A1)

1. **Scope:** The Charm method is a chemiluminescent end-point procedure for the determination of ALP activity applicable to milk, skimmed milk, semi-skimmed milk, cream, cheese, flavored milk, sour cream, and cottage cheese.
2. **References:** Chapter 3: Sampling Dairy and Related Products.
3. **Definitions:** *ALP activity:* International units (IU) in which 1 IU of enzyme activity is that amount of enzyme that catalyzes the transformation of 1 micromole of photo-activated substrate per minute per liter of sample (mU/L) as specified in ISO/DIS Draft Standard 11816.3 (IDF 155:Part 3).[12]
4. **Principle:** ALP activity is measured by chemiluminescence in which the enzyme catalyzes the transformation of a non-chemiluminscent ortho phosphoric monoester dioxetane substrate. The release of the phosphate radical gives rise to a rearrangement of the substrate into a luminescent product that emits light in direct proportion to the amount of ALP activity present in the sample.
5. **Reagents:** All reagents are available in kit form from Charm Sciences, Inc., Lawrence, MA 01843.
    1. **Reagent AP—ALP substrate** *(3-[2′-Spiroadamantanane]-4-methoxy-4-(3′-phosphate phenyl-1,2-dioxetane)* **in DEA Buffer in ready-to-use form.** Stable for 6 months in the refrigerator and 24 hours at 30°C.
    2. **Stopping solution** *(DEA Buffer pH 7.5).* Stable for 1 year in the refrigerator and 2 months at room temperature.
    3. **Calibration tables for preparation of calibrators.** Stable for 2 years in the refrigerator. Table contains 875 mU/L of ALP activity and is diluted in heated (negative) milk product to provide a calibration curve.
    4. **Diluent AP—Extraction diluent for cheese.** A pH-adjusted buffer.

Stable for 1 year in the refrigerator and 2 months at room temperature.

5. **Positive control**—when rehydrated with 5 mL milk contains 400 ± 50 mu/L phosphatase.

6. **Apparatus**
   1. Charm analyzer (Charm II 6000 or 6600, or Luminometer models K or T) that read light emission at 540 nm. Results of ALP activity are automatically calculated by the software or calculated manually.
   2. Cuvettes: 13- × 100-mm borosilicate glass with 13-mm caps or 2 mL microcentrufuge tubes with caps that fit the analyzer being used [14.060.6.1].
   3. Pipets: Fixed-volume positive displacement of 100 ± µL (0.1 mL) and fixed-volume reagent dispenser at 1.0 mL.
   4. Incubator block: Dry well set at 35° ± 0.5°C.
   5. Centrifuge capable of at least 2000 × g.

7. **Sampling:** All samples of milk and milk products must be held at 0° to 4.4°C or less from the time of collection until sampling and analysis. ALP must be measured within 48 hours of collection.

8. **Sample Preparation**
   A. **Fluid milk products, flavored dairy drinks, and cream:** Carefully mix and use aliquots directly in the assay.
   B. **For semi-solid dairy drinks** *(flavored milk and cream)* **Charm II 6000 or 6600 only:** Add equal parts sample and extraction diluent. Mix and centrifuge 1200 × g (flavored drinks only) for 3 minutes. Sample the supernatant directly.
   C. **For solid dairy products** *(cheese and butter):* Add 4 parts extraction diluent and 1 part of the sample. Mix or blend then centrifuge at 1200 × g for 3 minutes. Sample the supernatant directly.

9. **Procedure**
   A. Prepare negative control by heating product to 95° ± 1°C and holding for 1 minute and then rapidly cooling. With cheeses first extract 2.5 grams with 12.5 grams Diluent AP and then centrifuge.
   B. **Calibration:** Dilute the calibration tablet with prepared negative control to provide a calibration curve. Obtain a calibration curve or single-point calibration for each type of dairy product being tested. Obtain a new calibration curve with each new lot of reagents. For fluid milk products (and cream and flavored drinks with luminometor) add 1 tablet each to 2.5 mL, 5.0 mL, and 20.0 mL of the negative control. Mix well. This provides calibrators A, B, and C, which have respectively 350 mU/L, 175 mU/L, and 44 mU/L of ALP activity.

   For cream and flavored dairy products with Charm II 6000 and 6600, add 1 tablet to 5.0 mL, 10.0 mL, and 20 mL of the Diluent AP to give calibrators A, B, and C with ALP values of 350 mU/L, 175 mU/L, and 88 mU/L. Centrifuge flavored calibrators only for 3 minutes.

   For cheese and solid dairy products add 1 tablet to 12.5 mL of the Diluent AP and 2.5 g of cheese and homogenite, then centrifuge for 3 minutes. Use supernatant as 350 mU/kg calibrator. Calibrators are stable for 6 hours in the refrigerator or for 2 months frozen at ±15°C or lower.

C. **Controls:** Analyze a positive and negative control with every batch of test samples or at least once per shift. Each positive result should be repeated with additional controls as required.

1. **Negative control.** See 14.020 for preparation. Must test less than 44 mU/L for milks, 88 for creams and flavors, and 200 mU/L for cheeses.
2. **Positive control.** Must test 350 to 500 mU/L.
3. **Interfering substance and reagent control.** Not specified by the manufacturer.
4. **Microbial control.** See 14.020 for preparation and interpretation.
5. **Reactivated control.** See 14.020 for preparation and interpretation.

D. **Assay procedure**

1. Dispense 0.1 mL of the ALP substrate into labeled 13- × 100-mm test tubes. Add 0.1 mL of the sample or sample extract or calibrators A, B, and C to their respective labeled tubes. Mix all tubes.
2. Place all tubes into the incubator heating block and incubate for 3 minutes at 35° ± 1°C.
3. At the end of the incubation, add 1.0 mL of stopping solution to each tube. Cap and mix each tube by shaking.
4. Read and record the luminescence of each tube at 5-second intervals. Take all readings within 6 minutes of adding the stopping solution.

10. Calculation and Expression of Results: Results are automatically calculated by the software in the luminescence reader or may be calculated manually.

Record the relative light units (RLU) of calibrators A, B, and C. Average the results from triplicate assays of each calibrator. Plot the RLU's for each calibrator versus the mU/L ALP activity using best-fit analysis. Read the values of the unknown dairy samples off of the curve.

Values for cheeses are read using a single-point calibrator set point. Run a calibrator with 350 mU/L of ALP activity in triplicate. Compare the mean RLU obtained for the calibrator with the RLU values obtained for the unknown sample. If the unknown product RLU is less than the calibrator, the product is negative (below 350 mU/L); if the product is above the calibrator the product is positive (350 mU/L or more).

11. Precision: The absolute difference in 410 mU/L test results for duplicate assays within the same run does not exceed 253 mU/L for whole milk, 341 mU/L for skimmed milk, 320 mU/L for flavored (chocolate) milk, and 281 mU/L for cream.

12. Test Report: Test reports should identify the method used and the results obtained.

Each report should also contain the sample identification number, sample type, and sufficient information for complete sample traceability. Report all results as mU/L for fluid milk products or mU/kg for solid products. A report of 350 mU/L or more indicates improper pasteurization or contamination with raw milk.

14.070 Cited References

1. ANGELINO, P.D.; CHRISTEN, G.L.; PENFIELD, M.P.; BEATTIE, S. Residual alkaline phosphatase activity in pasteurized milk heated to various temperatures—measurement with the Fluorophos and Scharer rapid phosphatase tests. J. Food Prot. **62:**81-85; 1999.
2. ANONYMOUS. The colorimetric determination of phosphatase in milk, sigma tentative technical bulletin, No. 104M; September 1967, Sigma Chemical Company, St. Louis, MO 63178.
3. SKINNER, W.W., ed. AOAC. *Official and tentative methods of analysis of the association of official agricultural chemists*, 5th ed. Washington, DC: APAC; 1940.
4. APHA. *Standard methods for the examination of dairy products*, 7th ed. Washington, DC: APHA; 1939.
5. ASCHAFFENBURG, R.; MULLEN, J.E.C. A rapid and simple phosphatase test for milk. J. Dairy Res. **16:**58-67; 1949.
6. BABSON, A.L.; GREELEY, S.J. New substrate for alkaline phosphatase in milk. J. Assoc. Off. Anal. Chem. **50:**555-557; 1967.
7. BARBER, F.W.; FRAZER, W.C. The development of a positive phosphatase test in refrigerated pasteurized cream. J. Dairy Sci. **26:**343-352; 1943.
8. BUCK, T.C. False positive phosphatase test from a thermopile in pasteurized milk. Am. J. Public Health **32:** 1224-1236; 1942.
9. ECKER, K.F. Fluorometric analysis of alkaline phosphatase inactivation correlated to *Salmonella* and *Listeria* inactivation. J. Food Protection **55:**960-963; 1992.
10. FARKYE, N.Y.; IMAFIDON, G.I. Thermal denaturation of indigenous milk enzymes, Chapter 16, pp. 331-363, 1995. In *Heat-induced changes in milk*, 2nd ed. Brussels, Belgium: International Dairy Federation; 1995.
11. IDF STANDARD. Detection of phosphatase activity (screening method). Brussels, Belgium: International Dairy Federation; 1987: 82A.
12. IDF DRAFT STANDARD. Determination of alkaline phosphatase activity chemiluminescent method. Brussels, Belgium: ISO 11613-3 IDF 155-Part 3; 2003.
13. IDF STANDARD. Determination of alkaline phosphatase activity fluorometric method. Brussels, Belgium: International Dairy Federation; 1992: 155.
14. ISO STANDARD. Milk and milk products; determination of alkaline phosphatase activity using a fluorometric method. Brussels, Belgium: International Standards Organization, 1997: 11816-1.
15. KAY, H.D.; GRAHAM, W.R. Phosphorus compounds in milk. J. Dairy Res. **5:**63-74; 1933.
16. KAY, H.D.; GRAHAM, W.R. The phosphatase test for pasteurised milk. J. Dairy Res. **6:**191-203; 1935.
17. KAY, H.D.; NEAVE, F.K. Some results of the application of a simple test for efficiency of pasteurization. Lancet **ii:**1516-1518; 1935.
18. KLEYN, D.H. Rapid screening method for alkaline phosphatase activity in cheese: collaborative study. J. Assoc. Off. Anal. Chem. **61:** 1035-1037; 1978.
19. KLEYN, D.H.; LIN, S.H.C. Collaborative study of a new alkaline phosphatase assay system for milk. J. Assoc. Off. Anal. Chem. **51:**802-807; 1968.
20. KLEYN, D.H.; HUANG, C.L. Collaborative study of the spectrophotometric determination of phosphatase activity in milk utilizing a new alkaline phosphatase assay system. J. Assoc. Off. Anal. Chem. **55:**498-503; 1972.
21. KNIGHT, A.; FRYER, S.M. The development of heat-resistant phosphatase activity in raw milk. J. Society Dairy Tech. **42:**81-86; 1989.
22. LEAHY, H.W. A study of pasteurized milk in Rochester, N.Y. employing the phosphatase test. J. Milk Technology **2:**147-151; 1939.
23. MCCOMB, R.B.; BOWERS, G.N.; POSEN, S. *Alkaline phosphatase.* New York, NY: Plenum Press; 1979.
24. MURTHY, G.K.; COX, S. Evaluation of APHA and AOC methods for phosphatase in cheese. J. Assoc. Off. Anal. Chem. **71:**1195-199; 1988.

25. MURTHY, G.K.; KAYLOR, L.O. Evaluation of APHA and AOAC II methods for phosphatase in butter and differentiation of milk and microbial phosphatase by agarose-gel electrophoresis. J. Assoc. Off. Anal. Chem. **73:**681-687; 1990.
26. MURTHY, G.K.; MARTIN, R.; RHEA, U.S.; PEELER, J.T. Rapid colorimetric test for alkaline phosphatase in dairy products. J. Food Protection **42:**794-799; 1979.
27. MURTHY, G.K.; PEELER, J.T. Rapid methods for differentiating reactivated from residual phosphatase in milk and cream: Collaborative study. J. Assoc. Off. Anal. Chem. **62:** 822-827; 1979.
28. MURTHY, G.K.; PEELER, J.T. Collaborative study of rapid methods for alkaline phosphatase in milk and cream. J. Food Protection **42:**800-803; 1979.
29. MURTHY, G.K.; PEELER, J.T. Determination of alkaline phosphatase in casein: collaborative study. J. Assoc. Off. Anal. Chem. **64:**623-627; 1981.
30. NATIONAL CONFERENCE OF INTERSTATE MILK SHIPPERS (NCIMS). Resolution. October 1, 1995.
31. PRATT-LOWE, E.L.; GEIGER, R.M.; RICHARDSON, T.; BARRETT, E.L. Heat resistance of alkaline phosphatase produced by microorganisms isolated from California Mexican-style cheeses. J. Dairy Sci. **71:**17-23; 1988.
32. RICHARDSON, L.A.; MCFARREN, E.F.; CAMPBELL, J.E. Phosphatase reactivation. J. Dairy Res. **47:**205-210; 1964.
33. ROCCO, R.M. Fluorometric analysis of alkaline phosphatase in fluid dairy products. J. Food Protection **53:**588-591; 1990.
34. ROCCO, R.M. Fluorometric determination of alkaline phosphatase in fluid dairy products: Collaborative study. J. Assoc. Off. Anal. Chem. **73:** 842-849; 1990.
35. SCHARER, H. A rapid phosphomonesterase test for the control of dairy pasteurization. J. Dairy Sci. **21:**21-34; 1938.
36. SCHARER, H. Improvements in the rapid phosphatase test for detection of improper pasteurization of milk and its products. J. Milk Technology **1:**35-38; 1938.
37. SCHARER, H. Scharer modified phosphatase methods. J. Milk Food Technology **16:**86-88; 1953.
38. SCHARER, H. Method for detecting enzyme activity. United States Patent No. 2,359,052; Issued September 26, 1944.
39. SIMMONS, J.S.; GENTZKOW, C.J. Laboratory methods of the United States Army, 5th ed. Philadelphia, PA: Lea & Febiger; 1944: 297-298.
40. STIVEN, D. A simple method of conducting the phosphatase test. J. Dairy Res. **15:**57-61; 1947.
41. USDHEW. Milk ordinance and code, recommendations of the Public Health Service. Washington, DC: U.S. Department of Health, Education, and Welfare, Public Health Service; 1953.
42. WRIGHT, R.C.; TRAMER, J. Reactivation of milk phosphatase following heat treatment I. J. Dairy Res. **20:**177-188; 1953.
43. WRIGHT, R.C.; TRAMER, J. Reactivation of milk phosphatase following heat treatment II. J. Dairy Res. **20:**258-273; 1953.

14.080 Other References

Pre-study Report Committee Draft ISO/CD 11816-3/IDF 155-3 2003-02-17.

Chapter 15

Chemical and Physical Methods

R. Hooi, D. M. Barbano, R. L. Bradley, D. Budde, M. Bulthaus, M. Chettiar, J. Lynch, and R. Reddy
(E. A. Arnold, Tech. Comm.)

15.010 Introduction

This chapter contains methods used to determine the chemical constituents and physical properties of fluid milk and dairy products. The chapter has been revised to include additional methods and a method format that is consistent with other official references. Methods continue to be combined to reduce the amount of cross-referencing. Additionally, methods that were classified as C or D methods in prior editions of *SMEDP* have been deleted.

New methods have been added to this section, including aflatoxin assays; peroxide value for determination of oxidation in fats and oils; enzymatic testing for lactose and galactose; solubility and scorched particle tests in nonfat dry milk; Karl Fischer titration for total moisture in high lactose products; and additional nitrogen (protein) tests to include nonprotein nitrogen, casein, and whey protein nitrogen.

Additional sections have been added to this chapter to discuss the minerals in dairy products and their analysis as well as the appropriate uses of food additives in dairy products.

Methods continue to be added in recognition of the advancing complexity and sophistication of the dairy laboratory. The methods included were selected to meet the needs of typical dairy laboratories. Where possible, statistical performance parameters have been included with each method.

15.020 Acidity Tests

Titratable acidity is valuable for measuring the extent of growth of acid-producing bacteria in dairy products. In some cases it has also been used as a gauge for comparing organoleptic determinations. Its measurement is affected by any condition that causes a change in the state of calcium phosphate in the sample. Some of these factors are the amount of dilution of the sample, the speed of titration, the amount of indicator, and the temperature of the sample. All samples should be titrated as quickly as possible at room temperature, using exact amounts of sample, diluent, and reagents. Methods covered in the following sections include titration with an indicator, pH meter, potentiometry, and gold electrode.

This section covers acidity defined through titration and by use of a pH meter. In titratable acidity, the titration for acidity with a titrant (e.g., sodium hydroxide) using either an indicator (phenolphthalein), the pH to pH 8.3 method, or potentiometry is covered. Titration of a sample for acidity is determined by the measurement of a reagent called the titrant (in this case a base) needed to react stoichiometrically with the acid in a sample. pH is defined as: $pH = -\log [H^+]$ or negative log of the hydrogen ion concentration. Proper quantitative chemical analysis practices must be followed to produce results that are precise and accurate.

15.021 Acidity, Titratable—Phenolphthalein Indicator (Class O)[27,47,48]

1. **Scope:** This method is applicable to milk and milk products.
2. **References:** Chapter 2 on "Laboratory Quality Assurance and Safety." Chapter 3 on "Sampling Dairy and Related Products."
3. **Definition:** Titratable acidity is defined as the amount of titrant needed to react stoichiometrically with lactic acid in milk.
4. **Principle:** A standardized solution of sodium hydroxide (0.1N) is added to a specified volume of sample with added phenolphthalein indicator. The end point is reached when the color of the sample changes to a light pink.
5. **Reagents:** Unless otherwise specified, all chemicals are reagent or ACS grade.
   - 5.1 Phenolpthalein, 1%: Disssolve 1 g in 100 mL of 95% ethanol.
   - 5.2 Sodium hydroxide (NaOH): 0.1000N.
   - 5.3 Water (LG):
6. **Apparatus and Glassware:** All volumetric flasks, pipets, and burets are Class A unless otherwise specified.
   - 6.1 Balance: 0.1 gram sensitivity.
   - 6.2 Beakers: 100 mL, 250 mL.
   - 6.3 Buret: 25 mL, 1/10 mL subdivisions, class A preferred. An automatic zero buret may also be used.
   - 6.4 Casserole: Porcelain (crucible) 70 × 30 mm.
   - 6.5 Cylinder: Graduated, 100 mL.
   - 6.6 Electric mixer (blender): Hamilton Beach No. 936 or equivalent (replace steel disc with round Teflon stirrer, 3.25 cm in diameter × 0.64 cm thick) for use with dry milk and dry milk products.
   - 6.7 Flasks: Erlenmeyer, 125 mL; volumetric, 100 mL.
   - 6.8 Pipets: Standard milk, 17.6 mL, TC; standard cream, 9 mL, TC; volumetric, 25 mL.
   - 6.9 Stirring rod with policeman.
   - 6.10 Wash bottle.
7. **Sampling:** Chapter 3: Sampling Dairy and Related Products.

8. **Preparation of Test Sample**
   8.1 Mix milk, fluid ice cream, and sherbet mixes thoroughly by shaking or stirring gently. If milk is lumpy or frozen, heat it to 37° ± 10° before mixing gently.
   8.2 Frozen ice cream, sherbet, and similar samples should be warmed to room temperature and mixed thoroughly.
   8.3 The 17.6 mL TC milk pipet will deliver approximately 18 grams of whole milk or skim milk at 20°C. Rinsing will improve accuracy for viscous products. For greatest precision and accuracy, weigh all samples to 18.0 grams.

9. **Procedure:** Before beginning analysis review material safety data sheets on all chemicals and use appropriate safety equipment such as hoods, aprons, face shields, and glasses.
   9.1 **Milks; fluid whey; melted ice creams, sherbets, ices; mixes; and yogurts:** Measure a 9- or 18-gram sample into a 100-mL beaker or casserole using a pipet. Rinse the pipet with two volumes of LG water if the sample is measured volumetrically. Add rinse to the sample in the beaker and mix gently but thoroughly. If the sample is weighed, use a clean pipet, add twice the sample weight in LG water, and mix thoroughly. Add 0.5 mL of phenolpthalein indicator and titrate with 0.1N sodium hydroxide to the first permanent color change to pink (30 seconds). Use a constant amount of indicator because, as either a weak base or weak acid, its concentration will influence results.

   If the sample is dark in color (such as chocolate milk and mixes), it will be necessary, after adding LG water, to titrate with a pH meter to pH 8.3 (see method 15.023).

   9.2 **Dry buttermilk, dry whey, and whey concentrate products:** Weigh accurately 10 grams of dry buttermilk or buttermilk products, 6.5 grams of dry whey, or 10 grams of whey concentrate into a 100-mL beaker. Add 25 mL of LG water and stir slowly with a stirring rod to dissolve or suspend the sample. Transfer with the aid of a wash bottle to a 100 mL volumetric flask. Make to volume and mix well.

   Transfer 18 grams of rehydrated dry buttermilk, dry whey, or whey concentrate into an Erlenmeyer flask or casserole. Rinse the pipet with an equal volume LG water and add the rinse to the sample in the flask or the casserole.

   Add 0.5 mL of phenolphthalein indicator and titrate with 0.1N sodium hydroxide to the first permanent color change to pink (30 seconds).

   9.3 **Dry whole milk, nonfat dry milk, and malted milk products:** Weigh 10 grams of nonfat dry milk, or malted milk, or 13 grams of dry whole milk, into a 250-mL beaker. Add 100 mL of LG water to the sample and mix, using an electric mixer, for no more than 1 minute to avoid formation of excessive foam.

   Allow the sample to stand for 1 hour at room temperature. Gently but thoroughly mix the sample with a stirring rod. Transfer an 18-gram sample into an Erlenmeyer flask or casserole. Add 0.5 mL of phenolpthalein indicator and titrate with 0.1N sodium hydroxide to the first permanent color change to pink (30 seconds).

10. **Expression of Results**

Acidity is expressed as percentage of lactic acid (1 mL of 0.1 N Sodium hydroxide (NaOH) = 0.009 grams of lactic acid).

10.1 Calculations

10.1.1 For undiluted samples on an as-is basis:

$$\% \text{ acidity} = \frac{(\text{mL NaOH}) \times \dfrac{(\text{Normality of NaOH})}{(1000 \text{ mL of NaOH})} \times \dfrac{(1 \text{ mole lactic acid})}{(1 \text{ mole NaOH})} \times \dfrac{(90.08 \text{ g lactic acid})}{(1 \text{ mole of lactic acid})} \times 100}{\text{Sample weight titrated in grams}}$$

OR

$$\% \text{ acidity} = \frac{(\text{mL NaOH}) \times (\text{Normality of NaOH}) \times (.09) \times 100}{\text{Sample weight titrated in grams}}$$

OR

$$\% \text{ acidity} = \frac{(\text{mL NaOH}) \times (\text{Normality of NaOH}) \times 9}{\text{Sample weight in grams titrated}}$$

10.1.2 Reconstituted samples reported on a reconstituted basis: Samples are reconstituted to original solids content of raw material. See section 10.1.1 for long-form calculation.

$$\% \text{ acidity reconstituted basis} = \frac{(\text{mL NaOH}) \times (\text{Normality of NaOH}) \times 9}{\text{Weight in grams of reconstituted sample titrated}}$$

10.1.3 Dry powders: Samples are reconstituted to original solids content of raw material. See section 10.1.1 for long-form calculation.

$$\% \text{ acidity (powder basis)} = \frac{\% \text{ acidity reconstituted basis/grams of powder}}{\text{grams of powder plus grams water added}}$$

Example:

$$\frac{[(\text{mL NaOH}) \times (\text{Normality of NaOH}) \times 9]/[\text{Weight of reconstituted sample} \times \text{grams of solids}]}{\text{grams of reconstituted sample}}$$

11. **Precision and Performance Parameters**

11.1 Precision data available for evaporated milk indicate the mean variation is ± 0.02%. Higher variation can be expected when assaying reconstituted dry samples with subsequent reporting on the dry basis.

11.2 Estimated precision for duplicate samples reconstituted on a 10% basis is ± 0.01%.

12. **Test Report and Interpretation:** The test report shall identify the method used and results obtained. The report will also identify any variation in the test not specified in this method as well as problems that may have impacted the test result. Each sample will be described in such a manner as to ensure traceablity as to its origin.

15.022 Acidity, Potentiometric, pH, (Class O)[69]

1. **Scope:** This method is applicable to milk and milk products.
2. **References:** Chapter 2 on "Laboratory Quality Assurance and Safety." Chapter 3 on "Sampling Dairy and Related Products."

3. **Definition:** pH is defined as: pH = –log [H^+] or negative log of the hydrogen ion concentration.
4. **Principle**: pH is a measurement of hydrogen ion activity indicating acidity. The electric potential between a sensing electrode and reference electrode is determined by use of a pH probe and meter calibrated using buffers with defined pH values. The electrode of a standardized pH meter is inserted directly into a sample or dilution thereof and the pH is read directly from the meter. The pH measurement provides relative acidity or alkalinity values for samples at a given temperature.
5. **Reagents**: Unless otherwise specified all chemicals are reagent or ACS grade.
   5.1. Buffer solutions: pH 4.0; pH 5.0; pH 7.0; and pH 10.0.
   5.2. Potassium chloride, saturated (or recommended electrode fill solution): Used to refill electrodes.
   5.3. Potassium chloride solution: Dissolve 35 grams in 100 mL of LG water.
   5.4. Cleaning reagents: As specified by electrode manufacture.
   5.5. Water (LG).
6. **Apparatus and Glassware:** All volumetric flasks, pipets, and burets are Class A unless otherwise specified.
   6.1. Beakers: 30, 40, 50, and 400 mL.
   6.2. Centrifuge: For butter or margarine, any laboratory type.
   6.3. Electrodes: Glass and calomel or combination electrode.
   6.4. Funnel: Separatory type.
   6.5. pH meter.
   6.6. Pipet: 10 mL, large bore tip, for butter or margarine.
   6.7. Refrigerator or ice water bath: For butter or margarine.
   6.8. Thermometer: 0°C to 100°C, 1°C or smaller division.
   6.9. Tissue.
   6.10. Wash bottle: Plastic.
   6.11. Water bath: Thermostatically controlled, for butter or margarine.
7. **Sampling:** Chapter 3 on "Sampling Dairy and Related Products."
8. **Preparation of Test Sample:** Take a representative sample that has previously been mixed, stirred, ground, blended, or otherwise prepared in order to make sample uniform.
9. **Procedure:** Before beginning analysis review material safety data sheets on all chemicals and use appropriate safety equipment such as hoods, aprons, face shields, and glasses.
   9.1 **Care and use of electrodes**
      9.1.1 Handle carefully. The electrode is the most important and sensitive component used for pH measurements. Scratches and abrasions on the tip will modify the electrode's sensitivity and accuracy.
      9.1.2 Before using a new glass electrode, soak it for at least 2 hours in potassium chloride solution to ensure proper functioning.
      9.1.3 Keep the electrode exceptionally clean. Follow manufacturer's instructions with regard to cleaning, rinsing, and wiping probes between buffer solutions and samples.

9.1.4 When working with samples containing fatty substances, which may reduce the sensitivity of the electrode, it may be necessary to remove the built-up film from bulb. Follow manufacturer's instructions as to appropriate method. This may vary depending on the type and manufacture of probe. Fatty and protein deposits on electrodes are often evidenced by a slowed probe response time.

9.1.5 When using an electrode with a fill port, the protective sleeve on the glass electrode must be moved to ensure that potassium chloride can move through the wick.

9.2 **Combination electrode calls for the following additional procedures**

9.2.1 Vent the reference side of the electrode before use by removing the rubber cap at the filling tube. This permits the slow leakage of solution from the electrolyte bridge, thereby ensuring good electrical contact at the liquid junction and preventing contamination of the reference electrode.

9.2.2 Since the potassium chloride solution will diffuse outward, it is necessary to replace the saturated potassium chloride through the refill aperture. The solution should never fall more than 2.5 cm below the refill aperture.

9.2.3 Store the electrode by immersing the pH-sensitive tip in potassium chloride. This maintains the hydrated condition of the glass electrode and reduces leakage. Storing in LG water can result in a high-resistance junction, which may cause inefficiencies in operation. If electrodes are not to be used for several months, they may be stored dry. In this instance, the glass electrode must be hydrated in potassium chloride solution for a few days before reuse.

9.3 **Standardization of pH Meter**

9.3.1 The pH meter should be turned on for one half hour before use to stabilize. It is best to leave the pH meter turned on at all times with the proper line and surge protection.

9.3.2 The pH meter must be standardized with uncontaminated buffer solution before determinations are made. Buffer solutions must be capped when not in use to prevent evaporation and contamination. Never pour used buffer back into the stock bottle. Discard used solution at the end of the day.

9.3.3 Pour approximately 25 mL of buffer solution into a 50-mL beaker. Standardize the meter, using both a 7.0-pH and a buffer solution as close as possible to that of the sample being tested. Generate the slope of the calibration to determine the proper response of the meter and electrodes. Follow manufacturer's recommendations as to the appropriate slope.

9.3.4 The pH meter should be re-standardized periodically during each day. When the types of samples are being changed or when the meter has not been used for at least a half hour, it is advisable to repeat the regular standardization procedure.

9.4 **Sample preparation**

9.4.1 Assay liquid samples without further preparation.

9.4.2 Prepare dry products according to the procedure for titratable acidity (method 15.021).

9.4.3 Blend or grind cheese to provide for a uniform sample. The pH for a piece of cheese will vary throughout the sample. Pack the blended sample in a small container to ensure good electrode contact.

9.4.4 Butter and margarine require that the pH be determined on the serum phase and that this be separated from the fat phase. To prepare serum, heat about 115 g of butter or margarine in a 400-mL beaker to 46° to 52°C in a water bath, so that the fat melts and rises to the top while the serum goes to the bottom. (This may require 45 minutes to occur.) The sample should not be agitated during the heating. When separation is complete, remove the serum under the fat layer by pipet and transfer it to a 30-mL beaker or centrifuge tube. Centrifuge for 3 minutes in a Babcock type or other suitable centrifuge.

Place the beaker containing the serum in a refrigerator or in ice water for approximately 2 hours to permit any remaining fat to rise and solidify.

After the fat has formed a hard layer, plunge a pipet through it and draw off the serum. Transfer the serum to a clean 30-mL beaker, warm it to 25°C, and determine the pH.

Alternatively, after melting the butter or margarine, remove the serum under the fat layer by pipet and place it in a separatory funnel. Allow the fat to rise. Centrifuging the separatory funnel will speed separation. Drain the serum from below the fat in the separatory funnel, warm it to 25°C, and determine the pH.

9.5 **Determination**

9.5.1 Immerse the electrode directly into the sample so the pH sensitive bulb and reference junction make good contact with the sample. For cheese, make sure the sample is well packed and that the electrode makes direct contact with the cheese.

9.5.2 Take the temperature of the sample and set the sample temperature compensator to correspond with it, preferably at 25°C ± 3°C. If measurements are performed on samples at temperatures outside this temperature range, temper calibration buffers and the electrode to the same temperature (±3°C) as the sample. Use appropriate temperature-adjusted target pH specified by the calibration buffer supplier that is stated on the original buffer container for that temperature.

9.5.3 Activate the pH meter. Make sure the electrode contacts the sample for at least 45 seconds and until the reading stabilizes. Read the pH directly.

10. Expression of Results: Report the reading as pH units to the nearest 0.01 pH units.

11. **Precision and Performance Parameters**
    11.1 No precision data available; however it is estimated that duplicate assays should be within 0.03 pH units for liquids and 0.06 pH units for less homogenous samples such as cheese.

12. **Test Report and Interpretation:** The test report shall identify the method used and results obtained. The report will also identify any variation in the test not specified in this method as well as problems that may have impacted the test result. Each sample will be described in such a manner as to ensure traceablity as to its origin.

15.023 Acidity, Titratable, Potentiometric End Point (Class O)[27,47,48]

1. **Scope:** This method is applicable to milk and milk products.

2. **References:** Chapter 2 on "Laboratory Quality Assurance and Safety."
   Chapter 3 on "Sampling Dairy and Related Products."
   Chapter 15, methods 15.021 and 15.022.

3. **Definition:** Titratable acidity is defined as the amount of titrant needed to react stoichiometrically with lactic acid in milk to a final specified pH value.

4. **Principle:** A standardized solution of sodium hydroxide (0.1N) is added to a specified volume of sample until the final pH of the solution reads 8.3. The amount of titrant is then calculated to determine the acidity of the sample.

   Titratable acidity cannot always be tested with phenolphthalein because a product may have color such as flavored milks and viscous products that interferes with observation of the pink color. This method combines 15.021 and 15.022 of Chapter 15 to determine the end point. The object is to titrate a sample to an end point pH of 8.3 with the use of a pH meter.

5. **Reagents:** Unless otherwise specified all chemicals are reagent or ACS grade.
   5.1 Utilize same reagents as specified in methods 15.021 and 15.022 except for the reagent phenolphthalein.

6. **Apparatus and Glassware:** Unless otherwise specified all chemicals are reagent or ACS grade.
   6.1 Utilize same apparatus and glassware as methods 15.021 and 15.022.

7. **Sampling:** Chapter 3 on "Sampling Dairy and Related Products."

8. **Preparation of Test Sample**
   8.1 Mix milk, fluid ice cream and sherbet mixes thoroughly by shaking or stirring gently. If milk is lumpy or frozen, heat it to 37° ± 1°C before mixing gently.
   8.2 Frozen ice cream, sherbet, and similar samples should be warmed to room temperature and mixed thoroughly.
   8.3 The 17.6-mL TC milk pipet will deliver approximately 18 grams of whole milk or skim milk at 20°C. Rinsing will improve accuracy for viscous products. For greatest precision and accuracy, weigh all samples to 18.0 grams.

9. **Procedure:** Before beginning analysis, review material safety data sheets on all chemicals and use appropriate safety equipment such as hoods, aprons, face shields, and glasses.
   9.1 Set up and standardize pH meter as specified in section 9 of method 15.022.
   9.2 Use a glass and calomel electrodes or a combination electrode with calibration and precautions identified in the above sections. Note: During calibration, stir buffers the same way that the sample will be stirred.
   9.3 Immerse the electrode in the sample with the rinse water from the pipet. Use constant stirring while titrating but do not allow the stirrer bar to touch the electrodes.
   9.4 Add 0.1N sodium hydroxide to a pH of 8.3. Additions may be rapid to pH of approximately 7.6 and slow thereafter. Allow sufficient time for equilibration to occur.

10. **Expression of Results**
    10.1 Calculation: Calculate results as specified in section 10 of method 15.021.

11. **Precision and Performance Parameters**
    11.1 Precision data available for evaporated milk indicate the mean variation is ± 0.02%. Higher variation can be expected when assaying reconstituted dry samples with subsequent reporting on the dry basis.
    11.2 Estimated precision for duplicate samples reconstituted on a 10% basis is ±0.01%.

12. **Test Report and Interpretation:** The test report shall identify the method used and results obtained. The report will also identify any variation in the test not specified in this method as well as problems that may have impacted the test result. Each sample will be described in such a manner as to ensure traceablity as to its origin.

15.024 Acidity, pH, Gold Electrode/Quinhydrone (Class O)[71,83]

1. **Scope:** This method is applicable to natural cheese.
2. **References:** Chapter 2 on "Laboratory Quality Assurance and Safety." Chapter 3 on "Sampling Dairy and Related Products."
3. **Definition:** A gold wire in a standard solution of quinhydrone is used as a reversible electrode for pH determinations. pH is defined as: pH = –log $[H^+]$ or negative log of the hydrogen ion concentration.
4. **Principle:** A pH meter is set up with a gold electrode and a reference electrode to measure oxidation/reduction potential of samples. The oxidation/reduction potential is related to pH values by calibrating the meter and electrode with buffers of known pH values that correspond to specific millivolt readings at specified temperatures.
5. **Reagents:** Unless otherwise specified all chemicals are reagent or ACS grade.
   5.1 Buffer solutions: pH 4.0, pH 5.0, and pH 7.0.
   5.2 Potassium chloride (ACS), saturated solution: Weigh 50 grams of

potassium chloride into a pre-weighed 250-mL beaker and add 100 mL of LG water. Heat the solution to boiling to dissolve all the crystals. While the solution is hot, transfer it to a glass storage bottle. Allow it to cool, with crystals forming on the bottom of the bottle, before use.

5.3 Quinhydrone: 171° to 173°C melting point. *Caution: Quinhydrone is considered an acute health hazard.*

5.4 LG Water.

6. **Apparatus and Glassware:** Unless otherwise specified all chemicals are reagent or ACS grade.

6.1 Beakers: 50 mL, 100 mL.

6.2 Electrodes: Gold tip electrode used in conjunction with calomel electrode.

6.3 Mortar and pestle.

6.4 pH meter.

6.5 Soda straws: Plastic, 2 cm in length.

6.6 Thermometer: 0° to 100°C, 1°C or smaller divisions.

7. **Sampling:** Chapter 3 on "Sampling Dairy and Related Products."

8. **Preparation of Test Sample:** Take a representative sample that has previously been mixed, stirred, ground, blended, or otherwise prepared in order to make sample uniform.

9. **Procedure:** Before beginning analysis review material safety data sheets on all chemicals and use appropriate safety equipment such as hoods, aprons, face shields, and glasses.

9.1 **Care and use of electrodes**

9.1.1 **Calomel reference electrode:** Handle carefully; follow the manufacturer's instructions for care and maintenance.

9.1.2 **Gold electrode:** The wire tip of the gold electrode is soft and will break if repeatedly bent or flexed. Always use gentle pressure to force the electrode into solid samples.

Thoroughly clean the gold electrode assembly immediately after completing each calibration or measurement. Thoroughly wash the entire assembly at the end of each day of use.

Between measurements, store the clean gold electrode with the gold tip immersed in LG water that contains a few crystals of quinhydrone.

9.2 **Standardization of pH meter**

9.2.1 Insert a shorting strap between the electrode and the reference connection on the pH meter. Set the meter for millivolt (mV) readings and activate. The reading should be 0.0 mV.

9.2.2 Assemble the gold electrode and liquid sample tube by wetting the electrode stem with water and gently pushing the stem into the plastic calibration tube.

9.2.3 Pour 10 to 15 mL of a buffer solution of pH similar to that of samples to be tested into a 50-mL beaker. Add quinhydrone (the size of a pea) to the solution and stir rapidly to disperse. When enough quinhydrone disperses, a black solution results.

9.2.4 Immediately fill the quinhydrone electrode with well dispersed quinhydrone/buffer solution.

9.2.5 Fill the electrode assembly with enough buffer-quinhydrone mixture to immerse the gold wire completely.

9.2.6 Push the gold electrode stem into the plastic tube until the gold wire tip is at the bottom of the open tip of the tube.

9.2.7 Place the tip of the assembly in the buffer/quinhydrone mixture and withdraw the plunger until the gold wire is just below the top of the plastic tube. Remove the tip from the mixture and invert the assembly so that the open tip points upward.

9.2.8 Gently push the electrode stem into the tube until the air has been expelled and the liquid begins to overflow from the tip of the plastic tube. If necessary, repeat the air expulsion and filling steps. The tip should now be completely immersed in the mixture and should rest midway in the plastic calibration tube.

9.2.9 Insert the gold electrode lead into the reference electrode input and insert the calomel cell into the adapter input. Make sure electrode is plugged in before starting testing.

9.2.10 Immerse the filled gold electrode assembly and the tip of the calomel electrode in 25 mL to 50 mL of saturated potassium chloride solution in a 100-mL beaker.

9.2.11 During measurement, the gold tip must be entirely immersed in the quinhydrone mixture. A reading cannot be obtained if there is direct contact between the gold electrode and the potassium chloride solution.

9.2.12 Record the temperature of the remaining buffer/quinhydrone solution and the millivolt reading from the pH meter.

9.2.13 To determine the millivolt (MV) reading of the buffer at the temperature of the buffer/quinhydrone mixture, use

$$MV = 452.9 + 0.02t - pH\,[0.198322\,(t + 273)],$$

Where t = temperature in degrees Celsius (°C) of the buffer/quinhydrone solution. If the actual millivolt reading is more than ± 0.03 mV from the theoretical value, clean the electrode and repeat. The theoretical millivolt (MV) value is obtained by calculation using the above formula. Enter the temperature of the buffer/quinhydrone solution and the manufacturer's pH value for that temperature.

9.3 **Determination**

9.3.1 While preparing the cheese sample, immerse the tip of the calomel electrode in 25 mL to 50 mL of saturated potassium chloride solution in a 100-mL beaker.

9.3.2 Place approximately 5 grams of cheese at room temperature in a mortar.

9.3.3 Add 1 gram ± 0.2 gram of quinhydrone powder to the mortar and use the pestle to mix it thoroughly with the cheese. Record the temperature of the mixture.

9.3.4 Repeatedly press a section of plastic straw into the cheese/quinhydrone mixture until the straw is firmly packed.

9.3.5 With the plastic tube removed from the gold electrode, hold a gloved finger over one end of the straw and gently push the gold wire into the sample mixture until the tip is completely embedded.

9.3.6 Place the straw end of the electrode assembly into the beaker with the calomel electrode and saturated potassium chloride solution.

9.3.7 Lower the gold electrode so that only the bottom portion of the sample is in the potassium chloride mixture. The end of the gold wire must be above the potassium chloride solution.

9.3.8 Determine (within 90 seconds of adding quinhydrone to the cheese) and record the millivolt reading.

10. Expression of Results

10.1 Calculation:

$$pH = \frac{452.9 + 0.02t - mV}{0.198322\ (t + 273)}$$

Where t = temperature in degrees Celsius (°C) of the cheese/quinhydrone mixture, and

mV = millivolt reading (positive number)

If this method is to be used repeatedly, it is recommended that tables be prepared to convert millivolt to pH at different temperatures.

11. Precision and Performance Parameters

11.1 No precision data available; however, it is estimated that assays should be within 0.03 pH units for liquids and 0.06 pH units for less homogenous samples such as cheese.

12. Test Report and Interpretation: The test report shall identify the method used and results obtained. The report will also identify any variation in the test not specified in this method as well as problems that may have impacted the test result. Each sample will be described in such a manner as to ensure traceablity as to its origin.

15.030 Adulterant Tests

15.031 Vegetable Oil in Milkfat (Beta-sitosterol), (Class O)[11(970.50)]

1. **Scope:** This method is applicable to milk and milk products.
2. **References:** Chapter 2 on "Laboratory Quality Assurance and Safety." Chapter 3 on "Sampling Dairy and Related Products."
3. **Definition:** Vegetable oil in milkfat is defined as the amount of β-sitosterol in excess of 1 mg/100 gram of lipid.
4. **Principle:** The method involves complexing 3-β-OH sterols with digitonin, elution from a packed column, and gas chromatographic (GC) quantification.
5. **Reagents:** Unless otherwise specified all chemicals are reagent or ACS grade.

   5.1 **Benzene:** (CAUTION: This compound is a known carcinogen; use appropriate safety precautions to include hood and protective clothing and equipment.)

5.2 **Chloroform:** High-performance liquid chromatography (HPLC) grade. (CAUTION: This compound is a known carcinogen; use appropriate safety precautions to include hood and protective clothing and equipment.)

5.3 **Diatomaceous earth:** Celite 545 or equivalent.

5.4 **Digitonin**

5.5 **Dimethylsulfoxide (DMSO):** 99% plus purity. (CAUTION: Hazardous material, use appropriate safety equipment.)

5.6 **n-hexane:** Redistilled over potassium hydroxide. (CAUTION: Hazardous material, use appropriate safety equipment.)

5.7 **Sterol standards, campesterol, cholesterol, β-sitosterol:** Highest purity, suitable for gas chromatography.

6. **Apparatus and Glassware:** All volumetric flasks, pipets, and burets are Class A unless otherwise specified.

6.1 **Column:** Separation, 2 × 12 cm with a 5-mm inner diameter, outflow equipped with rubber tubing and a pinch clamp.

6.2 **Gas chromatograph:** Because of the wide variety of instruments available, only general operating specifications are needed. An automatic sampler is desirable because it will minimize errors involved with sample injection.

6.3 **Set temperatures**: (1) Flame ionization detector, 265° to 285°C, (2) Injection port, 265° to 285°C, (3) oven, 225° to 250°C.

6.4 **Column requirements, packed:** 3% JXR silicone on 100-120 mesh Gas-Chrom Q with carrier gas flow adjusted to give approximate retention times of cholesterol 16 to 18 minutes, campesterol 22 to 24 minutes, and β-sitosterol 28 to 30 minutes.

6.5 **Column requirements, capillary:** Coating is cross-linked 5% phenylmethyl silicone with splitter, and gas flow is adjusted to give approximate retention times of cholesterol 5.5 minutes, campesterol 7.0 minutes, and β-sitosterol 8.5 minutes.

6.6 **Pipet:** Pasteur, disposable.

6.7 **Tube:** Centrifuge, 50 mL, with Teflon-lined screw cap.

6.8 **Vial:** 2 mL, screw cap.

7. **Sampling:** Chapter 3 on "Sampling Dairy and Related Products."

8. **Preparation of Test Sample:** Take a representative sample that has previously been mixed, stirred, ground, blended, or otherwise prepared in order to make sample uniform.

9. **Procedure:** Before beginning analysis review material safety data sheets on all chemicals and use appropriate safety equipment such as hoods, aprons, face shields, and glasses.

9.1 Use heat to dissolve 300 mg of digitonin in 5 mL of water and add to 10 g of Celite. Mix thoroughly with a mortar and pestle. This packing material can be stored in an airtight glass container at 5°C for several months. Put a small amount of glass wool in the bottom of a 2 × 12 cm separation tube. Transfer 3 g of digitonin-Celite mixture to this tube and pack it firmly with a tamping rod so that the flow rate is 0.5 to 0.75 mL/minute. Saturate the digitonin-Celite with 5 mL of n-hexane. Allow the n-hexane to drain until it reaches the top of the packing. Use the column immediately and do not let it dry.

9.2 Dissolve about 0.9 g of lipid in 3 mL of n-hexane and add internal standard (see section 9.4). Quantitatively transfer the sample to the column using two 2-mL rinses of n-hexane with a disposable Pasteur pipet. Allow the solvent to enter the packing material by opening the pinch clamp. Wash the sample into the column using five 2-mL n-hexane rinses. After all the n-hexane has entered the column, wash with five 2-mL portions of benzene. When the last of the benzene is about 1 cm above the packing, remove the rubber tubing and rinse the inner and outer surfaces of the column tip with benzene to remove all traces of lipid. This minimizes interference from lipids and the resulting poor chromatograms. Discard the eluates of hexane and benzene.

9.3 Before benzene falls below the top of the packing, add 10 mL of DMSO to elute sterols. Collect DMSO eluate in a 50-mL screw cap (Teflon-lined) centrifuge tube. Add 3 mL of n-hexane to the eluate; shake and centrifuge. Carefully transfer the upper layer containing any sterols to another screw-cap centrifuge tube. Repeat the extraction of DMSO eluate in the first tube using two 4-mL portions of n-hexane and benzene (1:1); shake, centrifuge, and again carefully transfer the upper layer to the second centrifuge tube. Add 3 mL of water to the pooled upper layers in the second tube and centrifuge until clear. Remove the upper layer and evaporate it gently under nitrogen in a small beaker or tube. Transfer to a 2-mL vial with two 0.8-mL portions of chloroform. Evaporate the solvent and resuspend the residue in 0.1 mL of the chloroform for GC analysis.

9.4 **Internal standard:** Prepare a solution containing 1 mg of campesterol in 1 mL of chloroform. Add 0.5 mL of this solution to the column at the point in the procedure where the lipid sample is added to the digitonin-Celite column (section 9.2).

10. Expression of Results

10.1 **Calculations:** Identify the campesterol and β-sitosterol peaks from the chromatogram, and measure the peak heights. Calculate the milligrams of β-sitosterol per 100 g of lipid; correct the result using the internal standard:

$$\text{Mg of } \beta\text{-sitosterol per 100 g lipid} = \frac{H_i}{H_x} \times \frac{C_x}{C_i} \times \frac{S_x}{S_i} \times \frac{Q_i}{Q_x} \times 100$$

Where i = internal standard, campesterol;
x = β-sitosterol;
H = peak height, mm;
C = concentration of sterols, µg/µL;
S = peak height mm;
Q_I = concentration of campesterol µg/µL; and
Q = mg sample/µL.

10.2 Interpretation: Butteroil has trace amounts of β-sitosterol in the range of 0 to 1 mg/100 g of lipid while ice cream may have up to 4 mg/100 g of lipid as a result of the emulsifiers used.

11. **Precision and Performance Parameters:** No precision parameters available for this test.

12. **Test Report and Interpretation:** The test report shall identify the method used and results obtained. The report will also identify any variation in the test not specified in this method as well as problems that may have impacted the test result. Each sample will be described in such a manner as to ensure traceablity as to its origin.

15.032 Water, Added to Milk, Thermistor Cryoscope (Class A1)[10,28,36,41,46,78]

Cryoscope analysis to determine whether or not water (over and above the average normal level) has been added to milk has gained acceptance as a tool to monitor the quality of milk and some milk products. Some regulatory agencies have tolerances for added water, and penalties are imposed on producer supplies when a particular percentage is exceeded. Additional information such as dilution with processing, nutritional profiles of bovine dairy herds, and compliance with specifications for contracts can also be obtained with routine use of the milk cyroscope. The values obtained are certainly useful, but must be approached with caution on an individual basis. Many factors can affect individual readings, and an understanding of these factors should be behind any use of freezing point data. It can be a very good method for determining evidence of added water when the data obtained are carefully examined.

Several studies on herd raw milk have determined that the average freezing point of raw milk is nearly constant. This nearly constant value indicates that the solute (dissolved solids in the water phase) of normal milk does not differ from supply to supply. Pure water freezes at 0.0°C and pure product freezes at a specific point less than this (depressed), establishing a linear relationship between the concentration of no added water and the concentration of 100% water. It has been successfully applied to raw bulk tank milk, silo milk, skimmed milk (raw or pasteurized), homogenized whole milk, UHT-treated and sterilized milks, and concentrated milks. Determination of the freezing point for the absolute pure product (no added water) is vital to establishing the values corresponding to added water.

Pure water freezes at 0.0°C. Water with dissolved salt, sugars, etc., freezes at lower than this temperature, and it is generally recognized that the higher the concentration of solids dissolved in the water phase of milk, the lower the freezing point. The baseline freezing point value for average normal raw milk has been accepted to be 0.540°H. Values closer to zero, or higher than this, are often calculated to contain added water on a percentage basis by plotting points on a line from zero water to 100% water. Instruments used to obtain this information are calibrated with known concentrations of salt solutions (optional, sugar solutions). The concentrations of salt solutions are chosen to bracket the extremes of values that may be encountered when measuring samples. The value obtained from a milk cryoscope is generally a number in degrees Hortvet. The instrument supercools the test sample and, by using mechanical vibration, induces crystallization. The heat of crystallization causes a rise in sample temperature until the sample is at the precise point of freezing.

1. **Scope:** This method is applicable to raw commingled milk.
2. **References:** Chapter 2 on "Laboratory Quality Assurance and Safety." Chapter 3 on "Sampling Dairy and Related Products."
3. **Definition:** Water added to milk is defined as the amount of added water necessary to raise the freezing point of milk to a specified level.
4. **Principle:** Milk sample is supercooled, whereby mechanical vibration induces crystallization. The heat of crystallization causes a rise in sample temperature until the sample is at the precise point of freezing. At this point the temperature is determined.
5. **Reagents:** Unless otherwise specified all chemicals are reagent or ACS grade.
   - 5.1 **Commerical or prepared standards:** Values associated with either standard are –0.408C and –0.600C, respectively.
     - 5.1.1 **Salt solutions**: Equivalent to 7% and 10% sucrose (sucrose solutions acceptable alternative). 0.6892g and 1.0206 g of sodium chloride each made up to 100 mL with LG water.
     - 5.1.2 **Sucrose solutions:** 7% and 10%. 7.0000 g and 10.0000 g of sucrose, each made up to 100 mL of LG water.
   - 5.2 **Bath liquid:** (33% volume/volume aqueous solution of ethylene glycol or commercially available bath liquid).
   - 5.3 **LG water**
6. **Apparatus and Glassware:** All volumetric flasks, pipets, and burets are Class A unless otherwise specified.
   - 6.1 **Thermistor cryoscope:** Consists of a cooling bath, a precise thermistor probe (senses temperature changes less than 0.001°C), a stirrer, a mechanism to cause the supercooled sample to freeze, and a mechanism to display temperature.
   - **6.2 Pipets:** 2.0 mL.
   - **6.3 Cyroscope sample tubes**: Glass, uniformly thick throughout, and sized for the instrument.
   - **6.4 Sample tube rack (optional for automatic multisample system).**
   - **6.5 Continuous pipeting device (optional for multiple samples).**
   - **6.6 Drying oven**: For tubes after washing, optional.
7. **Sampling:** Chapter 3 on "Sampling Dairy and Related Products."
8. **Preparation of Test Sample:** Take a representative sample that has previously been mixed, stirred, or otherwise prepared in order to make sample uniform.
9. **Procedure:** Before beginning analysis review material safety data sheets on all chemicals and use appropriate safety equipment such as hoods, aprons, face shields, and glasses.
   - 9.1 **Instrument calibration**
     - 9.1.1 Instrument must be switched on for at least 12 hours prior to calibration. Position of probe, vibration amplitude of stirring wire, and temperature of cooling bath are as recommended by manufacturer.
     - 9.1.2 Follow manufacturer's recommendations for instrument calibration using known solutions. Standard solutions must give proper values prior to sample analysis.

9.1.3 Determine values on known samples daily. If instrument does not give proper results on standard solutions, results on samples will not be valid.

9.1.4 Follow the same procedure for standard analysis as for sample analysis.

9.1.5 With continuous use, run a calibration sample once per hour.

9.2 **Instrument check**

9.2.1 Check the level of coolant and temperature of cooling bath. (normal is –4° to –7°C).

9.2.2 Place the tip of the thermistor near the center of the 2-mL sample.

9.2.3 Adjust the stirrer and the freezer-vibrator to give good mixing and strong vibration for freezing.

9.2.4 Ensure that sample tubes are clean, lint-free, and unscratched to prevent prefreezing of the sample. Be sure tubes that have been washed are dry before introduction of sample.

9.2.5 If using cryoscope with rack and automatic sample advance, load samples a few at a time to avoid evaporation prior to sample analysis and keep temperature of samples delivered for analysis relatively constant.

9.2.6 Follow recommended maintenance guidelines in the instrument manual to ensure optimal test results.

9.3 **Determination**

9.3.1 Transfer 2 mL of a well-mixed sample to a test tube.

9.3.2 Cool and freeze the sample according to manufacturer's instrument instructions. Optionally, hold the sample in an ice water bath (0°-4.0°C) before testing, but avoid formation of condensate on walls of tube above the sample.

9.3.3 If sample prefreezes or does not freeze, prepare another sample and retest. When sample prefreezes, heat in water bath to 32°-38°C, mix well, and rerun procedure after cooling the sample in the ice water bath.

9.3.4 A single test gives an approximate freezing point. Second and third replicates establish more accurate freezing points.

9.3.5 Occasionally, sample will not freeze successfully when presented to the instrument even after the above precautions are taken. If this occurs obtain a new sample and test again.

9.4 **Troubleshooting**

Variations in results on individual milk samples may result from a number of factors independent of normal instrument variation.

9.4.1 The ash content of the sample will affect the freezing point.

9.4.2 Seasonal variations are generally slight, but real.

9.4.3 Herd health affects the freezing point.

9.4.4 Excess mineral supplements in the cow's diet or low carbohydrates will give altered freezing point values.

9.4.5 Breed of animals will sometimes change the value of the freezing point from the expected value for normal milk in a given market area.

9.4.6 High bacteria counts that may have resulted in some lactose fermentation will alter the normal freezing point. Samples with a titratable acidity value of over 0.18% will usually show a lower freezing point and should not be run.

9.4.7 Previously frozen samples will generally not give reliable readings.

9.4.8 Mastitic milk will not give normal freezing point values.

9.4.9 Contamination with soaps and or sanitizers may significantly alter the expected value.

9.4.10 Milk of a high colostrum content will often not freeze or will show unexpected results.

9.4.11 Adverse weather conditions, which are stressful situations to bovine herds, can alter the expected freezing point.

10. Expression of Results

10.1 **Calculation:** Calculate the added water as follows: 1% of added water raises the freezing point of milk about B/100.

$$\frac{(B\text{-}T) \times 100}{\%\ \text{added water}} = B$$

where B = base freezing point of normal samples
T = true freezing point of test sample

10.2 Conversion of different readings is done by the following:
Degrees Celsius = 0.96231 Degrees H – 0.00240
Degrees Hortvet = 1.03616 Degrees C – 0.00250

10.3 Optionally, read value from display and use linear conversion chart to calculate the percentage of added water.

11. Precision and Performance Parameters

11.1 **Repeatability:** Duplicate results on the same sample by same analyst in the same laboratory will not exceed 4 millidegrees C.

11.2 **Reproducibility:** Difference between tests on the same sample, by different analysts, in different laboratories, using different equipment, will not exceed 7 millidegrees C.

12. Test Report and Interpretation: The test report shall identify the method used and results obtained. The report will also identify any variation in the test not specified in this method as well as problems that may have impacted the test result. Each sample will be described in such a manner as to ensure traceablity as to its origin.

15.040 Ash Tests

15.041 Ash, Gravimetric (Class O)[6,11(954.46)]

1. **Scope:** This method is applicable to milk and milk products.
2. **References:** Chapter 2 on "Laboratory Quality Assurance and Safety." Chapter 3 on "Sampling Dairy and Related Products."
3. **Definition:** Ash is defined as the residue remaining after ignition at 550°C to constant weight (approximately 5 hours).
4. **Principle:** Ignition at 550°C will eliminate all organic matter, with the remaining material being primarily minerals.

5. **Reagents:** Unless otherwise specified all chemicals are reagent or ACS grade.
   5.1 Aqua regia solution: Mix three parts hydrochloric acid (HCL) with one part nitric acid (HNO_3) and dilute 1:1 with LG water. (Add acid to water.) CAUTION: Eye protection should be worn.
   5.2 Water (LG).
6. **Apparatus and Glassware:** All volumetric flasks, pipets, and burets are Class A unless otherwise specified.
   6.1 Balance: 0.1-mg sensitivity.
   6.2 Bunsen burner.
   6.3 Crucible: Porcelain, Coors No. 1 or platinum dish.
   6.4 Desiccator: Charged with efficient desiccant.
   6.5 Furnace: Muffle, thermostatically controlled.
   6.6 Hot plate: Thermostatically controlled.
   6.7 Marking ink: Permanent type for crucibles.
   6.8 Oven: Forced draft.
   6.9 Steam bath.
   6.10 Stirring rod with flat end.
   6.11 Tongs: For muffle furnace.
   6.12 Tripod: Iron.
   6.13 Wash bottle.
   6.14 Watch glass: Diameter larger than crucible.
7. **Sampling:** Chapter 3 on "Sampling Dairy and Related Products."
8. **Preparation of Test Sample:** Take a representative sample that has previously been mixed, stirred, ground, blended, or otherwise prepared in order to make sample uniform.
9. **Procedure:** Before beginning analysis review material safety data sheets on all chemicals and use appropriate safety equipment such as hoods, aprons, face shields, and glasses.
   9.1 **Preparation of crucible**
      9.1.1 Heat the side of the crucible to be marked over a low flame for a few minutes. Apply marking ink while the crucible is warm. Allow the ink to dry. Fire the crucible over the burner at a dull red heat and cool.
      9.1.2 Submerge the crucible carefully in aqua regia. CAUTION: Eye protection should be worn. Allow the crucible to remain in the aqua regia for several hours. Remove it and rinse it in LG water.
      9.1.3 Dry the crucible in an oven at 100°C. When it is dry, ignite it in a muffle furnace or over a burner to a dull redness. Cool it to room temperature. Place it in a desiccator until it is ready to use. Crucibles must be cleaned in aqua regia, dried, and ignited in this manner prior to each use.
   9.2 **Determination**
      9.2.1 Weigh accurately into a prepared, preweighed crucible 2 g of dry products or 10 g of other samples.
      9.2.2 Evaporate to dryness in a forced draft oven at 100°C, or place on a steam bath and dry for 1 hour. (Dry powders do not require this step.)

9.2.3 Transfer the crucible to the hood, place it on an iron tripod over a Bunsen burner, and slowly carbonize the sample. Heat cautiously to prevent spattering. (A few drops of olive oil may be added to reduce spattering.) Remove the burner if fat ignites, and smother the fire with a large watch glass. The flame should be adjusted to a height whereby carbonization is complete in about 30 minutes. The sample should not be carbonized to such a point where any part becomes white, but it should be smokeless.

9.2.4 Place the sample in a muffle furnace regulated at 540° to 550°C. Incinerate the sample until it is free of carbon and a light gray or white ash remains.

9.2.5 Remove the sample from the furnace and cool. Moisten the ash with a small amount LG water to form a paste, and gently crush the ash particles with a flat-end stirring rod. To remove any adhering ash particles, rinse the rod with a few milliliters of LG water and allow the rinsing to drain into the crucible.

9.2.6 Evaporate the sample solution on a steam bath. Remove the crucible and dry its contents on a hot plate regulated at 100° to 120°C. (If the hot plate is too hot, ash may spatter because of residual moisture present. After the sample has been partially dried, the temperature of the hot plate may be increased to ensure the thorough drying of the ash.)

9.2.7 Return the dried sample crucible to the muffle furnace, observing the same precautions as noted above, and ash again for 1 hour. Remove the crucible and cool to room temperature in a desiccator until an ambient temperature is reached. Reweigh.

10. Expression of Results

10.1 **Calculations**

$$\% \text{ ash} = \frac{\text{weight of residue} \times 100}{\text{weight of sample}}$$

11. Precision and Performance Parameters: No precision data available; however, it is estimated that duplicate samples tested by the same analyst, in the same laboratory, using the same equipment, should not exceed ± 0.05%.

12. Test Report and Interpretation: The test report shall identify the method used and results obtained. The report will also identify any variation in the test not specified in this method as well as problems that may have impacted the test result. Each sample will be described in such a manner as to ensure traceablity as to its origin.

15.042 Alkalinity of Ash (Class O)[6,11(941.07)]

1. Scope: This method is applicable to dry milk.

2. References: Chapter 2 on "Laboratory Quality Assurance and Safety." Chapter 3 on "Sampling Dairy and Related Products."

3. **Definition:** Alkalinity of ash is defined as the mL of 0.1N HCL required to neutralize the ash of 100 grams of dry milk. Typical non-fat dry milk has an alkalinity of ash of <100 mL per 100 gram of product.[69]

4. **Principle:** The measurement of alkalinity of ash is helpful in determining the use of sodium hydroxide or other similar products used to neutralize lactic acid that may have developed in the product due to microbiological growth. Low alkalinities are not significant but may indicate a high level of acid in the original product.

5. **Reagents:** Unless otherwise specified all chemicals are reagent or ACS grade.
   - 5.1 Calcium chloride solution, 40%: Dissolve appropriate amount of calcium chloride (40 g of anhydrous calcium chloride plus 60 g of LG water) in LG water. Add a few drops of phenolphthalein indicator and adjust to neutrality with 0.100N hydrochloric acid.
   - 5.2 Hydrochloric acid (HCL), 0.100N.
   - 5.3 Phenolphthalein indicator, 1.0%: Dissolve 1 g in 100 mL of 95% ethyl alcohol.
   - 5.4 Sodium hydroxide (NaOH), 0.100N.
   - 5.5 Water (LG).

6. **Apparatus and Glassware:** All volumetric flasks, pipets, and burets are Class A unless otherwise specified.
   - 6.1 Beaker: 400 mL.
   - 6.2 Buret: 50 mL, 0.1-mL divisions.
   - 6.3 Cylinder: Graduated, 50 mL.
   - 6.4 Pipet: Volumetric, 50 mL.
   - 6.5 Watch glasses: 90 mm.

7. **Sampling:** Chapter 3 on "Sampling Dairy and Related Products."

8. **Preparation of Test Sample:** Take a representative sample that has previously been mixed, stirred, ground, blended, or otherwise prepared in order to make sample uniform.

9. **Procedure:** Before beginning analysis review material safety data sheets on all chemicals and use appropriate safety equipment such as hoods, aprons, face shields, and glasses.
   - 9.1 **Preparation of crucible**
     - 9.1.1 Heat the side of the crucible to be marked over a low flame for a few minutes. Apply marking ink while the crucible is warm. Allow the ink to dry. Fire the crucible over the burner at a dull red heat and cool.
     - 9.1.2 Submerge the crucible carefully in aqua regia. CAUTION: Eye protection should be worn. Allow the crucible to remain in the aqua regia for several hours. Remove it and rinse it in tap water and then in LG water.
     - 9.1.3 Dry the crucible in an oven at 100°C. When it is dry, ignite it in a muffle furnace or over a burner to a dull redness. Cool it to room temperature. Place it in a desiccator until it is ready to use. Crucibles must be cleaned in aqua regia, dried, and ignited in this manner after each use.

9.2 **Determination**

9.2.1 Weigh accurately into a prepared, preweighed crucible 2 g of dry products or 10 g of other samples.

9.2.2 Evaporate to dryness in a forced draft oven at 100°C, or place on a steam bath and dry for 1 hour. (Dry powders do not require this step.)

9.2.3 Transfer the crucible to the hood, place it on an iron tripod over a Bunsen burner, and slowly carbonize the sample. Heat cautiously to prevent spattering. (A few drops of olive oil may be added to reduce spattering.) Remove the burner if fat ignites, and smother the fire with a large watch glass. The flame should be adjusted to a height whereby carbonization is complete in about 30 minutes. The sample should not be carbonized to such a point where any part becomes white, but it should be smokeless.

9.2.4 Place the sample in a muffle furnace regulated at 540° to 550°C. Incinerate the sample until it is free of carbon and a light gray or white ash remains.

9.2.5 Remove the sample from the furnace and cool. Moisten the ash with a small amount LG water to form a paste, and gently crush the ash particles with a flat-end stirring rod. To remove any adhering ash particles, rinse the rod with a few milliliters of LG water and allow the rinsing to drain into the crucible.

9.2.6 Evaporate the sample solution on a steam bath. Remove the crucible and dry its contents on a hot plate regulated at 100° to 120°C. (If the hot plate is too hot, ash may spatter because of residual moisture present. After the sample has been partially dried, the temperature of the hot plate may be increased to ensure the thorough drying of the ash.)

9.2.7 Return the dried sample crucible to the muffle furnace, observing the same precautions as noted above, and ash again for 1 hour. Remove the crucible and cool to room temperature in a desiccator until an ambient temperature is reached. Reweigh.

9.3 Moisten ash with a small amount of LG water and transfer the sample quantitatively to a 400-mL beaker.

9.4 Pipet 50 mL of 0.100N hydrochloric acid and add it to the sample in the beaker. Cover it with a watch glass and boil gently for 5 minutes. Avoid spattering. Allow the beaker to cool, and rinse the watch glass with freshly boiled LG water. Allow rinsings to drain back into the beaker.

9.5 Add 30 mL of 40% calcium chloride solution, gently stir, cover with a watch glass, and allow the sample to stand for 10 minutes.

9.6 Add 10 drops of phenolphthalein indicator solution and titrate with 0.100N sodium hydroxide to a faint pink end point that lasts 30 seconds.

10. **Expression of Results**

10.1 **Calculations**

All results are expressed as "milliliters of 0.1N hydrochloric acid per 100 g or dry milk." If exactly 2 g of sample is weighed out and the hydrochloric acid and sodium hydroxide solutions are exactly 0.1N, the calculation is simplified:

$$\text{mL } 0.1\text{N HCL}/100\text{g} = 50 \times (50 - \text{mL } 0.1\text{N NaOH}).$$

10.2 If the weight of the sample is not exactly 2 g and the solutions are not exactly 0.1N, the following formula is used:

$$\text{mL } 0.1\text{N HCL}/100\text{g} = \frac{1000 \times 50 \times (\text{N HCL}) - (\text{mL NaOH} \times \text{N NaOH})}{\text{weight of sample}}$$

11. **Precision and Performance Parameters**

11.1 No precision data are available for this assay; however, it is estimated that duplicate results should be within ± 15 mL.

12. **Test Report and Interpretation:** The test report shall identify the method used and results obtained. The report will also identify any variation in the test not specified in this method as well as problems which may have impacted the test result. Each sample will be described in such a manner as to ensure traceability as to its origin.

15.050 Chloride Tests

15.051 Chloride (Salt), Mohr Method (Class O)[25,65]

1. **Scope:** This method may be used for milk, cream, cottage cheese, whey, and similar products where the salt is easy to get into solution.
2. **References:** Chapter 2 on "Laboratory Quality Assurance and Safety." Chapter 3 on "Sampling Dairy and Related Products."
3. **Definition:** The chloride content as expressed by this method is the equivalent content of sodium chloride (salt).
4. **Principle:** Suspension of sample in water, followed by titration of chloride ion with standardized silver nitrate using potassium chromate as indicator.
5. **Reagents:** Unless otherwise specified all chemicals are reagent or ACS grade.

   5.1 Potassium chromate (K_2CrO_4), 10% aqueous solution.

   5.2 Silver nitrate ($AgNO_3$), 0.1000 or 0.1711 N:ACS.

   5.3 Water (LG).
6. **Apparatus and Glassware:** All volumetric flasks, pipets, and burets are Class A unless otherwise specified.

   6.1 Balance: 0.01-g sensitivity.

   6.2 Magnetic stirrer.

   6.3 Filter paper: Whatman No. 2 fluted, 12.5 cm.

   6.4 Buret: 50 mL, 0.1-mL divisions.

   6.5 Beaker: 250 mL.

   6.6 Flasks: Erlenmeyer, 125 mL; volumetric, 100 mL.

   6.7 Funnel.

6.8 Pipets: Mohr, 10 mL, graduated in 0.1 mL; standard cream, 9 mL, TC; volumetric, 25 mL.

6.9 Thermometer: 0° to 100°C.

6.10 Wash bottle.

7. **Sampling:** Chapter 3 on "Sampling Dairy and Related Products."

8. **Preparation of Test Sample:** Take a representative sample that has previously been mixed, stirred, ground, blended, or otherwise prepared in order to make sample uniform.

9. **Procedure:** Before beginning analysis review material safety data sheets on all chemicals and use appropriate safety equipment such as hoods, aprons, face shields, and glasses.

9.1 Transfer 9 g of milk, cream, or other liquid into a clean flask. Rinse a pipet with an equal volume of LG water into the same flask. Proceed with step 9.3 below.

9.2 Accurately weigh 10 g of cottage cheese or similar product into a 250-mL beaker. Add about 15 mL of warm LG water (50° to 55°C) and mix to a thin paste with a magnetic stirrer. Add about 25 mL of LG water and mix until the sample is dispersed.

Transfer the solution to a 100-mL volumetric flask. Rinse the beaker and stirrer bar with LG water several times and mix thoroughly. Filter through fluted filter paper and collect approximately 50 mL of filtrate. Pipet 25 mL of filtrate into a clean flask.

9.3 Add 1 mL of potassium chromate indicator. Titrate with 0.1N silver nitrate to the first visible pale red-brown color lasting 30 seconds. The end point is much sharper if the titration is conducted under a yellow light. (Alternatively, titrate with 0.1711N silver nitrate using 1 g of sample so that milliliters of titrant equal the percentage of salt.)

10. **Expression of Results**

10.1 **Calculations**

$$\% \text{ chloride} = \frac{\text{mL } AgNO_3 \times \text{N } AgNO_3 \times 0.0355 \times 100}{\text{weight of sample or aliquot}}$$

$$\% \text{ sodium chloride (salt)} = \frac{\text{mL } AgNO_3 \times \text{N } AgNO_3 \times 0.0585 \times 100}{\text{weight of sample or aliquot}}$$

The weight of 9 mL of sample is assumed to be 9 g. This is not exact, but the salt content of most dairy products is so low that any error due to this difference is beyond the accuracy of the test.

Aliquot weight is determined by dividing sample weight by dilution and multiplying by volume pipeted:

$$\frac{\text{g sample} \times \text{mL pipeted}}{\text{mL diluted sample}}$$

11. **Precision and Performance Parameters:**

11.1 No precision data available; however, it is expected that results should fall within ±0.1% for the average of duplicate values greater than 0.5% in chloride content.

12. **Test Report and Interpretation:** The test report shall identify the method used and results obtained. The report will also identify any variation in

the test not specified in this method as well as problems that may have impacted the test result. Each sample will be described in such a manner as to ensure traceability as to its origin.

15.052 Chloride (Salt) Volhard Method (Class O)[11(935.43),83]

1. **Scope:** This method is for cheese, processed cheese, cheese foods, and cheese spreads where salt may be bound within the matrix. It can also be used for most dairy foods, including whey and whey products, by adjusting the amount of silver nitrate to provide an excess. *Parts of this method are hazardous. Safety precautions must be taken to protect the analyst and to remove fumes.*
2. **References:** Chapter 2 on "Laboratory Quality Assurance and Safety." Chapter 3 on "Sampling Dairy and Related Products."
3. **Definition:** The chloride content as expressed by this method is the equivalent content of sodium chloride (salt).
4. **Principle:** Sample is digested with nitric acid in presence of silver nitrate, followed by titration of excess silver nitrate with standardized potassium thiocyanate using ferric ammonium sulfate as indicator.
5. **Reagents:** Unless otherwise specified all chemicals are reagent or ACS grade.
   - 5.1 Ferric ammonium sulfate, saturated: Standard indicator.
   - 5.2 Nitric acid: ACS, specific gravity (sp g) 1.42.
   - 5.3 Potassium permanganate, 5 % solution: ACS.
   - 5.4 Potassium thiocyanate (KSCN), 0.1000 or 0.1711N: ACS. NOTE: *Method performance will improve with use of lower normality solution.*
   - 5.5 Silver nitrate ($AgNO_3$), 0.1000 or 0.1711N: ACS. NOTE: *Method performance will improve with use of lower normality solution.*
   - 5.6 Sucrose.
   - 5.7 Water (LG).
6. **Apparatus and Glassware:** All volumetric flasks, pipets, and burets are Class A unless otherwise specified.
   - 6.1 Balance: 0.1-mg sensitivity.
   - 6.2 Beaker: 50 mL.
   - 6.3 Boiling chips.
   - 6.4 Burets: 50 mL, 0.1-mL subdivisions; 100 mL, for dispensing nitric acid.
   - 6.5 Cylinder: Graduated, 25 mL.
   - 6.6 Filter paper: Whatman No. 2 fluted, 12.5 cm.
   - 6.7 Flasks: Erlenmeyer, 250 mL; volumetric, 1000 mL.
   - 6.8 Funnel: 75 mm.
   - 6.9 Hood or adequate air exhaust area.
   - 6.10 Hot plate.
   - 6.11 Pipets: 5 mL, automatic; Mohr, 10 mL, 0.1-mL divisions.
   - 6.12 Stainless stirring rod with flat end.
   - 6.13 Thermometer: 0° to 100°C.
   - 6.14 Tongs.
   - 6.15 Wash bottle.

7. **Sampling:** Chapter 3 on "Sampling Dairy and Related Products."
8. **Preparation of Test Sample:** Take a representative sample that has previously been mixed, stirred, ground, blended, or otherwise prepared in order to make sample uniform.
9. **Procedure:** Before beginning analysis review material safety data sheets on all chemicals and use appropriate safety equipment such as hoods, aprons, face shields, and glasses.

9.1 Accurately weigh about 2 g of sample into a 250 Erlenmeyer flask. Add about 20 mL of warm (50° to 55°C) LG water, and break up the particles with the flat end of a stainless steel stirring rod until a uniform slurry is formed. Rinse rod with about 10 mL of warm (50° to 55°C) LG water into the flask.

9.2 Add exactly 25 mL of 0.1000N silver nitrate (amount of silver nitrate can vary depending on amount of chloride or salt anticipated) to the sample. Immediately add 10 mL of nitric acid and about 50 mL of LG water. Add one clean boiling chip. Place on a hot plate and boil the solution in an area where the exhaust system is adequate, preferably in a hood. CAUTION: *Eye protection needs to be worn and work must be done in a chemical fume hood.*

9.3 As the solution boils, add a sufficient amount (usually 15 mL) of potassium permanganate in 5-mL portions until the solution turns brown and remains brown for a least 5 minutes of gentle boiling. CAUTION: Adding potassium permanganate to the boiling solution is hazardous. Add the permanganate down the side of the flask in small portions. The direct addition of permanganate into the center of the boiling solution could cause the solution to "pop" and spray the analyst with hot acid.

9.4 Continue heating until the brown color disappears with a resulting clear, straw-colored solution. There will be white curdlike particles in the digestate that are silver chloride aggregates. This material will decompose on continued digestion. If the solution is not clear, add more 5-mL portions of potassium permanganate until the solution becomes clear, indicating the complete oxidation of organic material. If too much potassium permanganate is added to the solution and the brown color does not clear by boiling for 15 to 20 minutes, add a very small amount of sucrose to clear the solution.

9.5 Filter the hot solution through fluted filter paper into a clean 250-mL Erlenmeyer flask. Wash the filter paper thoroughly with hot LG water. Cool the solution to room temperature. Add 2 mL of ferric ammonium sulfate indicator and titrate the excess silver nitrate with either 0.1000 or 0.1711N potassium thiocynate (use the same normality solution that was used for the silver nitrate for ease in calculating) to the first pale red-brown color that lasts 30 seconds. Subtract the final titration obtained for the sample from the blank value obtained using 2 mL of LG water plus water in place of 2 g of sample.

10. **Expression of Results**

10.1 **Calculations**

$$\% \text{ chloride} = \frac{(\text{mL KSCN blank} - \text{mL KSCN sample}) \times 0.0355 \times 100}{\text{g sample}}$$

$$\% \text{ sodium chloride (salt)} = \frac{(\text{mL KSCN blank} - \text{mL KSCN sample}) \times 0.0585 \times 100}{\text{g sample}}$$

11. **Precision and Performance Parameters**

11.1 No precision data available; however, it is expected that results should fall within ± 0.1% for the average of duplicate values greater than 0.5% in chloride content.

12. **Test Report and Interpretation:** The test report shall identify the method used and results obtained. The report will also identify any variation in the test not specified in this method as well as problems that may have impacted the test result. Each sample will be described in such a manner as to ensure traceability as to its origin.

15.053 Chloride (Salt) Coulometric Titration (Class B)[58]

1. **Scope:** This method is applicable to cheese, whey, and other dairy products with added sodium chloride (salt).
2. **References:** Chapter 2 on "Laboratory Quality Assurance and Safety." Chapter 3 on "Sampling Dairy and Related Products."
3. **Definition:** The chloride content as expressed by this method is the equivalent content of sodium chloride (salt).
4. **Principle:** The salt content of a sample is determined by the titration of chloride with silver ions, which are generated coulometrically from the silver anode. The constant DC voltage applied across a pair of silver electrodes immersed in the diluted sample causes a release of silver ions into the mixture. The chloride ions present in the sample precipitate out as silver chloride. When all the chloride has reacted, the concentration of silver ions increases, causing the conductivity of the mixture to rise. Sensing electrodes detect the rise in conductance and stop the titration. Because titration of chloride ions is at a constant rate, the instrument calculates chloride levels directly from elapsed titration time.
5. **Reagents:** Unless otherwise specified all chemicals are reagent or ACS grade.

   5.1 Acetic acid: Glacial.

   5.2 Chloride standard solution: Recommended by instrument manufacturer.

   5.3 Nitric acid.

   5.4 Polyvinyl alcohol, 99% to 100% hydrolyzed.

   5.5 Silver electrode polish.

   5.6 Sodium chloride (NaCl).

   5.7 Water (LG).

   5.8 Acid buffer with chloride solution (commerically available solution may be used).

5.8.1 Prepare solution by adding 950 mL of 70°C LG water into a 1000-mL beaker. Place the filled beaker on the hot plate with a magnetic stirrer and add the stirrer bar.

5.8.2 Turn on the stirrer and add 2.25 g of polyvinyl alcohol. Stir constantly until the polyvinyl alcohol goes into the solution.

5.8.3 Turn off the heat but continue to stir the solution. Add 48 mL of glacial acetic acid, 0.04 g of sodium chloride, and 1.6 mL of nitric acid.

5.8.4 Allow the solution to cool, and transfer it to a clear, clean, screw-capped storage bottle.

6. **Apparatus and Glassware:** All volumetric flasks, pipets, and burets are Class A unless otherwise specified.

6.1 Balance: 0.1-mg sensitivity.

6.2 Beakers: 20 mL, 50 mL, 1000 mL.

6.3 Blender: Oster, Waring, or equivalent.

6.4 Bottle: Glass Storage, 1000 mL.

6.5 Chloride meter: Corning No. 926, Buchler No. 4-2500 or equivalent. Follow the manufacturer's instructions on meter preparation and calibration. The unit must be checked for calibration at least daily using a known chloride standard. If repeated tests of standards are not reproducible, check pipeting accuracy, condition of the buffer, and condition of the electrodes and stirrer. Inaccurate pipeting and dirty electrodes are the most frequent sources of poor reproducibility.

6.6 Filter paper: Whatman No. 2, fluted, or equivalent.

6.7 Flask: Volumetric, 100 mL.

6.8 Funnel.

6.9 Hot plate: With magnetic stirrer, thermostatically controlled at 70°C.

6.10 Pipets: 100 mL; volumetric, 1 mL, automatic pipeter, 100 mL.

6.11 Silver electrodes.

6.12 Stirring bar: Magnetic.

6.13 Stirring rod: Stainless steel, with flat end.

6.14 Wash bottle.

7. **Sampling:** Chapter 3 on "Sampling Dairy and Related Products."

8. **Preparation of Test Sample:** Take a representative sample that has previously been mixed, stirred, ground, blended or otherwise prepared in order to make sample uniform.

8.1 Liquid samples may be assayed directly unless the chloride level is not too high to be read on the meter. If the reading is too high, make a dilution to bring the sample within usage range.

8.2 **Cheese samples**

8.2.1 Prepare by weighing approximately 10 grams of cheese into a blender jar, adding 100 mL of LG water and blending for 1 minute, being careful not to leak water from the container during blending.

8.2.2 Pipet exactly 2 mL of nitric acid into the solution and stir.

8.2.3 Filter the solution by gravity into a clean beaker.

9. **Procedure:** Before beginning analysis review material safety data sheets on all chemicals and use appropriate safety equipment such as hoods, aprons, face shields, and glasses.
   9.1 Following the manufacturer's instructions, place the acid buffer into the beaker and immerse the electrode into the solution.
   9.2 Carefully pipet the required amount of sample into the buffer using the same pipet used for calibration.
   9.3 Start the instrument and record the stabilized reading.

10. **Expression of Results**
   10.1 **Calculations**

$$\%\ \text{chloride} = \frac{\text{reading} \times \text{dilution volume}^* \times 0.0355}{\text{mL pipeted} \times \text{g sample}}$$

$$\%\ \text{sodium chloride} = \frac{\text{reading} \times \text{dilution volume}^* \times 0.0585}{\text{mL pipeted} \times \text{g sample}}$$

* Cheese has three components: fat, solids, and moisture. Only the moisture content contributes to the dilution volume. The amount of water contributed by the cheese is added to the volume of the dilution water and the nitric acid to give the dilution volume. For example, 10 g of cheese with 35% moisture would have a dilution volume of $(0.35 \times 10) + 100 + 2 = 105.5$ mL.

11. **Precision and Performance Parameters**
   11.1 No precision data available; however, it is expected that results should fall within ± 0.1% for the average of duplicate values greater than 0.5% in sodium chloride content.

12. **Test Report and Interpretation:** The test report shall identify the method used and results obtained. The report will also identify any variation in the test not specified in this method as well as problems that may have impacted the test result. Each sample will be described in such a manner as to ensure traceability as to its origin.

15.060 Contaminant Tests

The contaminant tests in this section include quantitative and qualitative assays for aflatoxin and narrative discussions of pesticides, herbicides, and radionuclides in milk.

Aflatoxins

The molds *Aspergillus flavus* and *Aspergillus parasiticus* produce a group of highly toxic secondary metabolites that are referred to as aflatoxins (otherwise known as mycotoxins). The most common forms of aflatoxins are B_1, B_2, G_1, and G_2. Of these forms, aflatoxin B_1 is the most toxic and carcinogenic. Of major significance with respect to milk and dairy product is recognition of the fact that growth of *A. Flavus* and *A. Parasiticus* on animal feed can result in aflatoxin production. When consumed by dairy cattle, contaminated feed containing aflatoxin B_1 can be metabolized to aflatoxin M_1. M_1 is the hydroxylated metabolite of aflatoxin B_1 and resides primarily in the protein fraction of milk. M_1 was the first residue of aflatoxin to be found in the issue of dairy cows, and milk is one of the only foods known to be naturally contaminated with M_1. Allcroft and Roberts[2] report that excretion of M_1 in milk is proportional to the amount of B_1 ingested. M_1 disappears from milk within approximately 3 to 4 days following removal of a contaminated feed source. Applebaum et al.[9] discuss the association of aflatoxins with milk and dairy products. Wiseman and Marth[106] made ice cream and orange sherbet from milk naturally contaminated with aflatoxin M_1. The aflatoxin concentration remained unchanged in the ice cream during 8 months of frozen storage. Results obtained with sherbet were somewhat variable, but here too aflatoxin was detectable in the product that had been frozen for 8 months.

When milk contaminated with aflatoxin is used for cheese making,[51] the toxin will be present in the cheese and will persist during ripening and storage. Kiermeier[51] examined 19 varieties of cheese and found detectable levels of aflatoxin B_1 and/or G_1 in some varieties, demonstrating that mold growth and toxin production can occur on the surface of cheese. No acute health hazard has been associated with mold metabolites (mycotoxins) produced by *Penicillium roquefortii* and *Penicillium caseicolum* used in production of Camembert and blue cheese.

Occasionally, dried milk has been found to contain aflatoxin M_1.[72] Although the amount of toxin present in fluid milk is reduced somewhat by the drying process, a significant percentage of it appears to survive the process and will survive for extended periods in the dry product.

Other mycotoxins are produced by numerous other molds, but their significance in milk is not documented.

15.061 Aflatoxin, Vicam,® Quantitative, Affinity Chromatography (Class B)[33,44,94]

1. **Scope:** This method describes the quantitative measurement of aflatoxins in fluid milk and milk powder at the level of 0.05 ppb in fluid milks and 0.5 ppb in powdered milks. *CAUTION: Aflatoxins are known carcinogens. Handle with appropriate care, using protective gloves, lab coats, and equipment.*
2. **References**: Chapter 2 on "Laboratory Quality Assurance and Safety."
   Chapter 3 on "Sampling Dairy and Related Products."
3. **Definition:** Aflatoxin M_1 is the mass fraction of substances described in this procedure and is expressed in parts per billion.
4. **Principle:** Aflatoxin M_1 is isolated from the sample by passing the sample through an immunoaffinity column. The column contains antibodies that are bound on the side of the column. As the sample passes through the column, the antibodies selectively bind any aflatoxin M_1 present and form an antibody–antigen complex. Aflatoxin M_1 is then eluded from the column and assayed by fluorometric detection.
5. **Reagents:** Unless otherwise specified all chemicals are reagent or ACS grade.
   - 5.1 **Immunoaffinity columns:** For aflatoxin M_1 (Aflatest™, Vicam, Somerville, MA).
   - 5.2 **Methanol:** HPLC grade.
     - 5.2.1 Methanol diluted with LG water to 80%, and 10% methanol.
   - 5.3 **Bromine solution:** 0.001% made daily from concentrate (Aflatest™ Developer Solution).
   - 5.4 **Sodium chloride.**

5.5 **Water (LG).**

6. **Apparatus and Glassware:** All volumetric flasks, pipets, and burets are Class A unless otherwise specified.
   6.1 **Fluorometer:** Sequola–Turner (Mountain View, CA) Model 450 modified by manufacturer to increase sensitivity. Modification consisted of replacement of the lamp by a mercury lamp with a phosphor emitting at 365 nm. Excitation was set at 360 nm and emission at 450 nm by filters.
   6.2 **Fluorometer standards**: Aflatest™ P Calibration standards available through Aflatest™ Vicam, Sommerville, MA. Follow instructions for standardization of fluorometer using calibration standards.
   6.3 **Centrifuge:** capable to 2000 g.
   6.4 **Glass syringe and barrel:** 10 mL.
   6.5 **Pump assembly:** (Aflatest™ stand with syringe pump and coupling) for use in pushing sample through affinity column.
   6.6 **Cuvette:** 12 × 75 mm borosillicate glass tube.
   6.7 **Filter:** Whatman #4 filter or equivalent.
7. **Sampling:** Chapter 3 on "Sampling Dairy and Related Products."
8. **Preparation of Test Sample:** Work should be carried out with the exclusion of daylight.
   8.1 **Fluid milk:** Bring sample to room temperature, add 1 g of sodium chloride to 50 mL fluid milk and mix well. Centrifuge milk for 5 minutes at 2000 g. Remove fat layer with spatula and filter through Whatman #4 or equivalent.
   8.2 **Milk powders:** Weigh 11-g sample and add to 99 mL of LG water. Add glass beads to assist mixing and shake in a wide-mouth dilution bottle until sample is uniformily mixed. If sample is whole milk powder, follow preparation procedure as in 8.1 and remove fat as part of the preparation of sample.
9. **Procedure:** Before beginning analysis review material safety data sheets on all chemicals and use appropriate safety equipment such as hoods, aprons, face shields, and glasses.

   Work should be carried out with the exclusion of daylight.
   9.1 Pour or pipet 10 mL of prepared sample into glass syringe barrel reservoir with attached capped affinity column that is maintained in a vertical position.
   9.2 Remove column end cap. Push the 10 mL of sample through the affinity column by depressing the 10-mL syringe barrel. Use a steady flow rate of 1 to 2 drops per second.
   9.3 Wash the affinity column by pouring or pipeting 10 mL of 10% methanol into the syringe barrel. Push the 10% methanol solution through the aflatest column by depressing syringe barrel. Leave approximately 1 mL of solution in barrel reservoir.
   9.4 Wash the column with a second 10 mL of 10% methanol and leave 1 mL of solution in barrel reservoir again.
   9.5 Complete the washing with a third 10 mL of 10 methanol and depress plunger to completely discharge the washing solution from barrel reservoir.

9.6 Wipe off aflatest column with a tissue and place glass cuvette under outlet end of column.

9.7 Pipet 1.0 mL of 80% methanol into the syringe barrel and collect elute in the glass cuvette.

9.8 Add 1.0 mL of dilute aflatest developer directly to elute in the cuvette. Mix well.

9.9 Place cuvette in calibrated fluorometer.

9.10 Record digital readout in ppb total aflatoxins for the sample extracted.

10. **Expression of Results:** Sensitivity of test is 0.05 ppb. For fluid products report results that are less than 0.05 as <0.05 ppb. For powdered milk products multiply result times 10 and report lower level as <0.5 ppb.

11. **Precision and Performance Parameters:** Raw milk, containing no detectable aflatoxin by HPLC (detection level of 0.05 ppb), was spiked with known amounts of aflatoxin M_1. Spiking levels were 0.05 to 0.5 ppb. Recovery by VICAM®, as measured by HPLC, was linear (r = 0.994), with an average and standard deviation of individual sample recoveries of 97± 0.97%.

12. **Test Report and Interpretation:** The test report shall identify the method used and results obtained. The report will also identify any variation in the test not specified in this method as well as problems that may have impacted the test result. Each sample will be described in such a manner as to ensure traceability as to its origin.

15.062 Aflatoxin M_1, Snap® Qualitative (Class B)

1. **Scope:** This method describes the qualitative measurement of aflatoxins in raw commingled bovine milk at or above 0.5 ppb. *CAUTION: Aflatoxins are known carcinogens. Handle with appropriate care, using protective gloves, lab coats, and equipment.*

2. **References:** Chapter 2 on "Laboratory Quality Assurance and Safety." Chapter 3 on "Sampling Dairy and Related Products."

3. **Definition:** Aflatoxin M_1 is the mass fraction of substances described in this procedure and is expressed in parts per billion.

4. **Principle:** The SNAP Aflatoxin M_1 test is an enzyme-linked receptor binding assay that will detect Aflatoxin M_1. A preincubation step allows enzyme labeled conjugate "A" to bind with aflatoxin residue, if present, in the sample. Adding the sample to the SNAP device allows unbound enzyme-labeled conjugate "A" to bind to the sample spot while enzyme-labeled conjugate "B" binds to the control spot. The sample wicks along the flow matrix until it begins to turn the green activation circle white. The activator is depressed, puncturing the foil in the base of the device and allowing substrate to be absorbed and drawn across the sample and control spots in the results window. Substrate is cleaved by the enzyme portion of the conjugate to form a blue precipitate, causing color development. As a competitive assay, the SNAP test functions such that the more residue in the sample, the less color on the sample spot.

5. **Reagents:** Reagents are part of the test kit apparatus.

6. **Apparatus and Other Equipment**
   6.1 **SNAP Aflatoxin M_1 test kit** (Idexx Laboratories, Inc., One Idexx Drive, Westbrook, ME 04092). Kits contain 20 individual foil packets. Each foil packet contains a SNAP device, sample tube with reagent pellet, and a pipet. All materials must be refrigerated at 0°-7°C (32°-45°F). Tests may be kept at room temperature, 18°-29°C (64°-84°F), during the day of use. Remove only the number of tests to be used for the day.
   6.2 **Heater block** capable of maintaining an operating temperature of 45°C (113°F) ± 5°C or base unit including a SNAP heat block insert providing heat distribution with inset for sample tubes and SNAP devices.
   6.3 **Pipet,** single use 450 µL, with indicator line to measure amount of sample, supplied by manufacturer, or fixed-volume pipeter to dispense 450 µL.
   6.4 **Timer**

7. **Sampling:** Chapter 3 on "Sampling Dairy and Related Products."

8. **Preparation of Test Sample**
   8.1 Mix samples of milk by slowly inverting sample until material is uniform.

9. **Procedure:** Before beginning analysis review material safety data sheets on all chemicals and use appropriate safety equipment such as hoods, aprons, face shields, and glasses.
   9.1 Remove SNAP device, pipet, and sample tube from foil packet.
   9.2 Ensure that the heat block has been preheated and that the temperature has maintained 45°C (113°F) ± 5°C for at least five minutes.
   9.3 Verify that the reagent pellet is at the bottom of the sample tube (if not, tap tube to return pellet to the bottom).
   9.4 Place SNAP device(s) in heat block.
   9.5 Mix milk sample thoroughly.
   9.6 Remove and discard sample tube cap.
   9.7 Draw up milk sample (450 µL ± 50 µL) to the indicator line.
   9.8 Carefully add all of milk sample from pipette to tube.
   9.9 Shake sample tube to dissolve reagent pellet.
   9.10 Incubate sample tube in preheated heat block 45°C (113°F) ± 5°C for 5 minutes. (Incubation must occur for a minimum of 5 minutes and no longer than 6 minutes.)
   9.11 Pour entire contents of sample tube into sample well of SNAP device and discard tube. The sample will flow across the results window toward the green activation circle.
   9.12 When the green activation circle *begins* to disappear, push the activator firmly until it snaps flush with the body of the SNAP device. NOTE: When the edge of the circle nearest the sample well begins to turn from dark green to white, activation should occur. Do not let the circle completely disappear.
   9.13 Wait 4 minutes. SNAP device must remain in heat block during color development. Blue control and sample spots will develop during this time.

9.14 Remove the SNAP device and orient the device with the sample well to the left.

9.15 Visually read results immediately.

10. Expression of Results

10.1 If the sample spot is darker than or equal to the control spot the sample is negative.

10.2 If the sample spot is lighter than the control spot the sample is positive.

11. Precision and Performance Parameters: This is a qualitative assay; no precision data available for this assay.

12. Test Report and Interpretation: The test report shall identify the method used and results obtained. The report will also identify any variation in the test not specified in this method as well as problems that may have impacted the test result. Each sample will be described in such a manner as to ensure traceability as to its origin.

15.063 Aflatoxin M_1, Charm II® Method Qualitative, (Class B)

1. **Scope:** This method describes the qualitative measurement of aflatoxins in raw commingled bovine milk at or above 0.5 ppb. *CAUTION: Aflatoxins are known carcinogens. Handle with appropriate care, using protective gloves, lab coats, and equipment.*

2. **References:** Chapter 2 on "Laboratory Quality Assurance and Safety." Chapter 3 on "Sampling Dairy and Related Products."

3. **Definition:** Aflatoxin M_1 is the mass fraction of substances described in this procedure and is expressed in parts per billion.

4. **Principle:** The Charm Aflatoxin M_1 Test uses antibodies with specificity to the mycotoxins M_1 and B_1. The antibodies are added to a milk sample along with an exempt amount of [^{3}H] labeled aflatoxin (tracer). Any aflatoxin M_1 already in the milk competes for the binding sites with this tracer. The amount of tracer that binds to the antibody is measured and compared to a previously determined control point or to a standard curve. The greater the amount of tracer measured, the lower the Aflatoxin M_1 concentration in the sample. The lower the amount of tracer measured the greater the concentration in the sample.

5. **Reagents:** Use only reagents of recognized analytical grade, unless otherwise specified, and distilled or demineralized water or water of equivalent purity.

5.1 **Aflatoxin reagents:** Purple tracer reagent and white binding reagent packed in blister packs of 10 tests. Observe precautions and regulations for handling and disposing low levels of ^{3}H or ^{14}C radioactivity.

5.2 **Aflatoxin M_1 standard 0.25 ppb:** Positive control standard reconstituted with 50 mL negative milk or zero control to make a concentration of 0.25 ppb. Reconstituted shelf life of 48 hours at 0.4.4°C or 2 months at –15°C or lower.

5.3 **Reagent Af**: Store at room temperature.

5.4 **Zero control standard**: Powdered milk based buffer representative of commingled bovine milk from untreated herd. Reconstituted with 100 mL 37°C water.

6. **Apparatus and Glassware:** All volumetric flasks, pipets, and burets are Class A unless otherwise specified.
   6.1 **Charm II (6000 or 6600 models) analyzer.**
   6.2 **Optifluor scintillation fluid.**
   6.3 **Test tubes:** 13 × 100 test tubes, disposable, of borosilicate glass, of diameter 13 mm and length 100 mm with 13-mm caps.
   6.4 **Cotton swabs.**
   6.5 **Fixed-volume dispenser:** To dispense 5.0 mL.
   6.6 **Positive-volume dispenser:** To dispense 300 μL.
   6.7 **Incubator block**: For 13 × 100 test tubes, maintained at a temperature of 35° ± 2°C.
   6.8 **Centrifuge**: For 13 × 100 test tubes capable of 1200 g.
   6.9 **Test tube mixer (vortex).**
7. **Sampling:** Chapter 3 on "Sampling Dairy and Related Products."
8. **Preparation of Test Sample:** Take a representative sample that has previously been mixed, stirred, or otherwise prepared in order to make sample uniform. Carefully mix the laboratory sample and use aliquots as required.
   8.1 For all samples the sample must be centrifuged 1200 g for 3 minutes prior to testing the skim portion. This is included as the first step 9.2.1 of the procedure.
   8.2 For pasteurized and other dairy products, refer to General Sample Preparation and Test Validation Procedure for Charm II Test Antibiotic Analysis.
9. **Procedure:** Before beginning analysis review material safety data sheets on all chemicals and use appropriate safety equipment such as hoods, aprons, face shields, and glasses.
   9.1 **Calibration-Control Point**
      9.1.1 Establish a control point by testing a positive control 6 times and taking the average. For Charm II multiply the average by 1.15. This is the control point. All 6 tests should be less than the control point, or else redo control point determination.
      9.1.2 Determine a negative average by testing zero control 3 times and taking an average.
      9.1.3 Daily check control point and equipment operation by testing a positive and negative control. Negative control should be ± 30% of negative average and positive should be less than control point. Provided these conditions are met, 9.1.1 and 9.1.2 only need to be done with each new lot. If conditions are not met, recalibrate equipment and redo 9.1.1 and 9.1.2.
   9.2 **Determination**
      9.2.1 Fill labeled test tube ¾ full with milk (approx. 6 mL). Add 300 μL reagent Af, mix, and centrifuge 1200 g for 5 minutes. Remove from centrifuge and cool to 0°-4.4°C in ice bath.
      9.2.2 Label empty test tubes, one for each test sample, and add 1 white tablet to empty tube.

9.2.3 Add 300 µL water to each tube.

9.2.4 Break up tablets in tubes by mixing tubes 10 times/10 seconds on mixer in a rise and fall motion.

9.2.5 Draw 5.0 mL milk from below fat layer (tubes 8.2.1) using new pipet tip for each sample. Add drawn sample to appropriate labeled tubes.

9.2.6 Add purple tablet to each tube and mix 15 times/15 seconds on mixer in a rise and fall motion.

9.2.7 Incubate tubes for 3 minutes at 35° ± 2°C.

9.2.8 Remove tubes and centrifuge for 5 minutes.

9.2.9 Pour off milk. While still draining tubes, remove fat ring with 2 or more cotton swabs, continue until dry, do not touch pellet.

9.2.10 Using water pipet, add 300 µL of water to tubes and break up pellets using mixer.

9.2.11 Pellets must be completely suspended. Add 3 mL of scintillation fluid to each tube, cap, and vortex to mix.

9.2.12 Count tubes on scintillation counter for 1 minute using [^{3}H] channel. Record counts as counts per minute (CPM).

9.2.13 Control tests: Observe 8.1.3.

10. Expression of Results

10.1 If the CPM of the analyzer is more than (50 points greater than with Charm II) the control point, then the sample is negative (contains less than the ppb level used to calculate the control point).

10.2 If the CPM is less than or equal to the control point then the sample is presumptive positive.

10.3 If the CPM of a Charm II test is within 50 points of the control point the sample should be re-counted. If the recount is less than or equal to the control point the sample is presumptive positive. If the recount is greater than the control point the sample is negative.

10.4 Confirmation of presumptive positive samples should be performed by diluting the original sample 1 part to 1 part Zero Control Standard and retesting the sample along with positive and negative controls. Controls should meet conditions of 9.1.3. If conditions 9.1.3 are met and 10.2 is repeated with the diluted sample, the sample is positive at the U.S. level of 0.5 ppb. If 9.1.3 conditions are met and 10.1 conditions are met with the diluted sample, the sample is negative at the U.S. level of 0.5 ppb. If 9.1.3 conditions are not met, then the test is invalid (the equipment and test should be recalibrated before retesting the sample).

11. Precision and Performance Parameters

11.1 The Charm II Aflatoxin M_1 test has been verified to have at least 90/95% selectivity of negative samples (0/60 positives in a blind study) and minimum 90/95% sensitivity to Aflatoxin 0.25 ppb (0.5 ppb after sample dilution of confirmation procedure).

11.2 MRL levels of Aflatoxin M_1 are lower than U.S. levels. A procedural modification using a sequential format, called the extended aflatoxin assay, will detect these MRL levels.

12. **Test Report and Interpretation:** The test report shall identify the method used and results obtained. The report will also identify any variation in the test not specified in this method as well as problems that may have impacted the test result. Each sample will be described in such a manner as to ensure traceablity as to its origin.

15.064 Aflatoxin M_1, Charm® SL, Qualitative, (Class B)

1. **Scope:** This method describes the qualitative measurement of aflatoxins in raw commingled bovine milk at or above 0.5 ppb. *CAUTION: Aflatoxins are known carcinogens. Handle with appropriate care, using protective gloves, lab coats, and equipment.*
2. **References:** Chapter 2 on "Laboratory Quality Assurance and Safety." Chapter 3 on "Sampling Dairy and Related Products."
3. **Definition:** Aflatoxin M_1 is the mass fraction of substances described in this procedure and is expressed in parts per billion.
4. **Principle:** The Charm SL Aflatoxin M_1 Test uses antibodies with specificity to the mycotoxins M_1. The antibodies are bound to inert colored beads and applied to a test strip. When milk is added to the strip, the beads solubilize and travel with the flow front across a line containing aflatoxin M_1 (T-line) and across a line containing anti-antibody (C-line). If there is no aflatoxin in the milk, a majority of the beads will form a reddish line on the T-line. If there is aflatoxin in the milk, a majority of the beads will pass the T-line and be captured on the C-line. Comparing the darkness of the T versus the C line makes a qualitative visual determination of positive or negative. The reader can measure the T and C lines and delivers a ppt concentration of aflatoxin M_1 in the sample. A ppt concentration higher than 400 ppt is considered positive to assure high confidence at 500 ppt.
5. **Reagents:** Use only reagents of recognized analytical grade, unless otherwise specified, and distilled or demineralized water or water of equivalent purity.
   - 5.1 **Aflatoxin test strips**: Individual test strips are packaged in groups of 25 with desiccants in a moisture proof zip bag.
   - 5.2 **Aflatoxin M_1 standard 0.5 ppb**: Positive control standard reconstituted with 10 mL negative milk to make a concentration of 0.5 ppb (500 ppt).
   - 5.3 **Negative milk**: Raw milk identified as a strong negative by the test.
6. **Apparatus and Glassware:** All volumetric flasks, pipets and burets are Class A unless otherwise specified.
   - 6.1 **Strip incubator:** 56° ± 1°C with built in timer light.
   - 6.2 **Fixed-volume dispenser**: To dispense 300 µL.
   - 6.3 **ROSA reader or Lum-T**: With reader adapter.
7. **Sampling:** Chapter 3 on "Sampling Dairy and Related Products."
8. **Preparation of Test Sample**: Take a representative sample that has previously been mixed, stirred, or otherwise prepared in order to make sample uniform.
   - 8.1 No preparation of raw or pasteurized milk is required.

8.2 For powdered products, reconstitute to 10% solids, pH adjust to 6.8 with NaOH if needed, and centrifuge 1200 g for 3 minutes, test supernate.

9. **Procedure:** Before beginning analysis review material safety data sheets on all chemicals and use appropriate safety equipment such as hoods, aprons, face shields, and glasses.

9.1 Calibration strips and readers are precalibrated.

9.1.1 Positive control should be visually positive and yield a positive number (>400) by reader.

9.1.2 Negative control should be visually negative and yield a negative number (<200) by reader.

9.1.3 Daily check test and equipment operation by testing a positive and negative control. Conditions 9.1.1 and 9.1.2 must be met. If conditions are not met, equipment needs recalibrating; seek technical assistance.

9.2 **Determination**

9.2.1 Temperature indicator should be green at 55°C indicating the temperature is 56° ± 1°C. Shake milk sample. Place labeled test strip in strip incubator with flat side facing up. Use tab to peel tape back to edge of white label, exposing sample pad.

9.2.2 Slowly, to avoid spilling, pipet 300 µL milk or centrifuged sample into either side well of the sample pad compartment. Reseal tape over sample pad compartment by pressing. Close cover on incubator and tighten latch. Solid red timer light will automatically start when the lid is closed.

9.2.3 Incubate for 8 minutes (up to 10 minutes). Test light (green/blinking) will start blinking at 8 minutes.

9.3 Control tests: Observe 9.1.3.

10. **Expression of Results**

10.1 Remove test from incubator. Be careful to hold the sample pad in the down position as shown. Do not squeeze the sample pad. Visually inspect results by comparing test line (T) to control line (C). Read result as follows: Negative sample—(T) is darker/more than (C) or test line is the same as (C). Presumptive positive sample—(T) is clearly lighter/less than (C) or (T) is barely visible or partially or unevenly colored, or (T) is absent. Invalid sample if no (C) appears, or (C) is unevenly or partially colored. If invalid, retest the sample.

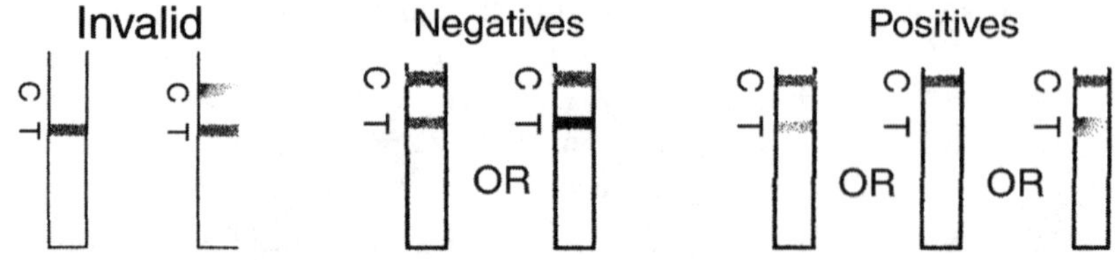

10.2 **Reader option:** Insert valid completed test strip into ROSA reader or Lum-T with imager (blister side down) as shown. Slide completely into slot (LED comes on in a strip imager for LUM-T).

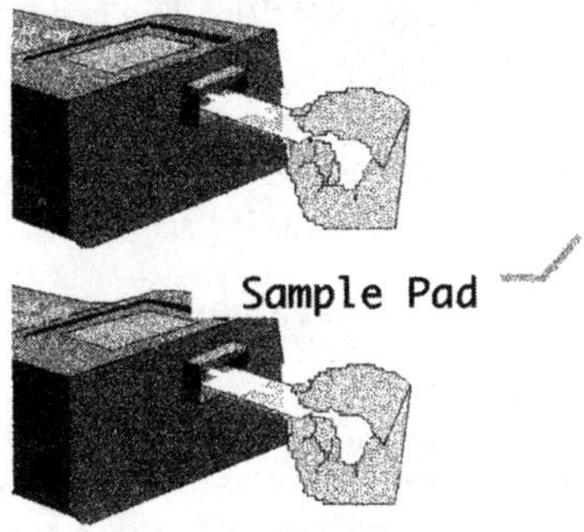

Read results on AFLA channel of ROSA Reader or LUM-T. If desired, enter Samp# and/or Oper# and press ENTER. A numerical value (Read:=) and an interpretation (Result:) are displayed on screen in 5 seconds. Results are in memory and may be subsequently recalled and downloaded to printer or computer. Reading is the approximate ppt level in the sample. If the ppt level exceeds 400 the reader will interpret the reading as positive.

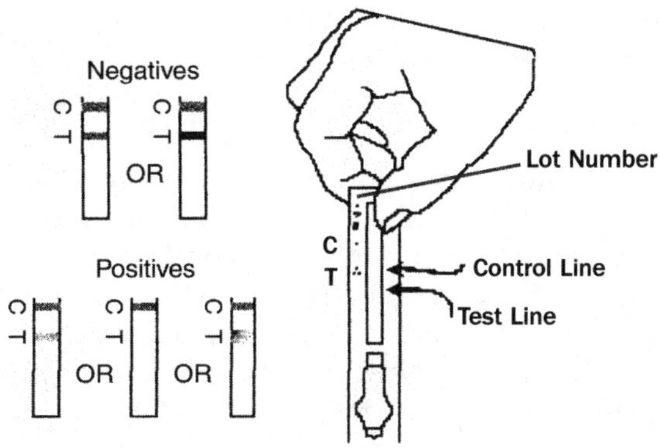

Repeat testing of presumptive positives with positive and negative control. If conditions 9.1.1 and 9.1.2 are met and sample retests positive, it is positive. If control conditions are met and the sample retests negative, the sample is negative. If control conditions are not met the test is invalid, disregard results and seek technical assistance.

11. Precision and Performance Parameters: The Charm SL Aflatoxin M_1 test has been verified to have at least 90/95% selectivity of negative samples (0/60 positives in a blind study) and minimum 90/95% sensitivity to Aflatoxin 0.50 ppb when positive is determined based on 400 ppt reading. (Charm Sciences internal data. Charm Sciences, Inc., 36 Franklin St., Malden, MA 02148.)

The ppt determination has been shown to have a CV of 10% at 500 ppt and 33% at 250 ppt. The ppt range is 0-500 and becomes nonlinear (flat) at higher concentrations. (Charm Sciences internal data.)

12. **Test Report and Interpretation:** The test report shall identify the method used and results obtained. The report will also identify any variation in the test not specified in this method as well as problems that may have impacted the test result. Each sample will be described in such a manner as to ensure traceablity as to its origin.

15.065 Pesticide and Herbicide Residues in Milk[26]

The purpose of this section is not to cover the details of pesticide and herbicide residue analysis but rather to provide the reader with an overview of the issues and resources available in the area of residue analysis.

Milk may be contaminated with one or more pesticide residues in the same sample. The common classes of pesticides include organophosphastes as well as organochlorines (chlorinated hydrocarbons) and carbamates. Residues of chlorinated hydrocarbon pesticides have received the greatest amount of attention in pesticide residue monitoring programs. Organochlorine residues are very stable, can accumulate in fatty tissue, are fat soluble, and very slowly metabolized by the bovine. They appear in milk, body fat, and excreta after ingestion. Organophosphate (e.g., parathion) pesticides are metabolized by the bovine; these metabolites are usually less toxic than the parent compounds, and they appear in milk and excreta. Pesticide residues that have been found in milk products include DDE (dichlorophenyl-dichloroethylene), dieldrin, lindane, methoxychlor, heptachlor epoxide, DDT (dichlorodiphenyltrichloroethane), hexachlorobenzene, and TDE (tetrachlorodiphenylethane). Since the banning of nonspecific uses of all organochlorine pesticides in general, and of DDT and aldrin/dieldrin in particular, the overall pattern of residues of these pesticides in milk has changed to levels at or below method sensitivity.

Residues of polychlorinated biphenyls (PCBs), while not pesticides, have also been and continue to be found in milk. These multicomponent and persistent industrial chemicals have been limited in permitted uses that have virtually eliminated them from consideration as contaminants.

The analytical methods for organochlorine chemicals are described in the AOAC's *Official Methods of Analysis*. Further information on pesticide analysis can also be found in the U.S. FDA's *Pesticide Analytical Manual* (*PAM*)[96] and in the U.S. EPA *Manual of Chemical Methods for Pesticides and Devices*[98] from AOAC. In these methods, qualitative and quantitative determinations are based on chromatographic principles that make possible the simultaneous determination of multiple residues present in the same sample. Extraction and cleanup procedures use solvent partitioning and column chromatography to quantitatively recover the chemicals sought. Subsequent chromatographic determinations require clean samples for analytical accuracy. These separation methods have been tested in interlaboratory collaborative studies with dairy products. More than 100 organochlorine pesticides and PCBs, certain parent organophosphate pesticides, and other nonpolar pesticides are completely or partially recovered by these methods. A compilation of how these chemicals behave in the methods is given in FDA's *PAM*. Detection of PCBs and organochlorine pesticide residues together in the same sample requires special additional procedures to separate before determination.

15.066 Radionuclides[35]

The importance of radioactive substances in dairy foods as a result of accidental spills, fallout from nuclear power plants, or weapons discharge has been established. In the food chain, milk is potentially a major source of radionuclides for children and a significant contributor to radioisotope ingestion by adults. Although several radionuclides are present in the event of a fallout, most of them either have a short half life or are not metabolized by the cow; only a few are found in measurable amounts. They are strontium 89, strontium 90, iodine 131, cesium 137, and barium 140. In the vicinity of a nuclear test site, however, iodine 133 ($^{t}\!/_{2}$ = 20.8 hours) and tritium 3 ($^{t}\!/_{2}$ = 12.3 years) may be found in milk. Around nuclear processing plants, zinc 65 ($^{t}\!/_{2}$ = 245 days) has also been found in milk. The amount of tritium 3 observed in milk is normally quite low, and its level is close to detection limit of 200 pCi/L.

The concentration of strontium 89, strontium 90, iodine 131, cesium 137, and barium 140 will reach levels of significance immediately following the use of nuclear weapons but will normally fall to lower levels. It is considered advisable to determine concentrations of these milk-borne fission materials to assess their dietary contribution to assist in evaluating the biological effects, if any, of man's ingestion of them. The building of nuclear power generating stations in milk production areas renders advisable the radioassay of milk for its environmental contaminants.

Sampling milk for analysis depends on whether samples are indicated and intended for determination of radionuclides 1) affected by farm practices, 2) in the vicinity of nuclear power generating stations, or 3) at the consumer level. To study the effect of farm practices on radionuclides in milk, samples are collected from individual cows or a portion of pooled milk is taken from the storage tank on the farm. Milk samples in the vicinity of nuclear power generating stations are taken from within a discrete geographical area, depending on meteorological conditions and the number of farms affected. To study market milk, samples at each location are composites of subsamples from each milk-processing plant, the quantity being proportional to the plant's average sales in the community served.

Frequency of sampling depends on the seriousness of the situation, whether it is warranted and the radionuclide considered for analysis. With iodine 131 ($^{t}\!/_{2}$ = 8.08 days), it is necessary to collect milk samples every day or at least once a week. With strontium 90 ($^{t}\!/_{2}$ = 28 years), it is necessary to collect samples at least every month.

15.070 Extraneous Material Tests

This section covers the procedures for determining extraneous material by sediment testing. Procedures for cheese, milk-quantitative, and milk-quantitative (Sani-guide method) are covered.

The principle of these methods is based on filtering a volume of sample through a filter (lintine disc) and comparing it to a set of known standards (photographs from USDA). The sediment test is designed to determine the amount of insoluble extraneous material in a representative sample. The findings of these tests in milk are important in determining cleanliness during the milking procedure. In cheese this test can be used to determine the introduction of extraneous material from milk as well as from the cheese making process.

15.071 Extraneous Material, Cheese (Class O)[84]

1. **Scope:** This method is applicable to natural and pasteurized cheese.
2. **References:** Chapter 2 on "Laboratory Quality Assurance and Safety." Chapter 3 on "Sampling Dairy and Related Products."
3. **Definition:** Extraneous material is defined as that material remaining after passing a solublized sample of cheese through a filter disc.
4. **Principle:** Cheese sample is digested with the aid of acid and enzyme, and passed through a filter disc. Disc is examined microscopically for presence of extraneous matter and compared to a standard.
5. **Reagents:** Unless otherwise specified all chemicals are reagent or ACS grade.
   - 5.1 **Pepsin (for processed cheese):** 1-10,000 granular. Refrigerate the pepsin. Remove it from the cooler before use and equilibrate it to room temperature before opening the container.
   - 5.2 **Pepsin-phosphoric acid (for processed cheese):** To approximately 200 mL of LG water in a 1,000-mL volumetric flask, add 20 mL of 85% phosphoric acid and 6.5 grams of pepsin. Swirl to dissolve the pepsin. Make up to volume with LG water. Filter the solution through a lintine disc before use.
   - 5.3 **Phosphoric acid:** 85% (for processed cheese).
   - 5.4 **Sodium citrate:** 10% for (natural cheese): Dissolve 100 grams of sodium citrate in a 1-L volumetric flask of LG water and dilute to volume. Filter through a lintine disc before use.
   - 5.5 **Water (LG):** Filtered through a lintine disc prior to use.
6. **Apparatus and Glassware:** All volumetric flasks, pipets, and burets are Class A unless otherwise specified.
   - 6.1 **Balance:** 0.1-g sensitivity.
   - 6.2 **Beakers:** 400 mL; 2 L, stainless steel or glass, with slotted cover for mechanical mixing or solid cover if magnetic stirrer is used.
   - 6.3 **Blender:** With 1-L jar.
   - 6.4 **Bottles:** Glass stoppered, wash bottle.
   - 6.5 **Cellophane envelopes:** 4 7.6 cm.
   - 6.6 **Extraneous material record cards.**
   - 6.7 **Filter flask:** With side arm, 1,000 mL or 2,000 mL.
   - 6.8 **Graduate:** 250 mL and 1,000 mL.
   - 6.9 **Hot plate:** Thermostatically controlled with stirrer apparatus.
   - 6.10 **Infrared lamp or forced air draft oven.**
   - 6.11 **Knife or spatula:** Stainless steel.
   - 6.12 **Lintine disc:** 3.1 cm diameter.
   - 6.13 **Microscope:** Minimum 12× magnification.
   - 6.14 **Pipet:** Mohr, 0.5 mL.
   - 6.15 **Standard test chart:** USDA Sediment Standard Chart for Milk and Milk Products, No. 7, CFR 58.2728.

6.16 **Suction (Vacuum) filtering apparatus:** To hold a 3.1-cm lintine disc.

6.17 **Thermometer:** 0° to 150°C.

7. **Sampling:** Chapter 3 on "Sampling Dairy and Related Products."

8. **Preparation of Test Sample**

   8.1 **Hard natural cheese:** Blend with an electric blender for a few seconds, pulsing the motor off and on during the mixing.

   8.2 **Soft natural and processed cheese:** Cut with a knife into 1.25 cm or smaller cubes.

9. **Procedure:** Before beginning analysis review material safety data sheets on all chemicals and use appropriate safety equipment such as hoods, aprons, face shields, and glasses.

   9.1 Place a 225-g sample into a 2-L stainless steel beaker containing 1,000 mL of 10% sodium citrate solution for natural cheese or 1,000 mL of pepsin-phosphoric acid solution for processed cheese.

   9.2 Place on a hot plate and mechanically agitate for 1 hour at 55°C (optimum temperature) ± 3°C for natural cheese or at 52°C (optimum temperature) ± 4°C for processed cheese. (If the sample is heated to more than 60°C, the protein will coagulate and produce a clot, which can clog the filter.) The beaker should be covered during agitation to prevent contamination.

   9.3 After 1 hour, remove and rinse the agitator with filtered LG water, allowing the rinsing to drain back into the sample beaker. Filter the solution (should take no more than 5 minutes) using medium suction (vacuum) through a lintine disc, waffle side up.

   9.4 Rinse the beaker with about 150 mL of filtered LG water and pour the rinsing through the same disc.

   9.5 Remove the disc from the filtering apparatus and dry it with an infrared lamp or in a forced air draft oven at 65°C for 20 minutes. The disc should be protected while drying to prevent contamination.

   9.6 Enclose the disc in a cellophane envelope and mount it on an extraneous material record card showing its identity.

   9.7 Examine the disc under a microscope using at least 12× magnification.

10. **Expression of Results:** Identify and record on the card the kinds of extraneous matter present using the appropriate USDA standard.[30]

11. **Precision and Performance Parameters:** This is an empirical test with no precision data available; however, for purposes of quality control it is recommended that duplicate analysis be performed on 10% of samples to provide a degree of confidence that the information can be replicated.

12. **Test Report and Interpretation:** The test report shall identify the method used and results obtained. The report will also identify any variation in the test not specified in this method as well as problems that may have impacted the test result. Each sample will be described in such a manner as to ensure traceablity as to its origin.

15.072 Extraneous Material, Milk Quantitative (Class O)[30,52,104,108]

1. **Scope:** This method is applicable to raw milk.
2. **References:** Chapter 2 on "Laboratory Quality Assurance and Safety." Chapter 3 on "Sampling Dairy and Related Products."
3. **Definition:** Extraneous material is defined as that material remaining after passing a sample of raw milk through a filter disc.
4. **Principle:** The laboratory version of the sediment test consists of passing a known volume of milk through a filter disc, observing the type and amount of residue, and comparing the disc with known standards to ascertain the types and amount of sediment present.
5. **Reagents:** Not applicable for this method.
6. **Apparatus and Glassware**
   - 6.1 **Mounting cards:** See section 6.4.
   - 6.2 **Sediment disc:** 3.18 cm in diameter mounted over a flat screen and with a filtration diameter of 2.86, 1.02, 0.51, 0.35, or 0.25 cm.
   - 6.3 **Standards:** Photographs of standard discs to be used in grading. Do not use soiled or faded photos. USDA Sediment Standard Chart for Milk and Milk Products No. 7, CFR 58.2729-CFR 58.2732 (available from Nelson-Jameson, Inc., USDA, Standardization Branch, Dairy Division, Agricultural Marketing Service, Washington, DC 20250).
   - 6.4 **Tester:** To hold the sediment disc. Before using, check the tester for precision (repeatability) of results and to ensure that no milk can bypass the disc. (Supplies available from Clark Dairy Supply Company, Inc., 430 E. Main St., Box 157, Greenwood, IN 46152; NASCO, 901 Janesville Ave., Ft. Atkinson, WI 53538, or 1524 Princeton Ave., Modesto, CA 95352; Sediment Testing Supply Company, 1512 W. Jarvis Ave., Chicago, IL 60626, Nelson-Jameson, or Weber Scientific, 2732 Kuser Road, Hamilton, NJ 08691).
7. **Sampling:** Chapter 3 on "Sampling Dairy and Related Products."
8. **Preparation of Test Sample:** Take a representative sample that has previously been mixed or otherwise prepared in order to make sample uniform.
9. **Procedure:** Before beginning analysis review material safety data sheets on all chemicals and use appropriate safety equipment such as hoods, aprons, face shields, and glasses.
   - 9.1 **Procedures available:** The source and volume of the sample determine both the filtering area and the procedure. Care should be taken in collecting a good representative sample.
     - 9.1.1 **Mixed-sample method**: Uses standard discs prepared from fine sediment mixtures for comparison. This method is used to assay sediment in milk from bulk milk tanks, tank trucks, storage tanks, processing equipment, and final containers.
     - 9.1.2 **Off-bottom method:** Intended to measure the amount of sediment in raw milk in cans. When the sediment apparatus is properly used, the assay effectively demonstrates unsanitary production of milk.

9.2 **Determination**

9.2.1 **Mixed samples:** Temper 470 mL of milk to 35°C to 38°C, and filter it through a disc of 1.02 cm in diameter when the disc is properly mounted in the tester. (Milk varies in its rate of flow through the disc, depending on temperature, solids [i.e., fat, protein, lactose] content, freezing, high acidity, extent of fat clumping, abnormal milk [such as colostrum], and amount of sediment in the sample). If the filtering diameter of the disc is less than 1.02 cm, adjust the sample size accordingly:

Filtering Diameter	Sample Size
0.51 cm	120 mL
0.35 cm	60 mL
0.25 cm	30 mL

9.2.2 **Off-bottom samples:** A tester is used to withdraw 0.47 L of milk from the bottom of the milk can. Collect the sample within the device while moving the suction end across the bottom or, if the bottom has a high center, around the circumference. Discharge the milk sample through the disc. Remove the disc from the tester and store it in a protective manner using a mounting card.

10. **Expression of Results**

10.1 Grade the disc by comparing it with standard discs. Indicate whether it was graded wet or dry. The character of the sediment may be determined by microscopic examination.

11. **Precision and Performance Parameters:** No precision data available for this assay.

12. **Test Report and Interpretation:** The test report shall identify the method used and results obtained. The report will also identify any variation in the test not specified in this method as well as problems that may have impacted the test result. Each sample will be described in such a manner as to ensure traceablity as to its origin.

15.073 Extraneous Material, Milk Qualitative, Sani-Guide (Class B)[104]

1. **Scope:** This is a screening test designed for use during the pumping of raw milk from farm bulk tanks and raw milk transport tanks to determine the amounts of coarse sediment. Because there is no control over the amount of milk that passes through the filter, this test is a qualitative test for insoluble extraneous material in raw milk. This determination is not a substitute for the sediment assay performed in the laboratory [see method 15.072].
2. **References:** Chapter 2 on "Laboratory Quality Assurance and Safety." Chapter 3 on "Sampling Dairy and Related Products."
3. **Definition:** Extraneous material is defined as that material remaining after passing a sample of raw milk through a filter disc.
4. **Principle:** Saniguide filter is placed in line and milk is pumped from one storage vessel to another. The filter is examined for the amount and type of extraneous material.

5. **Reagents:** Not applicable for this method.
6. **Apparatus and Glassware**
   6.1 Saniguide pipeline inserts: Available in diameters of 3.81, 5.08, and 7.62 cm (Kendall Company, Fiber Products Division, Walpole, MA 02081; or Nelson-Jameson, Inc.). Plastic filters are unsatisfactory for retaining coarse sediment for later evaluation.
   6.2 Saniguide grading chart [see section 6.1 for source].
7. **Sampling:** Chapter 3 on "Sampling Dairy and Related Products."
8. **Preparation of Test Sample:** Since the entire vessel sample passes through Saniguide, no sample preparation is necessary.
9. **Procedure**
   9.1 Place a Saniguide insert into the pipe connection between either the farm tank and hose connection or the bulk truck and pipeline connection from the pump. The insert serves as a gasket when it is properly positioned.
   9.2 When the tank or truck is empty, remove the Saniguide.
10. **Expression of Results**
    10.1 Grade the sediment disk by comparing it with the standard grading chart.
    10.1 If the Saniguide is left for the producer's evaluation, store refrigerated in a plastic bag designed for this purpose [see section 6.1 for supplies].
11. **Precision and Performance Parameters:** No precision data available for this assay.
12. **Test Report and Interpretation:** The test report shall identify the method used and results obtained. The report will also identify any variation in the test not specified in this method as well as problems that may have impacted the test result. Each sample will be described in such a manner as to ensure traceablity as to its origin.

15.080 Fat Determination Methods

15.081 Introduction

Over the years, much effort has been expended to increase the accuracy and applicability of the original Babcock method when used to determine the fat content of various types of milk, cheese, whey, and other related dairy foods. These refinements consist of the following: 1) Using LG water maintained at specified temperatures. 2) Controlling and standardizing the technique used in adding acid to the samples to produce the necessary heat for complete disintegration of the structure of the nonfatty material, while at the same time releasing liquefied fat for measurement. The technique involves rapid addition of acid accompanied by a smooth rotary swirling of the bottle by hand. Time allotted for adding acid to the sample should not exceed 20 seconds, as heat loss due to time lag causes the incomplete digestion of the sample, resulting in a cloudy fat column. 3) Using a mechanical shaker to aid in the digestion of the nonfatty materials and the quick release of fat. 4) Controlling the variability in temperature of the product-acid mixture. 5) Improving the accuracy of the glassware. 6) Using the cream method, which has been collaboratively studied and revised to make it more consistent with the method for milk. 7) Adjusting the centrifuge, adding water, and tempering bath temperatures to bring the results of the Babcock into closer agreement with the Mojonnier method over the full range of fat levels in different dairy foods (JAOACI 1997:80;845-859).

The Gerber method is included with no major revisions. The Gerber method is sometimes favored on certain fermented dairy products that contain high sugar contents because it may be easier to avoid having burnt particles in the fat column. The Roese-Gottlieb and Mojonnier methods are very similar and their primary difference is that in the Roese-Gottlieb the weight of the fat plus pan is determined after solvent evaporation, and then the fat is removed from the pan, the pan is dried, and the difference in weight is used to calculate fat content. This approach has not been collaboratively studied and is not used in common practice in laboratories because it takes extra time, introduces additional sources of error, and uses more solvent. The IDF and AOAC now have only one procedure that combines the best aspects of both methods and it has been collaboratively studied. That procedure will be reported as method 15.085–Mojonnier Method and is equivalent to AOAC 989.05 and IDF Provisional Standard 1D:1996. The Mojonnier ether extraction has been shown to be more precise than the Babcock and has been accepted by the dairy industry as a more accurate reference. The standard methods version of the Roese-Gottlieb procedure from the 16th edition has been surplused and is not included the 17th edition of *SMEDP*.

15.082 Babcock Fat, Milk (Class A1)

1. **Scope:** This method is applicable to raw milk.
2. **References:** Chapter 2 on "Laboratory Quality Assurance and Safety."
   Chapter 3 on "Sampling Dairy and Related Products."
3. **Definition:** Fat is the mass fraction of substances determined according to this procedure and is expressed as a percentage by mass.
4. **Principle:** Milk and concentrated sulfuric acid are mixed to produce an exothermic reaction that disintegrates the emulsion structure in milk to release free fat. The free fat is collected in the graduated portion of the neck of the Babcock bottle, which is calibrated to express the fat content of the product on a percentage fat by mass.
5. **Reagents:** Unless otherwise specified all chemicals are reagent or ACS grade.
   - 5.1 **Sulfuric acid (H_2SO_4):** Specific gravity 1.825 ± 0.005 at 20/20°C, unless otherwise noted, tempered to 21 ± 1°C. Each new lot should be compared to the previous lot.
   - 5.2 **Water:** Laboratory grade maintained at 51 ± 1°C, unless otherwise specified.
6. **Apparatus and Glassware:** All volumetric flasks, pipets, and burets are Class A unless otherwise specified.
   - 6.1 **Adjustable acid delivery system:** Calibrated to deliver the correct amount of acid to obtain the desired product-acid reaction temperature.

6.2 **Balance:** Sensitivity 0.01 g.

6.3 **Bottles, Babcock, milk bottle:** 0 to 8%: 18 g, 16 to 17 cm, with 0.1% divisions and calibration meeting AOAC specifications. For use with samples containing up to 8% fat. Calibrated portion of the neck must be at least 75 mm in length. It is highly recommended that Babcock bottles have etched and pigmented neck markings and be calibrated for improved accuracy. The procedure for verification of calibration accuracy of milk and cream bottles is described elsewhere (JAOACI 78:463-471) and is usually done by the manufacturer of the bottles or a certification laboratory. Width of markings on the neck will be no greater than 0.2 mm. (Forcoven Products, Inc. P.O. Box 1556, Humble, TX 77338; and Kimble Glass, Vineland, NJ.)

6.4 **Bottle holder:** For test bottles.

6.5 **Centrifuge:** Electrically heated to maintain air temperature of 46° to 51°C. The centrifuge should be equipped with a speed indicator (tachometer). Proper speed may be determined from Table 15.1. The diameter of the wheel is the distance between the inside bottom of opposite cups, as measured through the center of rotation of the centrifuge wheel while the cups are fully extended horizontally.

Table 15.1. Rotational Speed Required in a Babcock Centrifuge

Diameter of Wheel		Speed
inch	*cm*	*rpm*
10	25.4	1074
12	30.5	980
14	35.6	909
16	40.6	848
18	45.7	800
20	50.8	759
22	55.9	724
24	61.0	693

6.6 **Digital thermometer:** To measure the temperature of the product-acid reaction. Scale divisions at least every 1°C over the range from 85 to 120°C. The probe must have a small diameter (less than 0.5 mm) to ensure rapid response time, and its length should be such that the tip is approximately 1 cm above the bottom of the bottle when fully inserted. A simple check for accuracy of calibration can be done by placing the probe in boiling LG water. The temperature should be within 100° ± 1°C.

6.7 **Dividers:** For measuring the fat column.

6.8 **Pipet, milk:** Standard 17.6-mL milk pipet meeting AOAC specifications with a small rubber or plastic ring to allow air-flow out of the Babcock bottle and entry of milk into the bottle when the pipet is standing in the neck of the bottle during the release of milk.

6.9 **Reading light with magnification:** Light used as a background when measuring the fat column. Light should be diffuse (soft white) and provide illumination from angles above and below the level of the fat column. Bottle is held in front of the light and behind the magnification device such that the bottom and top meniscus of the fat column can each be centered in the field of the magnification device during placement of each caliper point. A magnification device must be used to aid reading.

6.10 **Shaker for test bottles:** Mechanical, variable speed, matched to the maximum capacity of the centrifuge.

6.11 **Thermometer, glass:** 0° to 110°C.

6.12 **Water bath:** For tempering samples before pipeting, with a thermometer to maintain samples at 38° ± 1°C.

6.13 **Water bath:** For test bottles; provided with a thermometer to maintain temperature of the fat columns at 48° ± 1°C. Must be deep enough so that water level is above the upper level of the fat column in the Babcock bottles.

7. **Sampling:** Chapter 3 on "Sampling Dairy and Related Products."

8. **Preparation of Test Sample:** Warm the fresh or preserved raw milk sample to 38° ± 1°C by means of the water bath. The level of the water should be at or above the milk level within the container. Mix the milk sample by inversion 10 times without causing frothing or churning. Inspect the container to ensure that there is no line of unmelted cream stuck to the side or inside the lid of the container. If there is a cream line, run hot (ca. 50° to 60°C) tap water on the outside surface of the container for 15 to 20 seconds to release the fat from the inside surface of the container so that it is dispersed in the sample immediately prior to pipeting the test portion (9.1). Mix the sample by inversion and pipet the test portion immediately. Do not allow test samples to remain in the water bath more than 15 minutes after reaching 38°C.

9. **Procedure:** Before beginning analysis review material safety data sheets on all chemicals and use appropriate safety equipment such as hoods, aprons, face shields, and glasses.

   9.1 **Determination of milk-scid reaction temperature:** The probe of the digital thermometer should be at room temperature immediately before insertion into the Babcock bottle. Prior to testing a group of samples, determine the correct amount of acid to be used by measuring the milk-acid reaction temperature. Start by adding 17.5 mL of 21° ± 1°C sulfuric acid to a Babcock milk bottle containing 17.6 mL of milk at the same temperature. Add the 17.5 mL of acid in one delivery so that all traces of milk are washed into the bulb. Cleanly layer the acid under the milk. Insert the digital thermometer probe full down the bottle neck, and immediately swirl the bottle manually until all traces of curd disappear. The desired peak reaction temperature, 108° ± 2°C, will occur very rapidly, approximately when the last trace of milk mixes with the acid during the manual swirling. If the observed reaction temperature is too low or too high, repeat the procedure described above and adjust the amount of sulfuric acid added until the milk reaction temperature is within the correct temperature range and the color of resulting fat column is a translucent golden yellow to amber. The amount of acid required may differ for different technicians with the same batch of acid and for different lots of acid.

Factors that influence milk-acid reaction temperature are the amount of acid added, the rate at which the milk-acid mixture is swirled, and the temperature of the milk and acid. This test takes practice to obtain good, clear, reliable fat columns. Two technicians in the same lab may need to use different amounts of acid to obtain the same reaction temperature because of person-to-person differences in swirling of the milk-acid mixture. Depending on the impurities in the acid and its specific gravity, the volume of acid required to achieve the desired reaction temperature may vary in extreme cases from approximately 14 to 19 mL.

9.2 **Test portion and pretreatment:** To the clean Babcock milk bottle add 17.6 ± 0.05 mL of the warmed milk sample using a Babcock milk pipet. Do not release the sample until the bulb of the pipet rests on the neck of the test bottle. After active flow has stopped (about 30 seconds) blow out the last drops from the pipet into the bottle, remove the pipet, and adjust the milk to 21 ± 1°C.

9.3 **Testing raw milk samples:** Hold the bottle at a slight angle and add the appropriate volume (as determined in 9.1) of 21° ± 1°C sulfuric acid in one addition, washing down all traces of milk into the bulb. The time for complete acid addition should not exceed 20 seconds. Immediately hand swirl the milk-acid mixture by the same technique used during the milk-acid reaction temperature measurement, until all traces of curd disappear. Shake on a mechanical shaker (6.10) at medium speed for 1 minute after the last bottle has been inserted in the mechanical shaker. The temperature of the milk plus acid in the first bottle should not be less than 50.5°C at the time the bottles are transferred into the centrifuge.

Place the bottles in a heated (48.5°C) centrifuge, counter balance, and turn on the centrifuge. After the proper speed (see Table 15.1) has been attained, centrifuge for 5 minutes. Gently stop the centrifuge and add hot (51°C) LG water until the bulb of each bottle is filled to within 0.6 cm of the base of the neck. Centrifuge for 2 minutes. Stop the centrifuge and again add hot (51°C) LG water until the liquid fat column approaches the top graduation of the scale. Centrifuge for 1 minute.

9.4 Reading the test result: Transfer the bottles to a water bath that will adjust the fat columns to 48° ± 1°C, and temper the bottles for a minimum of 5 minutes. The water level should be slightly above the level of the fat columns in the necks of the bottles. Remove the bottles one at a time from the water bath and quickly dry the bottle. Immediately (before the column cools and contracts significantly) measure (with the aid of a reading light and magnification) the fat column using dividers. Place the divider points on the vertical line on the bottle neck, with one point at the bottom of the lower meniscus and the other point at the top of the upper meniscus. Without changing the distance between the two points on the dividers, move the dividers down the bottle neck until the lower point rests in the horizontal graduation mark at 0%. Place the upper point against the bottle graduation and read the test in percentage fat by weight to the nearest 0.05%. The fat column at the time of measurement should be translucent, golden yellow or amber, and free of visible suspended particles.

Reject all tests that produce a cloudy fat column or show the presence of charred matter or curd, or where for any reason the reading is indistinct or uncertain. Repeat the test. Corrections can be made by adjusting the amount of acid added to obtain a milk-acid reaction temperature in the desired range of 108° ± 2°C.

10. Expression of Results

10.1 Results: Results are read directly from the bottle and expressed as percentage fat by weight to the nearest 0.05%.

11. Precision and Performance Parameters: The values for repeatability and reproducibility have been derived from the results of interlaboratory tests on raw milk in accordance with Horwitz.[38]

11.1 **Repeatability:** The absolute difference between the results of two single determinations, carried out simultaneously or in rapid succession by the same operator under the same conditions on identical test material, should not exceed 0.105 g of fat per 100 g of milk.

11.2 **Reproducibility:** The absolute difference between two single and independent results, obtained by two operators working in different laboratories on identical test material, should not exceed 0.133 g of fat per 100 g of milk.

11.3 **Method Performance Statistics** (for raw milk[14,59-61])

$s_r = 0.037$ $RSD_r = 0.901\%$ r value = 0.105
$s_R = 0.047$ $RSD_R = 1.147\%$ R value = 0.133

12. Test Report and Interpretation: The test report shall identify the method used and results obtained. The report will also identify any variation in the test not specified in this method as well as problems that may have impacted the test result. Each sample will be described in such a manner as to ensure traceablity as to its origin.

15.083 Babcock Method, Cream (Class A1), Cheese (Class B)[38,60,68]

1. **Scope:** This method is applicable to unhomogenized cream and cheese.
2. **References:** Chapter 2 on "Laboratory Quality Assurance and Safety."
   Chapter 3 on "Sampling Dairy and Related Products."
3. **Definition:** Fat is the mass fraction of substances determined according to this procedure and is expressed as a percentage by mass.
4. **Principle:** Cream or cheese and concentrated sulfuric acid are mixed to produce an exothermic reaction that disintegrates the emulsion structure to release free fat. The free fat is collected in the graduated portion of the neck of the Babcock bottle, which is calibrated to express the fat content of the product as a percentage fat by mass.
5. **Reagents:** Unless otherwise specified all chemicals are reagent or ACS grade.

5.1 **Sulfuric acid (H_2SO_4):** Specific gravity 1.825 ± 0.005 at 20/20°C, unless otherwise noted, tempered to 21° ± 1°C. Each new lot should be compared to the previous lot.

5.2 **Water:** Laboratory grade maintained at 51° ± 1°C, unless otherwise specified.

5.3 **Glymol (red or blue reader):** Specific gravity not to exceed 0.85, at 20/20°C.

6. Apparatus: All volumetric flasks, pipets, and burets are Class A unless otherwise specified.

6.1 **Adjustable acid delivery system:** Calibrated to deliver the correct amount of acid to obtain the desired product-acid reaction temperature.

6.2 **Balance:** Sensitivity 0.01 g.

6.3 **Bottles, Babcock, cream or cheese bottle:** 0 to 50%: 9 g, 15 to 17.0 cm, or 9 g, 21 to 22.9 cm, or 18 g, 21 to 22.9 cm, with 0.5% divisions. Cheese bottle, 0 to 10%, 0 to 20%, or 0 to 50% Paley bottle 9 g, 15.5 to 17.0 cm with side opening for addition of sample. All bottles with calibrations meeting AOAC specifications. For use with samples containing up to 50% fat. Calibrated portion of the neck must be at least 75 mm in length. It is highly recommended that Babcock bottles have etched and pigmented neck markings and be calibrated for improved accuracy. The procedure for verification of calibration accuracy of milk and cream bottles is described elsewhere (JAOACI 78:463-471) and is usually done by the manufacturer of the bottles or a certification laboratory. Width of markings on the neck will be no greater than 0.2 mm. (Forcoven Products, Inc. P.O. Box 1556, Humble, TX 77338; and Kimble Glass, Vineland, NJ.)

6.4 **Bottle holder:** For test bottles.

6.5 **Centrifuge:** Electrically heated to maintain air temperature of 46° to 51°C. The centrifuge should be equipped with a speed indicator (tachometer). Proper speed may be determined from Table 15.1. The diameter of the wheel is the distance between the inside bottom of opposite cups, as measured through the center of rotation of the centrifuge wheel while the cups are fully extended horizontally.

6.6 **Digital thermometer:** To measure the temperature of the product-acid reaction. Scale divisions at least every 1°C over the range from 85° to 120°C. The probe must have a small diameter (less than 0.5 mm) to ensure rapid response time, and its length should be such that the tip is approximately 1 cm above the bottom of the bottle when fully inserted. A simple check for accuracy of calibration can be done by placing the probe in boiling LG water. The temperature should be within 100° ± 1°C.

6.7 **Dividers:** For measuring the fat column.

6.8 **Reading light with magnification:** Light used as a background when measuring the fat column. Light should be diffuse (soft white) and provide illumination from angles above and below the level of the fat column. Bottle is held in front of the light and behind the magnification device such that the bottom and top meniscus of the fat column can each be centered in the field of the magnification device during placement of each caliper point. A magnification device must be used to aid reading.

6.9 **Shaker for test bottles:** Mechanical, variable speed, matched to the maximum capacity of the centrifuge.

6.10 **Thermometer, glass:** 0° to 110°C.

6.11 **Water bath:** For tempering cream samples before pipeting, with a thermometer to maintain samples at 38° ± 1°C.

6.12 **Water bath:** For test bottles; provided with a thermometer to maintain temperature of the fat columns at 48° ± 1°C. Must be deep enough so that water level is above the upper level of the fat column in the Babcock bottles.

7. **Sampling:** Chapter 3 on "Sampling Dairy and Related Products."

8. **Preparation of Test Sample:** Take a representative sample that has previously been mixed or otherwise prepared in order to make sample uniform.

8.1 **Cream:** Warm the fresh or preserved unhomogenized cream sample to 38° ± 1°C by means of the water bath. The level of the water should be at or above the milk level within the container. Mix the cream sample 10 times by inversion without causing frothing or churning. Inspect the container to ensure that there is no line of unmelted cream stuck to the side or inside the lid of the container. If there is a cream line, run hot (ca. 50° to 60°C) tap water on the outside surface of the container for 15 to 20 seconds to release the fat from the inside surface of the container so that it is dispersed in the sample immediately prior to weighing the test portion. Mix the sample by inversion and weigh the test portion immediately. Do not allow test samples to remain in the water bath more than 15 minutes after reaching 38°C.

8.2 **Cheese:** Shred cheese using a grater or blender.

9. **Procedure:** Before beginning analysis, review material safety data sheets on all chemicals and use appropriate safety equipment such as hoods, aprons, face shields, and glasses.

9.1 **Determination of cream-acid reaction temperature:** The probe of the digital thermometer should be at room temperature immediately before insertion into the Babcock bottle. Prior to testing a group of samples, determine the correct amount of acid to be used by measuring the cream-acid reaction temperature. Start by adding 9 mL of 21° ± 1°C sulfuric acid to a Babcock cream or cheese bottle containing 9 g of cream, or 16 mL of sulfuric acid to a bottle containing 18 g of cream. Add the 9 or 16 mL of acid in one delivery so that all traces of cream are washed into the bulb. Cleanly layer the acid under the sample in the Babcock bottle. Insert the digital thermometer probe full down the bottle neck, and immediately swirl the bottle manually until all traces of curd disappear. The desired peak reaction temperature is 93°-103°C for 30-45% cream (the lower the fat content, the higher the reaction temperature) and will occur very rapidly, approximately when the last trace of cream mixes with the acid during the manual swirling. If the observed reaction temperature is too low or too high, repeat the procedure described above and adjust the amount of sulfuric acid added until the sample reaction temperature is within the correct temperature range and the color of resulting fat column is a translucent golden yellow to amber. The amount of acid required may differ for different technicians with the same batch of acid and for different lots of acid.

Factors that influence the reaction temperature are the amount of acid added, the rate at which the cream-acid mixture is swirled, the temperature of the cream, water content of the cream, and the temperature of the acid. This test takes practice to obtain good, clear, reliable fat columns. Two technicians in the same lab may need to use different amounts of acid to obtain the same reaction temperature because of person-to-person differences in swirling of the cream-acid mixture. Depending on the impurities in the acid and its specific gravity, the volume of acid required to achieve the desired reaction temperature may vary.

9.2 **Test portion and pretreatment**

9.2.1 **Cream:** For each cream sample, accurately weigh 9 ± 0.03 g into a 9-g cream-test bottle or 18 ± 0.03 g into an 18-g cream-test bottle. Adjust the cream in the test bottle to 21° ± 1°C. Adjust the sulfuric acid to 21° ± 1°C. Weigh the cream into some additional bottles for use in determining the cream-acid reaction temperature.

9.2.2 **Cheese:** Weigh 9 g (± 0.01 g) of grated cheese into a 9-g cream or a 9-g Paley test bottle.

9.3 **Testing cream samples:** Warm sample, weigh cream into test bottle and adjust to 21° ± 1°C. Hold the bottle at a slight angle and add the appropriate volume (as determined in the cream-acid reaction temperature procedure) of 21° ± 1°C sulfuric acid in one addition, washing all traces of cream into the bulb. The time for the complete acid addition should not exceed 20 seconds. Immediately hand swirl the cream-acid mixture by the same technique used during the cream-acid reaction temperature measurement until all traces of curd disappear. Shake on a mechanical shaker at medium speed for at least 1 minute after the last bottle has been inserted in the mechanical shaker. Add 6 mL of 47°-52°C LG water to all bottles and then shake full set for 1 additional minute.

9.4 **Testing cheese samples:** Pipet about 10 mL of hot (60°C) LG water into the bottle containing the 9 g of cheese. Mix to suspend the cheese thoroughly before adding acid. Cool to 21° ± 1°C. Hold the bottle at a slight angle and add about 15 mL of sulfuric acid portion-wise (approximately 8, 4, and 3 mL), swirling by hand after each addition. The time for the complete acid addition should not exceed 20 seconds. Immediately swirl the bottle until all lumps of curd completely disappear. Shake on a mechanical shaker. For types of cheese where the fat is more difficult to release, shaking the bottles on the shaker after the hot water addition and longer shaking times after addition of sulfuric acid may be necessary to dissolve the curd and release the fat. This procedure was designed for cheeses that typically contain between 15 and 35% fat. It may be more difficult to achieve full release of fat from lower fat cheeses, and it may be necessary to use Babcock bottles with calibrated necks for lower range of fat concentrations (i.e., <20%).

9.5 **Centrifugation:** Place the bottles in a heated (48.5°C) centrifuge, counterbalance, and turn on the centrifuge. After the proper speed has been attained, centrifuge for 5 minutes. Stop the centrifuge and add warm (51°C) LG water until the bulb of each bottle is filled to within 0.6 cm of the base of the neck. Centrifuge for 2 minutes. Stop the centrifuge and again add warm (51°C) LG water until the liquid fat column approaches the top graduation of the scale. Centrifuge for 1 minute.

9.6 **Reading the test:** Transfer the bottles to a water bath that will adjust the fat column to 48.0° ± 1°C, and temper the contents for a minimum of 5 minutes. The water level should be slightly above the level of the fat column in the bottles. Remove a bottle from the water bath and quickly dry it. Carefully add two drops of glymol, allowing it to run down the inside neck of the bottle on to the top of the fat column. Using dividers, immediately measure the fat column from the bottom of the lower meniscus to the sharp line of demarcation between the glymol and the fat. The divider points must be in the vertical etched line to prevent any error in reading. Read the percentage of fat to the nearest 0.25% when using a 0% to 50% bottle. The column at the time of measurement should be translucent, golden yellow or amber, and free of visible suspended particles.

Reject all tests that produce a cloudy fat column or show the presence of charred matter or curd, or where, for any reason, the reading is indistinct or uncertain. Repeat the test. Corrections can be made by adjusting the amount of acid added to obtain a cream or cheese-acid reaction temperature in the desired range of 93°-103°C. Other factors that may cause problems are the way the bottle is swirled when the acid is added or the temperature of the sample and acid. This test takes practice to obtain good, clear, reliable fat columns.

10. Expression of Results

10.1 **Results:** Results are read directly from the bottle and expressed as percentage fat by weight to the nearest 0.25%.

11. Precision and Performance Parameters

11.1 **Repeatability:** *Cream:* The absolute difference between the results of two single determinations, carried out simultaneously or in rapid succession by the same operator under the same conditions on identical test material, should not exceed 0.73 g of fat per 100 g of cream.

Cheese: Collaborative study data are not available for repeatability.

11.2 **Reproducibility:** *Cream:* The absolute difference between two single and independent results, obtained by two operators working in different laboratories on identical test material, should not exceed 1.00 g of fat per 100 g of cream.

Cheese: Collaborative study data are not available for reproducibility.

11.3 **Method performance statistics (for unhomogenized cream at 30 to 45% fat):**

$s_r = 0.258$ $RSD_r = 0.687\%$ r value = 0.730
$s_R = 0.353$ $RSD_R = 0.940\%$ R value = 0.998

12. **Test Report and Interpretation:** The test report shall identify the method used and results obtained. The report will also identify any variation in the test not specified in this method as well as problems which may have impacted the test result. Each sample will be described in such a manner as to ensure traceability as to its origin.

15.084 Babcock Method, Pennsylvania and Roccal (Class B)[14,38,59-61,68,87]

1. **Scope:** A method is applicable for the determination of the total fat content of chocolate milk, ice cream, frozen desserts, skim milk, buttermilk, whey, and cottage cheese.
2. **References:** Chapter 2 on "Laboratory Quality Assurance and Safety." Chapter 3 on "Sampling Dairy and Related Products."
3. **Definition:** Fat is the mass fraction of substances determined according to this procedure and is expressed as a percentage by mass.
4. **Principle:** The regular Babcock test for some dairy products does not yield the total amount of milk fat in the product because, under the conditions of the test, it is impossible to centrifuge out all the fat. The Babcock test for skim milk will customarily read low by 0.07 to 0.10%, whereas the test for buttermilk may be 0.3% low. This situation led to modifications of the Babcock procedure that use ammonium hydroxide and/or alcohol to free the fat. Another procedure uses Roccal solution to free the fat. Thus modified, these procedures show somewhat better agreement with results of the Mojonnier ether extraction method.
5. **Reagents:** Unless otherwise specified all chemicals are reagent or ACS grade.

5.1 **Diluted sulfuric acid (H_2SO_4):** Specific gravity 1.73 ± 0.01 at 20/20°C, tempered to 21° ± 1°C. Mix 3.5 parts sulfuric acid with 1 part water. *CAUTION: Add acid to water, not water to acid.* Each new lot should be compared to the previous lot.

5.2 **Water:** Laboratory grade maintained at 51° ± 1°C, unless otherwise specified.

5.3 **Ammonium hydroxide (NH_4OH):** 28 to 29% ammonia.

5.4 **Normal butyl alcohol:** Boiling point 117°C.

5.5 **Roccal II**: 50% concentrate of benzalkonium chloride (United States Pharmacopoeia, or USP).

5.6 **Roccal solution:** Add 200 mL of concentrated sulfuric acid (sp. g 1.835 – 1.84, 20/20°C) to 5 mL of 50% Roccal II. Mix well and cool before using. The Roccal-sulfuric acid solution will keep for about 2 weeks. When a dark amber color appears, the Roccal has dissipated and will not be effective in testing. Discard the solution when it becomes yellow to brown.

6. **Apparatus and Glassware:** All volumetric flasks, pipets, and burets are Class A unless otherwise specified.
   - 6.1 **Adjustable acid delivery system:** Calibrated to deliver the correct amount of acid to obtain the desired product-acid reaction temperature.
   - 6.2 **Balance:** Sensitivity 0.01 g.
   - 6.3 **Bottles, Babcock**
     - 6.3.1 **Milk bottle:** 0 to 8%: 18 g, 16 to 17 cm, with 0.1% divisions and calibration meeting AOAC specifications. For use with samples containing up to 8% fat. Calibrated portion of the neck must be at least 75 mm in length. It is highly recommended that Babcock bottles have etched and pigmented neck markings and be calibrated for improved accuracy. The procedure for verification of calibration accuracy of milk and cream bottles is described elsewhere (JAOACI 78:463-471) and is usually done by the manufacturer of the bottles or a certification laboratory. Width of markings on the neck will be no greater than 0.2 mm. (Forcoven Products, Inc., P.O. Box 1556, Humble, TX 77338; and Kimble Glass, Vineland, NJ.)
     - 6.3.2 **Skim milk bottle:** 0 to 0.5%, 18 g, 15.2-17.0 cm, double necked, with 0.01% divisions. For use with samples containing less than 0.5%.
     - 6.3.3 **Ice cream bottle:** 0 to 20%, 9 g, 15.2-17.0 cm, with 0.2% divisions. For use with samples containing 5 to 20% fat.
     - 6.3.4 **Bottle, Paley:** 0 to 10%, or 0 to 20%: 9 g, 15.5-17.0 cm, with divisions and side opening for addition of sample.
     - 6.3.5 **Other bottles:** A wide variety of other Babcock bottles exist with general purpose of providing ease of use and a range of calibration that is appropriate for various products. This is particularly true as lower fat versions of traditional dairy foods have been developed. The construction, calibration, and design of these bottles should be consistent with the bottles listed above.
   - 6.4 **Bottle holder:** For test bottles.
   - 6.5 **Centrifuge:** Electrically heated to maintain air temperature of 46° to 51°C. The centrifuge should be equipped with a speed indicator (tachometer): Proper speed may be determined from Table 15.1. The diameter of the wheel is the distance between the inside bottom of opposite cups, as measured through the center of rotation of the centrifuge wheel while the cups are fully extended horizontally.
   - 6.6 **Digital thermometer:** To measure the temperature of the product-acid reaction. Scale divisions at least every 1°C over the range from 85° to 120°C. The probe must have a small diameter (less than 0.5 mm) to ensure rapid response time, and its length should be such that the tip is approximately 1 cm above the bottom of the bottle when fully inserted. A simple check for accuracy of calibration can

be done by placing the probe in boiling LG water. The temperature should be within 100° ± 1°C.

6.7 **Dividers:** For measuring the fat column.

6.8 **Pipet, milk:** Standard 17.6-mL milk pipet meeting AOAC specifications with a small rubber or plastic ring to allow air flow out of the Babcock bottle and entry of milk into the bottle when the pipet is standing in the neck of the bottle during the release of milk.

6.9 **Reading light with magnification:** Light used as a background when measuring the fat column. Light should be diffuse (soft white) and provide illumination from angles above and below the level of the fat column. Bottle is held in front of the light and behind the magnification device such that the bottom and top meniscus of the fat column can each be centered in the field of the magnification device during placement of each caliper point. A magnification device must be used to aid reading.

6.10 **Shaker for test bottles:** Mechanical, variable speed, matched to the maximum capacity of the centrifuge.

6.11 **Thermometer, glass:** 0° to 110°C.

6.12 **Water bath:** For tempering samples before pipeting, with a thermometer to maintain samples at 38° ± 1°C.

6.13 **Water bath:** For test bottles; provided with a thermometer to maintain temperature of the fat columns at 48° ± 1°C. Must be deep enough so that water level is above the upper level of the fat column in the Babcock bottles.

7. **Sampling:** Chapter 3 on "Sampling Dairy and Related Products."

8. **Preparation of Test Sample**

8.1 **Ice cream and frozen desserts:** Melt ice cream and frozen desserts at room temperature and, if necessary, heat to about 20°C to eliminate foam. Reduce any large particles in fruit and nut ice cream to a finely divided state with a blender.

8.2 **Chocolate milk, skim milk, buttermilk, and whey:** Warm the sample to 38° ± 1°C by means of the water bath (6.12). The level of the water should be at or above the milk level within the container. Mix the milk sample by inversion 10 times by inversion without causing frothing or churning. Inspect the container to ensure that there is no line of unmelted cream stuck to the side or inside the lid of the container. If there is a cream line, run hot (ca. 50° to 60°C) tap water on the outside surface of the container for 15 to 20 seconds to release the fat from the inside surface of the container so that it is dispersed in the sample immediately prior to pipetting the test portion. Mix the sample by inversion and pipet the test portion immediately. Do not allow test samples to remain in the water bath more than 15 minutes after reaching 38°C.

8.3 **Cottage Cheese:** Blend thoroughly a full retail carton of cheese or a representative sample of larger containers until the product is uniform and pourable. The final temperature of the mixed sample should not be more than 25°C.

9. **Procedure:** Before beginning analysis review material safety data sheets on all chemicals and use appropriate safety equipment such as hoods, aprons, face shields, and glasses.

9.1 **Test portion**

9.1.1 **Ice cream and frozen desserts:** Accurately weigh 9 g of well-mixed ice cream into a test bottle of the correct size (6.3). For typical ice cream a 0 to 20% Paley bottle is used. However, for lower fat frozen dessert products a 0 to 10% fat Paley bottle may be more appropriate. Precautions must be taken to keep the sample from separating before being sampled.

9.1.2 **Chocolate milk** *(Pennsylvania Method, see 9.2.1 and 9.2.2):* Accurately weigh 18 g of well-mixed chocolate milk into a Babcock bottle. For chocolate milk containing more than 1% fat, use 0 to 8% milk bottle and method 9.2.1.

For chocolate milk containing less than 1% fat use skim test bottle and a 9-g sample with method 9.2.2.

9.1.3 **Skim milk, buttermilk, and whey** *(Pennsylvania Method, see 9.2.2):* Add exactly 9 mL of skim milk or whey with a pipet through the large neck or weigh 9 g of buttermilk into a skim test bottle. Tip the bottle during sample addition to facilitate escape of air, thus preventing any tendency for the large neck to clog or overflow.

Roccal Method (see 9.2.3): Pipet 17.6 mL (18 g) of sample into a skim test bottle through the large neck, tipping the bottle to facilitate the escape of air, thus preventing any tendency for the large neck to clog or overflow. Blow the last drop out of the pipet.

9.1.4 **Cottage cheese** *(Pennsylvania Method, see 9.2.4):* Weigh 9 g (± 0.01 g) of well-mixed cottage cheese into a 0 to 10% Paley test bottle through the side opening.

9.2 Determination

9.2.1 **Method I** *(Pennsylvania Method):* **Chocolate milk, ice cream, and frozen desserts:** Holding the bottle at a slight angle, add 2 mL of ammonium hydroxide and rotate the bottle slowly to mix the reagent with the sample thoroughly. Add 3 mL of normal butyl alcohol and mix thoroughly by swirling the bottle. Hold the bottle at a slight angle and add about 17.5 mL of diluted sulfuric acid portion-wise (approximately 8, 5, and 4 mL), rotating the bottle to wash traces of the milk product from the neck. Manually shake between portions to mix the acid and the sample. The time for the complete acid addition should not exceed 20 seconds. Immediately swirl the bottle until all lumps completely disappear.

9.2.2 **Method I** *(Pennsylvania Method):* **Skim milk, lowfat milk, buttermilk, whey:** Add 7 to 9 mL of diluted sulfuric acid (5.1) to a skim milk test bottle. It may be necessary to vary the amount of acid to obtain a fat column of golden yellow to light amber color. Mix the contents of the bottle thoroughly and proceed as in 9.2.5, 9.2.6, and 9.2.7 with the following exception: Because a 9-mL sample was used in an 18-g bottle, double the reading from the neck of the bottle to obtain the percentage fat.

9.2.3 **Method II** *(Roccal Method):* **Chocolate milk, skim milk, buttermilk, or whey:** Add 12 mL of the Roccal-sulfuric acid solution in small portions instead of sulfuric acid alone. Proceed as in 9.2.5, 9.2.6,and 9.2.7.

9.2.4 **Method I** *(Pennsylvania Method):* **Cottage cheese:** Add 2 mL of ammonium hydroxide (5.3) through the side opening and mix thoroughly. Add 3 mL of normal butyl alcohol (5.4), again though the side opening. Tightly insert the rubber stopper and mix the sample and reagents thoroughly by rotating the bottle. Shake on a mechanical shaker for 3 minutes. Add 9 mL of diluted sulfuric acid (5.1) and mix the contents thoroughly for 3 minutes on a mechanical shaker. Add a small amount of hot (51°C) water to the bottle through the side opening to dislodge any fat adhering to the stopper area. Proceed as in 9.2.5, 9.2.6, and 9.2.7.

9.2.5 Place the bottles in a heated (48.5°C) centrifuge (6.5), counter balance, and turn on the centrifuge. After the proper speed (see Table 15.1) has been attained, centrifuge for 5 minutes. Gently stop the centrifuge and add hot (51°C) LG water until the bulb of each bottle is filled to within 0.6 cm of the base of the neck. Centrifuge for 2 minutes. Stop the centrifuge and again add hot (51°C) LG water until the liquid fat column approaches the top graduation of the scale. Centrifuge for 1 minute.

9.2.6 Transfer the bottles to a water bath (6.13) that will adjust the fat columns to 48 ± 1°C, and temper the bottles for a minimum of 5 minutes. The water level should be slightly above the level of the fat columns in the necks of the bottles. Remove the bottles one at a time from the water bath and quickly dry each one. Immediately (before the column cools and contracts significantly) measure (with the aid of a reading light and magnification) the fat column using dividers (6.7). Place the divider points on the vertical line on the bottle neck, with one point at the bottom of the lower meniscus and the other point at the top of the upper meniscus. Without changing the distance between the two points on the dividers, move the dividers down the bottle neck until the lower point rests in the horizontal graduation mark at 0%. Place the upper point against the bottle graduation and read the test in percentage fat by weight. The fat column at the time of measurement should be translucent, golden yellow or amber, and free of visible suspended particles.

9.2.7 Reject all tests that produce a cloudy fat column or show the presence of charred matter or curd, or where for any reason the reading is indistinct or uncertain. Repeat the test. Corrections can be made by adjusting the amount of acid added.

10. **Expression of Results**
    10.1 **Ice cream and frozen desserts:** Results are read directly from the bottle and are expressed as percentage fat by weight to nearest 0.25%.
    10.2 **Chocolate milk:** Results are read directly from the bottle and are expressed as percentage fat by weight to nearest 0.05%.
    10.3 **Skim milk, buttermilk, and whey:** In the case of a 9-g sample size, results are read directly from the neck of the skim test bottle to the nearest 0.01% fat and then multiplied by 2. In the case of a 17.6-mL (18-g) sample, the results are read directly from the neck of the skim test bottle to the nearest 0.01% fat.
    10.4 **Cottage Cheese:** Results are read directly from the bottle and are expressed as percentage fat by weight to the nearest 0.1%.
11. **Precision and Performance Parameters**
    11.1 **Repeatability:** Ice cream and frozen desserts, chocolate milk, skim milk, buttermilk, whey, and cottage cheese. No collaborative study data available.
    11.2 **Reproducibility:** Ice cream and frozen desserts, chocolate milk, skim milk, buttermilk, whey, and cottage cheese. No collaborative study data available.
12. **Test Report and Interpretation:** The test report shall identify the method used and results obtained. The report will also identify any variation in the test not specified in this method as well as problems that may have impacted the test result. Each sample will be described in such a manner as to ensure traceablity as to its origin.

15.085 Gerber Fat Method (Class O, B)[45,53,57]

1. **Scope:** This method is applicable to raw, pasteurized, homogenized, and composite (preserved) milks. When used for the analyses of whole milk, the method is Class O. When used for lowfat milk, skim milk, flavored milks, cream, and frozen desserts, the method is Class B. Frozen desserts may be tested by this method for in-plant production control.
2. **References:** Chapter 2 on "Laboratory Quality Assurance and Safety." Chapter 3 on "Sampling Dairy and Related Products."
3. **Definition:** Fat is the mass fraction of substances determined according to this procedure and is expressed as a percentage by mass.
4. **Principle:** Milk and concentrated sulfuric acid are mixed to produce an exothermic reaction that disintegrates the emulsion structure in milk. The exothermic reaction in combination of the isoamyl alcohol releases the fat. The fat is collected in the graduated portion of the neck of the Gerber bottle, which is calibrated to express the fat content of the product on a percentage fat by mass.
5. **Reagents:** Unless otherwise specified all chemicals are reagent or ACS grade.
    5.1 **Isoamyl alcohol (CP) (sp. g 0.184-0.816, 15.5/15.5°C):** Boiling point 128° to 133°C, free of water, acid, fat, and furfural. Store in tightly closed containers in the dark. Test each batch of isoamyl alcohol identified by the manufacturer as suitable for Gerber milkfat tests by

transferring 10 mL of sulfuric acid, 11 mL of LG water, and 1 mL of isoamyl alcohol to the test bottle. Shake and centrifuge the bottles as required in the test for fat in milk (9.1.4). If oily particles are recovered, discard the batch of isoamyl alcohol. Determine the fat in a single sample of milk in duplicate using both the old and new isoamyl alcohol. Determinations should agree within ± 0.05%.

5.2 Water (LG).

5.3 **Sulfuric acid (sp. g 1.820–1.825, 15/15.5°C):** Clean, colorless, free of fat.

5.4 **Sulfuric acid, diluted:** For use only for chocolate milk and frozen desserts. Prepare by slowly adding 94 parts by volume of cold sulfuric acid (5.3) to 6 parts by volume of cold water.

6. **Apparatus and Glassware:** All volumetric flasks, pipets, and burets are Class A unless otherwise specified.

6.1 **Balance:** 0.01 g sensitivity with a pan bottle support on the balance to provide firm vertical support for the bottles.

6.2 **Bottle support rack:** To hold bottles in a secure, vertical position. Stainless steel racks consisting of two perforated shelves and a solid bottom, supported by solid sides, provide convenience and durability. Optionally use racks with stainless steel "rapid clamp-on" covers to lock bottles securely when using shaking machines.

6.3 **Butyrometer:** Gerber, for milk, to meet International Standards Organization (ISO) Standard 2446, with lock stopper and key; for cream and frozen desserts, to meet requirements as described in *SMEDP*, 14th ed.

6.4 **Centrifuge:** For bottles, standard style, with disc and a trunnion head to rotate at 1,100 ± 100 rpm. Trunnion-head models are supplied with heaters to maintain internal temperature at approximately 60°C (temperature of butyrometer contents after centrifugation should be between 30° and 55°C). Check the operating speed of all Gerber centrifuges under full load at monthly intervals, or more often if necessary. Bottles should receive an acceleration of 350 ± 50 × g. See the manufacturer's instruction manual. Optionally use Babcock centrifuges for 22.8-cm bottles, equipped with heaters and cup adaptors for Gerber bottles, and operate at 1,100 ± 100 rpms (350 ± 50 × g).

6.5 **Desk reader (optional):** Improvised to expedite reading of fat columns. Models with a shielded tubular electric bulb standardize background illumination for the bottles.

6.6 **Milk test pipet:** Gerber, TC 11.07 mL at 20°C, to meet requirements as described in *SMEDP*, 14th ed. This has been the traditional pipet for use in the United States. ISO Standard 2446:1976, clause 6.1.2., states that the capacity of the pipet shall be such to yield a comparable result by the ether extraction method (15.086) using bulk whole milk. If adequate statistical comparison is made to show that a different pipet volume gives comparable results, a pipet of that volume should be used.

6.7 **Reagent dispensers:** 10 mL for sulfuric acid, 1 mL for isoamyl alcohol.

6.8 **Shaking machine (optional):** Standardizes conditions and saves time.

6.9 **Washing device (optional):** consisting of a rack and perforated cover to expedite washing. After reading, return bottles to the rack, remove the stoppers, and lock the rack cover; empty, wash, rinse, and drain bottles as a unit.

6.10 **Water bath:** With depth to permit vertical immersion of bottles to the terminal bulb, equipped to provide intermittent or constant agitation and to control temperature at 60° to 63°C.

7. **Sampling:** Chapter 3 on "Sampling Dairy and Related Products."

8. **Preparation of Test Sample:** Take a representative sample that has previously been mixed, stirred, or otherwise prepared in order to make sample uniform.

9. **Procedure:** Before beginning analysis review material safety data sheets on all chemicals and use appropriate safety equipment such as hoods, aprons, face shields, and glasses.

9.1 **Milk**

9.1.1 Measure 10 mL of sulfuric acid ± 0.2 mL at 15° to 21°C into a test bottle. From a well-mixed milk sample at not more than 24°C, withdraw a sample using an 11.07-mL pipet, with the top of the meniscus resting on the graduation line of the suction tube, and touch off any residue at the top.

9.1.2 For composite milk (preserved) and aged milks assay by heating the milk to 35° to 38°C. Thoroughly disperse all fat before transferring the test sample. Hold the test bottle at a 45° angle, with the plane of its flat glass column vertical to displace milk from the bulb and column with acid. (Use this method when test bottles are filled at one location and tests are completed at another.)

9.1.3 Allow the milk (from 9.1.1 and 9.1.2) to drain into the bottle slowly at first to prevent a violent reaction with the acid; then permit the pipet to empty normally. Wait a full 3 seconds after free flow stops and blow out the last drop. Add 1 mL of isoamyl alcohol and insert the lock stopper securely. With the stoppered end up, grasp the test bottle at the graduated column and shake it until the curd is completely digested. Holding the bottle (CAUTION: HOT) at the stopper and neck, invert it at least four times to mix the acid remaining in the bulb with the contents. Using a machine to shake filled, sealed test bottles secured in racks and equipped with quick-locking covers ensures the safe, rapid, uniform treatment and proper temperature for centrifuging.

9.1.4 Before the contents of the bottles have cooled below 60°C, place them in a centrifuge and counterbalance as needed. Before operating the machine, close the cover and lock. After the required speed is attained, centrifuge for 4 minutes. Stop the machine and place the bottles in a water bath at 60° to 63°C, leaving only the bulbs exposed. After at least 5 minutes in the bath, lock the stopper. Gently push the straight line at the bottom of the fat column upward so that it coincides with the nearest whole percent graduation mark; then promptly read the scale at the bottom of the meniscus at the top of the fat column to the nearest 0.05% graduation. Subtract the lower from the upper reading and record the difference as the fat content.

9.1.5 Repeat the tests where fat columns are imperfect. As fat cools in the column, the slope of the meniscus increases, tending to lower the percentage of fat reading. Soft, glareless background lighting and a desk reader stand, which are readily adjusted to bring the column to tester eye level, expedite rapid, accurate readings. Proper fat columns contain no light or dark particles or zones. They are pale to strong yellow in color.

9.2 **Cream:** Measure 10 ± 0.2 mL of sulfuric acid at 15° to 21°C into a cream test bottle. Place the bottle in the support on the balance and preweigh. Weigh 5 g of prepared cream sample into the bottle. Remove the bottle from the balance and add 5 mL of water at 15° to 21°C and 1 mL of isoamyl alcohol. Insert the lock stopper securely and proceed as with milk (9.1.2-9.1.5).

9.3 **Sweetened, flavored milks:** Measure 10 ± 0.2 mL of diluted sulfuric acid at 15° to 21°C into a milk test bottle. From a properly prepared sample at not more than 24°C, withdraw a sample using an 11.07-mL pipet, with the top of the meniscus resting on the graduation line of the suction tube. Touch off any residue at the tip; allow the sample to drain into the bottle slowly at first to prevent a violent reaction with the acid; then permit the pipet to empty normally. Wait a full 3 seconds after free flow stops and blow out the last drop. If the sample is viscous, preweigh the bottle and weigh 11.125 g of properly prepared sample into the bottle. Add 2 mL of isoamyl alcohol. Insert the lock stopper securely and proceed as with milk (9.1.2-9.1.5).

9.4 **Frozen desserts (Class B):** In-plant production control samples containing high concentrations of nonfat milk solids, sugars, stabilizers, and emulsifiers, as well as homogenizing treatment, make vigorous shaking necessary to liberate fat after the addition of reagents. Prolonged action of sulfuric acid and isoamyl alcohol appears to increase the solubility of alcohol in fat, often resulting in higher fat determinations than those by the ether extraction method (15.086). For this reason, use of the Gerber test for frozen desserts and mixes should be restricted to processing control tests. Where critical data are required, the ether extraction method is necessary.

Measure 10 ± 0.2 mL of diluted sulfuric acid at 15° to 21°C into an ice cream test bottle. Place the bottle in the support on the balance and preweigh. Weigh 5 g of a well-mixed sample into the bottle. Remove the bottle from the balance and add 5 mL of water and 1 mL of isoamyl alcohol. Insert the lock stopper securely and proceed as with milk (9.1.2-9.1.5), except that the bottle should be centrifuged for 5 minutes. Read the scale to the nearest 0.2% graduation and record the results. Recentrifuge without inverting the bottle, retemper, and reread the fat column. If the second reading differs by more than 0.2% from the first, the initial shaking was inadequate and the test must be repeated. When the second reading is less than 0.2% above the first, report the result of the first test.

10. Expression of Results

10.1 **Milk:** Read the scale at the bottom of the meniscus at the top of the fat column to the nearest 0.05% graduation (0.01% for skim milk). Subtract the lower from the upper reading and record the difference as fat content.

10.2 **Cream:** Read the scale to the nearest 0.5% graduation mark and record the results. Subtract the lower from the upper reading and record the difference as fat content.

10.3 **Sweetened, flavored milks:** Read the scale to the nearest 0.1% graduation mark. Subtract the lower from the upper reading and record the difference as fat content.

10.4 **Frozen desserts:** Read the scale to the nearest 0.2% graduation and record the results. Subtract the lower from the upper reading and record the difference as fat content.

11. Precision and Performance Parameters

11.1 **Milk:** No precision data are available for this assay; however, it is estimated that duplicate results should be within 0.1%.

12. Test Report and Interpretation: The test report shall identify the method used and results obtained. The report will also identify any variation in the test not specified in this method as well as problems which may have impacted the test result. Each sample will be described in such a manner as to ensure traceablity as to its origin.

15.086 Mojonnier Method, Milk and Cream (Class A1); Other Products (Class O)[42,53]

1. Scope: This procedure specifies the reference method for the determination of the fat content of milk and cream.

WARNING: The use of this method involves the use of hazardous materials, operations, and equipment. This method does not claim to address all the safety problems associated with its use. It is the responsibility of the user to establish safety and health practices and determine the applicability of regulatory limitations prior to use.

2. References: Chapter 2 on "Laboratory Quality Assurance and Safety." Chapter 3 on "Sampling Dairy and Related Products."

3. Definition: Fat is the mass fraction of substances determined according to this procedure and is expressed as a percentage by mass.

4. Principle: Extraction of an ammoniacal ethanolic solution of a weighed test portion with ethyl ether and petroleum ether. The ether is decanted into a dry weighing dish and the ether is evaporated. The extracted material is dried to a constant weight and the mass of the substances extracted determined.

5. Reagents: Unless otherwise specified all chemicals are reagent or ACS grade.

5.1 **Ammonia hydroxide:** Concentrated, specific gravity 0.9.
5.2 **Ethyl alcohol, 95%:** No residue upon evaporation.
5.3 **Ethyl ether:** Peroxide free, no residue upon evaporation.
5.4 **Petroleum ether:** Boiling point range 30°-60°C, no residue upon evaporation. Alternatively, pentane with a boiling point of 36°C may be used.
5.5 **Phenolphthalein indicator:** 0.5% (m/v) in ethyl alcohol.

6. **Apparatus and Glassware:** All volumetric flasks, pipets, and burets are Class A unless otherwise specified.
6.1 **Analytical balance:** To read to the nearest 0.1 mg. Accuracy upon verification should be within 0.2 mg. Check balance accuracy periodically and whenever balance is moved or cleaned. Keep a record of balance calibration checks.
6.2 **Calibration weights, class S:** Use to verify balance accuracy within the weight range of the empty flask and the flask plus sample, and the empty weighing dish and the dish plus extracted material.
6.3 **Centrifuge:** Capable of holding fat-extraction flasks and achieving a speed of approximately 600 rpm. Use of a centrifuge is optional but recommended.
6.4 **Corks:** High-quality natural cork stoppers, size 5 or appropriate size to fit fat extraction flask. Soak corks in water over several hours to improve seal. Additionally, dry corks should also be available for use when weighing the test portion (9.2.1, 9.2.2).
6.5 **Desiccator:** Room temperature. Use for cooling weighing dishes after the preliminary and final drying. Use coarse desiccant (mesh size 6-16) that contains a minimum of fine particles and changes color when moisture is absorbed.
6.6 **Fume Hood:** Explosion proof and capable of venting vapors heavier than air.
6.7 **Hot plate, steam bath, or other heating device:** For evaporation of ether at ≤100°C. *If an electrical hot plate is used, it must be explosion proof and rated for evaporating solvents such as ether. Carry out evaporation in a fume hood (6.6).*
6.8 **Mojonnier-type fat extraction flasks:** With volume of 21-23 mL in lower bulb plus neck at bottom of flask. Flask should have smooth, round opening at the top that will seal when closed with a cork.
6.9 **Tongs:** For handling weighing dishes.
6.10 **Vacuum or forced air oven:** Vacuum oven must be capable of maintaining a temperature between 70° and 75°C at >50.8 cm (20 in.) of vacuum. Forced air oven must be capable of maintaining a temperature of 100° ± 1°C.
6.11 **Water bath:** For tempering sample materials prior to weighing. The bath should have a thermometer and device to maintain sample materials at 38°C.
6.12 **Weighing dishes**: Metal, 8.5-9.5 cm diameter and 4.5-5.5 cm tall, or 250-mL glass beakers.

7. **Sampling:** Chapter 3 on "Sampling Dairy and Related Products."

8. Preparation of Test Sample

8.1 Warm the test sample to 38° ± 1°C by means of the water bath (6.11). Level of water should be at or above milk level. Mix test sample by inversion 10 times without causing frothing or churning. If a fat line remains on the inside surface of the container, run hot tap water (ca. 50°-60°C) over outside surface for 15-20 seconds. Mix test sample thoroughly by inversion and weigh test portion immediately. Do not allow test samples to remain in the water bath more than 15 min. after reaching 38°C.

8.2 Reliable value for fat content cannot be expected if fat droplets are floating on surface of sample, white particles are visible on the walls of the sample container, sample is churned, or sample contains a distinct smell of free fatty acids during or after sample preparation.

9. Procedure: Before beginning analysis review material safety data sheets on all chemicals and use appropriate safety equipment such as hoods, aprons, face shields, and glasses.

9.1 **Preparation of weighing dishes:** Number clean weighing dishes (6.12) and pre-dry in an oven (6.10) under the same conditions that will be used for final drying after fat extraction. Always use tongs (6.9) when handling the dried weighing dishes. Be sure that all surfaces where weighing dishes will be placed (e.g., hot plate, desiccator, etc.) are clean and free of particulates. At the end of oven drying, place the dishes in a room temperature desiccator (6.5) and cool to room temperature. On same day as fat extraction, weigh the dishes to the nearest 0.1 mg and record the weights. Check balance zero after weighing each dish. Protect the weighed dishes from contamination with extraneous matter.

9.1.1 **Maintenance of desicant:** To avoid negative blanks and maintain dry dishes, it is best to remove the desiccant from the desiccator and dry it with the empty weighing dishes each time before analysis. Remove the hot desiccant from the oven and place it into the desiccator; then place the hot dishes in the desiccator. Be sure the desiccator seals properly; this requires a desiccator with a vent or a rubber-gasketed door.

9.2 **Test portion and pretreatment**

9.2.1 **Milk:** Weigh an empty flask (6.8) with a clean, dry cork stopper (6.4). Remove stopper.

Mix the 38°C test sample as described (8) and immediately pipet ca. a 10-g test portion into the flask. Deliver the test portion as completely as possible into the lower (small) bulb of the extraction flask. Stopper the flask and weigh to the nearest 0.1 mg. Check balance zero between samples.

9.2.2 **Cream:** Weigh an empty flask (6.8) with a clean, dry cork stopper (6.4). Remove stopper.

Mix the 38°C test sample as described (8) and immediately pipet enough cream to yield 0.3-0.6 g of extracted fat (e.g., approximately 1 g 40% cream, 2 g 20% cream). Deliver the test portion as completely as possible into the lower (small) bulb of the extraction flask. Stopper the flask and weigh to the nearest 0.1 mg. Check balance zero between samples. Dilute test portion to approximately 10 mL with 20°-22°C water.

9.3 **Blank test:** Carry out two reagent blank tests each day tests are conducted using the same procedure and same reagents but replacing the test portion with 10 mL of water. Record the weight of any dry residue collected and use the average blank weight in the calculation of the percentage fat in the test samples (10.1). The reagent blank should contain no more than 0.0020 g residue. If residue is greater than 0.0020 g, the cause should be identified and corrected.

A negative blank indicates an error such as insufficient drying of the dish prior to the initial weighing, balance calibration shifting between weighing the empty dish and the dish after the final drying, or the desiccator not being properly sealed. The cause of negative blanks should be identified and corrected.

9.4 **Determination:** Carry out the determination without delay. Conduct extractions and ether evaporation in a fume hood (6.6).

9.4.1 Add 1.5 mL ammonia hydroxide (5.1) to the test portion (9.2.1 or 9.2.2) and mix thoroughly in the small bulb of the flask. Ammonia hydroxide neutralizes any acid present and dissolves casein.

9.4.2 Add 3 drops of phenolphthalein indicator (5.5) to help sharpen the visual appearance of the interface between the ether and aqueous layers during the extraction.

9.4.3 For the first extraction, add 10 mL of ethyl alcohol (5.2), stopper with a water-soaked cork (6.4), and shake the flask for 15 seconds.

9.4.4 Add 25 mL of ethyl ether (5.3), replace cork, and shake flask very vigorously for 1 min, releasing built-up pressure by loosening the cork as necessary.

9.4.5 Add 25 mL of petroleum ether (5.4), replace cork, and repeat vigorous shaking for 1 min.

9.4.6 Centrifuge (6.3) the stoppered flask at approximately 600 rpm for about 30 s to obtain a clean separation of the aqueous (bright pink) and ether phases. If a centrifuge is not available, allow the stoppered flask to stand for at least 30 min until the ether layer is clear and distinctly separated from the aqueous layer.

9.4.7 Remove the cork and carefully decant the ether solution into weighing dish prepared as in (9.1). When the ether solution is decanted into the dish, be careful not to pour over any suspended solids or aqueous phase. Ether can be evaporated at ≤ 100°C from the dish as described in 9.4.10 while the second extraction is being conducted. However, remove dish from hot plate (6.7) when decanting the ether.

9.4.8 Carry out a second extraction by repeating the operations described in 9.4.3 to 9.4.7 inclusive, except add 5 mL of ethanol (5.2) instead of 10 mL, and 15 mL each of ethyl ether

(5.3) and petroleum ether (5.4), instead of 25-mL portions. Rinse the inside of the neck of the extraction flask when adding the ethers. If the interface of the aqueous and ether layers is below the neck of the flask after centrifugation, add water to bring the level approximately halfway up the neck to enable the final decantation of ether to be as complete as possible. Add the water slowly down the inside surface of the flask so that there is minimum disturbance of the separation.

9.4.9 Carry out a third extraction without the addition of ethanol by repeating the operations described in 9.4.4 to 9.4.7. Again, use only 15 mL of ethyl ether (5.3) and 15 mL of petroleum ether (5.4). Rinse the inside of the extraction flask when adding the ethers. If necessary, raise the interface of the aqueous and ether layers by the addition of water (9.4.8).

9.4.10 Completely evaporate solvents collected in the weighing dish in a fume hood (6.6) on a hot plate (6.7) at ≤100°C. Avoid splattering.

9.4.11 Dry weighing dish with extracted fat to a constant weight in a forced air oven at 100° ± 1°C (≥30 min) or in a vacuum oven at 70°-75°C at >50.8 cm (20 in.) of vacuum for ≥7 min. (6.10).

9.4.12 Using tongs (6.9), remove weighing dish from oven and place in a desiccator (6.5) to cool to room temperature.

9.4.13 Weigh dry, cooled dish to the nearest 0.1 mg.

9.4.14 Visually inspect each dish after the final weighing to determine if any extraneous nonfat material is present. If foreign material is observed, make note of it and repeat the test for the sample.

10. Expression of Results

10.1 **Calculation:** Calculate the fat content of the test material using the following equation

$$w_f = \frac{(m_1 - m_2) - b}{m_0} \times 100\%$$

where

w_f is the percentage of fat by mass of the test material;

m_o is the numerical value of the mass, in grams, of the test portion (9.2.1 or 9.2.2);

m_1 is the numerical value of the mass, in grams, of the weighing dish and the extracted matter, determined in 9.4.13;

m_2 is the numerical value of the mass, in grams, of the empty sample weighing dish (9.1); and

b is the average numerical value of the mass, in grams, of any dry residue in the blank determination (9.3), where the mass of dry residue is calculated by subtracting the weight of the empty blank weighing dish (9.1) from the weight of the weighing dish and any extracted matter (9.4.13). If blanks are negative, use the negative number in the calculation. Cause of negative blanks and excessively high positive blanks should be identified and corrected.

10.1.1 Input parameter values and calculate result to at least 4 decimal places.

10.2 **Expression of results:** Round the final result to the nearest 0.001% (*m/m*) for milk and to the nearest 0.01% (*m/m*) for cream.

11. Precision and Performance Parameters: The values for repeatability and reproducibility limit for raw milk and unhomogenized, heat-treated cream (30-45% fat) are expressed for the 95% probability level and were derived from the results of inter-laboratory tests in accordance with [1].[11(989.05,995.19)]

11.1 **Repeatability**

11.1.1 **Milk:** The absolute difference between two independent single test results, obtained using the same method on identical test material in the same laboratory by the same operator using the same equipment within a short interval of time, should not be greater than 0.044% (*m/m*) for raw whole milk.

11.1.2 **Cream:** The absolute difference between two independent single test results, obtained using the same method on identical test material in the same laboratory by the same operator using the same equipment within a short interval of time, should not be greater than 0.35% (*m/m*) for unhomogenized, heat-treated cream.

11.2 **Reproducibility**

11.2.1 **Milk:** The absolute difference between two independent single test results, obtained using the same method on identical test material in different laboratories with different operators using different equipment, should not be greater than 0.056% for raw whole milk.

11.2.2 **Cream:** The absolute difference between two independent single test results, obtained using the same method on identical test material in different laboratories with different operators using different equipment, should not be greater than 0.43% for heat-treated cream.

11.3 **Method Performance Statistics**

11.3.1 **Milk:** The method performance statistics derived from the results of an inter-laboratory collaborative study[11(989.05),14] using raw whole milk are as follows (% fat, *m/m*):

$s_r = 0.015$ $RSD_r = 0.396\%$ r value = 0.044
$s_R = 0.020$ $RSD_R = 0.512\%$ R value = 0.056

11.3.2 **Cream:** The method performance statistics derived from the results of an interlaboratory collaborative study[11(995.19),70] using heat-treated cream with a fat content between 30 and 45% are as follows (% fat, *m/m*):

$s_r = 0.125$ $RSD_r = 0.330\%$ r value = 0.354
$s_R = 0.151$ $RSD_R = 0.398\%$ R value = 0.427

12. Test Report and Interpretation: The test report shall identify the method used and results obtained. The report will also identify any variation in the test not specified in this method as well as problems that may have impacted the test result. Each sample will be described in such a manner as to ensure traceability as to its origin.

Table 15.2. Suggested Sample Weights and Extraction Conditions for the Mojonnier Test Procedure[a,b]

Product	Sample Size (g)	60°C Water (mL)	Ammonium Hydroxide (mL)
Milk, skim milk, buttermilk, whey	10	0	1.5
Cottage cheese	7	2	3.0
Evaporated milk, unsweetened condensed milks, condensed skim milk, sweetened condensed milk, ice cream mix	5	5	1.5
Condensed buttermilk	3	7	1.5
Cream			
<25% fat	2	8	1.5
>25% fat	1	9	1.5
Butter, skim milk powder, whole milk powder	1	9	1.5
Cheese, buttermilk powder	1	9	3.0
Malted milk, milk chocolate	10	0	1.5

[a] For all products: *1st extraction:* sample (see table), warm water (see table), ammonium hydroxide (see table), 3 drops phenolphthalein indicator, 10 mL ethyl alcohol, 25 mL ethyl ether, 25 mL petroleum ether. *2nd extraction:* 5 mL ethyl alcohol, 15 mL ethyl ether, 15 mL petroleum ether. *3rd extraction:* 15 mL ethyl ether, 15 mL petroleum ether.

[b] Samples should be completely dissolved by the water and ammonium hydroxide before proceeding with the first extraction. For some products, such as cottage cheese and cheese, vigorous shaking may be necessary. Refrigerating the stoppered flask containing the test portion, water, and ammonium hydroxide overnight may also aid in dissolving the sample. An increase in the amount of ammonium hydroxide added (up to 3 mL total) may be necessary to obtain a pink aqueous layer if product tested is acidic.

Annex: Use of Mojonnier Ether Extraction with Dairy Products other than Milk or Cream

The Mojonnier method is often used to determine the fat content of dairy products other than milk and cream but collaborative studies have not yet been conducted (other than for milk and cream). Thus, method performance statistics are not available, and expected performance is only speculative. Nonetheless, the Mojonnier procedure, with product-specific modifications, has the potential to apply to the determination of fat in a wide variety of dairy products.

Sample preparation is a key consideration. The material must be completely dissolved in order to quantitatively recover the fat. For hard-to-digest materials, various techniques are used such as the addition of 60°C water, an increase in the amount of ammonium hydroxide added, extended shaking times, and allowing time for the test portion to dissolve. Additional ethyl alcohol is sometimes added if emulsion problems are observed during extraction. Sample size is also important. It is recommended that the test portion size not exceed 10 g and, for full fat products, the test portion weight should be chosen to yield 0.3-0.6 g of extracted fat. Suggested test portion weights and extraction conditions are given in Table 15.2. The conditions for the analysis of milk and cream are included for comparison.

Analysts should be wary of using the Mojonnier procedure to determine the fat content of novel dairy product formulations. If the ingredients, such as stabilizers and emulsifiers, are soluble in ether the fat test will be erroneously high.

15.090 Lactose and Galactose Tests

15.091 Lactose, HPLC Method (Class B)[11(984.22),50]

1. **Scope:** This method is applicable to raw and pasteurized milk.
2. **References:** Chapter 2 on "Laboratory Quality Assurance and Safety." Chapter 3 on "Sampling Dairy and Related Products."
3. **Definition:** The method uses high-pressure liquid chromatography (HPLC) to determine the hydrated lactose content of the milk sample.
4. **Principle:** The lactose content is determined by using an NH_3 analytical column (carbohydrate column), a refractive index detector, an acetonitrile/water 55:45 mobile phase, and a system flow rate of 2 mL/minute. Milk samples are treated with sulfuric acid to precipitate the protein, releasing the whey fraction. Chromatograms of samples are compared to those of standards and spiked samples and the concentration determined by comparing the peak heights and peak areas of the samples to those of the samples to those of the standards. Lactose is expressed as a percent. The filtered samples are analyzed using HPLC.
5. **Reagents:** Unless otherwise specified all chemicals are reagent or ACS grade.
   - 5.1 Water: Distilled or deionized, HPLC grade preferred.
   - 5.2 Sulfuric acid 0.9N: Prepared by addition of 5.0 mL concentrated sulfuric acid to about 150 mL of distilled water in 200 mL volumetric flask and dilute to volume with distilled water.
   - 5.3 α-lactose: Monohydrate.
   - 5.4 Acetonitrile: HPLC grade.
   - 5.5 0.5% α-lactose standard: Weigh exactly 0.5000 ± 0.0001 grams of α-lactose monohydrate. Transfer to 100 mL volumetric, add approximately 75 mL of distilled water, mix well, and add 1 mL of 0.9N sulfuric acid. Bring flask to volume with distilled water at 20°C. This is a 0.5% α-lactose standard. Prepare 0.2% and 0.1% α-lactose working standards by dilution.
   - 5.6 Acetonitrile/water 55:45 mobile phase: Measure 550 mL of acetonitrile to a 1-L Erlenmeyer flask containing 450 mL of distilled water. Mix well, final volume will be less than 1 L. Filter 55:45 acetonitrile/water solution through a 0.20 micron organic filter.
6. **Apparatus and Glassware:** All volumetric flasks, pipets, and burets are Class A unless otherwise specified.
   - 6.1 Analytical balance: Accuracy to 0.0001 grams.
   - 6.2 HPLC guard column: High-performance carbohydrate column insert. Waters Chromatography Company part number WATO96895 or equivalent.
   - 6.3 NH3 Analytical column: High-performance carbohydrate column (250 mm × 4.6 mm). Waters Chromatography Company part number WATO 46895 or equivalent.

6.4 HPLC pump: Waters Model 510 or equivalent.

6.5 HPLC autosampler: Waters Intelligent Sample Processor Model 712 or equivalent.

6.6 HPLC refractometer detector: Waters Model 410 Refractive Index or equivalent.

6.7 HPLC data handling system: Waters Millennium 2010 or equivalent.

6.8 Graduated cylinders: 1000 mL.

6.9 Erlenmeyer flasks: 50 mL, 1000 mL, and 2000 mL.

6.10 0.20 micron filters: Watman 25 mm CD/× (0.2 mm) or equivalent and disposable syringes.

6.11 Volumetric flasks: 100 mL and 200 mL.

6.12 Volumetric pipet: 5 mL and 10 mL as required for preparation of standards.

6.13 Transfer pipets: 1000 μL Eppendorf or equivalent.

6.14 Autosampler vials: Glass screw cap HPLC vials to fit autosampler.

7. **Sampling:** Chapter 3 on "Sampling Dairy and Related Products."

8. **Preparation of Test Sample:** Take a representative sample that has previously been mixed, stirred, or otherwise prepared in order to make sample uniform.

9. **Procedure:** Before beginning analysis review material safety data sheets on all chemicals and use appropriate safety equipment such as hoods, aprons, face shields, and glasses.

9.1 Tare clean, dry 100 mL volumetric flask on analytical balance.

9.2 Rapidly transfer approximately 9.5 grams of the prepared sample to the tared volumetric flask. Add additional sample dropwise (using a pasteur pipet) to reach exactly 10.0000 ± 0.0030 grams. Record weight. Spike one sample with 0.2500 ± 0.0001 mL of α-lactose and take it through the entire analysis as follows.

9.3 Add 1.0 mL 0.9N sulfuric acid to the 10 grams of milk in the flask. Swirl the flask to mix the sample. Precipitate will form.

9.4 Add approximately 50 mL distilled water to the milk acid mixture and swirl flask to mix the sample.

9.5 Dilute to volume (100 mL) with distilled water at 20°C, stopper the flask, and shake vigorously for 20 seconds. Asonicator may be used to ensure vigorous mixing and separation of the lactose.

9.6 Let stand for 3-5 minutes to settle.

9.7 Filter approximately 20 mL of sample into a 50-mL Erlenmeyer flask.

9.8 Set up HPLC equipment, including mobile phase, autosampler injector, guard column, analytical column, detector, and data handling system.

9.9 Adjust system to correct system conditions: Ambient temperature, flow rate 2.0 mL/minute. Injection volume 20 μL (for fixed-loop injectors use a 20-μL loop and program a 50-μL injection so loop "overfills." Run time should be approximately 3 minutes.

9.10 Allow the HPLC system to equilibrate to a stable baseline (takes about an hour). Note that the retention time for lactose should not vary by more than 0.5 minutes over the batch run.

9.11 Transfer clear liquid from Erlenmeyer flask in section 9.7 to autosampler vials and add to HPLC autosampler tray.

9.12 Place samples, duplicates, spikes and standards in the autosampler tray as follows: Blank and the three working standards should begin each run, one standard should follow every fourth sample throughout the run, and one midlevel standard should complete each run.

9.13 Place the loaded autosampler tray into the autosampler and begin operation according to instrument operating instructions.

9.14 Monitor the system during operation and observe for excessive back pressure which may indicate blockage of the guard column.

10. Expression of Results

10.1 Standards

10.1.1 Examine chromatograms to ensure lactose retention time has remained constant.

10.1.2 Determine peak height and peak area for all alpha-lactose standards (if standards other than 0.5% have been used, determine for each standard).

10.1.3 Calculate the average and standard deviation from the chromatograms.

10.1.4 Determine the coefficient of variation (CV) for both the peak height and peak area. This should be less than 0.8 for each parameter.

10.1.5 If the CV limit is exceeded, examine the data and eliminate any highly unusual sample injections. Recalculate the results. If the CV is still exceeded, the problem should be determined, corrected, and the analysis repeated.

10.2 Samples

10.2.1 Lactose in samples is calculated by comparing the peak height/peak area to that of the standards. The average standard peak height is used and the average standard peak area is used. Each sample result is compared to this average (peak height of sample to average peak height of standard, and peak area of sample to average peak area of standard). Lactose concentration is expressed as % lactose.

10.2.2 Determine α-lactose peak response in height or area for all samples. Calculate the lactose level in the sample extract as follows:

$$\%\ \text{lactose in sample extract} = \frac{\%\ \text{lactose in Std.} \times \text{Sample peak response}}{\text{Sample peak response}}$$

10.2.3 Determine lactose concentration in milk for each average value of sample extract.

$$\%\ \text{Lactose in Milk} = \frac{\%\ \text{Lactose in sample extract} \times \text{Dilution volume, mL}}{\text{Sample weight in grams}}$$

10.2.4 Sample results should be reported to three significant figures (to two decimal points).

10.2.5 Spike recovery,

$$\% = \frac{\text{Lactose in spiked sample} - \text{Lactose in sample} \times 100}{\text{Added lactose}}$$

10.3 Troubleshooting

10.3.1 Injectors need to be maintained and cleaned properly to ensure correct results.

10.3.2 CV values above those outlined in the method for peak height and peak area may indicate a problem with the guard column.

10.3.3 CV values above the values in the method on one of the parameters only may indicate an autosampler problem.

11. Precision and Performance Parameters

11.1 The method detection limit is 0.1%. Values less than this may be routinely obtained as analysts become proficient at the method.

11.2 Milk sample with normal lactose should provide a standard deviation of 0.05% lactose (entire run).

11.3 Standard deviations on duplicate samples should also show a standard deviation not to exceed 0.05% lactose.

11.4 Performance parameters for different analysts and different standards should be within this range.

11.5 Spike recoveries using the 0.4500 gram beta-lactose addition should be from 98.8% to 104.8% maximum.

12. Test Report and Interpretation: The test report shall identify the method used and results obtained. The report will also identify any variation in the test not specified in this method as well as problems which may have impacted the test result. Each sample will be described in such a manner as to ensure traceablity as to its origin.

15.092 Lactose/Galactose Enzymatic Method, Milk (Class A1), Other Dairy Products (Class B)[10(984.15),49]

1. **Scope:** This method is applicable to the determination of lactose and galactose in milk (Class A1) and other dairy products (Class B). Normally galactose is not present in fresh milk. Presence of galactose indicates that some of the lactose has been hydrolyzed. Typically only the first part of this test is performed for lactose determination.
2. **References:** Chapter 2 on "Laboratory Quality Assurance and Safety." Chapter 3 on "Sampling Dairy and Related Products."
3. **Definition:** This is an enzymatic UV method for the determination of lactose and galactose based on amount of NADH formed by enzymatic hydrolysis of lactose and galactose.
4. **Principle:** Lactose is hydrolyzed to glucose and galactose in the presence of β-galactosidase and H_2O. β-galactose is then oxidized by NAD to galactonic acid in presence of β-galactose dehydrogenase; the amount of NADH formed, stoichiometrically proportional to lactose content, is measured by absorbance *A* at 340 nm. To determine the lactose content, the lactose plus galactose assay (9.7) and a separate galactose assay (9.8) must be performed. The absorbance due to lactose is calculated by difference.
5. **Reagents:** Unless otherwise specified all chemicals are reagent or ACS grade.

   5.1 Carrez I solution: 3.60 g $K_4[Fe(CN)_6]$ (potassium ferrocyanide)• $3H_2O$/ 100 mL LG water.

   5.2 Carrez II solution: 7.20g $ZnSO_4$ (zinc sulfate) • $7H_2O$/100 mL H_2O

5.3 Sodium hydroxide 0.1 M.

5.4 Assay reagents: Kits are commercially available.

5.4.1 Solution 1: 610 mg lypophilisate consisting of citrate buffer (pH 6.6), NAD (35 mg), $MgSO_4$, and stabilizers. Dissolve lypophilisate in 7.0 mL redistilled H_2O before use.

5.4.2 Solution 2: About 1.7 mL enzyme suspension of β-galactosidase (ca. 100 U).

5.4.3 Solution 3: 34 mL solution consisting of potassium diphosphate buffer (0.51 mol/L, pH 8.6) and stabilizers.

5.4.4 Solution 4: About 1.7 enzyme suspension of galactose dehydrogenase (ca. 35 U).

5.5 Lactose and galactose standard solutions: In the range of 0.05% to 0.2% as required based on lactose and galactose content of the samples.

6. **Apparatus and Glassware:** All volumetric flasks, pipets, and burets are Class A unless otherwise specified.

6.1 Spectrophotometer: Spectrophotometer with a slit width ≤10 nm.

6.2 Cuvets: Glass or disposable plastic cuvets (1 cm light path).

6.3 Pipets: Capillary pipets or μL pipeter for transfer of volumes <1 mL and >1 mL.

6.4 Stirrer: Plastic or glass rod, 1 mm diameter.

6.5 Filter paper: Whatman #1, 15 cm.

7. **Sampling:** Chapter 3 on "Sampling Dairy and Related Products."

8. **Preparation of Test Sample:** Take a representative sample that has previously been mixed, stirred, or otherwise prepared in order to make sample uniform.

9. **Procedure**

9.1 Accurately weigh ca. 2 g milk or other dairy product into 100 mL volumetric flask, add ca 60-mL redistilled water, and mix. For milk, hold for 15 minutes at room temperature. Incubate cheese samples for 15 minutes at approximately 60°C.

9.2 Add 5 mL Carrez I solution and mix vigorously.

9.3 Add 5 mL Carrez II solution and mix vigorously.

9.4 Add 10 mL 0.1 M NaOH solution, mix vigorously, and cool to room temperature.

9.5 Dilute to volume at room temperature with redistilled water, mix, and filter through Whatman #1 filter paper. Use clear filtrate for the assay.

9.6 Label cuvets for 'blank,' 'standards,' and 'samples.'

9.7 **Determination of lactose and free galactose**

9.7.1 Pipet 0.20 mL of solution I into each cuvet. Pipet 0.05 mL solution 2 into each cuvet. Pipet 0.10 mL sample solution (filtrate) into sample cuvet and 0.10 mL lactose standards into standards' cuvet. Prepare a blank cuvet with solution 1 and solution 2 only.

9.7.2 Mix contents of all cuvets with stirrer and hold for 10 minutes at 20°-25°C. Pipet 1.00 mL of solution 3 into each cuvet. Pipet

2.00 mL of redistilled H_2O into blank cuvet and 1.90 mL redistilled H_2O into sample and standard cuvets.

9.7.3 Mix and hold ca. 2 minutes at 20°-25°C. Read absorbance (A_1) of each solution at 340 nm.

9.7.4 NADH is formed in the next step and is light sensitive. It is recommended that analysis from step 9.7.4 forward be performed in dim light.

9.7.5 Add 0.05 mL of solution 4 to each cuvet. Mix and hold at 20°-25°C for 20°-25 minutes (the time is dependant on the lactose content of the samples). Samples must be held until the A_2 value plateaus. For routine analysis, it may be desirable to extend the time up to 40 minutes to avoid re-assaying to assure that the A_2 value has plateaued.

9.7.6 Read the final absorbance (A_2) of the solution at 340 nm at 20-25 minutes (or longer).

9.7.7 Determine the absorbance differences ($A_2 - A_1$) for blanks, samples, and standards.

9.8 Determination of galactose: For all samples that may contain galactose, this step must be performed to get an accurate value for percent lactose. It must be noted that in milk, free galactose is not present and hence this step is not necessary.

9.8.1 Pipet 0.20 mL of solution 1 into each cuvet, including the blank cuvet. Pipet 0.10 mL of sample solution (filtrate) into sample cuvet and 0.10 mL of galactose standards into standards' cuvet. (Note: Solution 2 is not added for determination of galactose.)

9.8.2 Pipet 1.00 mL of solution 3 into each cuvet. Add 2.05 mL of redistilled water into blank cuvet and 1.95 mL of redistilled water into sample and standard cuvets.

9.8.3 Mix and hold approximately 2 minutes at 20°-25°C. Read absorbance (A_1) of each solution at 340 nm.

9.8.4 Add 0.05 mL of solution 4 to each cuvet. Mix and hold at 20°-25°C for about 20 minutes until the reaction has stopped (when A_2 value plateaus).

9.8.5 Read the final absorbance (A_2) of the solution at 340 nm at 20 minutes.

10. Expression of Results

10.1 Calculation of percent lactose (anhydrous)

Calculate C (grams lactose/L sample solution) = $(11.30/\varepsilon \times \Delta A_{lactose})$

Where ε is the extinction coefficient of NADH at 340 nm = 6.3 ($L \times mmol^{-1} \times cm^{-1}$). If lactose is to be calculated as lactose monohydrate, use 11.89 in place of 11.30.

10.1.1 Subtract the absorbance difference of the blank form the absorbance difference of the samples and standards.

The following equation depicts how the A values will be used in the calculation:

$$\Delta A_{lactose + galactose} = (A_2 - A_1)_{sample} - (A_2 - A_1)_{blank}$$

10.1.2 If the sample contains lactose and galactose, ΔA from (9.7.5) is actually equal to $\Delta A_{lactose + galactose}$. In order to determine lactose, $\Delta A_{galactose}$ (9.8.5) must be determined by repeating the above assay without adding solution 2 (β-galactosidase).

10.2 **Calculation of D-galactose**

C (grams D-galactose/L sample solution) = $(5.95/\varepsilon \times \Delta_{D\text{-}galactose})$. ΔA of the standard in the kit can be used to check the recovery percent.

If the sample had been diluted to bring the absorbances to the range of the standards, the result must be multiplied by the dilution factor. To calculate % lactose in the sample, the sample weight (2 g) and the volume (100 mL) to which it was made up must be used to get the final percent concentration of lactose and % D-galactose.

10.3 **Expression of results**

10.3.1 Grams of lactose anhydrous/100 g of sample or percent anhydrous lactose.

10.3.2 Grams of galactose/100 g of sample or percent galactose.

11. Precision and Performance Parameters

11.1 The method detection limit is 0.03% lactose and 0.02% galactose. The standard deviation on duplicate samples is 0.05%.

12. Test Report and Interpretation: The test report shall identify the method used and results obtained. The report will also identify any variation in the test not specified in this method as well as problems that may have impacted the test result. Each sample will be described in such a manner as to ensure traceablity as to its origin.

15.100 Minerals and Food Additives

15.101 Determination of Mineral Components and Heavy Metals in Milk Products

1. Introduction: Milk contains a number of minerals. Although the total concentration of minerals in dairy products is less than 1%,[3] minerals are important ingredients in terms of the role they play in vital physiological processes in our body. Milk is the best dietary source of calcium, and the calcium-to-phosphorus ratio in milk is conducive to optimal skeletal growth in the presence of nutrients like vitamin D, which promote calcium absorption. Thus the bioavailability of calcium from dairy products is excellent.[107] In normal milk, the important salts of calcium, sodium, potassium, and magnesium occur as phosphates, chlorides, citrates, and caseinates. The amount of salts present in milk can vary. For example, toward the end of lactation, the sodium chloride content increases and gives the milk a salty taste. Sodium intake is important from a nutritional labeling standpoint because dairy products contribute about 10% of the sodium in the total diet of adults.[107]

Mineral determination is also important to the dairy industry because minerals affect the physical characteristics and functionality of dairy products. For example, it is well known that gelling properties of whey protein isolate are affected by minerals. Calcium affects the texture of cheese. Sodium chloride influences the development of micro flora during cheese processing. Phosphate salts are added to processed cheese as emulsifiers to prevent fat and moisture separation.

The second group of minerals in dairy products consists of trace elements like iron, zinc, manganese, cadmium, and copper, which are found in "trace" concentrations (microgram per gram or parts per million). The trace element content of milk and other dairy products like cottage cheese, whey protein isolate, cheddar cheese, and yogurt can vary as a result of the stage of lactation, season, milk yield, amount of trace elements in feeds, handling of milk following pasteurization, storage conditions, analysis methods, and accuracy of analysis.

General methods for quantitating minerals use atomic absorption or emission at specific wavelengths. Dry ashing or wet digestion is used to destroy organic materials in dairy products before analysis. In the most commonly used atomic absorption spectrophotometry, a fine mist of digested sample solution is aspirated into the flame. The decrease in intensity of the radiation from a hollow cathode lamp due to absorption by specific atoms in the flame is measured. The concentration of the mineral is calculated by comparison to the absorption by standard solutions of the different metals of interest. In some procedures, diluted unfractionated samples are injected directly into the flame photometer.

The atomic absorption (AA) systems are capable of detecting 0.001 μgm/mL for some systems with 1 μgm/mL being most common.[75] In order to improve the precision, accuracy, speed, and sensitivity of these assays, a number of sample introduction techniques, sequential multi element analysis, automatic standard calibration, and sample dilution can now be quickly carried out in highly automated atomic absorption systems.

Inductively coupled plasma (ICP) atomic emission spectroscopy, in which light emitted by atoms in an inductively coupled plasma is measured and related to concentration is now gaining popularity. The method is more sensitive and has a broader linear range and the instrument is more expensive than the more commonly used atomic absorption spectroscopy. Phosphates can be determined by ICP; however, phosphates in dairy products are commonly determined by a reaction forming phosphomolybdate, which is reduced to a blue compound and determined by colorimetric quantitation using a spectrophotometer.

Full details for the determination of macro minerals and trace metals in all sorts of dairy products can be obtained by consulting the reference. It is important to note that the need for specialized equipment and elaborate sample preparation techniques makes it difficult to include mineral analysis under routine dairy analysis in all laboratories.

15.102 Food Additives in Dairy Products[11]

1. **Introduction:** Even though additives in dairy products are rarely thought of, several are allowed by the individual product's Standard of Identity. These additives can be separated into two broad categories: 1) functional (e.g., preservatives, acidulants, stabilizers, and emulsifiers) and 2) product enhancement (e.g., salt, sweeteners, colors, and spices).

   Occasionally the concentration of these components will need to be determined. Analyses can be performed for a number of reasons, including product quality issues, or to determine compliance with regulatory requirements. Approved methods exist for the determination of several additives in dairy and other food products.

Fluid milk standards allow the fewest additives. Vitamin A and D addition is optional in prescribed amounts as indicated in 21CFR131 (minimum addition of Vitamin A at 2000 IU per quart and Vitamin D at 400 IU per quart). Methods are published in AOAC for the determination of these vitamins in milk (Vitamin A: AOAC method 992.04, Vitamin D: AOAC method 992.26, 17th Edition). Due to the fact that these vitamins are fat soluble and can be toxic when consumed in high amounts, and that milk is a staple in most children's diet, it is important to monitor the concentration of these vitamins in fluid dairy products. Flavors and juices are allowable ingredients in fluid milks. Concentration levels of these ingredients usually cannot be analyzed, unless a particular chemical that is amenable to analysis is present.

The standards for cultured products listed in 21CFR131[24] allow for safe and suitable additives that improve texture, prevent syneresis, and extend shelf life. These additives would fall into the functional category and would include stabilizers, antimicrobial agents, and thickeners. The addition of flavoring components is also allowed. Again, as with milk, most of the functional additives have methods defined by AOAC, but the flavor ingredients are more difficult to quantitate, involving complex chromatographic procedures.

The cheese standards (21CFR133) allow for various additives, depending on the type of product. Natural cheeses, by and large, only allow for the addition of various dairy ingredients, enzymes (for culturing and flavor production), calcium chloride, salt, colors, and antimycotic addition only on sliced products. Processed cheeses allow for the addition of acidifying chemicals, emulsifying agents, flavors, fruits, vegetables, and meats in addition to those additives allowed in natural cheese. Sorbates and propionates are allowed for the control of mold and microbe contaminants in pasteurized process cheese and cheese food. These antimycotics can be quantitated using chromatographic methods outlined in AOAC method 974.10 (17th Edition). Other additives that are allowed are stabilizers, thickeners, and the preservative nisin in cheese spread, as well as anticaking agents in grated cheese.

The standard for ice cream in 21CFR135 allows for the broadest range of food ingredients of all of the dairy products. All safe and suitable ingredients can be used when producing an ice cream product. A safe and suitable ingredient is defined as one that 1) performs an appropriate function in the food, 2) is used at a level no higher than necessary to achieve its intended purpose, and 3) is not a food additive or color additive as defined in the regulations. No additives are prohibited or are specifically allowed by the standard of identity; therefore, there are no restrictions except those listed in the general food additive regulations.

15.110 Moisture and Solids Tests

For accurate analyses, only a vacuum oven or forced draft oven should be used. Each oven should be assessed for temperature variability across the oven. No oven with greater variation than ± 2°C should be used. For this reason no convection or gravity ovens can be used. These ovens are slow to respond to temperature change within the oven, such as when the door is opened to add samples. All ovens should be assessed for their ability to consistently yield the same results whether half or completely full of samples in moisture pans.

15.111 Moisture/Solids, Vacuum Oven (Class O)[11(926.08,927.05)]

1. **Scope:** This method is applicable to dried milk, cheese, and cheese products.
2. **References:** Chapter 2 on "Laboratory Quality Assurance and Safety." Chapter 3 on "Sampling Dairy and Related Products."
3. **Definition:** Moisture is defined as the weight loss on drying of the sample under conditions of the test.
4. **Principle:** A preweighed sample is dried at 100°C, under vacuum, reweighed, and calculated as percent moisture or solids.
5. **Reagents:** Not applicable for this method.
6. **Apparatus and Glassware:** All volumetric flasks, pipets and burets are Class A unless otherwise specified.
   - 6.1 **Moisture dishes:** Aluminum dish, 5.5 cm, or disposable, 5.5 cm, Dyna-dish or equivalent. Reusable aluminum moisture pans must have insert covers.
   - 6.2 **Balance:** 0.1-mg sensitivity, electronic.
   - 6.3 **Blender:** Oster or Waring, use sterilizable blender heads that are suitable for autoclaving and fit 120-, 240-, or 480-mL Mason jars, or equivalent.
   - 6.4 **Covers:** Whatman GF/A fiberglass, 5.5 cm or equivalent. Reusable aluminum insert covers.
   - 6.5 **Crucible tongs.**
   - 6.6 **Desiccator:** Filled with efficient indicating desiccant such as Drierite, 4-mesh calcium sulfate.
   - 6.7 **Mason jars:** Plastic or glass; 120, 240, or 480 mL, depending on sample size; with covers and cover bands.
   - 6.8 **Moisture trap:** Drying column or equivalent, 6.6 × 29 cm, containing efficient anhydrous calcium sulfate with indicator.
   - 6.9 **Rotameter:** 117 mL/min of air, Gilmont No. 11, 0 to 300 mL/min or equivalent.
   - 6.10 **Spatula.**
   - 6.11 **Steam bath.**
   - 6.12 **Thermometer: 0° to 110°C.**
   - 6.13 **Vacuum oven:** Equipped with air distribution manifolds at top and bottom. Equipment should be arranged so that moisture is removed from air entering the oven from the outside. Variation of temperature within oven must not exceed 2°C at 100°C setting. Ovens with glass doors have wide temperature ranges and are unsuitable. Use Lab-Line model 3623 or equivalent.
   - 6.14 **Vacuum pump:** Capable of maintaining a minimum vacuum of –86kPa, preferably –96kPa in the oven.

7. **Sampling:** Chapter 3 on "Sampling Dairy and Related Products."

8. **Preparation of Test Sample:** Take a representative sample that has previously been mixed, stirred, ground, blended, or otherwise prepared in order to make sample uniform.
   8.1 **Dried milk:** Mix sample by rolling and inverting container. Avoid weighing sample under conditions of high temperature or humidity. Use between 1 and 2 grams of sample.
   8.2 **Natural cheese:** Cheese samples should be placed immediately in a container with a tight-fitting lid. Mix the cheese with a blender for about 15 seconds. Turn the blender off intermittently and manually shake the samples and jar to help move larger particles toward the blade side of the mixer. Avoid prolonged mixing as generated heat causes fat separation and mashing of product occurs. Keep the sample jar covered at all times. Use between 2 and 3 grams of sample.
   8.3 **Processed cheese, cheese food, and block-style spreads:** Place the sample in a 120- to 480-mL sample jar and, with a blender, mix the cheese with short, intermittent blender action for about 10 seconds total time. Avoid prolonged mixing as generated heat causes fat separation. Keep the sample jar covered at all times. Avoid including the outer surface of the cheese in the sample. Use between 1 and 2 grams of sample and partially dry on steam bath before placing in oven.
   8.4 **Pourable cheese spreads**: With a spatula, thoroughly mix approximately 150 g of a cheese sample in a 240-mL sample jar. Keep the sample jar covered at all times. Use between 1 and 2 grams of sample and partially dry on steam bath before placing in oven.
   8.5 **Condiment cheese spreads**: To obtain a homogeneous sample, mix at least 150 g of cheese in a blender for 4- to 15-second periods. Keep the sample jar covered at all times. Avoid overheating the sample. Use between 1 and 2 grams of sample and partially dry on steam bath before placing in oven.

9. **Procedure:** Before beginning analysis review material safety data sheets on all chemicals and use appropriate safety equipment such as hoods, aprons, face shields, and glasses.
   9.1 **Preparation of moisture dishes and covers:** Dry the clean aluminum dishes (re-usable as well as disposable) and covers in a forced draft or vacuum oven for at least 3 hours at 100°C. Store dishes at room temperature in a clean desiccator until needed. Dry the fiberglass covers for the disposable dishes 1 hour at 100°C, and store in a clean desiccator until needed.
      9.1.1 Weigh at least two empty dishes per run to be used as blanks in the test.
   9.2 Accurately and quickly weigh the amount of sample as specified in section 8 into a preweighed dish on an analytical balance. Open the sample container only as necessary, and transfer the sample as quickly as possible. For soft cheeses or cheese of high moisture content, pre-dry on a steam bath as specified in section 8.
   9.3 Place the disposable dish containing sample, with its fiberglass cover on a metal shelf, in the vacuum oven for 5 hours set at 100°C. When

using re-usable dishes, offset the cover when placed in the oven. The temperature should be measured under vacuum by a thermometer in contact with the shelf of the oven. The temperature in the open space of the oven may be different.

9.4 Operate oven at a minimum vacuum of –86kPa, preferably –96kPa. During drying, admit into the oven a slow current of air (about 117 mL/min) dried by passing through the calcium sulfate moisture trap. Alternatively measure airflow by bubbling air through glycol solution at the rate of 2 bubbles per second before passing through drying agent.

9.5 After 4.75 hours ± 15 minutes, shut off the vacuum and slowly admit dry air into the oven. Using tongs, remove the dish from the oven and cool it in a desiccator for at least 30 minutes until the dish has reached room temperature.

9.6 Weigh back each dried sample containing dish.

10. Expression of Results

10.1 **Calculations**

A = Dish and sample weight in grams

B = Blank average in grams

C = Empty dish weight

D = Sample weight in grams

$$\% \text{ moisture} = \frac{A - B - C \times 100}{D}$$

% solids = 100% – % moisture.

11. Precision and Performance Parameters: No precision data available for this assay.

12. Test Report and Interpretation: The test report should identify the method used and results obtained. The report will also identify any variation in the test not specified in this method as well as problems which may have impacted the test result. Each sample will be described in such a manner as to ensure traceability as to its origin.

15.112 Moisture/Solids, Oven, Sand pan (Class O)[86]

1. **Scope:** This method is applicable to sweetened condensed milk.
2. **References:** Chapter 2 on "Laboratory Quality Assurance and Safety." Chapter 3 on "Sampling Dairy and Related Products."
3. **Definition:** Moisture is defined as the weight loss on drying of the sample under conditions of the test.
4. **Principle:** A preweighed sample is dried at 102°C, reweighed, and calculated as percent moisture or solids.
5. **Reagents:** Not applicable for this method.
6. **Apparatus and Glassware**

6.1 **Forced-draft oven:** Equipped with manifold air delivery system and controlled at 102° ± 2°C. Lab-Line model 3485M or equivalent.

6.2 **Glass rods:** Small, with flattened tips, 3 × 60 mm.

6.3 **Quartz sand or sea sand:** Particle size to pass through a sieve with 500-µm openings but retained by a sieve with 180-µm openings. Sand must pass on the following suitability tests:

6.3.1 Place approximately 20 g of sand in dish with a stirring rod. Put dish with sand, cover, and stirring rod in oven at 102°C for 2 hours. Remove dish to desiccator and allow to cool and weigh to nearest 0.1 mg.

6.3.2 Add 5 mL of water to dish containing sand and mix with stirring rod. Heat dish for a least 4 hours at 102°C in the oven. Move dish with cover and stirring rod to desiccator and allow to cool. Reweigh and the difference between the two weighings shall not exceed 0.5 mg.

6.4 **Aluminum moisture dishes:** 5.5-7 cm diameter disposable dish or equivalent. Height of 2-2.5 cm.

6.5 **Balance:** 0.1-mg sensitivity, electronic or equivalent.

6.6 **Crucible tongs.**

6.7 **Desiccator:** Filled with efficient indicating desiccant such as Drierite, 4-mesh calcium sulfate.

6.8 **Mason jars:** Plastic or glass; 120, 240, or 480 mL, depending on sample size; with covers and cover bands.

6.9 **Spatula.**

6.10 **Steam bath.**

6.11 **Thermometer:** 0° to 110°C.

6.12 **Water bath:** 30°-40°C.

7. **Sampling:** Chapter 3 on "Sampling Dairy and Related Products."

8. **Preparation of Test Sample:** Transfer contents of the container and mix thoroughly by use of a spoon or spatula. Use up-and-down and side-to-side motions, being sure to scrape sides and bottom of container. Transfer to a second container (mason jar) that has an air-tight lid.

Warm the mason jar containing sample in a water bath between 30° and 40°C. Cool sample to 20°-25°C and mix until sample is uniform.

9. **Procedure:** Before beginning analysis review material safety data sheets on all chemicals and use appropriate safety equipment such as hoods, aprons, face shields, and glasses.

9.1 **Preparation of sand pan:** Weigh approximately 25 g of sand into a previously dried moisture pan. Heat the open pan with sand and stirring rod in an oven at 102°C for at least 1 hour. Allow dish to cool in a desiccator for at least 45 minutes and reweigh.

9.2 Tilt the dish to one side and add approximately 2 g of sample on a clear space of the dish bottom. Replace lid on dish and rod and reweigh.

9.3 Add 5 mL of water to the test portion and mix with the stirring rod. Mix the diluted sample and the sand thoroughly and spread sample/sand mixture evenly across the bottom of the dish. Leave end of stirring rod in dish.

9.4 Heat the dish on the steam bath with as much of the bottom of the dish exposed to the steam as possible. Heat for 30 minutes. Stir the mixture frequently initially so that sample dries evenly. Sample will become crumbly.

9.5 Heat dish containing stirring rod and cover in the oven at 102°C for 2 hours.

9.6 Allow the dish to cool in the desiccator for at least 45 minutes and reweigh to the nearest 0.1 mg.

9.7 Reheat dish for 1 hour, cool in desiccator, and reweigh. Difference in weighings should not exceed 1 mg.

10. Expression of Results

10.1 **Calculations**

A = Dish and sample weight in grams

B = Blank average in grams

C = Empty dish weight

D = Sample weight in grams

$$\% \text{ moisture} = \frac{A - B - C \times 100}{D}$$

% solids = 100% – % moisture.

11. Precision and Performance Parameters

11.1 **Repeatability[43]:** The difference between two single results found on identical test material by one analyst should not exceed 0.40% in more than 1 in 20 cases.

11.2 **Reproducibility[43]:** The difference between two single and independent results found by two operators working in different laboratories shall not exceed 0.60% in more than 1 in 20 cases.

12. Test Report and Interpretation: The test report shall identify the method used and results obtained. The report will also identify any variation in the test not specified in this method as well as problems that may have impacted the test result.

Each sample will be described in such a manner as to ensure traceability as to its origin.

15.113 Moisture-Free, Vacuum Oven (Class O)[5,8]

1. **Scope:** This method is applicable to dried whey.
2. **References:** Chapter 2 on "Laboratory Quality Assurance and Safety." Chapter 3 on "Sampling Dairy and Related Products."
3. **Definition:** Free moisture is defined as the loss on drying of the sample under conditions of the test.
4. **Principle:** A preweighed sample is dried at 65°C, reweighed, and calculated as percent moisture.
5. **Reagents:** Not applicable for this method.
6. **Apparatus and Glassware.**

6.1 **Moisture dishes:** Aluminum dish, 5.5 cm, with insert cover or disposable, 5.5 cm Dyna-dish or equivalent with GF/A Whatman fiberglass filter, 5.5 cm.

6.2 **Balance:** 0.1-mg sensitivity, electronic.

6.3 **Crucible tongs.**

6.4 **Desiccator:** Filled with efficient indicating desiccant such as Drierite, 4-mesh calcium sulfate.

6.5 **Moisture trap:** Drying column or equivalent, 6.6 × 29 cm, containing efficient anhydrous calcium sulfate with indicator.

6.6 **Rotameter:** 117 mL/min. of air, Gilmont No. 11, 0 to 300 mL/min. or equivalent.

6.7 **Spatula.**

6.8 **Thermometer:** 0° to 110°C.

6.9 **Vacuum oven:** Equipped with air distribution manifolds at top and bottom. Equipment should be arranged so that moisture is removed from air entering the oven from the outside. Variation of temperature must not exceed 2°C at 100°C setting. Lab-Line model 3623 or equivalent.

6.10 **Vacuum pump:** Capable of maintaining a minimum vacuum of –86 kPa and preferably –96kPa in the oven.

7. **Sampling:** Chapter 3 on "Sampling Dairy and Related Products."

8. **Preparation of Test Sample:** Take a representative sample that has previously been mixed, stirred, ground, blended, or otherwise prepared in order to make sample uniform.

   Mix dry sample by rolling and inverting container. Avoid weighing sample under conditions of high temperature or humidity. Use between 1 and 1.5 grams of sample.

9. **Procedure:** Before beginning analysis review material safety data sheets on all chemicals and use appropriate safety equipment such as hoods, aprons, face shields, and glasses.

9.1 Preparation of moisture dishes and covers: Dry the clean aluminum dishes (re-usable as well as disposable) and covers in a forced draft or vacuum oven for at least 3 hours at 100°C. Store dishes at room temperature, in a clean desiccator, until needed. Dry the fiberglass covers for the disposable dishes 1 hour at 100°C, and store in a clean desiccator until needed.

9.2 Accurately and quickly weigh (to four decimal places) the amount of sample as specified in section 8 into a preweighed dish on an analytical balance. Open the sample container only as necessary, and transfer the sample as quickly as possible.

9.3 Place the disposable dish containing sample, with its fiberglass cover, on a metal shelf in the vacuum oven for 16 hours set at 65°C. When using re-usable dishes, offset the cover when placed in the oven. The temperature should be measured under vacuum by a thermometer in contact with the shelf of the oven. The temperature in the open space of the oven may be different.

9.4 Operate oven with a minimum vacuum of –86 kPa and preferably –96kPa. During drying, admit into the oven a slow current of air (about 117 mL/min) dried by passing through the efficient calcium sulfate moisture trap. Alternatively measure airflow by bubbling air through glycol solution at the rate of 2 bubbles per second before passing through drying agent.

9.5 After 16 hours, shut off the vacuum and slowly admit dry air into the oven. Using tongs, remove the dish from the oven and cool it in a desiccator for at least 30 minutes until the dish has reached room temperature.

9.6 Weigh back each dried sample containing dish to four decimal places.

10. **Expression of Results**

10.1 **Calculations**

A = Dish and sample weight in grams

B = Blank average in grams

C = Empty dish weight

D = Sample weight in grams

$$\% \text{ moisture} = \frac{A - B - C \times 100}{D}$$

% solids = 100% – % moisture.

11. **Precision and Performance Parameters:** No precision data available for this assay.

12. **Test Report and Interpretation:** The test report should identify the method used and results obtained. The report will also identify any variation in the test not specified in this method as well as problems that may have impacted the test result. Each sample will be described in such a manner as to ensure traceability as to its origin.

15.114 Moisture/Solids, Forced Draft Oven, Milk (Class A1), Other Products (Class B)[11(990.20),23,62]

1. **Scope:** This method is applicable to raw and processed milk, condensed milk, evaporated milk, cream, ice cream/frozen desserts, and other liquid dairy products.

2. **References:** Chapter 2 on "Laboratory Quality Assurance and Safety." Chapter 3 on "Sampling Dairy and Related Products."

3. **Definition:** Moisture/solids is defined as the mass/mass loss in weight on drying of the sample under conditions of the test.

4. **Principle:** A preweighed sample is dried, reweighed, and calculated as percent moisture or solids.

5. **Reagents:** Not applicable for this method.

6. **Apparatus and Glassware:** All volumetric flasks, pipets, and burets are Class A unless otherwise specified.

6.1 **Aluminum moisture dishes:** Disposable, ≥5 cm without cover, Dyna-dish or equivalent. Dishes must be manufactured by the "oil-free" process to allow for a more uniform spreading of the sample in the dish

6.2 **Balance:** 0.1-mg sensitivity, electronic, Mettler AE163 or equivalent.

6.3 **Blender:** Oster or Waring, use sterilizable blender heads that are suitable for autoclaving and fit 120-mL, 240-mL, or 480-mL mason jars, or equivalent.

6.4 **Crucible tongs.**

6.5 **Desiccator:** Filled with efficient indicating desiccant such as Drierite, 4-mesh calcium sulfate.

6.6 **Forced-draft oven:** Capable of rapid temperature recovery after sample loading and of maintaining 100° ± 1°C. To evaluate temperature recovery, heat empty oven to 100° ± 1°C and stabilize for 15 minutes. Turn oven off and fully open door for 2 minutes. Close oven door, turn oven back on, start timing, and record time for oven to reach 99°C. Time should be ≤7 minutes. Oven exhaust vent needs to be partially open for this test and when testing samples.

6.7 **Spatula.**

6.8 **Steam bath.**

6.9 **Thermometer:** 0° to 100°C.

6.10 **Water bath:** For tempering sample materials prior to weighing. The bath should have a thermometer and device to maintain sample materials at 38°C.

7. **Sampling:** Chapter 3 on "Sampling Dairy and Related Products."

8. **Preparation of Test Sample:** Mix the liquid sample by inversion 10 times without causing frothing or churning. Viscous samples, other than milk, may require stirring or blending to make uniform.

8.1 **Raw milk and cream:** Warm the test sample to 38° ± 1°C by means of the water bath (6.10). Level of water should be at or above milk level. Mix test sample by inversion 10 times without causing frothing or churning. If a fat line remains on the inside surface of the container, run hot tap water (ca. 50°-60°C) over outside surface for 15-20 seconds. Mix test sample thoroughly by inversion and weigh test portion immediately. Do not allow test samples to remain in the water bath more than 15 min after reaching 38°C. Weigh approximately 2-3 grams of sample.

8.2 **Natural cheese:** Cheese samples should be placed immediately in a container with a tight-fitting lid. Mix the cheese with a blender for about 15 seconds. Turn the blender off intermittently and manually shake the samples and jar to help move larger particles toward the blade side of the mixer. Avoid prolonged mixing as generated heat causes fat separation and mashing of product occurs. Keep the sample jar covered at all times. Use between 2-3 grams of sample.

8.3 **Evaporated and condensed milks:** Temper samples in a 60°C water bath. Remove and vigorously shake sample every 15 minutes. After 2 hours, remove sample from bath and allow to cool to room temperature. Thoroughly mix by stirring sample with spoon or spatula. Dilute 40 g of sample with 60 g of LG water and mix thoroughly. Weigh approximately 4-5 grams.

8.4 **Ice cream and frozen desserts:** Cut frozen blocks of product into approximately one-half pint pieces. Select 2-3 pieces at random, place in cup of high-speed blender and close tightly. Let samples soften at room temperature and mix (2 minutes for plain products and ≤7 minutes for those containing nuts or hard candy chips). Do not allow temperature to exceed 12°C at any time during softening and mixing steps. If allowed to stand, shake vigorously before removing sample. Weigh approximately 1-2 grams.

9. **Procedure:** Before beginning analysis review material safety data sheets on all chemicals and use appropriate safety equipment such as hoods, aprons, face shields, and glasses.

9.1 **Preparation of moisture dishes and covers:** Dry the clean aluminum dishes (re-usable as well as disposable) in the forced draft or vacuum oven for ≥2 hours at 100°C. Store dishes at room temperature, in a clean desiccator, until needed (dishes must be used within one week or re-dried).

9.1.1 Weigh at least two empty dishes per run to be used as blanks in the test.

9.2 Accurately and quickly weigh to four decimal places the corresponding sample as specified in section 8 into a preweighed dish on an analytical balance. When weighing warm samples do not chase drift of balance. Record sample weight immediately after weight stabilizes and just before the start of steady drift to lower numbers. Open the sample container only as necessary, and transfer the sample as quickly as possible. Predry samples of evaporated/condensed milk for 10-15 minutes on a steam bath and ice cream/frozen dessert and cream for 30 minutes. Expose the maximum surface of dish bottom to the steam.

9.2.1 For the direct forced air method for milk and cheese only, weigh up sample as in 9.2; however, do not steam dry the sample. Move directly to the step in 9.3.1.

9.3 Place the steam-dried disposable dish, containing sample, on a metal shelf in the forced air (mechanical convection) oven for 3.5 hours when testing ice cream/frozen dessert or cream. When testing raw milk or evaporated/condensed milk, place in 100°C oven for 3 hours. When using re-usable dishes, offset the cover when placed in the oven.

9.3.1 For the direct forced air method for milk only, heat sample in forced air oven set at 100°C ± 1°C for 4 hours. When testing natural cheese, place in 100°C oven for 24 hours.

9.4 After the specified time, using tongs, remove the dish from the oven and cool it in a desiccator for at least 30 minutes until the dish has reached room temperature.

9.5 Weigh back each dried sample containing dish.

10. Expression of Results

10.1 **Calculations**

A = Dish and sample weight in grams

B = Blank average in grams

C = Empty dish weight

D = Sample weight in grams

$$\% \text{ moisture} = \frac{A - B - C \times 100}{D}$$

% solids = 100% – % moisture.

11. Precision and Performance Parameters: Method performance for the direct oven solids test when testing milk only is: $S_r = 0.019$; $S_R = 0.042$; $RSD_r = 0.149\%$; $RSD_R = 0.327\%$; r – value = 0.054; and R – value = 0.118.

12. Test Report and Interpretation: The test report shall identify the method used and results obtained. The report will also identify any variation in the test not specified in this method as well as problems that may have impacted the test result. Each sample will be described in such a manner as to ensure traceablity as to its origin.

15.115 Moisture/Solids, Microwave Oven (Class B)[10(977.11),16,31,73]

1. **Scope:** This method is applicable to natural and processed cheese.
2. **References:** Chapter 2 on "Laboratory Quality Assurance and Safety." Chapter 3 on "Sampling Dairy and Related Products."
3. **Definition:** Moisture is defined as the weight loss on drying of the sample under conditions of the test.
4. **Principle:** Microwave energy is used to heat a sample to remove moisture. Balance built in the oven weighs the initial weight of the sample and calculates the moisture loss after completion of the operating cycle.
5. **Reagents:** Not applicable for this method.
6. **Apparatus and Glassware:** All volumetric flasks, pipets and burets are Class A unless otherwise specified.
   - 6.1 **Balance:** Built into oven.
   - 6.2 **Blender:** Oster or Waring or equivalent: use sterilizable blender heads that fit 120-, 240-, and 480-mL mason jars.
   - 6.3 **Filter pads:** Fiberglass (CEM Corp., P.O. Box 9, Indian Trail, NC 28079) or equivalent.
   - 6.4 **Mason jars:** 120, 240, or 480 mL, plastic or glass, with covers and bands.
   - 6.5 **Microwave oven:** CEM Corp. or equivalent.
7. **Sampling:** Chapter 3 on "Sampling Dairy and Related Products."
8. **Preparation of Test Sample:** From a representative portion of cheese, cut a 1.5- to 2-mm thick slice from the middle of the sample. Quickly cut a 4- to 4.5-mm circle with a cutter.
9. **Procedure**
   - 9.1 Place the cut circle of cheese between two fiberglass pads on the internally contained balance. The top pad prevents spattering. Locate the sample as near center on the pedestal as possible.
   - 9.2 Weigh the sample.
   - 9.3 Subject the sample to microwave energy for a time and at a power setting that gives results equivalent to those of the vacuum oven method (15.111).
   - 9.4 At the end of the test cycle, reweigh the filter pads and the residue of the sample. Some units allow the results to be read directly in percentage of moisture or solids.
10. **Expression of Results**
    - 10.1 **Calculations**

      If the unit does not autocalculate the final result, calculate as follows:

      $$\% \text{ moisture} = \frac{\text{Loss in weight} \times 100}{\text{Weight of sample}}$$

      $$\% \text{ solids} = 100 - \% \text{ moisture.}$$
11. **Precision and Performance Parameters:** No precision data are available for this assay. Factors that affect drying are time, sample size, position of the sample in the oven, and energy of microwaves. Microwave ovens vary from unit to unit. Power settings and time may vary from unit to unit and with the age of the unit.

12. **Test Report and Interpretation:** The test report shall identify the method used and results obtained. The report will also identify any variation in the test not specified in this method as well as problems that may have impacted the test result. Each sample will be described in such a manner as to insure traceablity as to its origin.

15.116 Moisture/Solids, Moisture Balance (Class B)[69(p296-7)]

1. **Scope:** This method is applicable to dry milk products.
2. **References:** Chapter 2 on "Laboratory Quality Assurance and Safety." Chapter 3 on "Sampling Dairy and Related Products."
3. **Definition:** Moisture is defined as the weight loss on drying of the sample under conditions of the test.
4. **Principle:** Infrared (or other applicable heat source) heating device is used to heat a sample to remove moisture. Balance built in the unit weighs the initial weight of the sample and calculates the moisture loss after completion of the operating cycle.
5. **Reagents:** Not applicable for this method.
6. **Apparatus and Glassware:** All volumetric flasks, pipets, and burets are Class A unless otherwise specified.
   - 6.1 **Moisture balance** with built-in infrared heating device and torsion balance.
   - 6.2 **Moisture pans** to fit balance.
7. **Sampling:** Chapter 3 on "Sampling Dairy and Related Products."
8. **Preparation of Test Sample:** Take a representative sample that has previously been mixed, stirred, ground, blended, or otherwise prepared in order to make sample uniform.
9. **Procedure**
   - 9.1 Follow the manufacturer's instructions to zero the balance.
   - 9.2 Distribute powder sample evenly on the moisture pan and weigh the sample.
   - 9.3 Adjust the power control and times for the specific materials being tested. The time required for heating in the moisture balance will vary depending on the amount of moisture in different types of samples. Once the correct drying time has been established for a product type, it is desirable to maintain this same drying time for all like samples tested. A setting of 80% power for 8 minutes has been suggested as a starting point, but this may vary with different types of samples and instruments.
   - 9.4 Charring of the sample may introduce significant error.
   - 9.5 It is recommended that an oven moisture test be used to correlate with this test.
   - 9.6 At the end of the set time, turn off the heat and reweigh.
10. **Expression of Results**

$$\% \text{ moisture} = \frac{\text{Loss in weight} \times 100}{\text{Weight of sample}}$$

$$\% \text{ solids} = 100 - \% \text{ moisture.}$$

11. **Precision and Performance Parameters:** No precision data available for this assay.

12. **Test Report and Interpretation:** The test report shall identify the method used and results obtained. The report will also identify any variation in the test not specified in this method as well as problems that may have impacted the test result. Each sample will be described in such a manner as to ensure traceablity as to its origin.

15.117 Karl Fischer Moisture (Class O)[11(977.10,984.20),99]

1. **Scope:** This method describes the procedure for determining moisture in dairy products that contain high lactose levels and low levels of moisture.
2. **References:** Chapter 2 on "Laboratory Quality Assurance and Safety." Chapter 3 on "Sampling Dairy and Related Products."
3. **Definition:** Moisture (water) determination by Karl Fischer titration is valuable for stability of dry dairy products with high levels of lactose. Oven methods are not as capable of measuring moisture because when bound to lactose it is not readily released except by vacuum oven drying at 100°C. Unfortunately, products that are dried using oven methods are losing weight due to loss of volatiles as well as water. In addition, some products are susceptible to degradation by the heat of oven methods.
4. **Principle:** The Karl Fischer volumetric method is used to determine the moisture (water) content of a sample by titration. A known amount of sample is added to methanol solvent and titrated with a standardized titrant containing sulfur dioxide and iodine. The titration reaction involves the reduction of iodine by sulfur dioxide in the presence of water.
5. **Reagents:** Unless otherwise specified all chemicals are reagent or ACS grade.
   - 5.1 **RO/DI water.**
   - 5.2 **Methanol** (CH_3 OH), anhydrous.
   - 5.3 **Formamide** ($HCONH_2$).
   - 5.4 **Chloroform** ($CHCl_3$).
   - 5.5 **Karl Fischer (KF) reagent**, single solution, 5 mg H_2O/mL, Pyridine free.
   - 5.6 **Sodium tartrate dihydrate** ($Na_2C_4H_4O_6 \bullet 2H_2O$).
   - 5.7 **Desiccant.**
6. **Apparatus and Glassware:** Unless otherwise specified all chemicals are reagent or ACS grade.
   - 6.1 **Balance**, accurate to ± 0.1 mg.
   - 6.2 **Volumetric Karl Fischer titrator.**
   - **6.3 Weighing vessels.**
   - 6.4 **Disposable syringe:** 3 to 5 mL used for weighing liquid samples.
7. **Sampling:** Chapter 3 on "Sampling Dairy and Related Products."
8. **Preparation of Test Sample:** Take a representative sample that has previously been mixed, stirred, ground, blended, or otherwise prepared in order to make sample uniform.

9. **Procedure:** Before beginning analysis review material safety data sheets on all chemicals and use appropriate safety equipment such as hoods, aprons, face shields, and glasses.

9.1 Set up the volumetric Karl Fischer titrator according to the owner's manual.

9.2 Change the desiccant on the KF unit as needed.

9.3 Titration vessel set-up.

9.3.1 Select the appropriate working solvent for the sample type to be analyzed.

9.3.2 A one-component working solvent, anhydrous methanol, is used to determine moisture in most powder and liquid samples.

9.3.3 A two-component working solvent of methanol: chloroform may be used to aid in the dissolution of fats. The methanol content should not be less than 35% by volume. Ratios used should be noted.

9.3.4 A two-component working solvent of methanol: formamide may be used to aid in the dissolution of carbohydrates and proteins. The formamide should not be more than 50% by volume. For lactose monohydrate, use between 4.5% and 5.5% formamide in methanol. For anhydrous lactose, use no more than 1% formamide in methanol. Ratios used should be noted.

9.3.5 Add enough working solvent to the titration vessel to cover the electrode. Apply moderate stirring, making sure the vortex is not directly under the electrode. It should be off to the side. This ensures good contact with the electrode probes.

9.3.6 Remove the excess water and atmospheric moisture from the working solvent and titration vessel by titrating working solvent with KF reagent. This should be done each time the titration vessel is filled with new working solvent and just prior to sample analysis.

9.3.7 **Determination of moisture factor.** Analyze approximately 45-65 mg of water (usually 5 drops from a syringe) three individual times to obtain an average (section 9.4 sample analysis). Use this average to determine the moisture factor of the KF reagent. The standard deviation of the mean should be less than 0.10.

$$\text{mg of water} = \frac{\text{Moisture factor}}{\text{mLs of KF reagent}}$$

The moisture factor will be used in the final moisture calculation. The moisture factor will vary between lots of KF reagent and should be determined with each day of use.

9.4 Sample analysis

9.4.1 Put a weighing vessel on the balance. Tare the balance.

9.4.2 Place an appropriate amount of sample in the weighing vessel and place on the balance.

9.4.3 *Whey powder, deproteinized whey powder, and lactose.* A sample between 0.5 and 1.0 gm is appropriate for most dairy powders. Use less sample if the moisture content is high. The weighed sample should contain 10 to 250 mg of water.

9.4.4 Tare the balance again. Remove the stopper from the top of the titration vessel then *quickly and carefully* place the sample into the titration vessel through the hole and replace the stopper. Special care is needed so that sample is not lost between weighing and transferring of sample into the titration vessel. Special care should be taken to get the sample *into the working solution* and not onto the side of the titration vessel. Any loss of sample during this step will result in inaccurate sample weight and the sample should be reanalyzed.

9.4.5 Place weighing vessel back onto the balance and record the weight to the nearest 0.1 mg.

9.5 Start the titration.

9.5.1 The KF unit will indicate when the titration is finished.

9.5.2 Record the volume of KF reagent used. The end point of the working solvent should be a light yellow or amber color. If the end point of the working solvent is too dark (similar to ice tea color or darker) there is too much iodine present and the titration will be inaccurate.

9.5.3 Change the working solvent in the titration vessel for every one to five samples. Working solvent may be changed more frequently if necessary. Frequency of changing the solvent is related to the sample matrix, the amount of moisture in the sample, and the number of samples analyzed.

9.5.4 Refill the burette between each sample titration.

10. Expression of Results

10.1 **Calculation**

$$\frac{(\text{mL of KF reagent}) \times \text{Moisture factor}}{\text{mg of sample}} \times 100 = \%\ \text{moisture}$$

10.2 **Detection limit:** Any result less than 0.01% will be reported as less than 0.01% moisture.

10.3 **Significant figures**

Range	Significant Figures
0.01-0.99	0.XX
1.00-9.99	X.XX
10.00-99.99	XX.XX

11. Precision and Performance Parameters: No precision data available for this assay.

11.1 For best precision, atmospheric moisture must be excluded from the system.

11.2 A sodium tartrate dihydrate standard must be analyzed with each day of analysis. The value obtained should be between 98 and 100.5% of the expected value of 15.66 (between 15.35 and 15.74). Duplicates should be within 0.20%.

12. Test Report and Interpretation: The test report shall identify the method used and results obtained. The report will also identify and variation in the test not specified in this method as well as problems that may have impacted the test result. Each sample will be described in such a manner as to ensure tractability as to its origin.

15.118 Moisture/Solids Refractometer (Class B)[74,105]

1. **Scope:** This method is applicable to whey and whey products.
2. **References:** Chapter 2 on "Laboratory Quality Assurance and Safety." Chapter 3 on "Sampling Dairy and Related Products."
3. **Definition:** Solids are defined as the measure of the degree of refraction in the sample, which is then calculated as percent solids.
4. **Principle:** Light ray is bent as it passes obliquely through the sample. The degree of refraction is measured and calculated as percent solids.
5. **Reagents:** Unless otherwise specified all chemicals are reagent or ACS grade.
   5.1 Ethanol or xylol: For cleaning prisms.
   5.2 Water (LG).
6. **Apparatus and Glassware:** All volumetric flasks, pipets, and burets are Class A unless otherwise specified.
   6.1 **Hand Refractometer:** Bausch and Lomb, with scale range from 40% to 85%; or Zeiss Model No. 0 – 85, with double scale, complete with stand or equivalent.
   6.2 **Light source (illuminator):** For refractometer.
   6.3 **Spoons:** Plastic, for transferring sample to prism.
   6.4 **Tissue:** Soft paper, for wiping refractometer prisms.
7. **Sampling:** Chapter 3 on "Sampling Dairy and Related Products."
8. **Preparation of Test Sample:** Take a representative sample that has previously been mixed, stirred, ground, blended, or otherwise prepared in order to make sample uniform.
9. **Procedure**
   9.1 Place one or two drops of the warm sample on the prism of the refractometer. Close the cover and immediately raise the refractometer to eye level and point it toward a strong source of light.
   9.2 Observe the intersection of the field—dividing line and the scale.
   9.3 Make the necessary temperature correction indicated on the thermometer on the side of the refractometer.
   9.4 Immediately after taking the refractometer reading, wash the prism thoroughly with LG water to remove the dairy product; then wipe the prism dry with a soft tissue. Allowing the product to dry on the prism is harmful to the surface of the prism.
   9.5 Do not touch the prism with a glass stirring rod, metal spoon, or other abrasive equipment.
   9.6 The test must be read quickly, as crystals may form upon cooling and inaccurate results may be obtained.
   9.7 Air incorporated in the sample will cause erroneous results. Samples must be thoroughly but carefully mixed.
10. **Expression of Results**
    10.1 **Calculations**

    % solids = reading on refractometer scale – temperature correction factor.

    % moisture = 100 – % solids.

11. **Precision and Performance Parameters:** No precision data are available for this method. The accuracy of the test is about ±0.5% to 0.6% if all the steps in the procedure are followed explicitly. Results should be compared with a reference method, and a correction should be made based on multiple tests. This method is applicable to all condensed dairy foods (in the 30% to 60% solids range). A correction factor must be applied to whey concentrate with a higher solids content.

12. **Test Report and Interpretation:** The test report shall identify the method used and results obtained. The report will also identify any variation in the test not specified in this method as well as problems that may have impacted the test result.

    Each sample will be described in such a manner as to ensure traceablity as to its origin.

15.119 Moisture/Solids, Lactometric Method (Class 0)[34,64,66,104]

1. **Scope:** This method is applicable to fluid milk.
2. **References:** Chapter 2 on "Laboratory Quality Assurance and Safety." Chapter 3 on "Sampling Dairy and Related Products."
3. **Definition:** Solids by the lactometric method is defined as the amount of solids present based on the density of the fluid milk.
4. **Principle:** Density of the fluid milk is determined, and, in conjunction with the fat, the total solids are calculated.
5. **Reagents:** Not applicable for this method.
6. **Apparatus and Glassware:** All volumetric flasks, pipets, and burets are Class A unless otherwise specified.
   - 6.1 **Flask:** 500 mL and 1,000 mL.
   - 6.2 **Lactometer cylinder:** Inside diameter is sufficiently greater than the largest diameter of the lactometer to permit free movement of the lactometer; cylinder must have the capacity to float the lactometer.
   - 6.3 **Lactometers:** Before use and as often as needed, test lactometers for accuracy by comparing them with instruments of known accuracy at 15.5°C at two different specific gravity levels. Use levels near the extremes that are expected. Discard lactometers that differ by more than 0.0001 specific gravity from that of the reference standard.
     - 6.3.1 **Large type:** Scale range from 26 to 37 degrees, smallest divisions 0.2. Total length 28.7 ± 1.1 cm; stem length 8.9 ± 0.2 cm; ballast length 1.7 ± 0.2 cm; stem diameter 0.60 ± 0.05 cm; bulb diameter 3.40 ± 0.05 cm; scale length 6.1 ± 1 cm; scale width 1.2 ± 0.2 cm.
     - 6.3.2 **Small type:** Scale range from 24.5 to 35 degrees, smallest divisions 0.5. Specifications in centimeters are approximate since certain tolerances are allowable for glass hydrometers. Dimensions are total length 15 cm, stem length 4.5 cm, stem diameter 0.5 cm, bulb diameter 3.5 cm, scale length 2.3 cm.
   - 6.4 **Tissue or soft cloth**
   - 6.5 **Water bath:** Adjustable to 39° ± 1°C and equipped with overflow tube or device to hold water at the proper level for heating milk sam-

ples; deep enough to bring water to within 5 cm of the top of the cylinder(s).

7. **Sampling:** Chapter 3 on "Sampling Dairy and Related Products."
8. **Preparation of Test Sample:** Take a representative sample that has previously been mixed or otherwise prepared in order to make sample uniform.
9. **Procedure:** Before beginning analysis review material safety data sheets on all chemicals and use appropriate safety equipment such as hoods, aprons, face shields, and glasses.

   9.1 Rapidly heat about 150 mL of milk for a small lactometer or 300 mL for a large lactometer to approximately 39°C by immersing the sample in a clean flask or jar in water at about 46°C. Gently swirl sample at intervals to prevent overheating. The flask should be loosely stoppered to reduce evaporation.

   9.2 Transfer the sample with minimal agitation to a lactometer cylinder held in a water bath at 39°C. The water should be to within 5 cm to the top of the cylinder. The lactometer itself should be preheated for not less than 3 minutes before use by immersion in a cylinder of water held in the same bath. Remove the lactometer and wipe it dry immediately before use.

      9.2.1 A large number of determinations can be done rapidly by using several lactometer cylinders in a constant temperature bath. The cylinder of milk can be held at this temperature for about 1 hour with only negligible change in specific gravity, provided that the milk is gently stirred before the lactometer is immersed. However, this long holding method is not suitable for use with milk that has oiled off or become rancid.

   9.3 Slowly immerse the lactometer in the milk sample. Take the reading at the top of the meniscus after the lactometer has come to rest. The stem of the lactometer must be clean and dry above the milk surface. Repeat readings by withdrawing the lactometer just enough to wipe the stem with a tissue or soft cloth; then slowly immerse the lactomeer to the reading point.

   9.4 Each lactometer degree on the scale is divided into 0.2 degrees for the large and 0.5 degrees for the small lactometer.

   9.5 Estimate the reading to 0.1 degrees for the large and 0.2 degrees for the small lactometer. Successive readings should agree by these same respective amounts if the temperature remains constant.

   9.6 Check the temperature of milk with an accurate thermometer at the time of the reading.

   9.7 Conduct the fat test by the Babcock test or its equivalent.

10. **Expression of Results**

    Calculations

    $$\text{Milk, \% total solids} = 1.33F + \frac{273L}{L + 1000} - 0.040, \text{ and}$$

    $$\text{Skim milk, \% total solids} = 1.33F + \frac{273L}{L + 1000}$$

    where F = % fat, and

    L = lactometer reading in degrees.

11. **Precision and Performance Parameters:** No precision data available for this assay.

12. **Test Report and Interpretation:** The test report shall identify the method used and results obtained. The report will also identify any variation in the test not specified in this method as well as problems which may have impacted the test result.

    Each sample will be described in such a manner as to ensure traceablity as to its origin.

15.120 Multicomponent Methods

Infrared (IR)[18-20,100] analysis of milk is based on absorption of IR energy at specific wavelengths by carbonyl groups in ester linkages of fat molecules, by peptide linkages between amino acids of protein molecules, and by hydroxyl groups in lactose molecules. The wavelength of light absorbance by the carbon hydrogen bond in fatty acids has been used to refine results of analyses of fat. It has been used both by itself and in conjunction with the ester linkage wavelength. Total solids may be determined by adding an experimentally determined factor to the percentage of fat, protein, and lactose.

Infrared spectroscopy is now the most widely used method of determining the compositional characteristics of fluid milk products. Properly calibrated and maintained instruments provide a rapid, reliable measurement of fat, protein, lactose, and solids, which can be used for payment, production control, and regulatory compliance. A broad range of samples can be run on the newer instrument models, and multiple calibrations can be stored to provide tests on a full range of sample types. Attention to maintenance and calibration as well as condition of sample presented to the instrument heavily impacts the reliability and accuracy of the data obtained from these machines. Proper protocols and following official procedures have demonstrated this equipment's accuracy and reproducibility to official analysis procedures. For regulatory or official analysis purposes, the chemical reference method is still the standard; under proper use, these instruments will not differ substantially from the chemical tests.

Near infrared (NIR) measurement systems use wavelengths in the overtone region (1400 to 2400 nm for reflectance and 650 to 1050 nm for absorption) of the mid-IR spectrum. Absorption in this region approximates the integral multiplier of frequencies of absorption in the mid-infrared spectrum. Because of the many overtones for each fundamental absorption wavelength, there is considerable overlaying of wavelengths of different molecular groups. Although wavelength selection to analyze for a specific component may be chosen to monitor absorption that is partial to a function of weight, it is difficult to assign the representative absorption to individual wavelengths. Instruments are available for both set numbers of wavelengths (four or more) usually used in reflectance applications to a spectrum of wavelengths used in absorption applications. Estimates of components' percentages are calculated using multiple linear regression for fixed number of wavelengths used in reflectance and partial least squares for spectrum analysis calibrations for absorption using samples of known composition.

Calibration of the instrument must be based on the same standard analytical reference method as required for mid-infrared absorption in the previous section. Thirty or more samples must be used to generate a calibration model for different components.

Modified Kohman method[69] incorporates using the same sample for moisture, fat, curd, and salt. The assay begins by first driving off the moisture by use of a hot plate, measuring the loss, and continuing on to removing the fat by ether extraction, measuring and weighing back dry residue with subsequent analysis of the final residue for salt (chloride). This multi-assay method is directly applicable to butter and margarine; however, this test may not be applicable to some of the reduced fat and lowfat spread products containing emulsifiers, stabilizers, and other atypical butter or margarine ingredients. To confirm the validity of this multicomponent method for a specific matrix, use appropriate wet chemistry methods.

15.121 Multicomponent Method, Infrared Milk Analysis: Fat, Protein, Lactose, Total Solids (Class A2)

1. **Scope**

1.1 The method described applies to the estimation of fat, protein, and, as appropriate, lactose content of unhomogenized bovine milk. Total solids, solids-not-fat, and other solids can be calculated from these primary values. The method may be applied for milks from other species (e.g., goat, ewe, buffalo, etc.) with a specific calibration for milk produced by that species.

For practical reasons (particularly for calibration) samples may be preserved with, for instance, 0.1% m/m potassium dichromate or 0.02-0.06% bronopol. Individual instrument response must be checked for all channels.

1.2 This method provides the operating conditions for instruments used for the rapid estimation of fat, protein, and lactose content of milk, based upon the measurement of absorption of mid-infrared radiation at sample and reference wavelengths which are specific to each primary component analyzed (i.e., fat, protein, and lactose). Estimates of the total solids, solids-not-fat, and other solids content of a milk sample are calculated by using the values for the primary components, plus either a constant value or variable function to account for the nonfat, non protein, non-lactose solids present in milk. The mid-infrared method is a secondary method and must be calibrated using milks that have values established for fat, protein, and lactose content that have been determined in advance by a reference chemical method. The typical reference methods are: fat (Mojonnier ether extraction 15.086), protein (Kjeldahl total protein 15.132 or true protein 15.133, and lactose enzymatic 15.092 or HPLC 15.091). The results of the reference tests must be on a mass/mass basis. In practice, infrared measurements are made using commercial automatic or semi-automatic instruments designed and optimized for milk analysis.

An important characteristic of this analysis is that the absorption of light at any wavelength is not solely by the targeted bonds. Water absorbs light strongly at most mid-infrared wavelengths. Each individual milk component can absorb some light at each of the wavelengths. Also, when two samples contain the same concentration of the component being measured (e.g., fat), but different concentrations of a second component in the background (e.g., protein), then the total concentration of water in the background is different between the two samples, and this will shift the level of signal at the wavelength at which the component (e.g., fat) is measured. Intercorrection factors are used to compensate for these influences of variation in the background.

When milk samples are pumped into the instrument, they pass through a homogenizer before they arrive at the cuvette where infrared light is passed through the sample. The efficiency of homogenization of samples is important for both repeatability and accuracy of analysis. The homogenizer needs to produce a consistent particle size distribution from sample to sample and must efficiently homogenize all samples. Homogenizer performance deteriorates with use and must be evaluated. New homogenizers should be evaluated to check for defects. Variation in milk temperature when it enters the homogenizer causes variation in the efficiency of homogenization. In general, when a homogenizer wears with use, its performance becomes more sensitive to variability in sample temperature. Declining homogenizer performance will cause poor repeatability on raw milk and will cause variability in accuracy due to shifts in calibration that are a function of differences in homogenizer performance from one run of calibration milks to another.

Any model of instrument that does not comply with the principle of analysis or that incorporates modifications that may change the principal performance characteristics of the apparatus (e.g., repeatability and accuracy), as well as the means of adjusting the calibration, will require a separate method description (e.g., PLS calibration using mid-FTIR).

2. **References:** Chapter 2 on "Laboratory Quality Assurance and Safety." Chapter 3 on "Sampling Dairy and Related Products."

3. **Definition**

3.1 **Infrared Instrument:** Proprietary apparatus that, when used under the conditions defined in this method, is calibrated to estimate the concentration of fat, protein, and lactose in milk, expressed in grams per 100 grams of milk. Further estimates of total solids, solids-not-fat, and other solids are made by calculation from the fat, protein, and lactose values.

3.2 **Uncorrected signal:** This is the primary signal (fat b = Fb_u, protein = P_u, lactose = L_u, and fat a = Fa_u) from the instrument that has been linearized and multiplied by a gain factor that controls the primary slope of each component (i.e., fat, protein, and lactose) measured by the instrument. All intercorrection factors are set to zero and the final (i.e., secondary) slope and bias are set to 1.0 and 0, respectively.

Example: $Fb_u = [(Fb_u) + P_u *(0) + L_u * (0)]\ 1.0 + 0$

3.3 **Intercorrected signal:** The intercorrected signal is the uncorrected signal that has been adjusted by using the intercorrection factors.

Example: $Fb_u = [(Fb_u + P_u*(P/Fb) + L_u * (L/Fb)]\ 1.0 + 0$

3.4 **Corrected signal:** This is the final calibrated value. The intercorrected signal for each component is multiplied by the secondary slope and a bias value is added. The slope and bias are established by linear regression of the intercorrected signals versus the chemical values for each component for a group of calibration samples. An equation for fat b corrected, protein corrected, lactose corrected, or fat a corrected, would be in the following form.

Example: $Fb_c = [Fb_u + P_u* (P/Fb) + L_u * (L/Fb)]$ Secondary slope + bias

4. **Principle:** After homogenization of the milk sample by the instrument, measurement occurs with an infrared spectrometer using a quantity of radiation absorbed by the sample at specific wavelengths of light. The wavelength of light is absorbed by a characteristic portion of the chemical structure of the component being measured and at a reference wavelength at which there is only a slight absorption by the component being measured. In practice instruments using optical filters do not select for a single wavelength of light, but instead a band of wavelengths approximately centered on the mean values below. Thus, when collecting complete spectral data from an FTIR to use with the classical approach to milk component analysis, it is necessary to select a band of wavelengths from the absorption spectra to approximately correspond to a band of wavelengths selected by an optical filter. Recommended bandwidths for fat b, fat a, protein, and lactose sample and reference wavelengths are approximately 0.03, 0.05, 0.06, and 0.14 μm, respectively. This will provide more analytical stability as other background factors from sample to sample shift slightly the wavelength of peak absorption by the compound of interest.

The carbonyl groups of the ester bonds of the glycerides absorb light at approximately a sample wavelength of 5.72 to 5.76 μm (traditionally referred to as the A filter) and a reference wavelength of approximately 5.58 and/or by the CH groups at approximately a sample wavelength of 3.48 to 3.51 μm (traditionally referred to as the B filter) and reference wavelength of approximately 3.57 μm, for the determination of the fat content.

The secondary amide groups of the peptide bonds absorb at approximately a sample wavelength of 6.46 to 6.60 μm and a reference wavelength of approximately 6.7 μm, for the determination of protein.

The hydroxyl groups of lactose absorb at approximately a sample wavelength of 9.47 to 9.61 μm and a reference wavelength of approximately 7.7 μm, for the determination of the lactose content.

Note: In some models of instruments (e.g., Dairylab 2) one reference filter wavelength (i.e., ca. 6.8 μm) is used in combination with each of the four sample wavelengths mentioned above. In general, the approach using separate reference filter wavelengths has been the preferred method for use in payment testing.

The primary signal from the detector for each channel (i.e., the combination of sample plus reference wavelength signal) is first linearized. The gain factor is then applied in order to adjust the level of sensitivity (i.e., the primary slope) of the signal from each channel. Finally the intercorrection factors are applied to produce an intercorrected signal for each channel (i.e., fat a, protein, lactose, and fat b). Adjustment (i.e., calibration) of the intercorrected signal with a linear secondary slope and bias adjustment based on the analysis of a set of calibration samples with established chemical values is done at least once on each day of testing.

5. **Reagents:** Unless otherwise specified all chemicals are reagent or ACS grade.

   Use chemicals that are specified for adjustment of linearity by each instrument manufacturer.

   5.1 **Water** (or solution recommended by the manufacturer) for zeroing the instrument. If the manufacturer recommends a mixture of Triton X-100 and water for setting the zero, then it is important to carefully control the concentration of Triton X-100 in the zeroing solution. If the concentration is accidentally made 10-fold higher in error, it will cause about 0.05 to 0.1 shift in fat b filter readings.

   5.2 **Cleaning solutions:** Use chemicals recommended by the instrument manufacturer.

6. **Apparatus**

   6.1 Commercial infrared spectrophotometers are available that are specifically designed and optimized for milk analysis. They may use either an electronic ratioing or a servo system to estimate transmitted radiation, and may produce the relevant wavelengths with a diffraction grating, by optical filters, or by a Fourier transformed interferogram. In the case of an instrument producing full spectral data from an interferogram, the scope of this method is limited to the specific wavelengths mentioned in section 4 of this method.

   6.2 **Water bath:** Sufficient size and thermal recovery capacity for tempering sample materials prior to analysis. The water in the bath should be continuously circulated and the level of water should be at or above the level of milk within the sample containers placed in the water bath. Typically, there will be continuous addition of cold samples and removal of warm samples from the water bath. The thermal mass should be sufficient to maintain the temperature of the water bath without overheating of samples that have reached the analysis temperature. The bath should have a thermometer and device to maintain sample materials at 40°C or 42°C. It may be necessary to set the temperature of the water bath at a slightly higher temperature to achieve the target temperature at the time of sample uptake by the instrument.

7. **Sampling:** Chapter 3 on "Sampling Dairy and Related Products."

8. **Preparation of Test Sample**

   8.1 Warm the test sample to at least 40°C by means of the water bath (6.2). For models of instrument without an in-line sample heater, it is better to warm the samples to 42°C. In-line sample heaters improve consistency of homogenization and stability of results if the temperature of all samples are adjusted in the flow system to about 42° to 43°C prior to entry of the sample into the homogenizer. This improves homogenization efficiency and instrument performance. Whichever sample temperature is selected as the target, it must be maintained in all samples within ± 1°C. Variability in sample temperature will cause poor precision and poor accuracy. If 42°C is selected as the target sample temperature, more care is needed to avoid excessive holding time (will cause oiling off) in the water bath after samples reach this temperature.

8.2 Level of water in the water bath should be at or above milk level. If the instrument is not equipped with an automatic sample mixer, mix the test sample 5X by inversion without causing frothing or churning. If a fat line remains on the inside surface of the container, run hot tap water (ca. 50°-60°C) over outside surface for 15-20 seconds to disperse the fat. Mix test sample thoroughly by inversion and analyze test portion immediately. Do not allow test samples to remain in the water-bath more than 15 min. after reaching 40°C. If the instrument is equipped with an automatic sample feed and mixer, then inversion and prior mixing of routine fresh milk samples should not be necessary. However, preserved calibration milks that have a compacted cream layer may require hand mixing by inversion (prior to the automatic mixer on the instrument) to achieve the desired repeatability and accuracy.

9. **Procedure:** Precalibration checks should be performed on all instruments (1). There are several aspects of the instrument's performance listed in this section (i.e., 9.1-9.8) that should be checked routinely and whenever a major repair has been made to the instrument. If the instrument cannot meet these performance criteria prior to calibration, the chances of the instrument meeting the performance criteria for repeatability and reproducibility are reduced. While any of these tests can be done at any time to spot check the performance of the instrument, when evaluating an instrument with the objective of setting linearity, setting primary slope, or setting intercorrection factors, the tests are listed below in the order that they should be conducted. The instrument should pass each pervious precalibration performance test before moving to the next test within section 9.1 to 9.9.

9.1 **Mechanical performance:** Each model of instrument has a liquid flow system that needs to be properly maintained. In some cases the instrument manufacturer has specifications and tests for flow volume at various points in the system. These volumes should be checked periodically and a record of these checks should be maintained.

One of the most important flow system checks is the sample uptake volume. On most newer instrument models, the sample uptake volume is able to be selected from the menu in computer software built into (or external to) the instrument. The actual volume uptake should be measured by using a 10-mL graduated cylinder containing 10 mL of water and manually activating the sample uptake system to measure the uptake volume. The volume taken up should be within 0.2 mL of the volume set. For most instruments, an uptake volume of at least 5 mL will be necessary (some models of instruments require up to 10 ml) to maintain acceptable purging efficiency. In general, as the uptake volume is increased the number of samples that the instrument will test per hour will decrease. Thus, increasing sample uptake volume will generally improve purging efficiency, but at the expense of reducing the testing speed.

9.2 **Homogenization efficiency**

9.2.1 **Conventional procedure:** Check the efficiency of the homogenizer by making two consecutive analyses, first with an unhomogenized whole milk sample, and second with the same whole milk sample after it has been homogenized through the instrument homogenizer. To collect the instrument homogenized milk sample, milk must be collected from the output of the instrument from only the lines that contain milk that has been through the homogenizer (i.e., not from bypass lines).

The difference between the two fat readings shall not exceed 0.05 g fat per 100 g of milk for a milk sample containing 3.5 g per 100 g of milk fat. To calculate the appropriate pass/fail criteria for milk fat concentrations other than 3.5%, multiply the actual fat content by 0.0143 to obtain the new criteria.

This procedure is not applicable with some instruments (e.g., Foss-Electric Model Milko-Scan 134).

CAUTION: The result of this test can be misleading, as an instrument in which the homogenizer does not work at all will give very little difference between the unhomogenized and homogenized portion of the same milk.

9.2.2 **Particle size procedure:** An alternative method homogenization check procedure using particle size analysis is described below.[80,81]

Measure the particle size distribution of an unhomogenized and instrument homogenized portion of the same whole raw milk sample. The production of the instrument homogenized milk is done as described above. The d(0.9) value for the unhomogenized milk will typically be about 5 to 6 µm. The d(0.9) for the instrument homogenized milk should be less than 1.7 µm. Typically, a new homogenizer will produce a d(0.9) of about 1.3 µm when milk temperature is 42°C. The d(0.9) value indicates the milk fat globule diameter at which 10% of the volume of fat contained in globules of diameters larger than this value. Large milk fat globules cause scattering of light and errors in analysis. It is expected that at lower milk temperature the homogenizer performance will not be as good as at higher temperature. The milk temperature used for this test should be the same as the normal temperature at which milk samples are tested on the instrument.

Regardless of the milk temperature, the d(0.9) achieved by the instrument homogenizer should be <1.7 μm. At d(0.9) values higher than this value (i.e., when more that 10% of the milk fat is contained in globules greater than 1.7 μm in diameter), the repeatability on unhomogenized milk will be unacceptable and the instrument's ability to properly homogenize high-fat milk samples during calibration will be compromised. The particle size analysis can be done with a preserved milk sample, as long as the preservative is completely dissolved. The samples can be cooled on ice, refrigerated, and shipped to an outside laboratory for particle size analysis within one week.

9.3 **Water repeatability:** A simple test of water repeatability can be done immediately after cleaning the cuvette and zeroing the instrument. Run 20 analyses for all components on 40°C water (or the solution that is used for zeroing the instrument) in the sample measure mode. The range among the 20 readings on each channel (e.g., fat b, lactose, protein, fat a) should be ≤0.04%. If the variation exceeds this value, there is a repeatability problem with instrument that needs to be identified and corrected. The problem is independent of milk and efficiency of homogenization and has some other mechanical or electrical origin within the instrument.

9.4 **Zero shift:** The purpose of the zero shift test is to determine the condition of the cuvette. When starting with a clean cuvette, the values established for a zeroing solution prior to running milk through the cuvette should agree well with values after running milk through the cuvette. If they do not, it is an indication that the windows of the cuvette are rapidly fouling and the zero setting on the instrument is shifting. Failure of this test is an indication that the cuvette needs to be changed.

Start with a cuvette that has just been cleaned. Zero the instrument. Run three measured cycles of water (or zeroing solution) to establish a mean initial zero value on each channel. Run 10 measure cycles of any milk sample through the instrument (raw or homogenized are acceptable). You do not have to collect data for the milk. Flush the milk out of the cuvette by running three measure cycles of water. Finally, run three additional measure cycles of water and collect the data for each channel. If the mean reading for water on any channel has shifted >0.02 from the original mean zero value, it is very likely that the cuvette needs to be replaced.

9.5 **Linearity:** The purpose of the linearity evaluation is to determine the amount of nonlinearity remaining (i.e., residual nonlinearity) in the uncorrected instrument signal prior to primary slope adjustment and intercorrection factor determination. If the amount of residual non-linearity is too large, then the standard deviation of the difference (SDD) between chemistry and instrument prediction will be too large when the calibration is evaluated. If the amount of residual nonlinearity is too large, the linearity should be adjusted and residual non-linearity reduced before any adjustment of primary slope or determination of intercorrection factors is carried out.

The quality of the linearized uncorrected signal on each channel should be checked periodically or when a replacement of a detector, light source, or filter is made. The linearity on each channel can be checked by making a series of weight/weight solutions that cover the range of concentration of each component that will be included in the calibration. The solutions are prepared, data collected, and a residual nonlinearity plot is constructed as described by Smith et al.[82] For payment testing, residuals that are ≤0.02% over the concentration range of calibration are achievable for each channel. The stock material for evaluation of linearity of the fat a and b channels is a homogenized half and half (10% fat) or homogenized light cream (ca. 18% fat) diluted to 6% fat with skim milk. The stock solution for the fat and protein channels is canned evaporated skim milk (ca. 7.1% true protein and 11% lactose). Weight/weight dilution of the stock solutions are done with water. If the instrument fails the residual linearity evaluation, then the linearity of the channel(s) that is not linear should be adjusted according to the manufacturer's instructions using weight/weight dilutions of the chemicals specified. For producer payment testing the concentration of the linearity adjustment solutions should cover only the range over which the calibration is expected to be used. Most instruments have the capability to set different linearity factors for different product calibrations. Thus, the linearity equation for a cream calibration would be expected to be different than one opitimized for producer payment testing on raw milk.

9.6 **Primary slope:** Once the residual nonlinearity of each channel has been verified to conform with established limits, then the gain (i.e., primary slope) of the uncorrected signal can be checked and adjusted. The purpose of checking and setting gain is to achieve a sensitivity of the response (i.e., primary slope) of the linearized uncorrected signal that is close to the magnitude of the change in chemistry of normal milk samples. This can be done for fat, protein, and lactose. For fat, two portions of the same skim milk can be adjusted to contain about 2 and 4% fat by addition of cream. Measure the fat content of each by a reference method to determine the difference in fat content between the two milks (e.g., 2.0%). Then measure the fat content (either with the a or b channel) of each sample on the instrument and collect the uncorrected signal, then calculate the difference between the uncorrected readings (for example 1.8%). The primary slope of the uncorrected reading for that channel is 0.9 (i.e., 1.8/2.0). Adjust the gain setting on the instrument to provide a difference of uncorrected readings of 2.0% between these two samples. This is called setting the primary slope to 1 (i.e., 2.0/2.0). This is done in a similar fashion for protein and lactose by adding milk powder for the protein channel or lactose for the lactose channel. This ensures that the sensitivity of the instrument is set appropriately on each channel.

9.7 **Milk repeatability:** The purpose of the milk repeatability check is to determine if the instrument is consistently obtaining the same test value on all test channels on the same milk sample.

The milk repeatability test is done first with raw milk. First zero the instrument. Next, run 18 measure cycles of raw milk. Be sure to prevent the milk sample temperature from decreasing while making the 18 readings. Discard the first reading on milk. The range of values on each channel for the 17 readings on milk should be ≤0.04%. If this is true, then the instrument has satisfactory repeatability on milk. If the range of values on any one or more channels is >0.04 on raw milk, then a homogenized milk repeatability test should be run, as described for the raw milk. If the instrument has satisfactory repeatability on homogenized milk but not raw milk, then the problem is probably in the homogenizer. If the instrument has poor repeatability on both raw milk and homogenized milk, then go back and review the data that were collected for water repeatability. It is probable that the instrument passed the water repeatability test by a narrow margin. If this is the case, then there is a mechanical or electrical problem. Air bubbles in the line or cuvette, or the detent locking the filter wheel into place for each filter reading may not be seating properly, may be causing the poor repeatability.

9.8 **Purging efficiency**

9.8.1 Twelve vials of distilled water or zero solution and 10 vials of homogenized, whole milk are prepared. Label the 10 vials of distilled water with #1, #2, #5, #6, #9, #10, #13, #14, #17, #18, #21, and #22. Label the 10 vials of homogenized whole milk with #3, #4, #7, #8, #11, #12, #15, #16, #19, and #20. Place the 10 vials of distilled water and 10 vials of homogenized, whole milk *in numerical order* along with several more (minimum of 5) vials of distilled water to use for setting and checking zeros in the water bath. Set the instrument to produce uncorrected data. Set the zero on all channels following the manufacturer's instructions. The infrared analyzer has an automatic mixing device that is used during daily operation; use it during the purging efficiency test to mix both the water and milk samples. Do not wipe off any excess water or milk that remains on the automatic mixer or the sample uptake tube between readings, unless this is done for all samples during normal routine operation. When the distilled water and homogenized, whole milk have reached 40°C, run 1 measure cycle on each of the 20 vials in numerical order. Running an alternating series of two water vials, two milk vials, two water vials, etc., *record the uncorrected readings from all channels* from each measure cycle on a data sheet. Calculate the purging efficiency (water to milk) and (milk to water) for each channel.

9.8.2 **Water to milk purging efficiency (P.E.)**

M1 = First milk sample readings
M2 = Second milk sample readings
W1 = First water readings
W2 = Second water readings
P.E. = (sum of M1–sum of W2) / (sum of M2–sum of W2) * 100

9.8.3 **Milk to water purging efficiency (P.E.)**

P.E. = (sum of M2–sum of W1) / (sum of M2–sum of W2) * 100

Purging efficiency should be ≥99.0%. If the purging efficiency is <99.0%, it indicates a problem with the flow system or, if the infrared analyzer has an automatic mixer, the mixer may have too much carryover from one vial to the next. If an automatic mixer was used and the instrument failed the purging efficiency test, then repeat the purging efficiency test using an inversion to manually mix the samples and run a set of samples in manual operation mode. If the instrument passes using manual mixing and operation, then the sample mixing device is carrying too much liquid from one sample to the next. Modify or replace the sample mixer.

9.8.4 **Causes of purging efficiency test failures**

Too much carry over from the automatic mixer: Repair/replace mixer.

Milk leaking backwards out of sample uptake tube into the next sample: This condition should be obvious when going from the milk to the water samples during the purging efficiency test. At the initiation of sample uptake you may see milk flow out of the uptake tube into the water. Repair sample uptake system.

Too little volume going through the cuvette: Be sure the instrument is within specifications on flow system volume checks. The in-line filter before the cuvette may be causing too much restriction of flow, or the back pressure valve on the cuvette exit line may not be operating correctly.

Sample intake volume set too low: Generally, the sample intake volume should be 5 mL or larger, depending on the instrument model. Gernerally, increasing sample uptake volume will improve purging efficiency.

9.9 **Intercorrection factors:** These are the coefficients in the equations to calculate the infrared intercorrected values for each filter combination.[13] The intercorrection factors that are used are fat on protein, fat on lactose, protein on fat, protein on lactose, lactose on fat, and lactose on protein. The intercorrection factors are influenced by the spectral characteristics of the filters in the instrument and chemical characteristics of the compounds being measured. If primary slope is maintained (i.e., if it is held near 1.0), then once the intercorrection factors are determined for an instrument they should remain constant until a filter is changed or the orientation of a filter in the light beam is changed. This is not common. The intercorrection factors can be determined by preparing and testing a set of intercorrection determination solutions on the instrument. The linearity and primary slope should be adjusted and within specifications before determination of intercorrection factors.

Some equipment manufacturers provide or recommend solutions to prepare and analyze to determine intercorrection factors. The USDA Federal Milk Market Infrared Milk Analysis Quality

Assurance Program (Carrollton, Texas) also has a recommended set of solutions for determination of intercorrection factors for infrared milk analyzers. Typical values for intercorrection factors when the primary slope on each channel is kept near 1.0 and the traditional sample filter and reference wavelengths that are used are:

Fat on protein	=	+ 0.05 to + 0.09
Fat on lactose	=	+ 0.02 to + 0.05
Protein on fat a	=	– 0.08 to – 0.17
Protein on fat b	=	– 0.01 to +0.02
Lactose on protein	=	+ 0.05 to + 0.09
Lacose on fat a	=	– 0.21 to – 0.28
Lactose on fat b	=	+0.03 to + 0.06

9.10 **Calibration:** Make (or purchase) a set of milk samples for calibration that have been tested by chemical methods for fat, protein, and lactose content by the reference chemical methods specified in section 1.1 of this method. The instrument will provide the best analytical performance and best agreement between laboratories when the chemical reference values for the calibration samples for protein are true protein and lactose are anhydrous lactose. The number of samples should be at least 10. Warm the samples as in Section 8. Collect three measure cycle readings on water to calculate a mean initial zero reading, then run three measure cycles from each calibration sample vial, and finally rinse the cuvette with three measure cycles of water and then collect three final water readings. First compare the initial mean zero to the final mean zero on each channel. If the mean zero on any channel has shifted by more than 0.02%, rezero the instrument and run a new set of calibration samples. If the mean ending zeros are satisfactory, then compare the second and third reading of each of the calibration milks. If the second and third reading of any sample differs by more than 0.04% run a repeat test on that sample. Once a satisfactory set of data has been collected, calculate an average of the second plus third intercorrected reading for each sample in the calibration set. Do a linear regression analysis of chemistry versus the average (i.e., of the second plus third readings) intercorrected instrument reading for each sample to calculate the secondary slope and bias adjustment for calibration of each channel (i.e., fat b, lactose, protein, fat a). This secondary slope and bias adjustment is the routine calibration adjustment of the instrument. Everything else is taken care of in precalibration.

After the slope and bias adjustment are made for each channel, the mean difference between instrument and chemical values will be zero on all channels. The standard deviation of the differences between instrument values after calibration adjustment and chemistry for the group of calibration samples should be calculated. There is a wide range of opinions on criteria for SDD values on calibration samples. Though many studies have been conducted and reported, most have lacked the control necessary to determine the true performance of the method because no precalibration evaluation or control of the instruments was done or reported. In many cases the performance of the chemical reference methods was not in compliance with established method performance criteria. In addition, calibration milk samples are not randomly selected milk samples from the population. Milks from farms are chosen in an attempt to achieve a wide range of concentration of each component. In some cases this selects for individual farms that have milk that is not typical of the population. In practice, a SDD of ≤0.03 on the fat b, protein, and lactose channels seems achievable with a sample set of 10 raw milk samples or more. The fat a channel is more variable and will generally have an SDD of ≤0.05.

Total solids can be calculated by adding the corrected value for fat, protein, and lactose for each sample and adding a constant value for ash. However, ash content of milk is not a constant. It is generally correlated with the protein content. Another approach (USDA, Federal Milk Markets) for adding a factor for ash is to use an equation to predict the ash content of each sample based on protein content. The prediction equation when using true protein for calibration is (0.0596 × % true protein) + 0.5279, and the prediction equation when using total nitrogen based protein is (0.0584 × % total protein) = 0.5309. Finally, the value for each calibration sample of the sum of the components (i.e., fat, protein, lactose, plus ash) can be used in a linear regression versus an oven drying reference value (15.114) for total solids for each sample to calculate a secondary slope and bias calibration adjustment for total solids. This produces a total solids prediction that is traceable back to a reference method (i.e., forced-air oven drying). Once this is done, solids-not-fat can be calculated by subtracting the instrument fat test from the total solids test, and the other solids can be obtained by subtracting the sum of fat and true protein from the total solids test. Both of these values are directly linked to instrument predictions that have a calibration reference to actual tests of calibration milk samples test by a reference method.

9.11 **Validation:** Validation of calibration accuracy and precision is something that should be done but is not routinely carried out in most milk analysis laboratories. To validate the calibration of an instrument, a group of randomly selected milks (e.g., 10 or more) should be tested by the reference chemistry methods and by the instrument. The mean difference (MD) and standard deviation of the difference (SDD) between instrument and chemistry should be calculated. The instrument is not expected to produce a zero mean difference on any small group of samples. Again, very little solid data are available to set criteria for validation. However, most state and federal regulatory agencies have guidelines for agreement with validation milk samples. Certainly, most laboratories should be able to achieve the AOAC standards of ≤0.05% for maximum mean difference and ≤0.06% SDD on fat, protein, and lactose or the ≤0.09% maximum mean difference and ≤0.12% SDD for total solids. In practice, instruments should perform much better than these values.

9.12 **Routine analysis of milk samples:** At the beginning of testing day, it would be normal practice to run a set of calibration samples and make any adjustment to slope and bias that may be necessary. In routine analysis, only one sip of each milk sample is analyzed. Generally, a pilot sample(s) is used to monitor the stability of the instrument at periodic intervals (maybe hourly or after some fixed number of analyses). An unhomogenized pilot sample is used to check both the instrument stability and the operator sample handling, and a homogenized sample provides an evaluation of instrument stability, independent of operator handling. A control chart of the uncorrected signals for the pilot sample(s) should be maintained; when the test of the pilot sample exceeds established control limits, the calibration samples should be tested to determine if changes in secondary slope and bias are needed.

10. **Expression of Results**
    10.1 Results are read directly off the machine or tabulated by computer program for the specific samples analyzed.

11. **Precision and Performance Parameters:** No collaborative study has been completed to move this method to an A1 classification and provide the repeatability and reproducibility statistics for this method. The traditionally accepted values for method performance are:

    Mean difference (MD) between instrument and reference method values for fat, protein, and lactose should be ≤0.05% and ≤0.09% for total solids. Standard deviation of the difference (SDD) between instrument and reference method values for fat, protein, and lactose should be ≤0.06% and ≤0.12% for total solids. In routine practice in milk-testing laboratories, the normal performance of the method should be well below these maximum values for MD and SDD.

12. **Test Report and Interpretation:** The test report shall identify the method used and results obtained. The report will also identify any variation in the test not specified in this method as well as problems that may have impacted the test result. Each sample will be described in such a manner as to ensure traceablity as to its origin.

15.122 Multicomponent Method, Near Infrared: Fat, Protein, Lactose, Total Solids (Class B)[101,102]

1. **Scope:** The method described applies to the estimation of fat, protein, and, as appropriate, lactose content of bovine milk. Total solids, solids-not-fat, and other solids can be calculated from these primary values. The method has applicability to other dairy products.

2. **References:** Chapter 2 on "Laboratory Quality Assurance and Safety." Chapter 3 on "Sampling Dairy and Related Products."

3. **Definition:** Proprietary apparatus that, when used under the conditions defined in this method, is calibrated to estimate the concentration of fat, protein, and lactose in milk, expressed in grams per 100 grams of milk. Further estimates of total solids, solids-not-fat, and other solids are made by calculation from the fat, protein, and lactose values.

4. **Principle:** The near infrared measurement system uses wavelengths in the overtone region (1400 to 2400 nm for reflectance and 650 to 1050 nm

for absorption) of the mid-IR spectrum. Absorption in this region approximates the integral multiplier of frequencies of absorption in the mid-infrared spectrum. Because of the many overtones for each fundamental absorption wavelength, there is considerable overlaying of wavelengths of different molecular groups. Although wavelength selection to analyze for a specific component may be chosen to monitor absorption that is partial to a function of weight, it is difficult to assign the representative absorption to individual wavelengths. Instruments are available for both set numbers of wavelengths (four or more), usually used in reflectance applications, to a spectrum of wavelengths, used in absorption applications. Estimates of components' percentages are calculated using multiple linear regression for fixed number of wavelengths used in reflectance and partial least squares for spectrum analysis calibrations for absorption using samples of known composition.

5. **Reagents:** Unless otherwise specified all chemicals are reagent or ACS grade.

   Use chemicals that are specified for adjustment of linearity by each instrument manufacturer.

   5.1 Wash solutions: As required or specified by manufacturer.

6. **Apparatus and Glassware**

   6.1 **Near infrared analyzer:** Depends on the supplier. Several manufacturers are available (e.g., reflectance instrument: Technicon Instrument Corp., 511 Benedict Avenue, Tarrytown, NY 10591; absorption instrument: CME Telemetrix Inc., 560 Parkside Drive, Waterloo, Ontario, Canada N2L 5Z4). Instrument should be plugged in and allowed to warm up to manufacturer-specified requirements prior to use. Individual near IR instrument used must meet the performance specifications in section 15.121 for mid infrared instruments in the previous section.

   6.2 **Water bath:** Capable of holding samples to 45° ± 1°C for melting and resuspending butterfat in raw milk samples prior to analysis. A second water bath may also be necessary to provide a constant sample temperature for analysis of 30° ± 5°C or as specified by the manufacturer. Water bath should be able to hold a temperature setting within ± 1°C.

   6.3 **Power supply:** Grounded and adequately protected to supply a constant power supply.

7. **Sampling:** Chapter 3 on "Sampling Dairy and Related Products."

8. **Preparation of Test Sample**

   8.1 Milk samples should not be sour and the fat should not be churned or oiled off. Samples that are not homogenous must be heated to 45° ± 1°C before analysis to melt the fat. Gently mix the samples by inverting six times, being careful not to incorporate air in churning of the sample. If the sample is more that 2/3 full, mix the samples by gently pouring from one container to another six times.

9. **Procedure**

   9.1 **Calibration of unit:** Calibration of the instrument must be based on the same standard analytical reference method as required for mid-infrared absorption in method 15.121. Thirty or more samples must be used to generate a calibration model for different components.

9.1.1 Different product/sample types will require different calibrations, as will different components.

9.1.2 Each instrument must be calibrated using at least 20 or more representative samples of the same type for each type of product/sample. (For example, butterfat for raw milk will require at least 20 raw milk samples with differing butterfat levels to calibrate for raw milk butterfat analysis.) For calibration purposes, do not use abnormal milk.

9.1.3 Analyze all calibration samples in duplicates using standard reference methods. [Mojonnier methods for fat (15.086), Kjeldahl for protein (15.131 or 15.132), and forced air oven for total solids (15.114)].

9.1.4 Commercially available standards may also be used for calibrations.

9.1.5 Following directions of the manufacturer's operating manual, analyze samples in duplicates with the instrument. Follow the manufacturer's instructions for determining wavelengths and coefficients to be used for each calibration.

9.1.6 After calibration, the calibration should be benchmarked with a set of samples. The results must meet the specifications provided in method 15.121.

9.1.7 Operating and maintenance instruction is provided in the operating manual. It may be necessary to analyze samples with one consistent sample temperature for both calibration and testing to provide for stable results.

9.1.8 Daily pilot/control preserved samples that were analyzed on the day of calibration or calibration check to make performance checks is recommended. If the results differ by more than the specifications in method 15.121, check the sample used and the instrument for stability. If warranted, adjust the instrument as necessary however it is recommended that slope/bias only be done with a set of six or more analyzed standard samples.

9.1.9 Clean, and perform preventive maintenance on the instrument as specified by the manufacturer.

10. Expression of Results

10.1 Results are read directly off the machine or tabulated by computer program for the specific samples analyzed.

11. Precision and Performance Parameters: No precision data available for this method.

12. Test Report and Interpretation: The test report shall identify the method used and results obtained. The report will also identify any variation in the test not specified in this method as well as problems that may have impacted the test result. Each sample will be described in such a manner as to ensure traceablity as to its origin.

15.123 Modified Kohman Method, Fat, Moisture, Chloride (Salt), in Butter and Margarine (Class O and Class B)[4,11(938.06,920.17),54,69,95]

1. **Scope:** This method is applicable to butter, margarine. and other high-fat spreads that do not incorporate water soluble emulsifiers, gums, or gelatin.

2. **References:** Chapter 2 on "Laboratory Quality Assurance and Safety." Chapter 3 on "Sampling Dairy and Related Products."

3. **Definition:** The chloride content as expressed by this method is the equivalent content of sodium chloride (salt).

   Moisture is defined as the loss in weight when sample is exposed to 232° ± 5°C and dried under conditions of this method.

   Fat is defined as the weight remaining after subtraction of the moisture, salt, and curd.

4. **Principle:** A weighed sample is heated to evaporate the moisture and then reweighed to determine the moisture lost. The fat is extracted with petroleum ether, and the remaining solids are weighed to determine the fat lost. The solids are then dissolved and the salt is determined by titration.

5. **Reagents:** Unless otherwise specified all chemicals are reagent or ACS grade.
   - 5.1 **Petroleum ether:** Boiling range 30° to 60°C.
   - 5.2 **Potassium chromate indicator:** 5% in LG water.
   - 5.3 **Silver nitrate:** 0. 1N.
   - 5.4 **Water (LG).**

6. **Apparatus and Glassware:** All volumetric flasks, pipets, and burets are Class A unless otherwise specified.
   - 6.1 **Balance:** 0.1 mg sensitivity for Class O assay, 500 g with 10.0 mg sensitivity for Class B.
   - 6.2 **Beaker:** 200 to 250 mL, 8.5 to 9.0 cm tall, 6.5 to 7.5 cm in diameter, aluminum with or without pouring spout. If this beaker cannot be obtained an alternative container is an aluminum enameled can available through Crown and Seal Company, Inc. Massilon, Ohio. Short can catalog number is A3310 with dimensions of 61 mm in height and 83 mm in diameter. Tall can catalog number is A3412 with dimensions of 85 mm in height and 83 mm in diameter.
   - 6.3 **Buret:** 25 or 50 mL, calibrated in 0.1-mL divisions.
   - 6.4 **Bunsen burner.**
   - 6.5 **Crucible:** Gooch.
   - 6.6 **Crucible tongs.**
   - 6.7 **Cylinder:** Graduated, 50 mL.
   - 6.8 **Desiccator:** With efficient desiccant.
   - 6.9 **Filter paper:** To fit Gooch crucible.
   - 6.10 **Flasks:** Erlenmeyer, 125 mL; filter, 500 mL; volumetric, 250 mL.
   - 6.11 **Hot plate:** Thermostatically controlled electric or a steam-heated hot plate with sensitivity of ± 3°C.
   - 6.12 **Oven:** Forced draft, 100°C.
   - 6.13 **Pipets:** Volumetric, 25 mL and pasteur, disposable.

6.14 **Stirring rods:** Glass, with rubber policeman.
6.15 **Vacuum flask:** 2-L Erlenmeyer.
6.16 **Wash bottle:** For petroleum ether.
6.17 **Water aspirator:** For vacuum source.

7. **Sampling:** Chapter 3 on "Sampling Dairy and Related Products."
8. **Preparation of Test Sample:** Take a representative sample that has previously been mixed, stirred, ground, blended, or otherwise prepared in order to make sample uniform. Temper samples to room temperature (20° to 25°C). Sample to be protected by the original wrapper or in a sealed container during tempering so that moisture is not lost.
9. **Procedure:** Before beginning analysis review material safety data sheets on all chemicals and use appropriate safety equipment such as hoods, aprons, face shields, and glasses.

9.1 **Procedure for moisture:** (Class O and Class B)

9.1.1 Using the analytical balance, weigh a clean, dry aluminum beaker tempered to room temperature (20° to 25°C).

9.1.2 Accurately weigh about 10 g of a well-mixed, tempered (20° to 25°C) sample into the aluminum beaker.

9.1.3 Using crucible tongs, place the aluminum beaker on the hot plate at 232° ± 5°C. Swirl the beaker constantly during heating to avoid the spattering and burning of milk solids. A mechanical shaker may be used.

Alternatively, heat sample over a Bunsen burner until sample bubbles vigorously. Rotate the beaker occasionally to avoid spattering or adjust the flame or temperature of hot plate low enough to avoid rapid boiling. When using a Bunsen burner, pass the beaker in and out of the flame to control boiling.

If aluminum cans are used it will be necessary to run blanks in these cans until there is no change in weight from one sample run to the next.

9.1.4 Continue evaporation until all foaming and bubbling has ceased and the milk solids take on a light brown (coffee) color. Care should be taken to obtain the same degree of color in each test.

9.1.5 Cool the beaker to room temperature in a desiccator.

9.1.6 Reweigh the beaker.

9.2 **Procedure for fat (Class O):** CAUTION: This procedure should take place in an exhaust hood. Do not use petroleum ether near an open flame or sparks.

9.2.1 Prepare the Gooch crucible by pressing the filter paper into it. Wash the filter paper twice with suction using 10 to 15 mL of petroleum ether per wash. Dry the crucible with suction for 15 seconds and then dry it in an oven at 100°C for a minimum of 15 minutes. Cool the crucible in a desiccator. Weigh the prepared crucible on the analytical balance.

9.2.2 Add about 125 mL of petroleum ether to the moisture-free residue in the aluminum beaker.

9.2.3 Use a glass rod to break up the residue in the beaker to ensure complete fat extraction. Rinse the rod with a few milliliters of petroleum ether before removing it from the beaker.

9.2.4 Transfer the dissolved fat and other solids into a preweighed, prepared Gooch crucible while applying suction. Use a wash bottle with petroleum ether to aid in the transfer.

9.2.5 Rinse the beaker twice with 25 mL of petroleum ether per rinse. Add rinse to the crucible so as to wash the solids into the crucible.

9.2.6 Dry the crucible with suction for 15 to 30 seconds after the last ether rinse has passed through.

9.2.7 Dry the crucible and its contents at 100°C for 15 minutes.

9.2.8 Cool the crucible to room temperature in a desiccator.

9.2.9 Reweigh the crucible and its contents on the analytical balance.

9.3 **Procedure for fat (Class B):** CAUTION: This procedure should take place in an exhaust hood. Do not use petroleum ether near an open flame or sparks.

9.3.1 Add about 100–125 mL of petroleum ether to the moisture-free residue in the aluminum beaker. Place aluminum cups containing ether on a platform adjusted to a 15-degree angle for 5-10 minutes to allow the curd to settle along the inside edge of the container.

9.3.2 Be careful not to disturb the curd that is settled along the inside edge of the container. On this first extraction, do not swirl the mixture. This will cause fat to collect on the upper portion of the container wall and make it difficult to extract all the fat from the sample.

9.3.3 Hook up a pasteur pipet to a hose and attach to the inlet of a 2-L vacuum flask.

9.3.4 Attach a second hose from the vacuum inlet of the flask to the water aspirator.

9.3.5 Turn on the aspirator until sufficient vacuum is generated.

9.3.6 Using the pasteur pipet vacuum assembly, draw the ether fat layer off without disturbing the solids at the base corner of the aluminum cup.

9.3.7 Repeat the extraction process (steps 9.3.1-9.3.6) two more times; this time mix with stirring rod or swirl the ether, fat, and curd in the container, let solids settle to edge, and draw off petroleum ether again.

9.3.8 Allow ether that is not drawn off by the vacuum pipet to evaporate from the aluminum cups while in the fume hood.

9.3.9 Dry the aluminum beaker containing solids at 100°C for 15 minutes.

9.3.10 Cool the aluminum beaker to room temperature in a desiccator.

9.3.11 Reweigh the aluminum beaker and its contents on the analytical balance.

9.4 **Procedure for salt (Class O)**

9.4.1 Transfer the filter paper and residue to a 250-mL volumetric flask with hot (65° to 70°C) LG water. Rinse the crucible three times and add the washings to the flask.

9.4.2 Cool the flask to room temperature and dilute to volume with LG water. Mix thoroughly. Because of the low levels of salt in the solution, the volume of the filter paper is not significant.

9.4.3 The salt will dissolve and the milk solids will settle in the flask.

9.4.4 Pipet 25 mL of this solution into a 125-mL Erlenmeyer flask.

9.4.5 Add 1 mL of 5% potassium chromate indicator. Titrate with 0.1N silver nitrate solution to the first visible pale red-brown color lasting 30 seconds. The end point is much sharper if the titration is conducted under a yellow light.

9.5 **Procedure for salt (Class B)**

9.5.1 Using a 250-mL volumetric flask, add 250 mL of hot (65° to 70°C) LG water to the aluminum beaker containing solids.

9.5.2 Allow sample and hot water containing aluminum beaker to cool to room temperature. Mix thoroughly.

9.5.3 The salt will dissolve and the milk solids will settle in the flask.

9.5.4 Pipet 25 mL of this solution into a 125-mL Erlenmeyer flask.

9.5.5 Add 2 mL of 5% potassium chromate indicator. Titrate with 0.1N silver nitrate solution to the first visible pale red-brown color lasting 30 seconds. The end point is much sharper if the titration is conducted under a yellow light.

Alternatively, rinse the aluminum beaker containing solids with 50 mL of distilled water and pour this into a 250-mL Erlenmeyer flask. Add 50 additional mL of distilled water to the flask, bringing the total volume to 100 mL.

Add 2 mL or 10 drops of 5% aqueous potassium chromate solution. Titrate with 0.1N silver nitrate solution until a brownish, red brick tinge persists for 30 seconds throughout sample.

10. Expression of Results

10.1 Calculations

$$\% \text{ moisture} = \frac{(B - D) \times 100}{C}$$

$$\% \text{ fat} = \frac{[(D - A) - (F - E)] \times 100}{C}$$

$$\% \text{ sodium chloride} = \frac{\text{mL AgN03} \times \text{N AgN03} \times \text{dilution volume} \times .0585 \times 100}{C \times \text{mL titrated}}$$

Alternatively, if the entire sample was titrated, the % sodium chloride can be calculated as follows:

% curd by difference = 100% – (% fat + % moisture + % sodium chloride)

where A = weight of beaker,

B = weight of beaker and sample,

C = weight of sample (B-A),

D = weight of beaker and moisture-free residue (fat, salt, milk solids),

E = weight of crucible (or beaker if using Class B method)
F = weight of crucible (or beaker) and solids (salt and milk solids).
0.0585 = milli-equivalents of sodium chloride.

11. **Precision and Performance Parameters:** No precision data available for this method.

12. **Test Report and Interpretation:** The test report shall identify the method used and results obtained. The report will also identify any variation in the test not specified in this method as well as problems that may have impacted the test result. Each sample will be described in such a manner as to ensure traceability as to its origin.

15.130 Protein/Nitrogen Tests

Since 1883, the Kjeldahl principle has been used as the standard method measuring total nitrogen in food and feed. With increasing emphasis being placed on the importance of protein in foods, however, more accurate, specific, and rapid methods have been developed. These methods must be calibrated against Kjeldahl results.

Two variations (traditional and block digestor equipment) of the macro Kjeldahl test are in common use in the dairy industry. Differences between the two are in how ammonia is removed from the digested sample by either boiling or by steam distillation. Apparatus for micro-Kjeldahl are available that use smaller sample size and shorter analysis times. However, the micro-Kjeldahl methods cannot achieve the within and between laboratory performance described for the methods detailed in this section.

As the value of protein increases and the technologies to fractionate milk proteins on commercial scale continue to develop, there will be a need for Kjeldahl methods to measure fractions of the total nitrogen content of milk. This section provides methods for determination of protein (nitrogen), non-protein nitrogen, noncasein nitrogen, casein, and true protein content of milk. The collaborative studies of these methods have been done on raw milk. Therefore, the within and between lab performance stated in the methods are for raw milk. Suggestions for modification of these methods for use on other dairy foods are included. In addition, the spectrophotometric method for the determination of undenatured whey protein nitrogen (WPN) in nonfat dry milk is included.

15.131 Protein, Kjeldahl Standard, Traditional Milk (Class A1), Other Products (Class O)[11(991.20),38]

1. **Scope:** This method is applicable for the determination of the total nitrogen content of milk.

2. **References:** Chapter 2 on "Laboratory Quality Assurance and Safety." Chapter 3 on "Sampling Dairy and Related Products."

3. **Definition:** Nitrogen content is the mass fraction of substances determined according to this procedure. It is expressed as a percentage by mass.

4. **Principle:** The principle is based on the digestion of a test portion with a mixture of concentrated sulfuric acid and potassium sulfate, using copper(II) sulfate as a catalyst to thereby convert organic nitrogen present to

ammonium sulfate. Excess sodium hydroxide is added to the cooled digest to liberate ammonia. Ammonia is distilled into an excess of boric acid solution and titrated with hydrochloric acid solution. Nitrogen is calculated from the amount of ammonia produced.

5. **Reagents:** Unless otherwise specified all chemicals are reagent or ACS grade.
   - 5.1 Potassium sulfate (K_2SO_4): Low in nitrogen content.
   - 5.2 Copper(II) sulfate solution: Dissolve 5.0 g of copper(II) sulfate pentahydrate ($CuSO_4 \cdot 5H_20$) in water and dilute to the mark in a 100-mL one-mark volumetric flask. Reagent is commercially available.
   - 5.3 Sulfuric acid: 95-98% (m/m), nitrogen free, P_{20} approximately 1.84 g/mL.
   - 5.4 Sodium hydroxide solution: Low in nitrogen, containing 50 g of sodium hydroxide (NaOH) per 100 g.
   - 5.5 Indicator solution: Dissolve 0.1 g of methyl red and dilute to 50 mL in 95% (V/V) ethanol. Dissolve 0.5 g of bromocresol green and dilute to 250 mL in 95% (V/V) ethanol. Mix 1 part of the methyl red solution with 5 parts of the bromocresol green solution or combine all of both solutions.
   - 5.6 Boric acid solution (with indicator): Dissolve 40.0 g of boric acid (H_3BO_3) in 1 L of hot water, allow to cool, bring to volume, add 3 mL of the indicator solution (5.5), mix, and store in a borosilicate glass bottle. The solution will be light orange in color. Protect the solution from light and sources of ammonia fumes during storage. Reagent is commercially available.
   - 5.7 Hydrochloric acid: Standard volumetric solution (HCl) = 0.1 ± 0.0005 mol/L (0.1 ± 0.0005 N).
   - 5.8 Ammonium sulfate [$(NH_4)_2SO_4$]: Minimum assay 99.9% on dried material.

     Immediately before use, dry the ammonium sulfate at 102° ± 2°C for not less than 2 hours and cool to room temperature in a desiccator.
   - 5.9 Tryptophan ($C_{11}H_{12}N_2O_2$) or lysine hydrochloride ($C_6H_{15}ClN_2O_2$): Minimum assay 99%. Do not dry in an oven before use.
   - 5.10 Sucrose: Nitrogen content not more than 0.002% (m/m). Do not dry in an oven before use.

6. **Apparatus and Glassware:** All volumetric flasks, pipets, and burets are Class A unless otherwise specified.
   - 6.1 Water bath: Maintained at a temperature of 38° ± 1°C.
   - 6.2 Kjeldahl flasks: Capacity 500 mL or 800 mL.
   - 6.3 Analytical balance: Readability to nearest 0.1 mg.
   - 6.4 Boiling aids: High-purity amphoteric alundum granules, plain, mesh size 10. Do not reuse. Glass beads of approximately 5 mm diameter are also used, but they do not promote as efficient boiling as the alundum granules and more foaming problems will be encountered during digestion with glass beads.
   - 6.5 Buret or automatic pipet: For delivering 1.0-mL portions of the copper sulfate solution (5.2).

6.6 Graduated measuring cylinders: Capacities 50 mL, 100 mL, and 500 mL.

6.7 Digestion apparatus: To hold the Kjeldahl flasks (6.2) in an inclined position (approximately 45°), with electric heaters and with a fume extraction system.

6.8 Distillation apparatus: Made of borosilicate glass or other suitable material, to which a Kjeldahl flask (6.2) can be fitted consisting of an efficient splash-head connected to an efficient condenser with straight inner tube and an outlet tube attached to its lower end; the connecting tubing and stopper(s) shall be close-fitting and preferably made of neoprene.

6.9 Conical flasks: Capacity 500 mL, graduated.

6.10 Burette: Capacity 50 mL, graduated at least every 0.1 mL, complying with the requirements of ISO 385, class A.

7. **Sampling:** Chapter 3 on "Sampling Dairy and Related Products."

8. **Preparation of Test Sample:** Warm the milk sample to 38° ± 1°C by means of the water bath (6.1). Gently mix the milk sample immediately prior to weighing the test portion (9.1).

9. **Procedure:** Before beginning analysis review material safety data sheets on all chemicals and use appropriate safety equipment such as hoods, aprons, face shields, and glasses.

9.1 **Test portion and pretreatment:** To the clean and dry Kjeldahl flask (6.2), add 5 to 10 boiling aids (6.4), 15 g of the potassium sulfate (5.1), 1.0 mL of the copper sulfate solution (5.2), approximately 5 ± 0.1 mL of the prepared test sample (8) weighed to the nearest 0.1 mg, and 25 mL of the sulfuric acid (5.3), using the acid to wash down any copper sulfate solution, potassium sulfate, or test portion left on the neck of the flask. Gently mix the contents of the flask. For advice on sample size to apply this method to dairy products other than milk, please see Annex section.

9.2 **Determination**

9.2.1 **Digestion:** Carry out digestion using a digestion apparatus (6.7) the heater source of which can be adjusted to bring 250 mL of water (including 5 to 10 boiling aids) with an initial temperature of 25°C to a rolling boil in approximately 5-6 min. To determine the maximum heater setting to be used during digestion, preheat the heat source at the heater setting to be evaluated. For an electric heater the preheat period shall be 30 min. Determine the heater setting that brings water from 25°C to a rolling boil in 5-6 min. for each of the heaters. This is the maximum heater setting to be used during digestion for each heater.

Turn on the fume extraction system (6.7) prior to beginning the digestion. Heat the Kjeldahl flask on the digestion apparatus (6.7) using a heater setting low enough such that charred digest does not foam up inside the neck of the Kjeldahl flask. Digest at this setting until white fumes appear (approximately 20 min.) in the flask. Increase the heater setting halfway to the maximum setting determined in 9.2.1 and continue heating for 15 min. At the end of 15 min. increase the heat to maximum setting determined in 9.2.1. After the digest clears (clear with light blue-green color) continue boiling for 1-1.5 h at maximum setting. If the liquid does not boil, the final burner setting may be too low. The total digestion time will be between 1.8 and 2.25 h.

To determine the specific boiling time required for analysis conditions in a particular laboratory using a particular set of apparatus for milk analysis, select a high-protein, high-fat milk sample and determine its protein content using different boil times (1-1.5 hours) after clearing. The mean protein result increases with increasing boil time, becomes consistent, and then decreases when boil time is too long. Select the boil time that yields the maximum protein result.

At the end of digestion, the digest shall be clear and free of undigested material. Allow the acid digest to cool to room temperature in open flasks in a separate hood over a period of approximately 25 min. If the flasks are left on the hot burners to cool, it will take longer to reach room temperature. The cooled digest (when cooled off the burners) should be liquid or liquid with a few small crystals at the bottom of the flask at the end of 25 min.

Note: Excessive crystallization after 25 min. of cooling is the result of undue acid loss during digestion and can cause low test values. Undue acid loss is caused by excessive fume aspiration or an excessively long digestion time caused by an incorrect maximum burner setting.

After the digest has cooled to room temperature (at least 20 min.), add 300 mL of water (for 800-mL flasks add 400 mL of water), using the water to wash down the neck of the flask. Mix the contents thoroughly and ensure that any crystals that separate out are dissolved. Add 5 to 10 boiling aids (6.4). Allow the mixture to cool to room temperature prior to distillation. Do not leave the *undiluted* digest in the flasks overnight. The undiluted digest may crystallize during this period and will be very difficult to get back into solution. Avoid this situation. Diluted digests may be stoppered and held for distillation at a later time.

9.2.2 **Distillation:** Turn on the condenser water for the distillation apparatus (6.8). Add 75 mL of sodium hydroxide solution (5.4) to the cooled, diluted digest by carefully pouring the solution down the inclined neck of the flask so as to form a layer at the bottom of the bulb of the flask. There should be a clean interface between the two solutions. Immediately after the addition of the sodium hydroxide solution to the Kjeldahl flask, connect it to a distillation apparatus (6.8), the tip of whose condenser outlet tube is immersed in 50 mL of the boric acid solution (5.6) contained in a conical flask (6.9).

Vigorously swirl the Kjeldahl flask to mix contents thoroughly (no separate layers of solution should be visible in the flask) and set the flask down on the burner. Turn on the burner to a setting high enough to boil the mixture. Continue distillation until irregular boiling (bumping) starts and then immediately disconnect the Kjeldahl flask and turn off the burner. Turn off the condenser water.

The distillation rate shall be such that approximately 150 mL of distillate are collected when irregular boiling (bumping) starts and the total volume of the contents of the conical flask will be approximately 200 mL. If the volume of distillate collected is less than 150 mL, then it is likely that less than 300 mL of water was added to dilute the digest. The efficiency of the condenser shall be such that the temperature of the contents of the conical flask does not exceed 35°C during the distillation when using a colorimetric end-point. Control of temperature of the distillate is a more important issue when using a pH end-point measured with a pH meter.

9.2.3 **Titration:** Titrate the boric acid receiving solution with the standard volumetric hydrochloric acid solution (5.7) to the first trace of pink. Estimate the buret reading *at least the nearest 0.05 mL*. A lighted stir plate may aid visualization of the end point. For advice on measuring pH with a pH meter to determine the endpoint of the titration, please see Annex section.

9.3 **Blank test:** Blanks should always be titrated using the same titrant as used for the samples. Carry out a blank test following the procedure described in 9.1 to 9.2.3, taking 5 mL of water with about 0.85 g of sucrose (5.10) instead of the test portion of milk. The same titrant solution and buret must be used for both the blanks and the samples.

The purpose of the sucrose in a blank or a recovery standard is to act as organic material to consume an amount of sulfuric acid during digestion that is roughly equivalent to a sample. If the amount of residual-free sulfuric acid at the end of digestion is too low, the recovery of nitrogen by both recovery tests 9.4.1 and 9.4.2 will be low. If the amount of residual acid present at the end of digestion is sufficient to retain all the nitrogen, but the temperature and time conditions during digestion were not sufficient to release all the nitrogen from a sample, then the nitrogen recovery in section 9.4.1 will be acceptable and the nitrogen recovery in section 9.4.2 will be low.

The titration volume for the blank should always be greater than 0.0 mL, and blanks within the same laboratory should be consistent across time. If the blank is already pink before the beginning of titration, there is something wrong. Usually, the conical flasks are not clean or water from the air that may condense on the outside of the condenser apparatus has dripped down into the collection flask to cause the contamination. Keep a record of blank values. If blank values change, identify the cause.

9.4 **Recovery tests**

9.4.1 The accuracy of the procedure should be checked regularly by means of the following recovery tests, carried out in accordance with 9.1 to 9.2.3.

9.4.2 Check that no loss of nitrogen occurs (delete as a result of excessive heat or mechanical leaks during distillation) by using a test portion of 0.12 g of ammonium sulfate (5.8) along with 0.85 g of sucrose (5.10). The ammonium sulfate recovery check does not give information about the capability of the digestion conditions to release nitrogen that is bound in the protein structures.

The percentage of nitrogen recovered shall be between 99.0 and 100.0% for all positions on the apparatus. Ammonium sulfate only is useful to determine if nitrogen loss has occurred or if the normality of the titrant is lower than the stated value in the case when recoveries exceed 100%. For recoveries less than 99%, the loss could be in the digestion or distillation. It is possible to use a mixture of ammonium sulfate and small amount of sulfuric acid (the amount of residual remaining at the end of a digestion) in a flask, dilute it with the normal volume of water, add the normal amount of sodium hydroxide, and distill. In this case, if the nitrogen recovery is still low by the same amount, the loss of nitrogen is in the distillation apparatus not the digestion. The probable cause is leaky tubing in a traditional system or the tips of the condensers not submerged under the surface of the boric acid early in the distillation. The apparatus should pass this test before going on to check recoveries by the procedure in 9.4.3.

9.4.3 Check the efficiency of the digestion procedure by using 0.16 g of lysine hydrochloride (5.9) or 0.18 g of tryptophan (5.9) along with 0.67 g of sucrose (5.10).

At least 98% of the nitrogen shall be recovered. If the recovery is lower than 98% after having a 99 to 100% recovery on ammonium sulfate, then the temperature or time of digestion is insufficient (follow procedure in 9.2.1, paragraph 3) or there is undigested sample material (i.e., char) on the inside of the flask. The final evaluation of performance is best done by participation in a proficiency testing system, where within and between laboratory statistical parameters are computed based on analysis of milk samples.

9.4.4 Lower results in either of the recovery tests (or higher than 100.0% in 9.4.2) will indicate failures in the procedure and/or inaccurate concentration of the standard volumetric hydrochloric acid solution (5.7).

10. Expression of Results

10.1 **Calculation of nitrogen content:** The nitrogen content, expressed as a percentage by mass, is equal to

$$\frac{1,4007\ (V_S - V_b)M}{W}$$

where

V_S is the volume, in milliliters expressed to at least the nearest 0.05 mL, of the standard volumetric solution of acid used in the determination (9.2.3);

V_b is the volume, in milliliters expressed to at least the nearest 0.05 mL, of the standard volumetric solution of acid used in the blank test (9.3);

M is the exact molarity, to four decimal places, of the standard volumetric solution of acid (5.7);

W is the mass, in grams to the nearest 0.1 mg, of the test portion (9.1).

Round the result to the nearest 0.0001% nitrogen.

10.2 **Calculation of crude protein content:** The crude protein content, expressed as a percentage by mass, is obtained by multiplying the nitrogen content (10.1) by 6.38 and expressing the result to the nearest 0.001% crude protein.

11. Precision and Performance Parameters: Note: The values for repeatability and reproducibility have been derived from the results of interlaboratory tests in accordance with IDF Standard 135A:1988.[15,42]

11.1 **Repeatability:** The absolute difference between the results of two single determinations, carried out simultaneously or in rapid succession by the same operator under the same conditions on identical test material, shall not exceed 0.0060 g of nitrogen per 100 g of milk (0.038 g crude protein per 100 g of milk).

11.2 **Reproducibility:** The absolute difference between two single and independent results, obtained by two operators working in different laboratories on identical test material, shall not exceed 0.0077 g of nitrogen per 100 g of milk (0.049 g crude protein per 100 g of milk).

11.3 **Method performance statistics:** For raw milk (expressed as protein):

$S_r = 0.014$, $RSD_r = 0.385\%$ $r - value = 0.038$

$S_R = 0.017$, $RSD_R = 0.504\%$ $R - value = 0.049$

12. Test Report and Interpretation: The test report shall identify the method used and results obtained. The report will also identify any variation in the test not specified in this method as well as problems that may have impacted the test result. Each sample will be described in such a manner as to ensure traceablity as to its origin.

Annex

Advice on Modification of the Total Nitrogen Procedure for Analysis of Other Milk Products When a Separate Standard for That Product Does Not Exist and Advice on Using a pH End Point for Titration Instead of a Colorimetric End Point

(Supplemental Information Not Part of the Official Method)

A.0 Introduction: The procedure described in 15.131 and 15.132 has been optimized and evaluated for the analysis of bovine milk. An analyst may desire to use the same procedure, with slight modification, for the determination of the nitrogen content of a range of milk products. However, the procedure and its performance for such uses have not been validated.

A.1 Procedure: Weigh, to the nearest 0.1 mg, the required mass of test portion (taken from an appropriately prepared test sample) as described below, and proceed with the determination of the nitrogen content using the method described in 9.1 to 10.2.

The amounts of sulfuric acid (5.3) and sodium hydroxide solution (5.5) used in the digestion and distillation process should not be changed. Changing the ratio of acid to other components by increasing the amount of acid decreases the initial boiling point of the mixture in the digestion and this is not recommended.

The appropriate sample size for a material can be estimated as follows: The optimal quantity of protein per flask is between 0.15 and 0.30 g per flask for any sample. Thus, for example, if an average cheddar cheese sample contains 24.00% protein, then the amount of cheddar cheese sample should be between 0.625 g and 1.25 g. The decision to use sample weights that average at the low end of the range or the high end of the range depends on how much acid the remainder of the sample components (i.e., fat and carbohydrate) will consume during the digestion. In the Part 1 method the analyst starts with 25 mL (approx. 46 g) of sulfuric acid. By the end of the digestion there needs to be about 15 g of sulfuric acid left in the flask to retain all the nitrogen. The analyst must remember that sulfuric acid is consumed by the sample and is also lost due to volatilization during the digestion. The loss by volatilization can be equal to the amount consumed by the organic matter in a sample. The final amount of residual acid will be a function of both of these processes. Excessive loss of acid by volatilization (caused by excessive aspiration of fumes during digestion or the necks of the flasks being too hot) can result in too little residual acid left at the end of digestion even though the sample size is correct. Too little residual acid will result in crystallization of the digest after 25 min. of cooling and low recovery of nitrogen.

Cream containing 40% fat is an example of a difficult product. In this case the protein or nitrogen content of the sample is low and the fat content is high. Assume an average cream sample contains about 40% fat, 1.9% protein, and 2.9% lactose. To achieve 0.15 g of protein in the flask, it would be necessary to use a cream sample of 7.89 g. This sample would contain 3.16 g of fat and the fat alone would consume 56.9 g (ca. 30.9 mL) of sulfuric acid in the digestion without allowing for any loss of sulfuric acid due to volatilization (based on the assumption that 1 g of fat will consume 18 g of sulfuric acid during the digestion). This is a case where the amount of sample must to be reduced to allow for an adequate amount of sulfuric acid to remain at the end of the digestion. In the case of sample materials like cream, it would also be best to use a titrant that has a lower concentration (e.g., 0.01 mol/L).

The amount of sucrose required for a blank or for recovery standards for products other than bovine milk can be determined as follows: First an estimate is required of the approximate fat, protein, and carbohydrate content for the type of sample material and the approximate sample size to be used in digestion. Second, during digestion 1 g of fat will consume about 18 g of sulfuric acid, 1 g of protein will consume about 9 g of sulfuric acid, and 1 g of carbohydrate will consume about 7 g of sulfuric acid. Based on this information the amount of acid consumed by a sample can be calculated, and the amount of sucrose required to consume the same amount of acid during the digestion can be calculated. This amount of sucrose should be used for the blank and the ammonium sulfate recovery standard. For the amino acid nitrogen recovery standard (9.4.2), reduce the amount of sucrose added to the flask by the amount of acid that would be consumed (calculated as protein) by the lysine hydrochloride or tryptophan. You should not assume that nitrogen recovery in the digestion for your apparatus is the same for products other than milk, without conducting recovery experiments to produce conditions that achieve similar levels of residual sulfuric acid at the end of digestion.

A.2 Titration End-Point by pH Measurement

Some laboratories use a pH meter to determine the end-point of the titration for Kjeldahl analysis. Use of a pH meter to determine titration end-point, instead of a color indicator, introduces several new sources of error into the method that may influence repeatability and reproducibility performance of the method. The sources of error are accuracy of the pH of reference buffers, response time of the electrode, accuracy of pH calibration of the pH meter, definition of the target pH for the end-point, and control of temperature of the distillates and the reference buffers. The approach of using a measured pH end-point determination was not included in previous collaborative studies[15,42] that established the performance statistics for these methods. A collaborative study of this method of end-point determination may be warranted, but first thorough ruggedness testing of the factors influencing the titration end-point determination by pH should be carried out.

In the short term the best advice for a laboratory that chooses to use a pH measurement for the Kjeldahl end-point is the following: Check recoveries and repeatability performance within your lab to ensure that the performance in your laboratory meets the criteria described in 15.131 or 15.132. If this is achieved, then the laboratory should participate in a multilaboratory proficiency test of the methods described in 15.131 and 15.132. A comparison of results should be made between laboratories that follow the procedure described in 15.131 or 15.132 of the standard versus laboratories that use a pH end-point. If the pH end-point is providing equivalent results to the colorimetric end-point, then laboratories using the pH end-point should be able to meet the performance criteria given in the method for between-laboratory reproducibility when their results are compared with a lab using a colorimetric end-point.

15.132 Protein, Kjeldahl, Block Digester Method Milk (Class A1), Other Products (Class O)

1. **Scope:** This method is applicable for the determination of the total nitrogen content of milk.
2. **References:** Chapter 2 on "Laboratory Quality Assurance and Safety." Chapter 3 on "Sampling Dairy and Related Products."
3. **Definition:** Nitrogen content is the mass fraction of substances determined according to this procedure. It is expressed as a percentage by mass.
4. **Principle:** Digestion of a test portion, using a block-digestion apparatus, with a mixture of concentrated sulfuric acid and potassium sulfate, using copper(II) sulfate as a catalyst to thereby convert organic nitrogen present to ammonium sulfate. Excess sodium hydroxide is added to the cooled digest to liberate ammonia. Ammonia is distilled using steam distillation (either manual or semi-automatic steam distillation) with an excess of boric acid solution and titrated with hydrochloric acid solution. Nitrogen is calculated from the amount of ammonia produced.
5. **Reagents:** Unless otherwise specified all chemicals are reagent or ACS grade.
   - 5.1 Potassium sulfate (K_2SO_4): Low in nitrogen content. This reagent in combination with the reagent in section 5.2 may be purchased commercially as tablets or packets.
   - 5.2 Copper(II) sulfate solution: Dissolve 5.0 g of copper(II) sulfate pentahydrate ($CuSO_4 \bullet 5H_2O$) in water and dilute to the mark in a 100-mL one-mark volumetric flask. This reagent in combination with the reagent in section 5.1 may be purchased commercially as tablets or packets.
   - 5.3 Sulfuric acid, 95-98% (m/m): Nitrogen-free P_{20} approximately 1.84 g/mL.
   - 5.4 Sodium hydroxide solution: Low in nitrogen, containing 50 g of sodium hydroxide (NaOH) per 100 g. Note: 40% (m/m) sodium hydroxide solution may be used instead of 50% (m/m), if plugging of the flow system in an automatic distillation unit is a problem.
   - 5.5 Indicator solution: Dissolve 0.1 g methyl red and dilute to 50 mL in 95% (V/V) ethanol. Dissolve 0.5 g bromocresol green and dilute to 250 mL in 95% (V/V) ethanol. Mix 1 part of the methyl red solution with 5 parts of the bromocresol green solution or combine all of both solutions. Reagent is commercially available.
   - 5.6 Boric acid solution (with indicator): Dissolve 40.0 g of boric acid (H_3BO_3) in 1 L of hot water, allow to cool, bring to volume, add 3 mL of the indicator solution (5.5), mix and store in a borosilicate glass bottle. The solution will be light orange in color. Protect the solution from light and sources of ammonia fumes during storage.
   - 5.7 Hydrochloric acid: Standard volumetric solution, (HCl) = 0.1 ± 0.0005 mol/L (or 0.1 ± 0.0005 N).
   - 5.8 Ammonium sulfate [$(NH_4)2SO_4$]: Minimum assay 99.9% on dried material. Immediately before use, dry the ammonium sulfate at

102° ± 2°C for not less than 2 h and cool to room temperature in a desiccator.

5.9 Tryptophan ($C_{11}H_{12}N_2O_2$) or lysine hydrochloride ($C_6H_{15}ClN_2O_2$): Minimum assay 99%. Do not dry in oven before use.

5.10 Sucrose: Nitrogen content not more than 0.002% (m/m). Do not dry in oven before use.

6. **Apparatus and Glassware:** All volumetric flasks, pipets, and burets are Class A unless otherwise specified.

6.1 Water bath: Maintained at a temperature of 38° ± 1°C.

6.2 Analytical balance: Readability to nearest 0.1 mg.

6.3 Digestion block: Aluminum alloy block or equivalent apparatus[15] (see collaborative study), fitted with an adjustable temperature control and device for measuring block temperature.

6.4 Digestion tubes: Suitable for use with the digestion block (6.3), of capacity 250 mL.

6.5 Exhaust manifold: Suitable for use with the digestion tubes (6.4).

6.6 Centrifugal scrubber apparatus: Filter pump, or aspirator, constructed of acid resistant material and for use with the mains water supply.

6.7 Buret or automatic pipet: For delivering 1.0-mL portions of the copper sulfate solution (5.2).

6.8 Graduated measuring cylinders: Capacities 25 mL, 50 mL, and 100 mL.

6.9 Distillation unit, manual or semi-automatic: For steam distillation; suited to accept 250-mL digestion tubes (6.4) and 500-mL conical flasks (6.10).

6.10 Conical flasks: Capacity 500 mL, graduated.

6.11 Burette: Capacity 50 mL, graduated at least every 0.1 mL, complying with the requirements of ISO 385, class A.

7. **Sampling:** Chapter 3 on "Sampling Dairy and Related Products."

8. **Preparation of Test Sample:** Warm the milk sample to 38° ± 1°C by means of the water bath (6.1). Gently mix the milk sample immediately prior to weighing the test portion (9.1).

9. **Procedure:** Before beginning analysis review material safety data sheets on all chemicals and use appropriate safety equipment such as hoods, aprons, face shields, and glasses.

9.1 **Test portion and pretreatment:** To a clean and dry digestion tube (6.4) add 12 g of potassium sulfate (5.1), 1.0 mL of the copper sulfate solution (5.2), approximately 5 ± 0.1 mL of the prepared test sample (8) weighed to the nearest 0.1 mg, and 20 mL of the sulfuric acid (5.3), using the acid to wash down any copper sulfate solution, potassium sulfate, or test portion left on the upper walls of the digestion tube. Gently mix the contents of the tube.

Note: The amount of acid used in block digestors is less than that used in the traditional system (15.131) because it was determined in the collaborative study[15] that volumes of acid greater than 20 mL in the block digestion systems gave excessive foaming problems during digestion and variable results. Users of block digestors must note that maintaining sufficient residual sulfuric acid at the end of digestion needs more attention by the analyst in block digestors than in traditional systems. Excessive acid loss due to over aspiration of fumes is more of concern in block digestors than traditional systems.

For advice on sample size to apply this method to dairy products other than milk, please see Annex in method 15.131.

9.2 **Determination**

9.2.1 **Digestion:** Set the digestion block (6.3) at a low initial temperature so as to control foaming (approximately 180°-230°C). Transfer the tubes to the digestion block and place the exhaust manifold (6.5), which is itself connected to a centrifugal scrubber or similar device (6.6), in the top of the tube. The aspiration rate of the centrifugal scrubber or similar device shall be just sufficient to remove fumes. The complete digestion apparatus may need to be kept inside a fume hood.

Digest the sample for 30 min. or until white fumes develop. Then increase the temperature of the digestion block to 410°-430°C and continue digestion of the sample until the digest is clear.

Note: It may be necessary to increase the temperature gradually over a period of approximately 20 min. to control foaming. In any event, do not let foam rise higher than 4-5 cm below the surface of the exhaust manifold inserted into the top of the digestion tubes.

After the digest clears (clear with light blue-green color) continue digestion at 410°-430°C for at least 1 h. During this period the sulfuric acid must be boiling. If visible boiling of the clear liquid is not apparent as bubbles forming at the surface of the hot liquid around the perimeter of the tube, then the temperature of the block may be too low. The total digestion time will be between 1.75 and 2.5 h.

To determine the specific boiling time required for analysis conditions in a particular laboratory using a particular set of apparatus, select a high-protein, high-fat milk sample and determine its protein content using different boil times (1-1.5 h) after clearing. The mean protein content increases with increasing boil time, becomes consistent, and then decreases when boil time is too long. Select the boil time that yields the maximum protein result.

At the end of digestion, the digest should be clear and free of undigested material. Remove the tubes from the block with the exhaust manifold in place and allow to cool to room temperature over a period of approximately 25 minutes. The cooled digest should be liquid or liquid with a few small crystals at the bottom of the tube.

Note: Excessive crystallization after 25 minutes is the result of undue acid loss during digestion and can cause low test values. Undue acid loss is caused by excessive fume aspiration or an excessively long digestion time caused by digestion for too long a period at temperatures below the maximum temperature of the analysis. To reduce acid loss, reduce the rate of fume aspiration.

After the digest has cooled to room temperature (at least 20 min.), remove the exhaust manifold and carefully add 85 mL of water to each tube, swirl to mix, and ensure that any crystals that separate out are dissolved. Do not leave the cooled, undiluted digests overnight before water addition because they may solidify and will be extremely difficult to get back into solution in water. Allow the contents of the tube to cool to room temperature.

9.2.2 **Distillation:** Turn on the condenser water for the distillation apparatus. Attach the digestion tube containing the diluted digest to the distillation unit (6.9). Place a conical flask (6.10) containing 50 mL of the boric acid solution (5.6) under the outlet of the condenser in such a way that the delivery tube is below the surface of the boric acid solution. Adjust the distillation unit to dispense 55 mL of sodium hydroxide solution (5.4).

Note: Where 40% (m/m) sodium hydroxide solution is used, the dispensed volume should be adjusted to be 65 mL. If the automatic delivery of sodium hydroxide solution is extremely variable due to partial plugging of the delivery tubing for the sodium hydroxide, then large variability in duplicate test results will occur.

Having due regard to the manufacturer's instructions, operate the distillation unit in such a way as to steam distill the ammonia liberated by addition of the sodium hydroxide solution, collecting the distillate in the boric acid solution. Continue with the distillation process until at least 150 mL of distillate has been collected. Remove the conical flask from the distillation unit.

9.2.3 **Titration:** Titrate the boric acid receiving solution (5.6) with the standard volumetric hydrochloric acid solution (5.7) to the first trace of pink. Take the buret reading to at least the nearest 0.05 mL. A lighted stir plate may aid visualization of the end-point. For advice on measuring pH with a pH meter to determine the end-point of the titration, please see Annex in method 15.131.

9.3 **Blank test:** Blanks should always be titrated using the same titrant as used for the samples. Carry out a blank test following the procedure described in 9.1 to 9.2.3, taking 5 mL of water with about 0.85 g of sucrose (5.10) instead of the test portion.

The purpose of the sucrose in a blank or a recovery standard is to act as organic material to consume an amount of sulfuric acid during digestion that is roughly equivalent to a sample. If the amount of residual free sulfuric acid at the end of digestion is too low, the recovery of nitrogen by both recovery tests 9.4.1 and 9.4.2 will be low. If the amount of residual acid present at the end of digestion is sufficient to retain all the nitrogen, but the temperature and time conditions during digestion were not sufficient to release all the nitrogen from a sample, then the nitrogen recovery in section 9.4.1 will be acceptable and the nitrogen recovery in section 9.4.2 will be low.

The titration volume of the blank should always be greater than 0.0 mL and blanks within the same laboratory should be consistent across time. If the blank is already pink before the beginning of titration, there is something wrong. Usually, the conical flasks are not clean or water from the air that may condense on the outside of the condenser apparatus has dripped down into the collection flask to cause the contamination. Keep a record of blank values. If blank values change, identify the cause.

9.4 **Recovery tests**

9.4.1 The accuracy of the procedure should be checked regularly by means of the following recovery tests, carried out in accordance with 9.1 to 9.2.3.

9.4.2 Check that no loss of nitrogen occurs by using a test portion of 0.12 g of ammonium sulfate (5.8) along with 0.85 g of sucrose (5.10).

The percentage of nitrogen recovered shall be between 99.0 and 100.0% for all positions on the digestion apparatus. Ammonium sulfate only is useful to determine if nitrogen loss has occurred or if the normality of the titrant is lower than the stated value in the case when recoveries exceed 100%. For recoveries less than 99%, the loss could be in the digestion or distillation. It is possible to use a mixture of ammonium sulfate and small amount of sulfuric acid (the amount of residual remaining at the end of a digestion) in a flask, dilute it with the normal volume of water, add the normal amount of sodium hydroxide, and distill. In this case, if the nitrogen recovery is still low by the same amount, the loss of nitrogen is in the distillation apparatus not the digestion. The probable cause is leaky tubing in the distillation system or the tip of the condenser was not submerged under the surface of the boric acid early in the distillation. In older steam distillation systems that have had heavy use, it has been found the erosion of the glass parts by the hot sodium hydroxide inside the distillation system of the apparatus can result in small pin-hole leaks or cracks in the glass and loss of ammonia through these leaks. This is very difficult to detect, but this has been documented as the cause of low recoveries in some labs with older steam-distillation equipment. The apparatus should pass this test before going on to check recoveries by the procedure in 9.4.3.

9.4.3 Check the efficiency of the digestion procedure by using 0.16 g of lysine hydrochloride (5.9) or 0.18 g of tryptophan (5.9) along with 0.67 g of sucrose (5.10).

At least 98.0% of the nitrogen shall be recovered. If the recovery is lower than 98% after having a 99 to 100% recovery on ammonium sulfate, then the temperature or time of digestion is insufficient (follow procedure in 9.2.1, paragraph 5) or there is undigested sample material (i.e., char) on the inside of the flask. The final evaluation of performance is best done by participation in a proficiency testing system where within and between laboratory statistical parameters are computed based on analysis of milk samples.

9.4.4 Lower results in either of the recovery tests (9.4.2 and 9.4.3) will indicate failures in the procedure and/or inaccurate concentration of the standard volumetric hydrochloric acid solution (5.7).

10. Expression of Results

10.1 **Calculation of nitrogen content:** The nitrogen content, expressed as a percentage by mass, is equal to

$$\frac{1{,}4007\,(V_S - V_b)M}{W}$$

where

V_S is the volume, in milliliters expressed to at least the nearest 0.05 mL, of the standard volumetric solution of acid used in the determination (9.2.3);

V_b is the volume, in milliliters expressed to at least the nearest 0.05 mL, of the standard volumetric solution of acid used in the blank test (9.3);

M is the exact molarity, to four decimal places, of the standard volumetric solution of acid (5.7); and

W is the mass, in grams to the nearest 0.1 mg, of the test portion (9.1).

Round the result to the nearest 0.0001% nitrogen.

10.2 **Calculation of crude protein content:** The crude protein content, expressed as a percentage by mass, is obtained by multiplying the nitrogen content (10.1) by 6.38 and expressing the result to the nearest 0.001% crude protein.

11. Precision and Performance Parameters: Note: the values for repeatability and reproducibility have been derived from the results of interlaboratory tests in accordance with IDF Standard 135A:1988.[15,42]

11.1 **Repeatability:** The absolute difference between the results of two single determinations, carried out simultaneously or in rapid succession by the same operator under the same conditions on identical test material, shall not exceed 0.0060 g of nitrogen per 100 g of milk (0.038 g crude protein per 100 g of milk).

11.2 **Reproducibility:** The absolute difference between two single and independent results, obtained by two operators working in different laboratories on identical test material, shall not exceed 0.0077 g of nitrogen per 100 g of milk (0.049 g crude protein per 100 g of milk).

11.3 **Method performance statistics:** For raw milk (expressed as protein):

$S_r = 0.014$, $RSD_r = 0.385\%$ r – value = 0.038

$S_R = 0.017$, $RSD_R = 0.504\%$ $R - \text{value} = 0.049$

12. **Test Report and Interpretation:** The test report shall identify the method used and results obtained. The report will also identify any variation in the test not specified in this method as well as problems that may have impacted the test result. Each sample will be described in such a manner as to ensure traceablity as to its origin.

15.133 Protein-Nitrogen (True Protein) Method, Direct and Indirect (Class A1)[11(991.22, -.23),15,17]

1. **Scope:** This method is applicable for the determination of protein nitrogen (true protein) content of raw milk.
2. **References:** Chapter 2 on "Laboratory Quality Assurance and Safety." Chapter 3 on "Sampling Dairy and Related Products."
   Chapter 15, methods 15.131 and 15.132.
3. **Definition:** The protein-nitrogen content is the mass fraction of substances determined according to the procedure specified in this method or by subtracting the result from method 15.135 from the results of method 15.131 or 15.132.
4. **Principle:** Precipitation of protein from a test portion by addition of trichloroacetic acid solution such that the final concentration of trichloroacetic acid in the mixture is approximately 12%. Separation of the protein precipitate by filtration. (The filtrate will contain the non-protein nitrogen contents.) Determination of the nitrogen content of the precipitate by the procedure described in method 15.131 or 15.132 is the direct method for true protein determination. Alternatively, a classical indirect determination of the true protein nitrogen content of a milk can be calculated by subtracting the value obtained for the non-protein nitrogen content of milk (determined using method 15.135) from the crude protein nitrogen content of the same sample (determined using method 15.131 or 15.132).
5. **Reagents:** Unless otherwise specified all chemicals are reagent or ACS grade.

   The reagents specified for the determination of total nitrogen by the method described in method 15.131 or 15.132 together with the following are required.

   5.1 **Trichloroacetic acid solution:** Dissolve 15.0 g of trichloroacetic acid (CCl_3COOH) in water and dilute to the mark in a 100-mL one-mark volumetric flask. Do not use concentrations of trichloroacetic acid and volumes of solutions other than those specified, because the performance of the method with respect to mean value and performance characteristics will be different.
6. **Apparatus and Glassware:** All volumetric flasks, pipets, and burets are Class A unless otherwise specified.

   6.1 Pipet: Capacity 5 mL.

   6.2 Filter funnel: Glass, diameter 75 mm.

   6.3 Filter paper: Diameter 15 cm, nitrogen-free, Whatman No. 1 or equivalent.

6.4 Automatic pipet: Piston pump pipet for delivering 10-mL portions of the trichloroacetic acid solution (5.1).

7. **Sampling:** Chapter 3 on "Sampling Dairy and Related Products."

8. **Preparation of Test Sample:** Warm the sample to 38° ± 1°C by means of the water bath. Gently mix the sample immediately prior to weighing the test portion (9.1).

9. **Procedure:** Before beginning analysis review material safety data sheets on all chemicals and use appropriate safety equipment such as hoods, aprons, face shields, and glasses.

9.1 **Test portion:** Weigh approximately 5 ± 0.1 mL, to the nearest 0.1 mg, of the prepared sample (8) into a Kjeldahl flask or digestion tube. Immediately add 5 ± 0.1 mL of water to the Kjeldahl flask or digestion tube, rinsing any milk on the neck of the flask or tube to the bottom.

9.2 **Determination**

9.2.1 Add 40 ± 0.5 mL of the trichloroacetic acid solution (5.1) to the flask or tube and swirl to mix the contents. Let the flask or tube stand for approximately 5 min. to allow the precipitate to settle (the precipitation must be done in the Kjeldahl flask or tube). Pour the mixture from the Kjeldahl flask or digestion tube through a filter paper (6.3) and collect the filtrate. Some of the precipitate will remain in the Kjeldahl flask or digestion tube and some will be collected on the filter paper. It is not necessary to remove all of the precipitate from the flask.

Immediately after pouring the mixture and so as not to allow any precipitate to dry on the neck of the Kjeldahl flask or digestion tube, add by means of an automatic pipet (6.4) 10 mL of the trichloroacetic acid solution, using the solution to rinse any precipitate from the neck of the flask or tube down into the bottom. Swirl to mix the contents. Pour the mixture from the flask or tube through the same filter paper, adding the filtrate to that collected previously. Again, immediately rinse the neck of the flask or tube with a further 10 mL of trichloroacetic acid solution. Swirl to mix the contents and again pour the mixture from the flask or tube through the same filter paper, adding the filtrate to that collected previously. The filtrate shall be clear and free of particulate matter.

Note: At this point, the filtrate is no longer needed and may be discarded in an appropriate manner.

9.2.2 Wearing gloves, carefully remove the filter paper from the filter funnel and fold the paper to enclose the precipitate. If any precipitate remains on either the inner or outer lip of the Kjeldahl flask or digestion tube, wipe with the folded filter paper so that any precipitate adheres to the paper and then drop the filter paper into the Kjeldahl flask or digestion tube.

9.2.3 Add boiling aids, potassium sulfate, copper catalyst solution, and sulfuric acid. Determine the nitrogen content of the precipitate and filter paper by the procedure described in methods 15.131 or 15.132.

9.3 **Blank test:** Carry out a blank test, taking a filter paper (6.3) washed with trichloroacetic acid solution (5.1) instead of the test portion. Keep a record of blank values. If blank values change, identify cause.

10. Expression of Results

10.1 **Calculation of protein-nitrogen content:** The protein-nitrogen content, expressed as a percentage by mass, is equal to

$$\frac{1{,}4007\,(V_S - V_b)M}{W}$$

where

V_S is the volume, in milliliters expressed to at least the nearest 0.05 mL, of the standard volumetric solution of acid used in the determination;

V_b is the volume, in milliliters expressed to at least the nearest 0.05 mL, of the standard volumetric solution of acid used in the blank test;

M is the exact molarity, to four decimal places, of the standard volumetric solution of acid; and

W is the mass, in grams to the nearest 0.1 mg, of the test portion.

Round the result to the nearest 0.0001% nitrogen.

10.2 **Calculation of "protein equivalent":** The protein-nitrogen content, expressed as "protein equivalent," is obtained by multiplying the protein-nitrogen content (10.1) by 6.38. This corresponds to the true protein content of milk.

11. Precision and Performance Parameters: Note: The values for repeatability and reproducibility have been derived from the results of interlaboratory tests in accordance with IDF Standard 135A:1988.[17,42]

11.1 **Repeatability:** The absolute difference between the results of two single determinations, carried out simultaneously or in rapid succession by the same operator under the same conditions on identical test material, shall not exceed 0.0038 g of protein-nitrogen per 100 g of milk (0.024 g of true protein per 100 g of milk).

11.2 **Reproducibility:** The absolute difference between two single and independent results, obtained by two operators working in different laboratories on identical test material, shall not exceed 0.0092 g of protein-nitrogen per 100 g of milk (0.059 g of true protein per 100 g of milk).

11.3 **Method performance statistics:** For raw milk (expressed as protein):

Indirect method:

$S_r = 0.014$, $RSD_r = 0.483\%$ $r - \text{value} = 0.040$

$S_R = 0.031$, $RSD_R = 1.051\%$ $R - \text{value} = 0.080$

Direct method:

$S_r = 0.008$, $RSD_r = 0.285\%$ $r - \text{value} = 0.024$

$S_R = 0.021$, $RSD_R = 0.702\%$ $R - \text{value} = 0.059$

12. Test Report and Interpretation: The test report shall identify the method used and results obtained. The report will also identify any variation in the test not specified in this method as well as problems that may have impacted the test result. Each sample will be described in such a manner as to ensure traceablity as to its origin.

15.134 Undenatured Whey Protein Nitrogen (Class O)

1. **Scope:** This method is applicable to nonfat dry milk.
2. **References:** Chapter 2 on "Laboratory Quality Assurance and Safety." Chapter 3 on "Sampling Dairy and Related Products." Chapter 15, methods 15.131 and 15.132.
3. **Definition:** Undenatured whey protein nitrogen is defined as the amount of undenatured whey protein present in the nonfat dry milk powder expressed as nitrogen in milligrams per gram.
4. **Principle:** The nonfat dry milk is rehydrated, heated in a saturated sodium chloride solution, and filtered. The filtrate contains the undenatured whey proteins as well as the non-protein nitrogen fractions. The filter contains the casein and denatured whey protein fractions. The filtrate is diluted in a saturated salt solution and acidified, and the solution is measured spectophometrically. The transmittance obtained is compared to a standard curve that plots Kjeldahl nitrogen values from standards against transmittance for those standards.
5. **Reagents:** Unless otherwise specified all chemicals are reagent or ACS grade.
   - 5.1 Sodium chloride.
   - 5.2 Sodium chloride, saturated solution: Dissolve 1000 g of sodium chloride in 2000 mL of LG water and heat the mixture to near boiling while frequently stirring to ensure complete saturation. Cool to room temperature and filter through S&S No. 605 pleated filter paper and store the filtrate at room temperature.
   - 5.3 Hydrochloric acid (HCL): Add 23 mL of concentrated reagent grade HCL to 77 mL of LG water.
   - 5.4 LG water.
   - 5.5 Standard reference samples: Low-heat nonfat dry milk (NDM) and high-heat NDM (available from American Dairy Products Institute, 130 North Franklin Street, Chicago, IL 60606).
6. **Apparatus and Glassware:** All volumetric flasks, pipets, and burets are Class A unless otherwise specified.
   - 6.1 Balance: 0.1 mg accuracy.
   - 6.2 Corks: Rubber to fit 25- × 150-mm test tubes.
   - 6.3 Cuvets: Sufficient size to handle a minimum of 15 mL of solution.
   - 6.4 Filter Paper: S&S No. 602, 9 cm or equivalent; S&S No. 605, 15 cm pleated or equivalent.
   - 6.5 Flask: Erlenmeyer, 500 mL.
   - 6.6 Funnels: Short stem, diameter 50 mm, stem length 65 mm; short stem, diameter 90 mm, stem length 65 mm.
   - 6.7 Pipets or pipeters: Ostwald-Folin type, 1, 2, 3, 4, and 5 mL; volumetric, 5, 10, 20, and 100 mL.
   - 6.8 Spectrophometer or colorimeter: Spectronic 20 or equivalent.
   - 6.9 Test tubes: 25 × 150 mm, screw cap type acceptable.

6.10 Water bath: Controlled at 37° ± 1°C.

6.11 Watch glasses: To fit over 90-mm diameter funnel.

7. **Sampling:** Chapter 3 on "Sampling Dairy and Related Products."

8. **Preparation of Test Sample:** Take a representative nonfat dry milk powder sample that has previously been mixed, stirred, ground, blended, or otherwise prepared in order to make sample uniform.

9. **Procedure:** Before beginning analysis review material safety data sheets on all chemicals and use appropriate safety equipment such as hoods, aprons, face shields, and glasses.

9.1 Weigh 2 grams of nonfat dry milk (NDM) into a 25- × 150-mm test tube.

9.2 Add 20 mL of LG water and mix thoroughly.

9.3 Add 8 grams of sodium chloride granules from section 5.1, shake, and place in 37°C water bath for 30 minutes.

9.4 Shake samples 8-10 times during the first 15 minutes of incubation time to ensure complete saturation of the sample with sodium chloride. Allow samples to remain undisturbed the last 15 minutes of incubation.

9.5 At the end of the 30-minute incubation, shake mixture without cooling, and pour through a S&S No. 602 9-cm filter paper. Refilter through the same filter paper if the first portion of filtrate is cloudy.

9.6 Pipet 1 mL of the filtrate into a cuvette and dilute with 10 mL of saturated sodium chloride solution. Stopper the cuvette and mix by slowly inverting once.

9.7 Add 2 drops (delivered from a 5-mL volumetric pipet or an equivalent volume) of the HCl solution to develop the turbidity. Stopper the cuvette and mix the acid with the diluted filtrate by slowly inverting twice. Invert slowly to prevent the formation of foam or bubbles.

9.8 Within 5-10 minutes of adding the acid, invert cuvette once again and measure the turbidity in the instrument with the wavelength set at 420 nanometers.

9.9 Adjust the instrument to 100% transmittance with a diluted casein-free filtrate made by diluting 1 mL of the original filtrate with 10 mL of saturated sodium chloride solution. Check the day-to-day reproducibility of the spectrophotometer by following the manufacturer's recommendations.

9.10 Make duplicate determinations on each filtrate.

10. **Expression of Results**

10.1 **Calculation:** For each transmittance reading, obtain a value for WPN from the standard curve. Take an average of the duplicates and report as milligrams of WPN per gram NDM.

10.2 **Standard curve preparation**

10.2.1 Mix 20 grams of each of the standard low-heat and high-heat NDM with exactly 200 mL of LG water in a 500-mL Erlenmeyer flask.

10.2.2 Add 80 grams of sodium chloride crystals to flask, stopper, and shake for 1 minute.

10.2.3 Incubate flask for 30 minutes at 37°C. Shake mixture from 8 to 10 times during the first 15 minutes to ensure complete saturation of sodium chloride. Allow flasks to remain undisturbed the last 15 minutes of incubation.

10.2.4 After the 30-minute incubation pour sample from flask into an S&S No. 605 pleated filter (15 cm). If the first portion of the filtrate is cloudy, refilter through the same filter. Filter until approximately 100 mL of filtrate has been collected. Cover filters with watch glasses to prevent evaporation during filtration.

10.2.5 Pipet proportions of low-heat and high-heat filtrates into 25- × 150-mm test tubes as follows:

Tube number	Low-Heat Filtrate	High-Heat Filtrate
1	10	0
2	8	2
3	6	4
4	4	2
5	2	8
6	0	10

10.2.6 Stopper the tubes containing the combined filtrates and mix by slowly inverting the tubes twice.

10.2.7 Pipet 1 mL of the mixed filtrates into cuvettes, dilute with 10 mL of saturated sodium chloride solution. Proceed as in sections 9.6, 9.7, 9.8, 9.9, and 9.10.

10.2.8 Plot the standard curve using the WPN/gram values provided with the standards on the horizontal axis and percent transmittance as the vertical axis on 8 ½ × 11 inch graph paper (1 mg WPN equals 1 inch, 10% transmittance equals 1 inch).

10.2.9 It is essential that the difference in transmittance readings between the low-heat and high-heat filtrates be at least 35%.

10.3 **Moisture-corrected values:** Whey protein nitrogen (WPN) values given by the reference samples are obtained by a modified Kjeldahl analysis and have been corrected to a 3.16% moisture content.[6] To correct the WPN value of nonfat dry milk to a 3.16% moisture content, use the following equation.

$$\text{WPN @ 3.16\% moisture} = \frac{[100 + (\text{\% moisture} - 3.16\%)]\ [\text{WPN value}]}{100}$$

11. Precision and Performance Parameters: No precision data available for this test.

12. Test Report and Interpretation: The test report shall identify the method used and results obtained. The report will also identify any variation in the test not specified in this method as well as problems that may have impacted the test result.

Each sample will be described in such a manner as to ensure traceability as to its origin.

12.1 When interpreting the WPN values keep in mind that as the heat increases in the processing of nonfat dry milk the WPN value will decrease. Typically, low-heat nonfat dry milk has a WPN of at least 6 mg of WPN/gram on nonfat dry milk. High-heat powder typically has a WPN value of less than 1.5 WPN/gram of nonfat dry milk.

15.135 Non-Protein Nitrogen, Kjeldahl (Class A1)

1. **Scope:** This method is applicable to raw milk.
2. **References:** Chapter 2 on "Laboratory Quality Assurance and Safety." Chapter 3 on "Sampling Dairy and Related Products."
   Chapter 15, methods 15.131 and 15.132.
3. **Definition:** Non-protein nitrogen is defined as the mass fraction of substances determined according to the procedure specified in this method. It is expressed as a percentage by mass.
4. **Principle:** Precipitation of protein from a test portion by addition of trichloroacetic acid solution such that the final concentration of trichloroacetic acid in the mixture is approximately 12%. Removal of the precipitated milk protein by filtration, the remaining filtrate containing the non-protein nitrogen components. Determination of the nitrogen content of the filtrate by the procedure described in 15.131 or 15.132.
5. **Reagents:** Unless otherwise specified all chemicals are reagent or ACS grade.

   The reagents specified for the determination of total nitrogen by the method described in 15.131 or 15.132, with the exception of 0.10 mol/L (0.10 N) hydrochloric acid, together with the following, are required.

   5.1 **Trichloroacetic acid solution:** Dissolve 15.0 g of trichloroacetic acid (CCl_3COOH) in water and dilute to the mark in a 100-mL one-mark volumetric flask. Do not use concentrations of trichloroacetic acid and volumes of solutions other than those specified, because the performance of the method with respect to mean value and between laboratory performance characteristics will be different.

   5.2 **Hydrochloric acid:** Standard volumetric solution c(HCl) = 0.01 ± 0.0001 mol/L (0.01 ± .0001 N).
6. **Apparatus and Glassware:** All volumetric flasks, pipets, and burets are Class A unless otherwise specified.

   The equipment specified in 15.131 or15.132 together with the following are required.

   6.1 Conical flasks: Capacity 125 mL.

   6.2 Pipets: Capacities 10 mL and 20 mL.

   6.3 Filter funnel: Glass or plastic, diameter 75 mm.

   6.4 Filter paper: Diameter 15 cm, nitrogen-free, Whatman No. 1 or equivalent.

   6.5 Beaker: Capacity 50 mL.
7. **Sampling:** Chapter 3 on "Sampling Dairy and Related Products."
8. **Preparation of Test Sample:** Warm the sample to 38° ± 1°C by means of the water bath. Gently mix the sample immediately prior to weighing the test portion (9.1).

9. **Procedure:** Before beginning analysis review material safety data sheets on all chemicals and use appropriate safety equipment such as hoods, aprons, face shields, and glasses.

9.1 **Test portion:** Pipet 10.0 ± 0.1 mL of the prepared test sample (8) into a preweighed conical flask (6.1) and reweigh, recording the weights to the nearest 0.1 mg.

9.2 **Determination**

9.2.1 Add 40 mL of trichloroacetic acid solution (5.1) to the flask and weigh the flask and contents to the nearest 0.1 mg. Swirl to mix. Let the flask stand for approximately 5 min. to allow the precipitate to settle. Filter the contents of the flask through a filter paper (6.4) and collect the entire filtrate in a clean, dry conical flask (6.1). The filtrate should be clear and free of particulate matter. If it is not, repeat the process of precipitation and filtration with a new test portion of milk. If duplicate tests are to be done, then separate precipitations and filtrations should be done.

9.2.2 Swirl the filtrate to ensure that it is mixed and then pipet 20 mL of the filtrate into a 50-mL beaker (6.5) and weigh. Pour the filtrate from the beaker into a Kjeldahl flask or digestion tube containing boiling acid, potassium sulfate, and copper sulfate solution as specified in 15.131 or 15.132. Immediately reweigh the empty beaker.

9.2.3 Add the appropriate amount of sulfuric acid to the Kjeldahl flask or digestion tube and continue with the digestion and distillation procedure specified in 15.131 or 15.132.

9.2.4 Titrate the liberated ammonia, using the 0.01 mol/L standard volumetric hydrochloric acid solution (5.2) as titrant (instead of the 0.1 mol/L hydrochloric acid solution as used in 15.131 or 15.132).

9.3 **Blank test:** Digest, distill, and titrate a blank comprising about 0.1 g of sucrose and 16 ± 0.5 mL of trichloroacetic acid solution (5.1).

Blanks should always be titrated with the same solution used to titrate samples. Keep a record of blank values. If blank values change, identify the cause.

10. **Expression of Results:** Where the total nitrogen content of the milk sample has previously been determined, the true protein-nitrogen content can be calculated as the difference between the total nitrogen content and the non-protein nitrogen content.

10.1 **Calculation of non-protein nitrogen content:** The non-protein nitrogen content, expressed as a percentage by mass, is equal to

$$\frac{1.4007(V_S - V_b)M}{W_f \times W_m/(Wt - 0.065\ W_m)}$$

where

V_S is the volume, in milliliters expressed at least to the nearest 0.05 mL, of the standard volumetric solution of acid used in the sample determination (9.2.4);

V_b is the volume, in milliliters expressed at least to the nearest

0.05 mL, of the standard volumetric solution of acid used in the blank test (9.3);

M is the exact molarity of the standard volumetric solution of acid (5.2);

W_f is the mass, in grams to the nearest 0.1 mg, of 20 mL of filtrate (9.2.2);

W_m is the mass, in grams to the nearest 0.1 mg, of the test portion of milk (9.1);

Wt is the mass, in grams to the nearest 0.1 mg, of the test portion of milk plus 40 mL of trichloroacetic acid solution (9.2.1).

Round the result to the nearest 0.0001% nitrogen.

Note: The factor 0.065 in the denominator assumes that milk contains about 3.5% fat and 3.0% true protein (thus 0.035 + 0.030). The factor may need to be adjusted if liquid dairy products of significantly different composition are analyzed (for example, concentrated or fractionated skim or whole milk products, etc.).

10.2 **Calculation of "protein equivalent":** The non-protein nitrogen content, expressed as "protein equivalent," is obtained by multiplying the nonprotein nitrogen content (10.1) by 6.38. Round the result to nearest 0.001% protein.

11. **Precision and Performance Parameters:** Note: The values for repeatability and reproducibility have been derived from the results of interlaboratory tests in accordance with Horwitz[38] and Barbano et al.[15]

11.1 **Repeatability:** The absolute difference between the results of two single determinations, carried out simultaneously or in rapid succession by the same operator under the same conditions on identical test material, should not exceed 0.0025 g of non-protein nitrogen per 100 g of milk (0.016 g of non-protein nitrogen on a protein equivalent basis per 100 g of milk).

11.2 **Reproducibility:** The absolute difference between two single and independent results, obtained by two operators working in different laboratories on identical test material, should not exceed 0.0052 g of non-protein nitrogen per 100 g of milk (0.033 g of non-protein-nitrogen on a protein equivalent basis per 100 g of milk).

11.3 **Method performance statistics** (for raw milk[17]).

$s_r = 0.006$	$RSD_r = 2.817\%$	r value = 0.016
$s_R = 0.012$	$RSD_R = 5.707\%$	R value = 0.033

12. **Test Report and Interpretation:** The test report shall identify the method used and results obtained. The report will also identify any variation in the test not specified in this method as well as problems that may have impacted the test result. Each sample will be described in such a manner as to ensure traceablity as to its origin.

15.136 Casein Nitrogen/Protein, Indirect, Kjeldahl (Class A1)[11(998.05-.07),15,38,40,77]

1. **Scope:** This method is applicable to fresh raw milk. Casein nitrogen will decrease with milk storage time due to casein breakdown even at 4°C.

The casein nitrogen of heat-treated milk will be artificially high because of whey protein denaturation.

2. **References:** Chapter 2 on "Laboratory Quality Assurance and Safety." Chapter 3 on "Sampling Dairy and Related Products." Chapter 15, methods 15.131 and 15.132.

3. **Definition:** Non-casein nitrogen is the mass fraction of substances determined according to the procedures specified in this method. Protein nitrogen is the mass fraction of substances determined according to the procedures specified in methods 15.131 or 15.132.

   The difference between the two values is the casein nitrogen and is expressed as a percentage by mass.

4. **Principle:** Determination of total nitrogen content of a test portion by the procedure described in 15.131 or 15.132 of the total nitrogen method. Precipitation of casein from a separate test portion by addition of acetic acid and sodium acetate solutions such that the final pH of the mixture is approximately 4.6. Removal of the precipitated milk casein by filtration, the remaining filtrate containing the non-casein nitrogen components. Determination of the nitrogen content of the filtrate by the procedure described in 15.131 or 15.132 of the total nitrogen method. Calculation of casein nitrogen content as the difference between total nitrogen content and non-casein nitrogen content.

5. **Reagents:** Unless otherwise specified all chemicals are reagent or ACS grade.

   The reagents specified for the determination of total nitrogen by the method described in method 15.131 or 15.132, together with the following, are required.

   5.1 Acetic acid solution, 10% (v/v): Pipet 10.0 mL of glacial acetic acid (CH_3COOH) into a 100-mL volumetric flask and dilute to the mark.

   5.2 Sodium acetate solution, 1N: Dissolve 8.20 g of sodium acetate (CH_3COONa) or 13.60 g of sodium acetate trihydrate ($CH_3COONa \bullet 3H_2O$) in water and dilute to the mark in a 100-mL volumetric flask. Prepare weekly.

6. **Apparatus and Glassware:** All volumetric flasks, pipets, and burets are Class A unless otherwise specified.

   Usual laboratory equipment and the equipment specified in 15.131 or 15.132, together with the following, are required.

   6.1 Water bath: Maintained at a temperature of 38° ± 1°C.
   6.2 Volumetric flasks with stoppers: Capacity 100 mL, class A.
   6.3 Serological pipet: Capacity 10 mL.
   6.4 Graduated measuring cylinder: Capacity 100 mL.
   6.5 Volumetric pipets: Capacities 1 mL and 50 mL, class A.
   6.6 Filter funnel: Glass or plastic, diameter 75 mm.
   6.7 Filter paper: Diameter 15 cm, nitrogen-free, Whatman No. 1 or equivalent. Pleat before use.
   6.8 Conical flasks or equivalent: Capacity 100 mL.

7. **Sampling:** Chapter 3 on "Sampling Dairy and Related Products."

8. **Preparation of Test Sample:** Warm the milk sample to 38° ± 1°C by means of a water bath (6.1). Gently mix the milk sample immediately

prior to weighing the test portion (9.1.1, 9.2.1).

9. **Procedure:** Before beginning analysis review material safety data sheets on all chemicals and use appropriate safety equipment such as hoods, aprons, face shields, and glasses.

9.1 **Total nitrogen determination**

9.1.1 Determine the total nitrogen content of the test sample (8) as described in 15.131 and 15132.

9.2 **Non-casein nitrogen determination**

9.2.1 Test portion: Pipet (6.3) 10.0 mL of the prepared test sample (8) into a preweighed 100-mL volumetric flask (6.2) and reweigh, recording the weights to the nearest 0.1 mg.

Note: Additional samples may be weighed at this point, but the additions of water, acetic acid solution, and sodium acetate solution plus filtration should occur within 15 minutes of weighing the milk. This minimizes proteolytic degradation of casein during sample preparation.

9.2.2 Add 75 mL (6.4) of 38°C water to the flask. Pipet (6.5) 1 mL of acetic acid solution (5.1) into flask. Stopper and swirl to mix. Incubate flask for 10 minutes in a 38°C water bath (6.1). Pipet (6.5) 1 mL of sodium acetate solution (5.2) into flask. Swirl to mix. Cool contents of flask to 20°C. Dilute to the mark with 20°C water. Stopper and invert to mix. Let precipitate settle. Filter the contents of the flask using a filter funnel (6.6) and a pleated filter paper (6.7) and collect entire filtrate in a conical flask (6.8). The filtrate should be clear and free of particulate matter. If it is not, repeat the process of precipitation and filtration with a new test portion.

9.2.3 Swirl the filtrate to ensure that it is mixed and then pipet (6.5) 50 mL of it into a Kjeldahl flask or digestion tube containing boiling aid, potassium sulfate, and copper solution as specified in 15.131 and 15.132.

9.2.4 Add the appropriate amount of sulfuric acid to the Kjeldahl flask or digestion tube. Digest, distill, and titrate as specified for milk in 15.131 or 15.132 of the total nitrogen method. Flask or tube may be stoppered after the addition of sulfuric acid, and digested, distilled, and titrated at a later time. When using 15.132 of the total nitrogen, caution should be taken to provide gradual heating if the digest foams excessively. The total digestion time may be longer than for milk total nitrogen.

9.2.5 **Blank test:** Digest, distill, and titrate a blank comprised of 50 mL of water, 0.5 mL of acetic acid solution (5.1), and 0.5 mL of sodium acetate solution (5.2).

10. **Expression of Results**

10.1 **Calculation of non-casein nitrogen content:** The non-casein nitrogen content, expressed as a percentage by mass, is equal to

$$\frac{1.4007 \times (V_S - V_b) \times M \times 2 \times 0.994}{W_m}$$

where

V_S is the volume, reported to a least the nearest 0.05 milliliters, of the standard volumetric solution of acid used in the determination (15.131 or 15.132);

V_b is the volume, reported to a least the nearest 0.05 milliliters, of the standard volumetric solution of acid used in the blank test (15.131 or 15.132);

M is the exact molarity, reported to four decimal places, of the standard volumetric solution of acid (15.131 or 15.132); and

W_m is the mass, in grams reported to four decimal places, of the test portion of milk (9.2.1).

Round the result to the nearest 0.0001%.

Note: The factor 0.994 in the numerator assumes that milk contains about 3.7% fat and 2.6% casein. The factor may need to be adjusted if liquid dairy products of significantly different composition are analyzed[77]: Factor = 1 − (0.11 × %fat/100) + (0.07 × %casein/100).

10.2 **Calculation of non-casein protein:** The non-casein nitrogen content, expressed as noncasein protein, is obtained by multiplying the noncasein nitrogen content (10.1) by 6.38. Round the result to the nearest 0.001%.

10.3 **Calculation of casein nitrogen:** The casein nitrogen content, expressed as a percentage by mass, is equal to total nitrogen content (9.1) minus non-casein nitrogen content (10.1). Round the result to the nearest 0.0001%.

10.4 **Calculation of casein protein:** The casein content, expressed as casein protein, is obtained by multiplying the casein nitrogen content (10.3) by 6.38. Round the result to the nearest 0.001%.

11. Precision and Performance Parameters

11.1 **Repeatability:** The absolute difference between the results of two single non-casein nitrogen determinations, carried out simultaneously or in rapid succession by the same operator under the same conditions on identical test material, should not exceed (expressed as % nitrogen) 0.0043 g of non-casein nitrogen per 100 g of milk, or (expressed as % protein) 0.028 g of casein protein per 100 g of milk.

The absolute difference between the results of two single indirect casein nitrogen determinations, carried out simultaneously or in rapid succession by the same operator under the same conditions on identical test material, should not exceed (expressed as % nitrogen) 0.0064 g of indirect casein nitrogen per 100 g of milk, or (expressed as % protein) 0.041 g of indirect casein protein per 100 g of milk.

11.2 **Reproducibility:** The absolute difference between the results of two single and independent non-casein nitrogen determinations, obtained by two operators working in different laboratories on identical test material, should not exceed (expressed as % nitrogen) 0.0072 g of non-casein nitrogen per 100 g of milk, or (expressed as % protein) 0.046 g of non-casein protein per 100 g of milk.The absolute difference between the results of two single and independent indirect casein determinations, obtained by two operators working in different laboratories on identical test material, should not exceed (expressed as % nitrogen) 0.0096 g of indirect casein nitrogen per 100 g of milk, or (expressed as % protein) 0.062 g of indirect casein protein per 100 g of milk.

11.3 **Method performance statistics**[63] (expressed on a protein basis):

Non-casein protein

$s_r = 0.010$	$RSD_r = 1.287\%$	r value = 0.028
$s_R = 0.016$	$RSD_R = 2.146\%$	R value = 0.046

Casein protein, indirect

$s_r = 0.015$	$RSD_r = 0.560\%$	r value = 0.041
$s_R = 0.022$	$RSD_R = 0.840\%$	R value = 0.062

12. **Test Report and Interpretation:** The test report shall identify the method used and results obtained. The report will also identify any variation in the test not specified in this method as well as problems that may have impacted the test result. Each sample will be described in such a manner as to ensure traceablity as to its origin.

15.137 Casein Nitrogen/Protein, Direct, Kjeldahl (Class A1)[11(998.05-.07),15,38,40,77]

1. **Scope:** This method is applicable to fresh raw milk. Casein nitrogen will decrease with milk storage time due to casein breakdown even at 4°C. The casein nitrogen of heat-treated milk will be artificially high because of whey protein denaturation.

2. **References:** Chapter 2 on "Laboratory Quality Assurance and Safety."
Chapter 3 on "Sampling Dairy and Related Products."
Chapter 15, methods 15.131 and 15.132.

3. **Definition:** Casein nitrogen/protein is the mass fraction of substances determined according to the procedures specified in this method. It is expressed as a percentage by mass.

4. **Principle:** Precipitation of casein from a test portion by addition of acetic acid and sodium acetate solutions such that the final pH of the mixture is approximately 4.6. Separation of the precipitated milk casein by filtration. (The filtrate will contain the non-casein nitrogen contents). Determination of the nitrogen content of the precipitate by the procedure described in 15.131 or 15.132 of the total nitrogen method.

5. **Reagents:** Unless otherwise specified all chemicals are reagent or ACS grade.

The reagents specified for the determination of total nitrogen by the method described in method 15.131 or 15.132, together with the following, are required.

5.1 Acetic acid solution, 10% (v/v): Pipet 10.0 mL of glacial acetic acid (CH_3COOH) into a 100-mL volumetric flask and dilute to the mark.

5.2 Sodium acetate solution, 1N: Dissolve 8.20 g of sodium acetate (CH_3COONa) or 13.60 g of sodium acetate trihydrate ($CH_3COONa \bullet 3H_2O$) in water and dilute to the mark in a 100-mL volumetric flask. Prepare weekly.

5.3 Buffer solution: Pipet 1.0 mL of acetic acid solution (5.1) and 1.0 mL of sodium acetate solution (5.2) into a 100-mL volumetric flask and dilute to the mark.

6. Apparatus and Glassware: All volumetric flasks, pipets, and burets are Class A unless otherwise specified.

Usual laboratory equipment and the equipment specified in 15.131 or 15.132, together with the following, are required.

6.1 Water bath: Maintained at a temperature of 38° ± 1°C.

6.2 Bottle-top dispensers: For delivering 70-mL portions of water and 30-mL portions of buffer solutions (5.3).

6.3 Pipets: Capacity 1 mL.

6.4 Filter funnel: Glass or plastic, diameter 75 mm.

6.5 Filter paper: Diameter 15 cm, nitrogen-free, Whatman No. 1 or equivalent. Pleat before use.

7. Sampling: Chapter 3 on "Sampling Dairy and Related Products."

8. Preparation of Test Sample: Warm the milk sample to 38° ± 1°C by means of a water bath (6.1). Gently mix the milk sample immediately prior to weighing the test portion (9.1).

9. Procedure: Before beginning analysis review material safety data sheets on all chemicals and use appropriate safety equipment such as hoods, aprons, face shields, and glasses.

9.1 **Test portion:** Weigh approximately 5 g of the prepared test sample (8), to the nearest 0.1 mg, into a Kjeldahl flask or digestion tube. This may be done by weighing directly into the flask or tube, or determining the difference between the weight of a small container containing approximately 5 g of the test sample and the weight of the container after the test portion is poured into the flask or tube.

Immediately add 70 mL of water by means of a bottle-top dispenser (6.2), rinsing any milk on the inside neck to the bottom of the flask or tube.

Note: Additional samples may be weighed at this point, but the additions of acetic acid solution and sodium acetate solution plus filtration should occur within 15 min. of weighing the milk and adding the water. This minimizes proteolytic degradation of casein during sample preparation.

9.2 **Determination**

9.2.1 Pipet (6.3) 0.75 mL of acetic acid solution (5.1) into Kjeldahl flask or digestion tube (avoid getting the acetic acid solution on neck of the flask or tube during addition). Swirl to mix. Let the flask or tube stand at room temperature for 10 minutes. Pipet (6.3) 0.75 mL of sodium acetate solution (5.2) into the Kjeldahl flask or digestion tube. Swirl to mix. Let precipitate settle. Pour mixture from the Kjeldahl flask or digestion tube through a filter funnel (6.4) containing pleated filter paper (6.5) and collect the filtrate. Some of the precipitate will remain in the Kjeldahl flask or digestion tube and some will be collected on the filter paper. It is not necessary to remove all the precipitate from the flask or tube. Filter completely before next pour.

Immediately after pouring the mixture and so as not to allow any precipitate to dry on the neck of the Kjeldahl flask or digestion tube, add by means of a bottle-top dispenser (6.2) 30 mL of buffer solution (5.3), using the solution to rinse any precipitate from the neck of the flask or tube down onto the bottom. Swirl to mix the contents. After the liquid from the first pour has completely filtered, pour the buffer rinse from the flask or tube through the same filter paper, adding the filtrate to that collected previously. Use the same side of the neck of the flask for all pour-overs to reduce area to which precipitate can adhere. Again, immediately rinse the neck of the flask or tube with an additional 30 mL of buffer solution. Swirl to mix the contents. After the first buffer rinse has filtered completely, pour the second buffer rinse from the flask or tube through the same filter paper, adding the filtrate to that previously collected. The filtrate should be clear and free of particulate matter. If particulates appear, recycle filtrate through the same filter paper or repeat the test.

Note: At this point, the filtrate is no longer needed and may be discarded in an appropriate manner.

9.2.2 Carefully remove the filter paper, after it has dried slightly, from the filter funnel and fold the paper to enclose the precipitate. Ensure that no precipitate on the filter paper is lost. If any precipitate remains on either the inner or outer lip of the Kjeldahl flask or digestion tube, wipe with the folded filter paper so that any precipitate adheres to the paper and then drop the filter paper into the Kjeldahl flask or digestion tube.

9.2.3 Add boiling acid, potassium sulfate, copper solution, and the appropriate amount of sulfuric acid to the Kjeldahl flask or digestion tube as specified in 15.131 or 15.132. Digest, distill, and titrate as specified in 15.131 or 15.132. Flask or tube may be stoppered after the addition of sulfuric acid and digested, distilled, and titrated at a later time.

9.3 **Blank test:** Digest, distill, and titrate a blank containing filter paper (6.5) instead of the test portion.

10. Expression of Results

10.1 **Calculation of casein nitrogen content:** The casein nitrogen content, expressed as a percentage by mass, is equal to

$$\frac{1.4007 \times (V_S - V_b) \times M}{W_m}$$

where

V_S is the volume, reported to at least the nearest 0.05 milliliters, of the standard volumetric solution of acid used in the determination (15.131 or 15.132);

V_b is the volume, reported to at least the nearest 0.05 milliliters, of the standard volumetric solution of acid used in the blank test (15.131 or 15.132);

M is the exact molarity, reported to four decimal places, of the standard volumetric solution of acid (15.131 or 15132); and

W_m is the mass, in grams reported to four decimal places, of the test portion of milk (9.1).

Round the result to the nearest 0.0001%.

10.2 **Calculation of casein protein:** The casein nitrogen content, expressed as casein protein, is obtained by multiplying the casein nitrogen content (10.1) by 6.38.

11. Precision and Performance Parameters

11.1 **Repeatability:** The absolute difference between the results of two single direct casein nitrogen determinations, carried out simultaneously or in rapid succession by the same operator under the same conditions on identical test material, should not exceed 0.0068 g of casein-nitrogen per 100 g of milk, or (expressed as % protein) 0.044 g of direct casein protein per 100 g of milk.

11.2 **Reproducibility:** The absolute difference between the results of two single and independent direct casein nitrogen results, obtained by two operators working in different laboratories on identical test material, should not exceed 0.0113 g of direct casein nitrogen per 100 g of milk or (expressed as % protein) 0.072 g of direct casein protein per 100 g of milk.

11.3 **Method performance statistics** (for raw milk[63]).

Casein protein, direct method

s_r = 0.015	RSD_r =0.597%	r value =0.044
s_R= 0.025	RSD_R =0.988%	R value = 0.072

12. Test Report and Interpretation: The test report shall identify the method used and results obtained. The report will also identify any variation in the test not specified in this method as well as problems that may have impacted the test result. Each sample will be described in such a manner as to ensure traceablity as to its origin.

15.140 Rancidity Tests

15.141 Acid Degree Value Method (Class O)[29,37,85,90]

1. **Scope:** This method is applicable to raw and pasteurized milk, cream, and other non-homogenized dairy products.
2. **References:** Chapter 2 on "Laboratory Quality Assurance and Safety." Chapter 3 on "Sampling Dairy and Related Products."
3. **Definition:** Acid degree value (ADV) is defined as the milliliters of 1N base required to neutralize the acids in 100 g of fat. The result is expressed as milliequivalents of free fatty acids per 100 g of milk fat.
4. **Principle:** Fatty acids are released from glycerides when milk fat undergoes hydrolysis. One measure of this is the ADV. Normal raw milk has been reported to have an ADV of 0.25 to 0.40. When the ADV reaches about 1.2, discriminating evaluators may detect the lipolyzed or rancid flavor by taste or smell. Hydrolytic rancidity is enhanced by the presence of moisture, high temperatures, and the presence of lipolytic enzymes.
5. **Reagents:** Unless otherwise specified all chemicals are reagent or ACS grade.

5.1 **Bureau of Dairy Industry (BDI) reagent:** 30 g of Trition X-100 and 70 g of sodium tetraphosphate (or sodium hexametaphosphate if uncaked) made to 1-L with LG water. Stir and warm to dissolve the sodium tetraphosphate.

5.2 **Fat solvent:** Four parts petroleum ether (ACS, boiling point 30° to 60°C) to one part n-propanol (analytical reagent [AR] by volume).

5.3 **Methyl alcohol, aqueous:** Mix equal volumes of absolute methanol (reagent grade) and LG water.

5.4 **Phenolphthalein, 1%:** Dissolve 1 g in 100 mL of absolute methanol (reagent grade).

5.5 **Potassium hydroxide, alcoholic (KOH):** Prepare 0.02N of potassium hydroxide in absolute methanol (reagent grade). Standardize the solution frequently against standard potassium acid phthalate. Protect the solution from air and absorption of CO_2 from the air.

6. **Apparatus and Glassware:** All volumetric flasks, pipets, and burets are Class A unless otherwise specified.

6.1 **Babcock test bottle:** 18 g, 8% milk; or 9 g, 20% ice cream; or 9 g, 50% cream.

6.2 **Centrifuge:** to accommodate test bottles at proper Babcock centrifugal force [15.8.A.1.f]. An unheated centrifuge is satisfactory.

6.3 **Flask:** 500-mL Erlenmeyer.

6.4 **Microburet:** 5-mL capacity, 0.01-mL divisions.

6.5 **Pipet:** 10 mL, may be automatic.

6.6 **Syringe, hypodermic:** 50 mL, graduated and fitted with a No. 15 needle; a standard 17.6-mL "to contain" (TC) milk pipet can be used as an alternative.

6.7 **Syringe, tuberculin:** 1 mL with a 10-cm, 14-gauge needle.

6.8 **Water baths:** one boiling, with rack to hold test bottles; one controlled at 57° ± 3°C.

7. **Sampling:** Chapter 3 on "Sampling Dairy and Related Products."

8. **Preparation of Test Sample:** Mix samples of milk or cream by slowly inverting sample until material is uniform. Extremely viscous cream may need to be heated up to 38°C for 15 minutes to uniformly mix.

9. **Procedure:** Before beginning analysis review material safety data sheets on all chemicals and use appropriate safety equipment such as hoods, aprons, face shields, and glasses.

Note: For better precision and accuracy, all steps using 0.02 N KOH solution should be blanketed with dry nitrogen or flushed continuously with dry nitrogen to prevent absorption of CO_2 from the air during handling of the KOH or during the titration.

9.1 Using a 50-mL syringe (or milk pipet), place 35 mL of milk or cream in each Babcock bottle.

9.2 Add 10 mL of BDI reagent and mix thoroughly.

9.3 Place the bottles in a bath of gently boiling water that covers their bases. Agitate the contents thoroughly after 5 minutes and again after 10 minutes in the bath. The bottles should remain in the boiling water at least 5 minutes more to ensure clean fat separation. Total time is 15 to 20 minutes.

9.4 Remove the bottles and centrifuge for 1 minute [15.8.A.1.f]

9.5 Add enough aqueous methyl alcohol to bring the fat column well within the graduated portion of each bottle neck.

9.6 Centrifuge again for 1 minute.

9.7 Place the bottle in a water bath (57° ± 3°C) for 5 minutes. The water level should be above the fat column.

9.8 Transfer 1 mL of fat at 57°C from each test bottle to a 50-mL Erlenmeyer flask, using the 1-mL syringe. Weigh the fat transferred.

9.9 Dissolve the fat in 5 mL of fat solvent and add five drops of 1% phenolphthalein.

9.10 Titrate to the first faint but definite color change with standardized alcoholic potassium hydroxide solution using a 5-mL microburet. If turbidity develops in the solvent-fat mixture during titration, 2 or 3 mL of additional solvent should clear the mixture.

9.11 Make blank titrations on the fat solvent (in the absence of fat) using 5 drops of phenolphthalein indicator.

10. Expression of Results

10.1 **Calculation**

$$\text{ADV} = \frac{(\text{mL KOH for sample} - \text{mL KOH for blank}) \times \text{N} \times 100}{\text{Weight of fat}}$$

where N = normality of methanolic KOH solution.

ADV should be reported only to the second decimal place.

10.2 **Interpretation:** Suggested values for the interpretation of ADV are as follows:

Less than 0.7 = Normal
0.7 to 1.1 = Slightly hydrolyzed
1.2 to 1.4 = Definitely hydrolyzed
Greater than 1.4 = Extremely hydrolyzed

11. Precision and Performance Parameters: No precision data available for this assay.

12. Test Report and Interpretation: The test report shall identify the method used and results obtained. The report will also identify any variation in the test not specified in this method as well as problems that may have impacted the test result. Each sample will be described in such a manner as to ensure traceablity as to its origin.

15.142 Peroxide Value (Class O)[7,11]

1. **Scope:** This method is applicable to all normal fats and oils, including margarine. The method is highly empirical and any variation the test procedure may cause variation of results.

2. **References:** Chapter 2 on "Laboratory Quality Assurance and Safety." Chapter 3 on "Sampling Dairy and Related Products."

3. **Definition:** Peroxide value is defined as the milliequivalents of peroxide per 1000 grams of sample.

4. **Principle:** This method determines all substances in terms of milliequivalents of peroxide per 1000 grams of sample, which oxidize potassium

iodide under the conditions of the test. These are assumed to be peroxides or other similar products of fat oxidation.

When the double bonds of unsaturated fats become oxidized, peroxides are among the products formed. Peroxides liberate iodine from potassium iodide added to the test system. The amount of iodine liberated is a measure of peroxide and correlates to the degree of oxidation experienced by the fat.

5. **Reagents:** Unless otherwise specified all chemicals are reagent or ACS grade.
   5.1 **Acetic acid-chloroform solution:** Mix 3 volumes of acetic acid with 2 volumes of chloroform.
   5.2 **Starch solution, 1%:** Mix approximately 1 g soluble starch with enough cold water to make thin paste, add 100 mL of boiling water, and boil approximately 1 minute while stirring.
   5.3 **Sodium thiosulfate solutions:** 0.1N and 0.01N. For 0.01N, dilute 0.1N with freshly boiled and cooled water.
   5.4 **Potassium iodide solution, saturated:** Dissolve excess KI in freshly boiled water. Excess solid must remain. Store in dark. Test daily by adding 0.5 mL to 30 mL acetic acid-chloroform solution, and 2 drops 1% starch solution. If solution turns blue, requiring greater than 1 drop of 0.1N sodium thiosulfate solution to discharge color, prepare fresh solution.

6. **Apparatus and Glassware:** All volumetric flasks, pipets, and burets are Class A unless otherwise specified.
   6.1 **Balance:** 0.1-mg sensitivity.
   6.2 **Beakers:** 400 and 600 mL.
   6.3 **Buret:** Class A microburet, 10 mL, or Class A buret, 50 mL.
   6.4 **Flask:** Flask, 250-mL glass-stoppered Erlenmeyer.
   6.5 **Pipets:** Mohr or equivalent to measure 0.5 mL and 10 mL.

7. **Sampling:** Chapter 3 on "Sampling Dairy and Related Products."

8. **Preparation of Test Sample:** Take a representative sample that has previously been mixed, stirred, ground, blended, or otherwise prepared in order to make sample uniform.
   8.1 If necessary, prepare sample (i.e., margarine) by melting completely on hot plate at low heat while stirring or heat in air oven at 60°-70°C (avoid excessive heat and long exposure greater than 40°C).
   8.2 When completely melted, hold in warm place until aqueous portion and most of solids have settled. Decant oil into clean beaker and filter through a Whatman No. 4 or equivalent paper. Do not reheat unless necessary to obtain clear filtrate.

9. **Procedure:** Before beginning analysis review material safety data sheets on all chemicals and use appropriate safety equipment such as hoods, aprons, face shields, and glasses.
   9.1 Weigh 5.00 ± 0.05 g sample into 250-mL glass-stoppered Erlenmeyer.
   9.2 Add 30 mL acetic acid-chloroform solution and swirl to dissolve.
   9.3 Add 0.5 mL saturated KI solution with Mohr pipet and let stand with occasional shaking for one minute.

Table 15.3. Sample Size and Normality of Titrant for Use with Hypochlorite Sanitizers

Expected Chlorine Concentration	Sample Size (mL)	N of Sodium Thiosulfate Titrant
Less than 10 ppm	400	0.01
10 to 50 ppm	200	0.01
50 to 100 ppm	100	0.01
100 to 200 ppm	50	0.01
200 to 500 ppm	25	0.01
Greater than 500 ppm	50	0.10

9.4 Add 30 mL water and slowly titrate with 0.1N sodium thiosulfate, with vigorous shaking until yellow is almost gone.

9.5 Add approximately 0.5 mL of 1% starch solution and continue titration, shaking vigorously to release all iodide from chloroform layer, until blue just disappears.

9.6 If less than 0.5 mL 0.1N sodium thiosulfate solution is used, repeat determination with 0.01N sodium thiosulfate.

9.7 Conduct blank determinations daily (must be ≤0.1 mL 0.1N sodium thiosulfate). Subtract blank determination from sample titration.

10. **Expression of Results**

10.1 **Calculations:** Peroxide value (milliequivalent peroxide/kg sample) =

$$\frac{S - B \times N \times 1000 \text{ g sample}}{\text{Sample weight (g)}}$$

where S = titration volume of sample
B = titration volume of blank
N = normality of sodium thiosulfate solution

11. **Precision and Performance Parameters:** No precision data available for this assay.

12. **Test Report and Interpretation:** The test report shall identify the method used and results obtained. The report will also identify any variation in the test not specified in this method as well as problems that may have impacted the test result. Each sample will be described in such a manner as to ensure traceablity as to its origin.

15.150 Sanitizer Tests

15.151 Chlorine, Available (Class O)[11(922.08)]

1. **Scope:** This method is applicable to calcium hypochlorite, sodium dichloroisocynaurate, commercially prepared solutions of sodium hypochlorite, and chlorine sanitizing solutions.

2. **References:** Chapter 2 on "Laboratory Quality Assurance and Safety." Chapter 3 on "Sampling Dairy and Related Products."

3. **Principle:** Glacial acetic acid is used in this procedure to liberate chlorine in the sample. Potassium iodide is used as a replacement for chlorine for easier indicator detection using starch. The titrant used is sodium thio-

sulfate. The following reaction occurs in a sample with sodium hypochlorite:

$$\text{Glacial acetic acid} + NaClO \rightarrow Cl_2^{o}$$
$$KI + Cl_2^{o} \rightarrow 2KCl + I_2^{o}$$
$$I_2^{o} + \text{Starch solution} \rightarrow \text{Blue color for titration}$$

4. **Definition:** Available chlorine is defined as the amount of chlorine as determined under conditions of the test as specified.

5. **Reagents:** Unless otherwise specified all chemicals are reagent or ACS grade.
   5.1 Acetic acid: Glacial, ACS.
   5.2 Potassium iodide solution, 10%: Weigh 10 g of potassium iodide into a 50 mL beaker and dissolve with LG water. Transfer to a 100-mL volumetric flask and bring to volume with LG water. Mix thoroughly. Store in a dark place when not in use and discard when solution develops a yellow color.
   5.3 Sodium thiosulfate ($Na_2S_2O_3$), 0.01N or 0.1N solution: See Table 15.3.
   5.4 Starch, 0.5%: Make a thin paste from 2.5 g of soluble potato starch and a little cold LG water. Stir in 500 mL of boiling LG water and allow to stand overnight. Use the clear supernatant liquid. To preserve the starch solution, add 1.25 g of salicylic acid.
   5.5 Water (LG).

6. **Apparatus and Glassware:** All volumetric flasks, pipets, and burets are Class A unless otherwise specified.
   6.1 Balance: 0.1 gram sensitivity.
   6.2 Beaker: 50 mL.
   6.3 Buret: 50 mL, 0.1-mL divisions.
   6.4 Cylinder: Graduated, 10 mL.
   6.5 Flasks: Erlenmeyer, 250 or 500 mL; volumetric, 100 or 1,000 mL.
   6.6 Pipets: Mohr, 10 mL, graduated in 0.1-mL divisions; volumetric, 25, 50, 100, and 200 mL.

7. **Sampling:** Chapter 3 on "Sampling Dairy and Related Products."

8. **Preparation of Test Sample:** Take a representative sample that has previously been mixed, stirred, blended, or otherwise prepared in order to make sample uniform.

9. **Procedure:** Before beginning analysis review material safety data sheets on all chemicals and use appropriate safety equipment such as hoods, aprons, face shields, and glasses.
   9.1 Into an Erlenmeyer flask of appropriate size, pipet the correct amount of sample as indicated in Table 15.3.
   9.2 Add 10 mL of potassium iodide solution and 5 mL of glacial acetic acid. Swirl to mix. A yellow color after addition of the acid indicates the presence of chlorine.
   9.3 Titrate the liberated iodine immediately upon the addition of acid using the sodium thiosulfate solution of required normality (Table 15.3) until a pale yellow color is reached.
   9.4 Add 1 mL of starch indicator and titrate until the blue color disappears for at least 30 seconds. If, after adding the acid, a solution is

Table 15.4. Volumes and Concentrations of Potassium Iodide (KI) and Nickel Nitrate for Use in Preparing Standard Solutions

Final Volume[a] (mL)	Final (KI) Concentration (mg/L)	Take (KI) Volume (mL)	Of (KI) Concentration (mg/L)	Plus 2 M Nickel Nitrate (mL)
25	8000	20	10000	0
100	1000	10	10000	1
100	100	10	1000	1
100	10	1	1000	1
1000	1	1	1000	10
500	2	1	1000	5
500	4	2	1000	5
500	8	4	1000	5
500	16	1	8000	5
500	32	2	8000	5
500	64	4	8000	5
500	128	8	8000	2.5

[a] Obtained by diluting with double deionized water.

very pale yellow in color, immediately add the starch indicator and then titrate until the solution remains colorless for 30 seconds. Adding the starch indicator too early will allow decomposition of the starch indicator and indistinct end points.

9.5 Determine a blank titration value using a volume of distilled water corresponding to that of the sample. If a blue color results, titrate with 0.01N sodium thiosulfate to the same end point as the sample.

9.6 Before calculating the available chlorine, subtract the result of the blank titration from the result of the sample titration. If the blank requires more than 0.2 mL of 0.01N sodium thiosulfate solution per 50 mL of water, examine the reagents and equipment for the source of contamination.

10. Expression of Results

10.1 Available chlorine

$$(\text{mg/L or PPM}) = \frac{\text{mL}\ (Na_2S_2O_3) \times \text{N}\ (Na_2S_2O_3) \times 0.0355 \times 10^6}{\text{mL sample}}$$

11. Precision and Performance Parameters: No precision data available for this test.

12. Test Report and Interpretation: The test report shall identify the method used and results obtained. The report will also identify any variation in the test not specified in this method as well as problems that may have impacted the test result. Each sample will be described in such a manner as to ensure traceablity as to its origin.

15.152 Iodine, Selective Ion Procedure (Class B)[22]

1. Scope: This method is applicable to raw milk. This method has product limitations as described by LaCroix and Wang.[56]

2. **References:** Chapter 2 on "Laboratory Quality Assurance and Safety." Chapter 3 on "Sampling Dairy and Related Products."
3. **Definition:** Iodide is determined using ion-selective electrode and method of known addition. Nickel nitrate is added to reduce interferences to iodide response of electrode.
4. **Principle:** This procedure uses direct potentiometry for the determination of iodide with an iodide sensitive electrode.
5. **Reagents:** Unless otherwise specified, all chemicals are reagent or ACS grade.
   5.1 Nickel nitrate: 2 M solution prepared with double-deionized water.
   5.2 Potassium iodide solution: 10,000 mg/L, 0.02 M in nickel nitrate. Weigh 13.1 g of potassium iodide in a 150-mL beaker. Dissolve in about 50 mL of double deionized water and transfer quantitatively (with rinsing) to a 1,000 mL stoppered volumetric flask using double deionized water.
   5.3 Prepare a set of standard potassium iodide solutions according to Table 15.4.
   5.4 Water: Double deionized of at least 1 megohm resistivity.
6. **Apparatus and Glassware:** All volumetric flasks, pipets, and burets are Class A unless otherwise specified.
   6.1 Balance: 50-mg sensitivity beakers: 150 and 250 mL.
   6.2 Iodide ion selective electrode: Orion [1 to 5×10^{-8} M; 127,000 to 5×10^{-3} ppm] or equivalent; reference, double junction, double function, Graphic Controls PHE 54473 or equivalent.
   6.3 Flasks: Stoppered, volumetric, 50, 100, 500, and 1,000 mL.
   6.4 Magnetic stirrer.
   6.5 Magnetic stirring bars: Teflon coated, 10×25 mm.
   6.6 Millivolt meter: Orion 701A or equivalent.
   6.7 Pipets: Volumetric, 2, 4, 5, 6, 10, and 40 mL.
7. **Sampling:** Chapter 3 on "Sampling Dairy and Related Products."
8. **Preparation of Test Sample:** Take a representative sample that has previously been mixed, stirred, ground, blended, or otherwise prepared in order to make sample uniform.
9. **Procedure:** Before beginning analysis review material safety data sheets on all chemicals and use appropriate safety equipment such as hoods, aprons, face shields, and glasses.
   9.1 **Calibration of electrodes**
      9.1.1 After assembling the meter and electrodes according to the manufacturer's instructions, set the electrodes in the 10 mg/L of potassium iodide standard (100 mL in a 150-mL beaker stirred with a magnetic stirrer).
      9.1.2 Set the meter to read in absolute millivolts, and allow the electrode to reach equilibrium (5 minutes is sufficient). The reading should be between –100 and –90 mV and steady (with no more than ± 0.1-mV variation).
      9.1.3 Repeat with 1 and 100 mg/L of standards. The reading for the 1-mg/L standard should be about 59.2 mV more than that for

the 10-mg/L standard, and the readings for the 100 mg/L should be about 59.2 mV less. Since a negative ion is being measured, the potential will get smaller as the concentration increases.

9.1.4 If the readings for all three standards are displaced by the same amount from what is expected, check the lower half of the reference electrode for the electrolyte level and change or add as necessary.

9.1.5 If the readings show more than 0.1-mV fluctuation, check the electrical ground on the meter and the electrode connections.

9.1.6 If the readings are steady but the change in reading is much less than 59.2 mV for a tenfold change in iodide concentration, polish the iodide ion selective electrode as recommended in the manual. When the electrodes are functioning properly, proceed to measure the potential for the eight standards (1 to 128 mg/L).

9.1.7 For a twofold change in iodide concentration, the potential should change 17.8 mV ($59.2 \times \text{Log } 2$), and the potential for the eight standards, 1 to 128 mg/L, should fall on a straight line when plotted on a semilog paper (concentration on the log scale). Any suspect standard should be replaced because the concentration reported in milk will be in error in proportion to the error in the standard added to the milk during determination.

9.2 **Determination in milk**

9.2.1 Weigh duplicate 100-g sample into 250-mL beakers.

9.2.2 Read the potential (E_1) of the milk directly while stirring with a magnetic stirrer after adding 1 mL of 2 M nickel nitrate solution.

9.2.3 Record E_1 and add 10 mL of a standard whose concentration is at least 10 times and not more than 20 times the concentration of the iodide in the milk estimated from E_1.

9.2.4 Consult the graph prepared during the calibration process. Read the potential (E_2) after adding the standard and record $E_2 - E_1$ as E.

10. Expression of Results

10.1 **Calculations**

10.1.1 For measurements made at 25°C, consult the table in the Orion (or equivalent Iodide ISE) manual to find the Q value that corresponds to the E measured in the sample.

10.1.2 Note that, for duplicate samples, E is allowed to vary by as much as 10 mV, but generally E will duplicate within 0.5 mV.

10.1.3 The concentration of iodide in milk in µg/kg is $1{,}000 \times Q \times C$, where C is the concentration of the standard (in milligrams per liter) used to obtain E_2.

11. Precision and Performance Parameters: No precision data for this assay.

12. Test Report and Interpretation: The test report shall identify the method used and results obtained. The report will also identify any variation in the test not specified in this method as well as problems that may have impacted the test result. Each sample will be described in such a manner as to ensure traceablity as to its origin.

15.160 Vitamins A, D2, and D3 in Milk Products, HPLC Method (Class O)[1,12,21,39,76,79,88,89,91-93]

1. **Scope:** This method is applicable to raw and pasteurized skim, reduced fat, and whole milks.
2. **References:** Chapter 2 on "Laboratory Quality Assurance and Safety." Chapter 3 on "Sampling Dairy and Related Products."
3. **Definition:** Vitamin A is measured as µg/mL and reported as international units (IU) per quart. One IU of vitamin A is the activity of 0.3 µg of all-trans-retinol, 0.344 µg of all-trans-retinyl acetate, 0.55 µg of all-trans-retinyl palmitate, 0.6 µg of β-carotene, or 1.2 µg of other provitamin carotenoids.

   Vitamin D is measured as µg/mL and reported as IU per quart. One µg of vitamin D_2 or D_3 is equivalent to 40 IU of biopotency.
4. **Principle:** The vitamins A and D in milk are isolated from milk by alkaline saponification followed by liquid-liquid extraction with n-hexane. The vitamins extracted into hexane are concentrated by evaporation. Vitamin A in the hexane extract is measured directly by HPLC with UV detection. The vitamin D analysis is carried out by further purifying the extract, using silica cartridge and solid-phase extraction. The eluent form the silica cartridge is concentrated and injected on to the C-18 column to determine vitamin D by HPLC with UV detection.
5. **Reagents:** Unless otherwise specified all chemicals are reagent or ACS grade equivalent.
   - 5.1 All-trans retinol.
   - 5.2 Ergocalciferol (Vitamin D_2).
   - 5.3 Cholecalciferol (Vitamin D_3).
   - 5.4 Pyrogallol.
   - 5.5 Potassium hydroxide.
   - 5.6 Sodium sulfate: anhydrous.
   - 5.7 Phenolphthalein: 1% solution.
   - 5.8 n-hexane: HPLC grade or equivalent.
   - 5.9 Acetonitrile: HPLC grade or equivalent.
   - 5.10 Chloroform: HPLC grade or equivalent.
   - 5.11 Ethyl acetate: HPLC grade or equivalent.
   - 5.12 Methanol: HPLC grade or equivalent.
   - 5.13 Reagent alcohol/ethyl alcohol.
   - 5.14 Iso-propyl alcohol: HPLC grade or equivalent.
   - 5.15 Distilled water.
   - 5.16 Ultra-pure nitrogen gas: Air Products UN 1066 or equivalent.
   - 5.17 HPLC grade water.
6. **Apparatus and Glassware:** All volumetric flasks, pipets, and burets are Class A unless otherwise specified.
   - 6.1 Volumetric flasks: 10 and 25 mL, low actinic (amber) and/or clear.
   - 6.2 Graduated cylinders: 10, 25, 50, and 100 mL.

6.3 Erlenmeyer flasks: 50 or 125 mL, low actinic or clear (with foil).
6.4 Pear-shaped or boiling flasks: 125, 250, or 500 mL.
6.5 Seperatory funnels: 125 and 250 or 500 mL, low actinic or clear.
6.6 Funnels.
6.7 Volumetric pipets: Assortment of sizes. 0.5, 1.0, 2.0, and 15 mL.
6.8 Graduated centrifuge tubes: 15 mL.
6.9 Eppendorf or equivalent pipeters: 10-100 µL and 100-1000 µL.
6.10 Solvent filtration: 0.2 µm , "66" nylon filters (0.2 × 47 mm), (Supelco Inc., Bellefonte, PA) or equivalent.
6.11 Solvent filtration apparatus: Supelco Inc., Bellefonte, PA, or equivalent.
6.12 Syringe filters: Gelman Acrodisc 13-mm, 0.2-µm or equivalent.
6.13 Disposable syringes.
6.14 Pasteur pipets and rubber bulbs.
6.15 Glass wool.
6.16 Hamilton microliter syringes: 20/100 µL or equivalent [for manual injections].
6.17 High-performance liquid chromatograph (HPLC): Hewlett-Packard 1050 system or equivalent.
6.18 Liquid chromatography vials: Clear glass or amber colored or equivalent.
6.19 Perkin-Elmer Lambda 2 Spectrophotometer or equivalent.
6.20 Quartz cuvettes.
6.21 Columns and cartridges.
6.22 Analytical column: Supelcosil LC-18, 250 × 4.6 mm, 5 µm (Supelco Inc., Bellefonte, PA) or equivalent.
6.23 Guard column: Supelguard LC-18, 20 × 4.6 mm, 5 µm (Supelco Inc., Bellefonte, PA) or equivalent.
6.24 Supelco Supelguard column holder or equivalent.
6.25 Analytical column: Vydac 201TP54 C_{18} 5 µM, 250 × 4.6 mm (Separations Group Inc.) or equivalent.
6.26 Guard column: Vydac 201 TP, 5 µm, 20 × 4.6 mm (Separations Group Inc., CA) or equivalent.
6.27 Vydac guard column holder or equivalent.
6.28 All-Tech Extract Clean Silica columns: 200 mG/3 mL (All-Tech Inc., Deerfield, IL) or equivalent.
6.29 Precolumn filters: Ultra-low dead volume with 0.5-µm frits.
6.30 Rotary evaporator: Buchi 461 water bath or equivalent.
6.31 Solvent evaporator: Zymark Turbo LV (optional).
6.32 Analytical scale: Ohaus, Analytical Plus, or equivalent.
6.33 Laboratory shaker: Labline model or equivalent (optional).
6.34 Water bath (optional).

7. **Sampling:** Chapter 3 on "Sampling Dairy and Related Products."

8. **Preparation of Test Sample:** Take a representative sample that has previously been mixed, stirred, or otherwise prepared in order to make sample uniform. Additionally, the exposure of samples to UV light must be prevented during collection, storage, and analysis of the samples to reduce the effect on isomerization of vitamins A and D.

9. **Procedure**

9.1 **Preparation of vitamin A standards**

9.1.1 **Preparation of vitamin A (all-trans retinol):** Weigh approximately 20-30 mg into 25-mL low-actinic volumetric flask. In place of low-actinic (amber) volumetric flask use clear glass flask with aluminum foil wrapper to prevent exposure to light. Note exact weight. Dissolve in iso-propyl alcohol (IPA) or hexane. Make up the volume to 25 mL with IPA. This is the vitamin A stock solution. Dilute vitamin A stock solution with IPA or hexane to such an extent that the resulting solution should have an absorbance between 0.2 and 0.8.

9.1.2 Obtain absorbance spectra and absorbance values according to directions of specific spectrometer using quartz cuvettes. Calculate vitamin A concentration (µg/mL) using the absorbance values at l_{MAX}, using equations (1) and (2).

9.1.3 Store vitamin A solutions at –20°C or below. For a accurate quantification of vitamin A, absorbance in the standard solutions is determined just before spiking the milk samples and before preparation of standards for calibration. Antioxidants such as BHT or ascorbic acid may be used to increase the stability. Even if the antioxidants are used, concentration must be validated.

9.2 **Preparation of vitamin D standards**

9.2.1 **Preparation of vitamin D_2 standard:** *Vitamin D_2 ergocalciferol:* Weigh approximately 20-30 mg into 10-mL low actinic volumetric flask. Dissolve in Reagent alcohol (95% ethyl alcohol) [EtOH] or methanol (MeOH). Make up the volume to 10 mL with EtOH or MeOH. This is vitamin D_2 stock solution. Dilute vitamin D_2 stock solution to such an extent that the resulting solution should have an absorbance between 0.2 and 0.8 with EtOH or MeOH. Obtain spectral scan for D_2 working solution and note absorbance value at l_{MAX}, i.e., at 264-265 nm. Calculate vitamin D_2 concentration in D_2 using equations in (1) and (2).

9.2.2 **Preparation of vitamin D_3 standard:** Repeat procedures 9.2 with vitamin D_3 and calculate concentration of vitamin D_3 stock solution.

9.3 **Preparation of reagents**

9.3.1 **Ethanolic potassium hydroxide:** Prepare fresh daily. Weigh 70 g of potassium hydroxide (KOH) into a 1-L Erlenmeyer flask. Place the flask in an ice water bath on a stir plate. Add stir bar. Add 155 mL of EtOH and 25 mL of distilled water. Cover the flask with a beaker or foil. Stir until the KOH is completely dissolved.

9.3.2 **Ethanolic pyrogallol:** Prepare fresh daily. Weigh 2.5 g of pyrogallol into a 25-mL flask. Dissolve in EtOH. Make up the volume to 25 mL with EtOH.

9.4 **Saponification of milk samples**

9.4.1 Temper milk sample to room temperature (20°-25°C).

Measure 15 mL of the milk into a 50- or 125-mL low actinic flask or into a flask wrapped with aluminum foil. Prepare two samples for each type of milk: control milk, and spiked milk, whole milk control and spiked whole milk, or skim milk control and spiked skim milk.

9.4.2 Measure appropriate amount and dilutions of vitamins A, D_2, and D_3 spiking solutions to each of the spiked milks. The approximate spike amounts should be around 9.0 µg of vitamin A, 0.16 µg of D_2 and D_3, approximately the same amounts of vitamins as expected in 15 mL of milk samples.

9.4.3 Reagent blank (optional): Prepare a blank sample (no milk added) with 15 mL distilled water and vitamin A, D_2, and D_3 spike solutions.

9.4.4 Measure 1.5 mL of ethanolic pyrogallol into each flask, including blank, and mix thoroughly.

9.4.5 Place the flasks in an ice bath. Slowly, transfer 15 mL of ethanolic KOH into each flask. Mix and cover the flasks with a glass-stoppered lid. Ice bath prevents rise in temperature.

9.4.6 Flush each flask with ultra-pure nitrogen gas for 1-2 min. Initially, gently mix the contents in the flask. If the flask size is greater than 50 mL, N_2 flushing should be longer (at least 2 min.). Cover the flask immediately with a lid.

9.4.7 Saponify at room temperature, in the dark, overnight (18-24 h). If the room temperature fluctuates use constant temperature water bath set about 25° ± 1°C.

9.5 **Liquid-liquid extraction of saponified milk samples**

9.5.1 All extractions must be carried out in a hood. Decrease illumination in the laboratory to reduce the chances of exposure to light. Use low actinic glassware (amber) wherever possible. In absence of low actinic glassware, use aluminum foil as a wrapper.

9.5.2 Swirl to mix the saponification flask and transfer the contents to a low actinic separatory funnel.

9.5.3 Add 15 mL distilled water to the saponification flask, swirl to mix, and transfer to separatory funnel. Add 5 mL EtOH to the saponification flask, swirl to mix, and transfer to separatory funnel.

9.5.4 Add 45 mL hexane to the saponification flask, swirl to mix, and transfer to separatory funnel. Shake the funnel vigorously for at least 1 min., venting occasionally by lifting the lid. If the saponification of samples is incomplete, emulsions may form in the separatory funnel. Break the emulsions with small amounts of EtOH (2-3 mL). Let phases separate for at least 2-3 minutes with the lid off.

9.5.5 Draw off the aqueous phase (lower layer) into a separate flask. Pour the hexane layer into another 250 or 500 mL low actinic (separatory) flask.

9.5.6 Transfer the aqueous layer back to the first separatory funnel.

9.5.7 Repeat steps 9.5.4 and 9.5.5 two more times (total of three extractions), pooling all the non-saponifiable hexane extracts in the second separatory funnel.

9.5.8 Add 15-20 mL of distilled water to the pooled hexane, shake vigorously for 30 sec. Let phases separate for 2-3 min. Draw off and discard the aqueous layer.

9.5.9 Add 50 mL of 5% KOH solution to the pooled hexane, and shake vigorously for 1 min. Let phases separate for 2-3 min. Draw off and discard the aqueous layer.

9.5.10 Wash the extract with distilled water (100 mL × 2), and let phases separate for 2-3 min. Draw off and discard the aqueous layer. Repeat washing one more time with 100 mL 55% EtOH. Let phases separate for 15 min. Draw off and discard all the traces of aqueous layer after the final wash. Test the washes for neutrality with 1 percent phenolphthalein solution. It is critical that the hexane extract should be neutral.

9.5.11 Layer a funnel with a small amount of glass wool and place a 1 inch layer of anhydrous sodium sulfate on top of the wool in the funnel. Place the funnel on a 250 or 500 mL pear shaped/boiling flask. Drain the pooled hexane extracts through sodium sulfate. After all the hexane extract is passed through, rinse the separatory funnel with 10 mL hexane and pass through sodium sulfate. Wash the sodium sulfate layer with 10 mL more of hexane. Press out hexane from sodium sulfate into the flask.

9.5.12 Drying: Rotavap and slowly evaporate hexane to almost complete dryness. During this entire drying step Rotovap water bath should not exceed 40°C and the flask or the rotavaporator water bath must be covered with aluminum foil.

9.5.13 Immediately add about 3-5 mL hexane to the flask with a Pasteur pipet and swirl vigorously to dissolve all the non-saponifiable material from the sides of the flask. Let all the hexane collect at the bottom cone for few seconds. With the aid of pasture pipet, transfer extract to a 15-mL centrifuge (graduated and calibrated) tube or a 10-mL vol. flask. Repeat washing with hexane successively, collecting all the hexane extracts in the centrifuge tubes or flasks.

9.5.14 If the volume of hexane is not exactly 10 mL, make up the volume or dry with gentle stream of N2 gas to obtain exactly 10 mL.

9.5.15 Remove 0.25 or 0.5 mL of the hexane from 9.5.14, and filter through a 0.2-micron filter into an amber LC vial. The amount of extract taken out is critical for final calculation of "D" results. Cap the vial, label it as "A" for analysis and store at less than –20°C till used. The HPLC analysis must be carried out within 24 h, preferably immediately.

9.5.16 Dry the remaining 9.75 or 9.5 mL of hexane extract with gentle stream of N2 to about 1 mL. Protect from light until used. Optionally, use Turbovap to dry.

9.6 Analysis for vitamin A

9.6.1 Prepare vitamin A standards to contain a range so that all the test sample values fall in this range. Extrapolation of the standard curve for calculations is not advisable. Analyze by HPLC by preparing a sequence with standards interspersed with sample vials from 9.5.15 with following HPLC conditions.

9.6.2 HPLC system and HPLC conditions: Hewlett-Packard 1050 LC with DAD and Hewlett-Packard 3D Chemstation or equivalent.

Guard column:	SupelGuard.
Analytical column:	Supelcosil LC-18; 250 × 4.6 mm.
Temperature:	Ambient temperature.
Mobile phase:	Methanol: water (95:5); isocratic. 1.5 mL/min.
Cleaning cycle:	Incorporate a cleaning cycle at regular intervals by consulting the column manufacturer. Replace guard column at regular intervals.

9.6.3 Identify all-trans-retinol by comparison of the retention times of the standard compound, either as reference standards or in spiked samples, with those of any similar peaks in the sample. Identification is accepted if peak retention time and shape are similar to the standard or spiked sample. Additionally, entire spectra or spectral ratios at different wavelengths of the sample peak and standard peaks may be compared for confirmation of the all-trans-retinol peak in the sample. The use of diode array technology lends additional confidence in the analysis.

9.7 Analysis for vitamin D

9.7.1 Condition the silica cartridge (All-Tech Extract-Clean Silica, 200 mg/3.0 mL) with at least 2 column volumes of hexane (5-7 mL). The cartridge should appear translucent. Do not let the cartridge dry before applying samples.

9.7.2 Thoroughly mix hexane extract (9.5.16) by vortexing vigorously. Let all the non-saponifiable dissolve in hexane. Allow a few seconds to drain all the hexane to the bottom of the tube. With the aid of a Pasteur pipet, transfer the extract to the silica cartridge. Let the extract pass through the column by gravity.

9.7.3 Pipet 2 mL of hexane to centrifuge tube, vortex, and transfer the wash to the silica cartridge. Let hexane pass through by gravity.

9.7.4 After all the hexane passed through, gently dry cartridge with slight positive pressure. Apply 1 mL of hexane:chloroform (22:78) mixture. Pass the mixture with a slight positive pressure. After most of the hexane:chloroform mixture is passed through, apply maximum vacuum pressure to dry the SPE cartridge. Continue drying the SPE cartridge for 1-2 min.

9.7.5 Elute vitamins D_2 and D_3 from silica cartridge with 1 mL of MeOH. Elute by applying a slight positive pressure (approximately 5 inches of Hg for 5-10 sec.). Collect the elute in a clean graduated centrifuge tube.

9.7.6 Immediately cool the MeOH elute from 9.7.5 at –20°C for about 15 min.

9.7.7 After cooling, centrifuge the MeOH elutes at 0°C for 10 min. at 3500 rpm using IEC Centra-8R.

9.7.8 Transfer the supernatent without disturbing the pellet into a graduated test tube. If the amount of MeOH elute collected is less than 1.00 mL, make up volume to 1.00 mL. The final volume must be exactly 1.00 mL to be correct in HPLC quantitation. Filter through a 0.2-µm filter into a low actinic LC vial.

9.7.9 Prepare vitamin D standards to contain a range so that all the test sample values fall in this range. Extrapolation of the standard curve for calculations is not advisable. Analyze by HPLC, by preparing a sequence with standards interspersed with sample vials from 9.7.8 with HPLC conditions described below in 9.7.10. If vitamin D2 is used as internal standard, follow procedure outlined by Hager et al.[32] to prepare standards and construct calibration curve.

9.7.10 HPLC conditions: Hewlett-Packard 1050 LC with DAD and Hewlett-Packard 3D Chemstation or equivalent.

Pre-column filter:	Ultra-low dead volume with 0.5-mm replaceable frits.
Guard column:	Vydac C18 201 TP, 5 µM 20 × 4.6 mm.
Analytical column:	Vydac 201TP54 C18,5 µM, 250 × 4.6 mm.
Temperature:	Ambient is suitable but if the room temperature fluctuates, controlling the separation temperature is helpful.
Mobile phase:	The objective is to separate all the interference peaks from D_2 and D_3 retention times. An interference peak is observed at the place D_2 retention time in some cases. Usually, this interference is a very small peak, but separating all the interferences from D_2 is critical for internal standard techniques. However, if the interference peak is less than 10% of the target analyte, it can be ignored and does not affect the results significantly.
Mobile phase 1:	Acetonitrile: Methanol (80:20); isocratic. 0.7 mL/min. as mobile phase. Adjust percentage of methanol if required.
Mobile phase 2:	Alternatively, use acetonitrile: chloroform: ethyl acetate (88:4:8) at 1.2

mL/min. as mobile phase. Several other laboratories are successfully using this mobile phase to quantitate vitamin D_3 by using D_2 as internal standard.

Cleaning cycle: Incorporate a cleaning cycle during each injection (100% ethyl acetate @ 2.5 mL/min. for 5 min.). At regular intervals replace pre-column filters and the guard columns. At regular intervals (for every 10-12 milk samples), clean the analytical column thoroughly by reverse flushing the column with 2-3 column volumes of the following: water, MeOH, MeOH, ethyl acetate, and chloroform. Consult the column manufacturer's technical service in implementing a cleaning cycle.

9.7.11 Identify vitamins D_2 and D_3 by comparing the retention times of the standard compound, either as reference standards or in spiked samples, with those of any similar peaks in the sample. Identification is accepted if peak retention time and shape are similar to the standard or spiked sample. If in doubt include the chromatogram from the reagent blank and compare the retention times and peak characteristics of the sample and standard.

10. Expression of Results

10.1 From the above HPLC analysis of vitamin A standards, obtain a regression equation by plotting peak height vs. µg of all-trans-retinol. Using the regression equation and peak heights of CM (control milk) and SM (spiked milk) samples, calculate µg of all-trans-retinol in control and spiked samples.

10.2 From the above HPLC analysis of vitamin D standards, obtain a regression equation, either by plotting peak area vs. µg of vitamin D_3 or by plotting ratios of D_3 and D_2 and peak areas of respective standards for internal standard techniques. Calculate µg of vitamin D_3 in control and spiked samples.

All qualitative and quantitative data must be recorded. Calculate percent recovery of all-trans-retinol and vitamin D_3 for each type of milk, using equation (3). Adjust vitamin values in control samples for dilution factor and for serving size. Unless otherwise requested all results must be reported unadjusted but along with the percent recovery values.

Equation (1)

$A = \varepsilon bc$ OR $c = \frac{A}{\varepsilon b}$

where A = absorbance at λ_{MAX}

ε = Molar absorptivity coefficient

(liters*mole^{-1}*cm^{-1})
b = Light path, cm
c = Concentration, moles*liter^{-1}

Equation (2)

$$c,\ \mu g/mL = \frac{\text{A at 325 nm}}{e,\ L \times moles^{-1} \times cm^{-1} \times 1\ cm} \times \text{Mol. Wt., gm} \times moles^{-1}\ \frac{10^{6}\ \mu G}{gm} \times \frac{10^{-3}\ L}{1\ mL}$$

Equation (3)

$$\frac{\text{Retinol}_{\text{spiked}}\ \text{Retinol}_{\text{ctrl}}}{\mu\text{g of retinol spiked}} \times 100 = \text{Percent recovery}$$

11. **Precision and Performance Parameters:** No precision data available for this assay.
12. **Test Report and Interpretation:** The test report shall identify the method used and results obtained. The report will also identify any variation in the test not specified in this method as well as problems that may have impacted the test result. Each sample will be described in such a manner as to ensure traceablity as to its origin.

15.170 Functional Tests

15.171 Solubility Index (Class O)[6]

1. **Scope:** This method is applicable to dry whole milk, nonfat dry milk, dry buttermilk, and dry buttermilk product.
2. **References:** Chapter 2 on "Laboratory Quality Assurance and Safety." Chapter 3 on "Sampling Dairy and Related Products."
3. **Definition:** Solubility index is defined as the amount of sediment remaining after solublization of the milk product under conditions of the test.
4. **Principle:** A sample of dried milk product is resolublized in water and centrifuged in a graduated tube, and the amount of sediment is measured.
5. **Reagents:** Unless otherwise specified all chemicals are reagent or ACS grade.
   - 5.1 Defoaming agent: Antifoam B emulsion, A5757 (Sigma Chemical Co., St. Louis, MO).
   - 5.2 Water (LG).
6. **Apparatus and Glassware:** All volumetric flasks, pipets, and burets are Class A unless otherwise specified.
   - 6.1 Balance: 500-g capacity and 0.1-g or better sensitivity.
   - 6.2 Blender or mixer: Waring, 7-speed commercial blender with glass container and blending assembly (Waring catalog #7012G; Waring model #31BL42).
   - 6.3 Centrifuge: Of required rpm with cups to accommodate conical centrifuge tubes. Steam turbine or heated Babcock centrifuge should not be used. The required rpm should be determined with test samples and with the door of the centrifuge closed. The following table gives the required rpm for different diameters of the head.

10-inch diameter	1075 rpm	18-inch diameter	800 rpm
12-inch diameter	980 rpm	20-inch diameter	759 rpm
14-inch diameter	909 rpm	22-inch diameter	724 rpm
16-inch diameter	848 rpm	24-inch diameter	695 rpm

The diameter of the head is the distance between the inside bottoms of the opposite cups measured through the center of rotation of the centrifuge head while the cups are horizontally extended.

6.4 Centrifuge tubes: Conical and graduated as follows:
From 0 to 1.0 mL in 0.1-mL divisions,
From 1.0 to 2.0 mL in 0.2-mL divisions,
From 2.0 to 10.0 mL in 0.5-mL divisions,
From 10.0 to 20.0 mL in 1.0-mL divisions,
And a 50.0-mL mark at least $^1/_2$ inch from the top of tube.

6.5 Siphon tube: Glass (for siphoning milk from the centrifuge tube).

6.6 Thermometer: 0° to 100°C

7. **Sampling:** Chapter 3 on "Sampling Dairy and Related Products."

8. **Preparation of Test Sample:** Take a representative sample that has previously been mixed, stirred, ground, blended, or otherwise prepared in order to make sample uniform.

9. **Procedure:** Before beginning analysis review material safety data sheets on all chemicals and use appropriate safety equipment such as hoods, aprons, face shields and glasses.

9.1 Add 20 g of nonfat dry milk, dry buttermilk, or dry buttermilk product or 26 g of dry whole milk to 200 mL of water at a temperature of 75°F (24°C) in the glass mixing container.

9.2 Place the glass container on the mixer and mix for exactly 90 seconds at the #1 speed setting of the Waring blender. If there is an immediate need for re-use of the mixing container, the entire mixed sample may, at this point, be transferred to a suitable tumbler.

9.3 Allow sample to stand for a period of at least 5 minutes but not to exceed 15 minutes.

9.4 Mix sample thoroughly with a spoon for 5 seconds and immediately fill the conical centrifuge tube to the 50-mL mark with rehydrated sample.

9.5 Centrifuge sample for 5 minutes at the required rpm.

9.6 Immediately siphon off the supernatant liquid to within 5 mL of the surface of the sediment level, using care not to disturb the sediment layer.

9.7 Add about 25 mL water at a temperature of 75°F (24°C) and mix the contents of the tube gently to disperse the sediment. If sediment does not dislodge, use a wire to disperse.

9.8 Fill the tube to the 50-mL mark with water at 75°F (24°C). Invert several times to mix the contents thoroughly.

9.9 Centrifuge again at the required rpm for 5 minutes.

9.10 After centrifuging, remove the conical tube and hold in a vertical position with the upper level of the sediment on a level with the eye. The sediment is easily distinguished when the tube is held between the eye and a strong source of light.

10. **Expression of Results:** Report to the nearest graduated scale division the milliliters of sediment in the tube.
11. **Precision and Performance Parameters:** No precision data available for this assay.
12. **Test Report and Interpretation:** The test report should identify the method used and results obtained. The report will also identify any variation in the test not specified in this method as well as problems that may have impacted the test result. Each sample will be described in such a manner as to ensure traceability as to its origin.

15.172 Scorched Particles (Class O)[6]

1. **Scope:** This method is applicable to dry whole milk, nonfat dry milk, dry buttermilk, and dry buttermilk product by spray process as well as the roller process.
2. **References:** Chapter 2 on "Laboratory Quality Assurance and Safety." Chapter 3 on "Sampling Dairy and Related Products."
3. **Definition:** Scorched particles are defined as the colored insoluble particle residue remaining on a filter disc after filtration of a resolubilized dry milk powder.
4. **Principle:** A sample of dried milk product is resolublized in water and filtered through a filter disc, and the material remaining on disc is visually compared to a specified standard.
5. **Reagents:** Unless otherwise specified all chemicals are reagent or ACS grade.
   - 5.1 Defoaming agent: Antifoam B emulsion, A5757 (Sigma Chemical Co., St. Louis, MO).
   - 5.2 Water (LG): Sediment free.
   - 5.3 Sodium citrate: 10% solution. Dissolve 100 g of sodium citrate in LG water and make up to 1 L. Filter through a cotton disc before using.
   - 5.4 Sodium hexametaphosphate (Calgon powder unadjusted): 2% solution. Dissolve 20 g of unadjusted Calgon in LG water and make up to 1 L. Filter cold through a cotton disc before using.
   - 5.5 Tetra sodium salt of ethylenediamine tetra-acetic acid (EDTA): 10% solution. Dissolve 100 g of the chemical and make up to 1 L. Filter cold through a cotton disc before use.
6. **Apparatus and Glassware:** All volumetric flasks, pipets, and burets are Class A unless otherwise specified.
   - 6.1 *ADPI Scorched Particle Standards for Dry Milks:* Photoprint published by the American Dairy Products Institute.
     - 6.1.1 The intensity of color in the ADPI *Scorched Particle Standards for Dry Milks* photoprint may fade over a period of time, depending on exposure to light and the method of handling/storage. To minimize fading when not in use, the photoprint should be stored in a dark place (i.e., desk or file drawer), ideally between two sheets of black construction paper. Periodic replacement is recommended. If it is noted that a standard photoprint has faded, it should be replaced with a new standard.

6.2 Balance: 500-g capacity and 0.1-g or better sensitivity.

6.3 Blender or mixer: Waring blender, or similar type.

6.3.1 Malted milk-type mixers and the solubility index mixer do not always give comparable results. Waring blender with worn or bent shaft should be replaced since metal particles may be produced, giving false scorched particle readings.

6.4 Pipet or pipeter: Capable of measuring 0.5 mL of Antifoam.

6.5 Thermometer: 0° to 100°C

6.6 Scorched particle filtering discs: Cotton discs 1.25-inch diameter, or cotton pads mounted on test cards for use with the aspirator-type tester.

6.7 Scorched particle disc test cards: Needed for individual discs only.

6.8 Scorched particle tester: Aspirator, or pressure type, 1.125-inch filtering diameter.

7. **Sampling:** Chapter 3 on "Sampling Dairy and Related Products."

8. **Preparation of Test Sample:** Take a representative sample that has previously been mixed, stirred, ground, blended, or otherwise prepared in order to make sample uniform.

9. **Procedure:** Before beginning analysis review material safety data sheets on all chemicals and use appropriate safety equipment such as hoods, aprons, face shields, and glasses.

9.1 **Water disc method, spray process for dry milk Products**

9.1.1 Measure 250 mL sediment-free water in Waring blender jar. Start the mixer and add 25 g of nonfat dry milk (NDM), dry buttermilk, or dry buttermilk product, or 32.5 g dry whole milk. Add 20 g of NDM, dry buttermilk, or dry buttermilk product or 26 g of dry whole milk to 200 mL of water at a temperature of 75°F (24°C) in the glass mixing container.

9.1.2 Add approximately 0.5 mL of Antifoam B emulsion, A5757, and mix for 60 seconds in the blender. Filter the entire solution through a standard cotton disc, using an aspirator or pressure type tester.

9.1.3 Rinse the mixing container and tester with approximately 50 mL of sediment-free water, also passing this through the cotton disc.

9.1.4 If re-liquefied sample is allowed to stand before filtering, stir vigorously just before pouring it into the tester. Do not allow samples to stand uncovered.

9.1.5 Remove the filter disc, place it in a scorched particle disc test card, and dry at 30°-40°C in a dust-free atmosphere.

9.2 **Calgon method, roller process for dry whole milk and NDM**

9.2.1 Measure 250 mL of the 2% Calgon solution, heated to 80°C, into a Waring blender jar. Turn on the mixer and add 17 g of well-mixed sample of nonfat dry milk (NDM) or 22 g of dry whole milk.

9.2.2 Add approximately 0.5 mL of Antifoam B emulsion A5757, and mix for 30 seconds in the blender. Filter immediately through a standard cotton disc, using an aspirator or pressure-type tester.

9.2.3 Rinse the mixing container and tester with approximately 25 mL of sediment-free water, also passing this through the cotton disc. Place the disc in a scorched particle disc test card and dry at 30°-40°C in a dust-free atmosphere.

9.3 **Sodium citrate method, roller process for dry whole milk and NDM**

9.3.1 Measure 200 mL of hot (80°-90°C) 10% sodium citrate solution into a Waring blender jar. Turn on mixer and add 17 g of well-mixed sample of NDM or 22 g of dry whole milk.

9.3.2 Add approximately 0.5 mL of Antifoam B emulsion, A5757, and mix for 30 seconds in the blender. Filter the entire solution through a standard cotton disc, using an aspirator or pressure-type tester.

9.3.3 Rinse the mixing container and tester with hot sediment-free water, also passing this through the cotton disc. Place the disc in a scorched particle disc test card and dry at 30°-40°C in a dust-free atmosphere.

9.4 EDTA method, roller process for dry buttermilk and dry buttermilk product

9.4.1 Place approximately 300 mL of a hot (80°-85°C) 10% solution of tetra sodium salt of ethylenediamine tetra acetic acid (dispersing agent) in the mixing jar of the high-speed mixer.

9.4.2 Turn on the mixer and add 17 g of dry buttermilk. Add a few drops of Antifoam B emulsion, A5757.

9.4.3 Mix 8-10 seconds.

9.4.4 Add additional hot solution of the dispersing agent to the mixer until the volume of sample solution is approximately 500 mL.

9.4.5 Agitate the sample solution for an additional 45 seconds and filter immediately through a 1.25-inch cotton disc. Rinse mixing container with hot water, passing all rinsings through the filter disc. Filter the entire solution through a standard cotton disc, using an aspirator or pressure-type tester.

10. Expression of Results: Compare the dry disc, placed on a table and viewed from directly above, with the ADPI *Scorched Particle Standards* photoprint under uniform, indirect light. Any test falling between two standard discs should be assigned the higher disc's letter. (Example: a disc showing more scorched particles than standard disc A but less than B should be assigned a B, and similarly for the other discs.)

11. Precision and Performance Parameters: No precision data available for this assay.

12. Test Report and Interpretation: The test report should identify the method used and results obtained. The report will also identify any variation in the test not specified in this method as well as problems that may have impacted the test result. Each sample will be described in such a manner as to ensure traceability as to its origin.

15.180 Cited References

1. ALBALA-HURTADO, S; NOVELLA-RODRIGUEZ, S.; VECIANA-NOGUES, M.T.; MARINE-FONT, A. Determination of vitamins A and E in infant milk formulae by high-performance liquid chromatography. J. Chromatogr. A. **778:**243-246; 1997.
2. ALLCROFT, R.; ROBERTS, B.A. Toxic groundnut meal: the relationship between aflatoxin B_1 intake by cows and excretion of afltoxin M_1 in milk. Vet. Rec. **82**:116-118: 1968.
3. ALPHA-LAVAL. Dairy Handbook. Lund, Sweden: Alpha-Laval Food Engineering AB. p. 23.
4. AMERICAN BUTTER INSTITUTE. Laboratory manual—methods of analysis, Chicago, IL: American Butter Institute. 1947.
5. AMERICAN DAIRY PRODUCTS INSTITUTE. Bulletin No. W-16. Chicago, IL: ADPI.
6. AMERICAN DAIRY PRODUCTS INSTITUTE. *Standards for Grades of Dry Milk, including Methods of Analysis.* Bulletin 916. Chicago, IL: ADPI; 1990.
7. AMERICAN OIL CHEMISTS SOCIETY. Official methods and recommended practices, 5th ed. Champaign, IL: AOCS; 1997.
8. ANDERSON, B.A.; BERLIN, E. Moisture Analysis and Estimation of Crystalline Alpha Lactose in Whey Powders. J. Dairy Science **57:**786-792; 1974.
9. APPLEBAUM, R.S.; BRACKETT, R.E.; WISEMAN, D.W.; MARTH, E.H. Aflatoxin: toxicity to dairy cattle and occurrence in milk and milk products—a review. J. Food Prot. **45**:752-777; 1982.
10. ASSOCIATION OF OFFICIAL ANALYTICAL CHEMISTS. *Official Methods of Analysis of AOAC International.* 16th ed. Washington, DC: AOAC; 1995.
11. ASSOCIATION OF OFFICIAL ANALYTICAL CHEMISTS. *Official Methods of Analysis of AOAC International.* 17th ed. Gaithersburg, MD: AOAC International, 2000.
12. BALL, G.F.M. Fat-soluble vitamin assays in food analysis. A comprehensive review. New York: Elsevier Applied Science. 1988.
13. BARBANO, D.M.; CLARK, J.L. Infrared milk analysis: Challenges for the future. J. Dairy Sci. **72:**1627-1636; 1989.
14. BARBANO, D.M.; CLARK, J.L.; DUNHAM, C.E. Comparison of the Babcock and ether extraction methods for determination of fat content of milk: Collaborative Study. JAOAC **71:**898-914; 1988.
15. BARBANO, D.M.; CLARK, J.L.; DUNHAM, C.E.; FLEMING, J.R. Kjeldahl method for determination of total nitrogen content of milk: collaborative study. JAOAC **73:**849-859; 1990.
16. BARBANO, D.M.; DELLA VALLE, M.E. Microwave drying to determine the solids content of milk and cottage and cheddar cheese. J Food Prot. **47**:272-278; 1984.
17. BARBANO, D.M.; LYNCH, J.M. Direct and indirect determination of true protein content of milk by Kjeldahl analysis: collaborative study. J. Assoc. Off. Anal. Chem. **74:**281-288; 1991.
18. BIGGS, D.A. Infrared estimation of fat, protein and lactose in milk: Evaluation of multispec instrument. JAOAC **62:**1202-1210; 1979.
19. BIGGS, D.A. Milk analyses with the infrared milk analyzer. J. Dairy Sci. **50:**799-803; 1967.
20. BIGGS, D.A. Performance specifications for infrared milk analysis. JAOAC **62:**1211-1214; 1979.
21. BRUBACHER, G.; MULLER-MULOT, W.; SOUTHGATE, D.A.T. Methods for the determination of vitamins in foods. New York: Elsevier Applied Science. 1986.
22. BRUHN, J.C.; FRANKE, A.A. An indirect method for the estimation of the iodine content in raw milk. J. Dairy Science. **61:**1557-1560; 1978.
23. CLARK, J.L.; BARBANO, D.M.; DUNHAM, C.E. Comparison of two methods for determining total solids content of raw milk: Collaborative Study. JAOAC **72:**712-718; 1989.
24. CODE OF FEDERAL REGULATIONS. 21CFR (sections 131, 133, 135), 2000, Washington, DC: Office of Federal Register, National Archives.
25. COTLOVE, E. Determination of the true chloride content of biological fluids and tissues: II. Analysis by simple, nonisotopic methods. Anal Chem. **35:** 101-105; 1963.
26. DE VRIES, J. *Food Safety and Toxicity*, CRC Press, 1997.

27. DOAN, F.J.; LARSON, B.L.; WINDER, W.C.; LEEDER, J.C. Procedures for making acidity tests of fluid milk products. J Dairy Science. **40:**1643-1644;1957.
28. ENGLAND, C.W.; NEFF, M. The accuracy of cryoscopic methods. JAOAC **46:**1043-1049; 1963.
29. FRANKEL, E.N.; TARASSUK, N.P. Inhibition of lipase and lipolyusis in milk. J. Dairy Sci. **42:**409-419;1959.
30. GORHAM, R.J. FDA Tech bulletin no.1, Principles of food analysis for filth decomposition and foreign matter. Washington, DC: FDA, 1985.
31. GREEN, W.C.; PARK, K.K. Comparison of AOAC, microwave and vacuum oven methods for determining total solids in milk. J Food Prot. **43:**782-783; 1980.
32. HAGER, A.F.; MADSEN, L.; WALES, L.; BRADFORD, H.B., Jr. Reversed-phase liquid chromatographic determination of vitamin D in milk. JAOAC Intl. **77:**1047-1051; 1994.
33. HANSEN, T.J. Affinity column cleanup and direct fluorescence measurement of aflatoxin M1 in raw milk. J. Food Protection, **53:**75-77; 1990.
34. HEINEMANN, B.J.; COSIMINI, J.; JACK, E.L.; WILLINGHAM, J.J.; ZAKARIASEN, B.M. Methods of determining the percent total solids in milk by means of the lactometer. J Dairy Sci. **37:**869-876; 1954.
35. HELRICH, K., ed. *Official methods of analysis*, 15th ed. Washington, DC: AOAC; 1990.
36. HENNINGSON, R.W. The variability of the freezing point of fresh raw milk. JAOAC **46:**1036-1042; 1963.
37. HERRINGTON, B.L. Lipase: a review. J. Dairy Sci. **37:**775-789; 1954.
38. HORWITZ, W. Guidelines for collaborative study procedures to validate characteristics of a method of analysis. JAOAC **71:**160-171; 1988.
39. INDYK, H; WOOLLARD, D.C. The determination of vitamin D in fortified milk powders and infant formulas by HPLC. J. Micronutr. Anal. **1:**121-141; 1985.
40. INTERNATIONAL DAIRY FEDERATION. IDF Standard 29:1964—Determination of the casein content of milk. Brussels, Belgium: IDF; 1964.
41. INTERNATIONAL DAIRY FEDERATION. IDF Standard 108:1982. Brussels, Belgium: IDF; 1982.
42. INTERNATIONAL DAIRY FEDERATION. IDF Standard 135A:1988—Milk and milk products: precision characteristics of analytical methods; Outline of collaborative study procedure. Brussels, Belgium: IDF; 1988.
43. INTERNATIONAL DAIRY FEDERATION, IDF Standard 15B:1991. Brussels, Belgium: IDF; 1991.
44. INTERNATIONAL DAIRY FEDERATION. IDF Standard 171:1995. Determination of aflatoxin M1 content; cleanup by immunoaffinity chromatography and determination by HPLC. Brussels, Belgium: IDF; 1995.
45. INTERNATIONAL ORGANIZATION FOR STANDARDIZATION. Milk—determination of fat content—Gerber butyrometers. International Standard ISO 488-1983(E). Geneva, Switzerland. 1983.
46. INTERNATIONAL ORGANIZATION FOR STANDARDIZATION. Milk—determination of freezing point—thermistor cryoscope method; ISO 5764. Geneva, Switzerland. 2000.
47. JAOAC. **30:**130; 1947.
48. JAOAC. **34:**239; 1951.
49. JAOAC. **67:**637; 1984.
50. JAOAC. **67:**899; 1984
51. KIERMEIER, F. The significance of aflatoxins in the dairy industry. Intern. Dairy Fed. Doc. No. 30; 1974.
52. KIHLSTRUM, E.E.; DELHEY, R.W., Farm bulk tank sediment testing. J. Milk Food Technology. **28:**108-112; 1960.
53. KLEYN, D.H.; TROUT, J.R.; WEBER, M. Determination of fat in raw milk: comparison of Mojonnior (ether extraction) and Gerber method. JAOAC **71:**851-853; 1988.
54. KOHMAN, E.F. Rapid and accurate method of butter analysis for factory control work. Ind. Eng. Chem. **11:**36; 1919.
55. KURAMOTO, S.; JENNESS, R.; COULTER, S.T.; CHOI, R.P. Standardization of the Harland–Ashworth test for whey protein nitrogen. J Dairy Science. **42:**28; 1959.

56. LACROIX; WANG. J. Food Protect. **43:**672- 675; 1980.
57. LEVOWITZ, D. An appraisal of the Gerber test for milkfat in milk and market milk products. J. Milk Food Technol. **23:**69-72; 1960.
58. LINGANE, J.J. Automatic coulometric titration with electrolytically generated silver ion: determination of chloride, bromide, and iodide iions. Anal. Chem. **26:**622-626; 1954.
59. LYNCH, J.M.; BARBANO, D.M.; HEALY, P.A.; FLEMING, J.R. Performance evaluation of the Babcock and ether extraction methods: 1989 through 1992. JAOACI **77:**976-981; 1994.
60. LYNCH, J.M.; BARBANO, D.M.; FLEMING, J.R. Comparison of Babcock and ether extraction methods for determination of fat content of cream: collaborative study. JAOACI. **79:**907-916; 1996.
61. LYNCH, J.M.; BARBANO, D.M.; FLEMING, J.R. Modification of Babcock method to eliminate fat testing bias between the Babcock and ether extraction methods (modification of AOAC official methods 989.04 and 995.18): collaborative study. JAOACI. **80:**845-859; 1997.
62. LYNCH, J.M.; BARBANO, D.M.; FLEMING, J.R. Performance evaluation of direct forced air total solids and Kjeldahl total nitrogen methods: 1990-1995. JAOACI **80:**1038-1043;1997.
63. LYNCH, J.M., BARBANO, D.M., FLEMING, J.R. Indirect and direct determination of the casein content of milk by Kjeldahl nitrogen analysis: Collaborative study. JAOAC International **81:**763-774; 1998.
64. MADDEN, D.E.; BRUNNER, J.R. Comparative accuracy of small lactometers for determining the total solids of individual cows' milk. J Dairy Sci. **41:**783-788; 1958.
65. MARSHALL, R.T., ed. *Standard Methods for the Examination of Dairy Products*. 16th ed. Washington, DC: APHA; 1992.
66. MARTH, E.H., ed. *Standard Methods for the Examination of Dairy Products.* 15th ed. Washington, DC: APHA; 1978.
67. MARTH, E.H. Dairy products. In: BEUCHAT, L.R., ed. *Food and beverage mycology,* 2nd ed. New York: Van Nostrand Reinhold Co.; 1987:175-209.
68. MCKINLEY, M.R.; ARNOLD, R.E.; ROSENBURY, J.B.; BORN, E.C.; DUNHAM, C.E.; PARK, D.L. Evaluation of the Babcock method for the determination of milkfat. JAOAC **58:**949-956;1975.
69. MILK INDUSTRY FOUNDATION. *Methods of analysis of milk and its products.* Washington, DC: Milk Industry Foundation. 3rd printing, 1964.
70. MOJONNIER, T.; TROY, H.C. *Technical control of dairy products.* Chicago, IL: Mojonnier Bros. Co.; 1925.
71. OLSON, N.F. Measuring cheese acidity—the relationship of titratable acidity and pH in cheese making. Dairy Field, Jan. 1976: 32-34
72. PAUL, R.; KALRA, M.S.; SINGH, A. Incidence of aflatoxins in milk and milk products. Ind. J. Dairy Sci. **29**:318-321; 1976.
73. PIEPER, H.; STUART, S.A.; RENWICK, W.R., Jr. Microwave technique for rapid determination of moisture in cheese. **60:**1392-1396; 1977.
74. POMERANZ, Y., MELOAN, C.E. *Food analysis: theory and practice.* Westport CT: AVI Publishing Co., Inc. 1982.
75. POMERANZ, Y.; MELOAN, C.E. *Food analysis: theory and practice.* 2nd edition. AVI Publishing Co., 1987.
76. REYNOLDS, J.N.; JUDD, H.J. Rapid procedure for the determination of vitamins A and D in fortified skimmed milk powder using high-performance liquid chromatography. Analyst. **109:**489-492; 1984.
77. ROWLAND, S.J. *J Dairy Res.* **9:**42-46; 1938.
78. SHIPE, W.F. Report on cryoscopy of milk. JAOAC **41:**262-267; 1958.
79. SLIVA, M.G.; GREEN, A.E.; SANDERS, J.K.; EUBER, J.R.; SAUCERMAN, J.R. Reversed-phase liquid chromatographic determination of vitamin D in infant formulas and enteral nutritionals. JAOAC International **75:**566-571; 1992.
80. SMITH, E.B.; BARBANO, D.M.; LYNCH, J.M.; FLEMING, J.R. Performance of homogenizers in infrared milk analyzers: A survey. JAOAC Int. **76:**1033-1041; 1993.
81. SMITH, E.B.; BARBANO, D.M.; LYNCH, J.M.; FLEMING, J.R. Effect of infrared analyzer homogenization on repeatability. JAOAC **77:**1217-1223; 1994.

82. SMITH, E.B.; BARBANO, D.M.; LYNCH, J.M.; FLEMING, J.R. A quantitative linearity evaluation method for infrared milk analyzers. JAOAC **76:**1300-1308; 1993.
83. SOMMER, H.H.; WINDER, W.C. *The physical chemistry of dairy and food products.* Madison, WI: University of Wisconsin; 1978.
84. SPICER, D.W.; PRICE, W.V. A test for extraneous matter in cheese. J. Dairy Science. **21:**1-6; 1938.
85. SPEER, J.F., Jr.; WATROUS, G.H., Jr.; KESLER, E.M. The relationship of certain factors affecting hydrolytic rancidity in milk. J. Milk Food Technol. **21:**33-37; 1958.
86. STEIGER, G.; MARTENS, R. 1988. Bulletin of the IDF No. 235, pp. 13-19.
87. SWOPE, W.D. The Pennsylvania methods for determining the percentage of fat in dairy products. State College, PA: Pennsylvania Agric. Exper. Sta. Bull. 412; 1941.
88. TEE, E.-S.; LIM, C.-L. The analysis of carotenoids and retinoids: A review. Food Chemistry. **41:**147-193; 1991.
89. THIEX, N.; SMALLIDGE, R.; BEINE, R. Sources of error in vitamin A analysis. JAOAC International. **79:**1269-1275; 1996.
90. THOMAS, E.L.; NIELSEN, A.J.; OLSON, J.C., Jr. Hydrolytic rancidity of milk: a simplified method for estimating the extent of its development. Amer. Milk Rev. **17:**50-52, 85; 1955.
91. THOMPSON, J.N. Review: Official methods for measurement of vitamin A. JAOAC International. **69:**727-738; 1986.
92. THOMPSON, J.N.; DUVAL, S. Determination of vitamin A in milk and infant formula by HPLC. J. Micronutr. Anal. **6:**147-159; 1989.
93. THOMPSON, J.N.; HATINA, G.; MAXELL, W.B., DUVAL, S. High performance liquid chromatographic determination of vitamin D in fortified milk, margarine and infant formulas. JAOAC International. **65:**624-631; 1982.
94. TRUCKSESS, et al. Immunoaffinity column coupled with fluorometry solution or liquid chromatography postcolumn derivatization for determination of aflatoxins in corn, peanuts and peanut butter: Collaborative study. JAOAC. **74:** 1991.
95. U.S. DEPARTMENT OF AGRICULTURE. Laboratory methods and procedures. In: "DA Instruction 918-RL" pages C12-1 through C12-5 (Revised January 2, 2001), Washington, DC: USDA, Agricultural Marketing Service, Dairy Programs, Dairy Grading Branch.
96. U.S. DEPARTMENT OF HEALTH AND HUMAN SERVICES. Food and Drug Administration, *Pesticide Analytical Manual*, Volumes I to V, 1999.
97. U.S. DEPARTMENT OF HEALTH AND HUMAN SERVICES. Pasteurized Milk Ordinance. Public Health Service/Food and Drug Administration. Publication 229, 1995.
98. U.S. ENVIRONMENTAL PROTECTION AGENCY. *Manual of Chemical Methods for Pesticides and Devices*. Arlington, VA: AOAC. 1992.
99. U.S. PHARMACOPOEIA. Vol. 23. National Formulary Vol. 18, 1995. Method 921 Water Determination pp. 1840-1841. and Water in Lactose, pp. 2257-2258.
100. VAN DE VOORT, F.R. Evaluation of Milk: Scan 104 infrared milk analyzer. JAOAC **63:**973-980; 1980.
101. VAN DE VOORT, F.R.; ELKASHEF, A.A.; BLAIS, J.S. Interlaboratory assessment of dry calibration milk powders for calibrating infrared milk analyzers. JAOAC **74:**1-8; 1991.
102. VAN DE VOORT, F.R.; ELKASHEF, A.A.; MILLS, B.L. Dry calibration milks for infrared milk analyzers. JAOAC **73:**688-692; 1990.
103. WATSON, N.E. Determination of sediment in milk in farm tanks and/or plant storage tanks and tank trucks. J. Milk Food Technology. **19:**228-229; 1956.
104. WATSON, P.D. Determination of the solids of milk by a lactometric method at 102°F. J Dairy Sci. **40:**394-402; 1957.
105. WEBB, B.H., JOHNSON, A.H., ALFORD, J.A. *Fundamentals of dairy chemistry.* 2nd ed. Westport, CT: AVI Publishing Co., Inc. 1974.
106. WISEMAN, D.W.; MARTH, E.H. Stability of aflatoxin M_1 during manufacture and storage of ice-cream and sherbet. Z. Lebensm. Unters. Forsch. **177:**22-24; 1983.
107. WONG, N.P. *Fundamentals of dairy chemistry.* 3rd edition. New York: Van Nostrand Reinhold, Agricultural Research Service, USDA. 1988; 372-384.

108. WRIGHT, E.O.; CLARK, W.S., Jr.; WEBBER, R.W.; ARLEDGE, W.L.; ROMAN, M.H.; HOTCHKISS, D.K. A collaborative study to determine the feasibility of using 0.40, 0.20, 0.14, and 0.10 inch diameter discs to measure sediment in fluid milk. J. Milk Prot. **40:**41; 1977.

Chapter 16

Milk and Milk Products Standards

D. Lewis, D. Spomer, M. Smith, and W. Clark
(R. T. Marshall, Tech. Comm.)

16.010 Introduction

This chapter is a compilation of U.S. and international milk product standards. It covers the nutritional, compositional, and microbiological requirements of 12 separate product categories. Section 16.020 focuses on labeling regulations of the U.S. It describes the federal requirements for nutrition information for food labeling purposes. Section 16.030 identifies U.S. compositional and physical parameter requirements while 16.040 identifies international compositional and physical parameter requirements. 16.050 provides microbiological specifications for those products for which specifications have been established.

The U.S. tabulated specifications reflect regulations in the FDA's Pasteurized Milk Ordinance, Dry Milk Ordinance, and Compliance Policy Guides. Information on dairy product standards is also available in FDA's Title 21, Code of Federal Regulations (CFR) and USDA's Title 7, CFR.

The international tabulated specifications reflect the standards of the U.N.-based Codex Alimentarius Commission or Codex. Codex is the principal international organization for establishing food standards that protect public health and facilitate trade.

Country-specific information is available in the *United States Dairy Export Manual*. Copies can be obtained on a fee basis from the U.S. Dairy Export Council, 2101 Wilson Boulevard, Suite 400, Arlington, VA 22201, Telephone: (703) 528-3049, Fax: (703) 528-3705.

16.020 Nutrition and Labeling Requirements

Congress provided for the establishment of definitions and standards of identity for particular foods in the Federal Food Drug and Cosmetic Act of 1938. FDA has established a number of standards of identity for milk and milk products and these are found in 21 CFR Parts 131 (milk and cream), 133 (cheese and related cheese products), and 135 (frozen desserts). Foods

Table 16.1. Nutrient Content Claims for Fat Content

Nutrient Content Claim	Synonyms	Fat Content
Fat free	Free of fat, no fat, zero fat, without fat, nonfat, trivial source of fat, negligible source of fat, dietary insignificant source of fat, or, in the case of milk products, skim	< 0.5 g of fat per RACC*
Lowfat	Low in fat, contains a small amount of fat, low source of fat, little fat	≤ 3 g of fat per RACC
Reduced fat	Reduced in fat, fat reduced, less fat, lower fat, lower in fat	Food contains at least 25% less fat per RACC than an appropriate reference food
Light	Lite	Contains at least 50% less fat per RACC than an appropriate reference food if the food derives 50% or more of its calories from fat

*Reference Amount Customarily Consumed
Source: Table 1. U.S. Food and Drug Administration. Code of Federal Regulations Title 21, Sub-Parts 101.56, 62.

that are defined by a standard of identity must be labeled according to the standard.

More recently, the Nutrition Labeling and Education Act (NLEA) of 1990 established labeling requirements for virtually all processed foods. The NLEA includes policy issues governing nutrition labeling, serving sizes, nutrient content claims, and health claims. Nutrition labeling has become mandatory on most foods except raw fruits, vegetables, and seafood. The food label content panel, which reflects changing health concerns of the nation, features information on the amount of cholesterol, saturated fat, carbohydrates, calories, and calories from fat contained in a serving of food. Under the NLEA, standardized reference amounts are set for 131 food categories in quantities customarily consumed and that are expressed on the label in common household measures. To communicate effectively, every manufacturer and marketer must use descriptors having only one meaning defined by FDA. The regulations spell out what terms may be used to describe the level of nutrients in a food and how they can be used.

NLEA policy concerning nomenclature permits foods to be named by use of a defined nutrient content claim (e.g., reduced fat or lowfat) and a standardized term (e.g., milk or cottage cheese) provided that in terms of shelf life and sensory, physical, functional, and nutritional characteristics, it is equivalent to the standardized food (see Table 16.1). The compositional specifications compiled in this chapter are standardized legal requirements that can be modified in accordance with NLEA regulations.

Standard serving sizes are the basis of reporting nutrient content in foods. NLEA defines serving size as the amount of food customarily eaten at one time. The serving sizes that appear on food labels are based on FDA and USDA established lists (see Table 16.2). They are expressed in both common household and metric measures.

Table 16.2. Reference Amounts Customarily Consumed per Eating Occasion

Product Category	Reference Amount	Label Statement
Cheese, cottage	110 g	__ cup (__ g)
Cheese used primarily as an ingredient (e.g., dry cottage cheese, ricotta cheese)	55 g	__ cup (__ g)
Cheese, grated, hard (e.g., Parmesan, Romano)	5 g	__ tbsp (__ g)
Cheese, all others except those listed as separate categories—cream includes cream cheese and cheese spread ure)	30 g	__ piece(s) (__ g) for distinct pieces; __ tbsp(s) (__ g) for cheese and cheese spread; 1 oz (28 g/visual unit of meas- for bulk
Cream, fluid	15 mL	1 tsp (15 mL)
Cream, powder	2 g	__ tsp (__ g)
Cream, half & half	30 mL	2 tbsp (30 mL)
Eggnog mL)	120 mL	__ cup (120 mL); 4 fl oz (120
Milk, condensed, undiluted	30 mL	2 tbsp (30 mL)
Milk, evaporated, undiluted	30 mL	2 tbsp (30 mL)
Milk, milk-based drinks (e.g., instant breakfast, meal replacement, cocoa)	240 mL	1 cup (240 mL); 8 fl oz (240 mL)
Shakes (e.g., dairy shake mixes)	240 mL	1 cup (240 mL); 8 fl oz (240 mL)
Sour cream	30 g	__ tsp (__g)
Yogurt	225 g	__ cup (__ g)
Ice cream, frozen yogurt, sherbet, all types, bulk and novelties (e.g., bars, sandwiches, cones)	__ cup—includes the volume for coatings and wafers for the novelty type varieties	__ piece(s) (__ g) for individually wrapped or packaged products; __ cup (__ g) for others
Butter	1 tbsp	1 tbsp (__ g); 1 tbsp (15 ml)

Source: Table 2. U.S. Food and Drug Administration. Code of Federal Regulations Title 21, Sub-Part 101.12.

16.030 Compositional Specifications

Table 16.3. Fluid Milk/Half and Half/Cream

Product	Milkfat % Min.	Milkfat % Max.	SNF % Min.
Whole milk	3.25	—	8.25
Reduced fat milk		2.44	8.25
Lowfat		1.25	8.25
Fat free		0.2	8.25
Half and half	10.5	18.0	—
Cream	18.0	—	—
Light cream	18.0	30.0	—
Light whipping cream	30.0	—	—
Heavy cream	36.0	—	—

Source: U.S. Food and Drug Administration. Code of Federal Regulations Title 21, Sub-Part 131.

Table 16.4. Concentrated Milks

Product	Milkfat % Min.	Total Milk Solids % Min.
Evaporated	6.5	23.0
Sweetened condensed	8.0	28.0

Source: U.S. Food and Drug Administration. Code of Federal Regulations Title 21, Sub-Part 131.

Table 16.5. Cultured/Acidified Products

Product	Milkfat % Min.	SNF % Min.	Titratable Acidity % Min.
Cultured milk	3.25	8.25	—
Sour cream	18.0	—	0.5
Acidified milk	3.25	8.25	0.5
Acidified sour cream	18.0	—	0.5

Source: U.S. Food and Drug Administration. Code of Federal Regulations Title 21, Sub-Part 131.

Table 16.6. Frozen Desserts

Product	Milkfat % Min.	Total Milk Solids % Min.
Ice cream and frozen custard	10.0	20.0
Goat's milk ice cream	10.0	20.0

Sources: U.S. Food and Drug Administration. Code of Federal Regulations Title 21, Sub-Part 151.

Table 16.7. Yogurt

Product[1]	Milkfat %		SNF %
	Min.	Max.	Min.
Nonfat	—	0.5	8.25
Lowfat	0.5	2.0	8.25
Regular	3.25	—	8.25

[1]Yogurt is exempt from the Nutrition Labeling and Education Act.
Source: U.S. Food and Drug Administration. Code of Federal Regulations Title 21, Sub-Part 131.

Table 16.8. Butter/Butteroil/Anhydrous Milkfat

Product	Milkfat % Min.	SNF % Min.
Butter	80.0	—
Butteroil	99.6	0.3
Anhydrous milkfat	99.8	0.1

Source: U.S. Department of Agriculture. Code of Federal Regulations Title 7, Sub-Part 58.305 and 345.

Table 16.9. Dry Products

Product	Milkfat %		Moisture %	Titratable Acidity %		Solubility Index, mL		Scorched Particles, mg
Dry milks	*Min.*	*Max.*	*Max.*	*Min.*	*Max.*	*Min.*	*Max.*	*Max.*
Nonfat								
Extra grade	—	1.25	4.0	—	0.15	—	1.25	15.0
Standard grade	—	1.5	5.0	—	0.17	—	2.0	22.5
Instant	—	1.25	4.5	—	0.15	—	1.0	15.0
Dry whole	—	—	—	—	—	—	—	—
Extra grade	26.0	40.0	4.5	—	—	—	1.0	15.0
Standard grade	26.0	40.0	5.0	—	—	—	1.5	22.5
Dry buttermilk[1]	—	—	—	—	—	—	—	—
Extra grade	4.5	—	4.0	0.1	0.18	—	1.20	15.0
Standard grade	4.5	—	5.0	0.1	0.2	—	2.0	22.5
Dry cream	40.0	75.0	5.0	—		—	—	—
	Milkfat %		**Moisture %**	**Protein %**			**Free Acid/mL**	**Extraneous Materials/mg**
Edible dry casein (Acid)	*Min.*	*Max.*	*Max.*	*Min.*			*Max.*	*Max.*
Extra grade	—	1.5	10.0	95.0[2]			0.20	15.0
Standard grade	—	2.0	12.0	90.0[2]			0.27	22.5
	Milkfat %		**Moisture %**	**Titratable Acidity %**		**Lactose %**		**Scorched Particles/mg**
Dry whey products	*Min.*	*Max.*	*Max.*	*Min.*	*Max.*	*Min.*	*Max.*	*Max.*
Dry whey	—	—	—	—	—	—	—	—
Sweet type	—	1.5	5.0	—	0.16	—	—	15.0
Acid type	—	1.5	5.0	0.35	—	—	—	15.0
*Reduced lactose	0.2	4.0	6.0	—	—	—	60.0	—
*Reduced minerals	0.2	4.0	6.0	—	—	—	85.0	—
*Whey protein								
Whey protein concentrate	0.2	10.0	6.0	—	—	—	60.0	—
Whey protein isolate[3,4]	—	1.0	4.5	—	—	—	—	15.0
*Lactose	—	—	6.0	—	—	98.0	—	—

[1] Dry buttermilk ≥ 30% protein; Dry buttermilk products < 30% protein.
[2] Protein on the dry basis (nitrogen x 6.38).
[3] Whey protein isolate—92% protein on dry basis.
[4] Commercial standard.

Sources: *U.S. Food and Drug Administration. Code of Federal Regulations Title 21, Sub-Part 184.1979a, 1979b, 1979c, 168.122.

U.S. Department of Agriculture. Standards and specification for dairy products. Agriculture Marketing Service Dairy Division Dairy Standardization Branch. Washington, DC.

American Dairy Products Institute. Ingredient description brochure, 1992.

Table 16.10. Selected U.S. Natural Cheeses

Product	Milkfat[1] %		Moisture %	
	Min.	Max.	Min.	Max.
Natural cheeses				
Asiago (Fresh)	50	—	—	45
Blue	50	—	—	46
Brick	50	—	—	44
Cheddar	50	—	—	39
Colby	50	—	—	40
Cottage	4[2]	—	—	80
Cream	33[2]	—	—	55
Edam	40	—	—	45
Gorgonzola	50	—	—	42
Gouda	46	—	—	45
Gruyere	45	—	—	39
Limburger	50	—	—	50
Monterey	50	—	—	44
Mozzarella	45	—	52	60
Low moisture	45	—	45	52
Part skim	45	—	52	60
Low moisture, part skim	30	45	45	52
Muenster	50	—	—	46
Neufchatel	20[2]	33	—	65
Parmesan	32	—	—	32
Provolone	45	—	—	45
Romano	38	—	—	34
Roquefort	50	—	—	45
Swiss	43	—	—	41

[1] Fat on a dry basis unless otherwise specified.

[2] Fat content is percent by weight of the finished food.

Source: U.S. Food and Drug Administration. Code of Federal Regulations Title 21, Sub-Part 133.

Table 16.11. Pasteurized Process Cheeses

Product	Milkfat[1] % Min.	Moisture % Min.	Moisture % Max.
Made from single variety of cheese	Minimum milkfat of the variety of cheese used, but not less than 47%		The maximum moisture content of the variety of cheese used plus 1%, but not greater than 43%
Pasteurized process washed curd or pasteurized process Colby cheese	Minimum milkfat of the variety of cheese used, but not less than 47%		40
Pasteurized process gruyere cheese	45		44
Pasteurized process limburger cheese	50		51
Pasteurized process Swiss cheese			44
Pasteurized process cheese made from Swiss and gruyere	45		44
Pasteurized process cheese made from 2 varieties of cheese	Arithmetic average of minimum milkfat of the cheese varieties used, but not less than 47%		The arithmetic average of the maximum moisture content of the cheese varieties used plus 1%, but not greater than 43%
Pasteurized process cheese made from 2 or more varieties of cheddar, Colby, washed curd, or granular cheese	Arithmetic average of minimum milkfat of the cheese varieties used, but not less than 47%		40
Pasteurized process cheese food	23[2]		44
Pasteurized process cheese spread	20[2]	44	60

[1] Fat on a dry basis unless otherwise specified.
[2] Fat content is percent by weight of the finished food.
Source: U.S. Food and Drug Administration. Code of Federal Regulations Title 21, Sub-Part 133.

Table 16.12. Cold Pack Cheeses

Product	Milkfat[1] % Min.	Moisture % Max.
Made from single variety of cheese	Minimum milkfat of the variety of cheese used, but not less than 47%	Maximum moisture content of the variety of cheese used with no added water permitted
Cold pack Swiss cheese	43	41
Cold pack gruyere cheese	45	39
Made from Swiss and gruyere cheese	45	Arithmetic average of the maximum moisture of the cheese varieties used
Made from 2 varieties of cheese	Arithmetic average of the minimum milkfat of the cheese varieties used, but not less than 47%	Arithmetic average of the maximum moisture of the cheese varieties used, but not greater than 42%
Made from 2 varieties of cheddar, washed curd, Colby, and granular cheese	Arithmetic average of the minimum of the cheese varieties used, but not less than 47%	

[1] Fat on a dry basis.
Source: U.S. Food and Drug Administration. Code of Federal Regulations Title 21, Sub-Part 133.

16.040 International Compositional Specifications

Table 16.13. Butter/Milkfat Products

Product	Milkfat % Min.	SNF % Max.	Water Content % Max.
Butter	80.0	2.0	16.0
Butteroil	99.6	—	—
Anhydrous butteroil	99.8	—	0.1
Anhydrous milkfat	99.8	—	0.1
Milkfat	99.6	—	—
Ghee	99.6	—	—

Source: Codex Alimentarius Commission. ALINORM 99/11, pp. 38, 41, 45, and 49.

Table 16.14. Concentrated Milks

Product	Milkfat %		Total Milk Solids %	Milk Protein in SNF %
	Min.	*Max.*	*Min.*	*Min.*
Evaporated milk	7.5	—	25.0	34.0
Evaporated skimmed milk		1.0	20.0	34.0
Evaporated partly skimmed milk	1.0	7.5	20.0	34.0

	Milkfat %	SNF %	Milk Protein in SNF %
	Min.	*Min.*	*Min.*
Evaporated high-fat milk	15.0	11.5	34.0

	Milkfat %		Milk Solids %	SNF %	Milk Protein in SNF %
	Min.	*Max.*	*Min.*	*Min.*	*Min.*
Sweetened condensed milk	8.0		28.0		34.0
Sweetened condensed skimmed milk	—	1.0	24.0	—	34.0
Sweetened condensed partly skimmed milk	1.0	8.0	24.0	20.0	34.0
Sweetened condensed high fat	16.0	—	—	14.0	34.0

Source: Codex Alimentarius Commission. ALINORM 99/11, pp. 38, 41, 45, and 49.

Table 16.15. Dry Products

Product	Milkfat %		Moisture %	Protein in MSNF	Solubility Index mL	Scorched Particles mg	Titratable Acidity %
Dry Milks	***Min.***	***Max.***	***Max.***	***Min.***	***Max.***	***Max.***	***Max.***
Skimmed milk		1.5	5.0	34.0	1.0	15.0	18.0
Partly skimmed	1.5	26.0	5.0	34.0	1.0	15.0	18.0
Whole milk	26.0	42.0	5.0	34.0	1.0	15.0	18.0
Cream powder	42.0		5.0	34.0	—	—	—

	Milkfat %	Moisture %	Protein %	Casein %	Lactose %	Ash %		Sediment mg/25g	Free Acid %	pH
Edible Caseins	***Max.***	***Max.***	***Min.***	***Min.***	***Max.***	***Min.***	***Max.***	***Max.***	***Max.***	***Max.***
Rennet casein	2.0	12.0	84.0	95.0	1.0	7.5	—	15.0		—
Acid casein	2.0	12.0	90.0	95.0	1.0	—	2.5	22.5	.27	—
Caseinates	2.0	8.0	88.0	95.0	1.0	—		22.5 spray 81.5 roller	—	7.5

	Milkfat %	Moisture %	Protein %	Lactose %	Ash %	pH (in 10% solution)
Dry Whey	***Max.***	***Max.***	***Min.***	***Min.***	***Max.***	
Whey powder	2.0	5.0	11.0	61.0	9.5	> 5.1
Acid whey powder	2.0	4.5	10.0	61.0	15.0	≤ 5.1

Source: Codex Alimentarius Commission. ALINORM 99/11, pp. 38, 41, 45, & 49.

16.050 Microbiological Specifications

Table 16.16. Action Levels for All Dairy Products

	Action Level[1]
Microorganisms	
Salmonella	≥ 1 positive unit
Campylobacter coli	Do.
Campylobacter jejuni	Do.
Escherichia coli 0157-H7	Do.
Listeria monocytogenes	Do.
Yersinia enterocolitica	Do.
Toxins	
Aflatoxin M_1	≥ 0.5 ppb
Staphylococcal enterotoxin	Positive

[1] Criteria for direct seizure and citation.

Source: U.S. Food and Drug Administration. Part II Compliance policy guides, Chapter 5: Foods Sec. 527.300, Pathogens in Dairy Products. U.S. Food and Drug Administration. Part II Compliance policy guides, Chapter 5: Foods Sec. 527.400, Whole Milk, Low Fat Milk, Skim Milk - Aflatoxin M_1.

Table 16.17. Fluid Milk Product

	Coliform/mL Max.	SPC/mL Max.	Somatic Cell Count/mL Max.
Raw milk			
Grade A producer milk	—	100,000	750,000[1]
Grade A commingled milk	—	300,000	—
*Manufacturing grade producer milk	—	500,000	750,000[1]
*Manufacturing grade commingled milk	—	1,000,000	—
Pasteurized	—	—	—
Fluid milk and milk products	10	20,000	—
Cultured products	10	—	—

[1] For goat's milk SCC/mL is 1,000,000 max.

Source: U.S. Department of Health and Human Services. Grade A pasteurized milk ordinance: Recommendations of the Public Health Service/FDA. Publication No. 299:14.

*U.S. Department of Agriculture. Milk for manufacturing purposes and its production and processing: Recommended requirements.

Table 16.18. Condensed and Dry Milk/Condensed and Dry Whey/Dry Casein

Product	SPC/g Max.	Coliform/g Max.	DMC millions/g Max.
Condensed milk	30,000	10	—
Nonfat dry milk	—	—	—
Grade A	30,000	10	—
Extra grade	40,000	10	100
Instant	30,000	10	75
Standard grade	75,000	10	100
Dry whole milk	—	—	—
Extra grade	30,000	10	100
Standard grade	50,000	10	100
Dry buttermilk	—	—	—
Grade A	30,000	10	—
Extra grade	50,000	10	—
Standard grade	200,000	10	—
Dry buttermilk products	—	—	—
Grade A	30,000	10	—
Edible dry casein (Acid)	—	—	—
Extra grade	30,000	Negative/0.1 g	—
Standard grade	100,000	2 /0.1 g	—
Grade A condensed whey	30,000	10	
Condensed whey	30,000	10	—
Dry whey	—	—	—
Grade A	30,000	10	—
Extra grade	30,000	10	—
Dry whey products	—	—	—
Grade A	30,000	10	

Sources: U.S. Department of Agriculture. Standards and specification for dairy products.
U.S. Department of Health and Human Services. Grade A condensed and dry milk ordinance.

Table 16.19. Cheese and Cheese Products

Microorganism	Regulatory Action Level [1]
Enteropathogenic *E. coli*	> 1,000/g
E. coli	> 10,000/g and unsanitary conditions

[1] Criteria for direct seizure and citation. For further information reference FDA's latest regulation on permissible levels of these microorganisms.

Source: U.S. Food and Drug Administration. Part II Compliance policy guides, Chapter 5: Foods Sec. 527.300, Pathogens in Dairy Products.

16.060 Cited References

1. CODEX ALIMENTARIUS COMMISSION. Joint FAO/WHO Food Standards Programme, Codex Alimentarius Commission, ALINORM 99/11. Rome: Food and Agriculture Organization of the United Nations; 1999: 38, 41, 45, 49.
2. U.S. DEPARTMENT OF AGRICULTURE. Code of Federal Regulations Title 7. Agricultural Marketing Service. Part 58. *Grading and Inspection, General specifications for approved plants*. Washington, DC: U.S. Govt. Print. Off.; 1998.
3. U.S. DEPARTMENT OF AGRICULTURE. *Milk for manufacturing purposes and its production and processing: Recommended requirements.* Washington, DC: U.S. Govt. Print Off.; 1996.
4. U.S. DEPARTMENT OF AGRICULTURE. *Standards and specification for dairy products.* Agricultural Marketing Service Dairy Division Dairy Standardization Branch. Washington, DC: U.S. Govt. Print. Off.
5. U. S. DEPARTMENT OF HEALTH AND HUMAN SERVICES. *Grade A pasteurized milk ordinance:* Recommendations of the Public Health Service/FDA. Publication No. 229: 14. Washington, DC: U.S. Govt. Print. Off.; May 1997.
6. U.S. DEPARTMENT OF HEALTH AND HUMAN SERVICES. *Grade A condensed and dry milk ordinance.* Center for Food Safety and Applied Nutrition. Washington, DC. 1995.
7. U.S. FOOD AND DRUG ADMINISTRATION. Code of Federal Regulations Title 21 Parts 100-169. Washington, DC: U.S. Govt. Print. Off.; 1998.
8. U.S. FOOD AND DRUG ADMINISTRATION. *Part II Compliance policy guides*, Chapter 5: Foods Sec. 527.300, Pathogens in Dairy Products. Washington, DC: U.S. Govt. Print. Off.; 1996.
9. U.S. FOOD AND DRUG ADMINISTRATION. *Part II Compliance policy guides*, Chapter 5: Foods Sec. 527.400, Whole Milk, Low fat Milk, Skim Milk–Aflatoxin M_1. Washington, DC: U.S. Govt. Print. Off.; 1996.

INDEX

(Page numbers followed by *t* indicate tables; those followed by *f* indicate figures.)

A

B

D

E

F

G

H

N

O

Q

T

U

V

W